Cardiology

An International Perspective

VOLUME 1

Cardiology

An International Perspective

EDITED BY

E. I. CHAZOV

V. N. SMIRNOV

AND

R. G. OGANOV

*USSR Cardiology Research Center
Moscow, USSR*

VOLUME 1

SPRINGER SCIENCE+BUSINESS MEDIA, LLC

Library of Congress Cataloging in Publication Data

World Congress of Cardiology (9th: 1982: Moscow, R.S.F.S.R.)
Cardiology, an international perspective.

"Proceedings of the Ninth World Congress of Cardiology, held June 20-26, 1982, in
Moscow, USSR"—T.p. verso.
Includes bibliographical references and index.
1. Cardiology—Congresses. 2. Cardiovascular system—Diseases—Congresses. I.
Chazov, E. I. II. Smirnov,V. N. (Vladimir Nikolaevich), date-   . III. Oganov, R. G.
IV. Title. [DNLM: 1. Cardiology—congresses. W3 W0537 9th 1982c/WG 100 W925
1982c]

| RC666.2.W67   1982 | 616.1'2 | 84-9776 |

ISBN 978-1-4757-1826-3   ISBN 978-1-4757-1824-9 (eBook)
DOI 10.1007/978-1-4757-1824-9

Proceedings of the Ninth World Congress of Cardiology,
held June 20-26, 1982, in Moscow, USSR

PREFACE

Once in four years, cardiologists of the world united into the
International Society and Federation of Cardiology come together
to discuss the most pressing problems of cardiovascular pathology,
sum up the accomplishments of the intervening years, and set
directions for future research and exploitation of the existing
knowledge. Not too much time passed since the I Paris Congress of
International Foundation of Cardiology in 1950, but since then we
have been witnessing a real information explosion. Extraordinary
amounts of new knowledge, accumulated during the past three decades,
has revolutionized our understanding of major cardiovascular diseases
as well as approach to their treatment and diagnosis.

The IX World Congress of Cardiology, held in Moscow in June 20-26,
gathered 5,099 delegates from 78 countries. In the course of the
Congress, prominent scientists presenting 21 lectures on topical
problems of theoretical and practical cardiology; 900 papers were
heard at 37 Symposia and 58 Free Communication Sessions. The papers
and discussions demonstrated an increased contribution of fundamental
research to clinical arsenal. Another feature of modern biomedical
research is that it makes use of the latest accomplishments in
other fields of science and technology: physics, chemistry, elec-
tronics, etc. Of late, a new research discipline, called molecular
cardiology, has formed. By elucidating the most subtle basic
mechanisms whereby pathological processes develop, it is expected to
afford ultimate control of cardiovascular diseases.

The Congress demonstrated that new knowledge about the diagnosis and
treatment is being successfully introduced into clinical practice.
New, mainly non-invasive, sensitive diagnostic techniques to study
the heart and vessels function have appeared. Already existing
angiographic and nuclear techniques are being further elaborated.
Taking together the growing amount of relevant information and the
development of new devices, techniques and effective drugs, the
chances of successful treatment and reduction of cardiovascular
mortality have been greatly improved. Considerable progress has
been made by preventive cardiology through intensive investigation
of prevalence and changes in the incidence of cardiovascular

diseases as well as factors that may influence these two. Large-
scale cooperative programs to control arterial hypertension and
coronary heart disease are being developed and implemented.

On the whole, the IX Congress in Moscow showed that modern cardiology
is a rapidly advancing science with great potential and feasible
prospects.

Academician Eugeni I Chazov

CONTENTS

SYMPOSIA

1   THE PROBLEM OF MILD HYPERTENSION

VOLUME 2

28   ECHOCARDIOGRAPHY

29   RADIONUCLIDE VENTRICULOGRAPHY AND PERFUSION
SCINTIGRAPHY — ADVANTAGES AND SHORTCOMINGS

30   RADIONUCLIDE TECHNIQUES FOR MEASURING
BLOOD FLOW

LECTURES

ARE THERE MARKERS FOR THE PHYSIOPATHOLOGY
OF ESSENTIAL HYPERTENSION?

Alberto Zanchetti

Istituto di Clinica Medica IV, Università di
Milano, and Centro di Fisiologia Clinica e
Ipertensione, Ospedale Maggiore, C.N.R.
Milan, Italy

INTRODUCTION

Widespread interest for the physiopathology of hypertension has undoubtedly been raised by the hope of understanding the error or the errors of regulation by which higher blood pressure values are attained, but this cognitive interest has often been coupled with the hope that improved physiopathologic understanding might result in improved management of hypertension. This practical interest is linked with the belief that qualitatively or, at least, quantitatively different mechanisms underlie the rise in blood pressure in different patients. The hope of learning the best individual treatment for a given physiopathological profile requires a process of simplification, that is the identification of simple but meaningful indices, or markers, from which a more complex functional pattern can be described. The question mark in the title of this lecture "Are there markers for the physiopathology of essential hypertension?" has been placed to signify the uncertainty as to whether any of the markers that have been proposed and used really measures the function we assume that it measures, whether other functional variables have a fixed relation with the supposed marker and can be inferred from measurement of the latter, and finally whether useful therapeutic guidelines can be derived from its measurement. We shall see that it is not easy to get rid of these question marks.

MARKERS OF SYMPATHETIC ACTIVITY

Measuring sympathetic activity in man has been, and still is, one of the most elusive undertakings in the clinical physiology of hypertension. Two main approaches have been followed, 1) that of assessing cardiovascular reflexes tonically regulating sympathetic activity in order to identify a primary or secondary disturbance in sympathetic regulation, and 2) that of measuring plasma catecholamines as an index of a possible increase in transmitter release from sympathetic postganglionic endings.

Cardiovascular Reflexes and Hypertension

Interest has been concentrated upon reflexes originating from low pressure and high pressure cardiovascular receptors. Limited information is available about low pressure receptor reflexes, but it has been suggested[1] that an exaggerated sympathetic vasoconstrictor response to withdrawal of the tonic inhibition from low pressure cardiopulmonary receptors occurs in borderline hypertension. A greater amount of attention has been concentrated on high pressure, or arterial (sino-aortic), receptor reflexes. Sleight[2], by studying the bradycardic and tachycardic reflex responses to injection of pressor and depressor drugs, has introduced the concept of baroreflex resetting accompanying human hypertension, resetting being characterized by a raised threshold and a diminished sensitivity. My group[3,4] has explored pressor and depressor responses to carotid sinus manipulation by the neck pressure chamber. Figure 1 illustrates the differences in the baroreflex responses we observed in a group of normotensive subjects and in two groups of moderate and severe hypertensives. The pressor response to reduction in carotid transmural pressure (that means baroreflex deactivation) was greatest in the normotensive group, decreased in moderate hypertensives, and was lowest in severe hypertensives. On the contrary, the depressor response to increased carotid transmural pressure (i.e., baroreflex stimulation) was lowest in normotensives, intermediate in moderate hypertensives and greatest in severe hypertensives. This resetting of baroreflexes, marking the progressive rise in arterial pressure, consists in an upward shift of the baroreceptor threshold without a real loss in reflex sensitivity, and allows maintenance of sympathetic activity, as well as its modulation, in hypertension. Available evidence, however, is that baroreflex resetting is secondary to the rise in pressure[5], and cannot be used as a marker of primary changes characterizing the development of hypertension. We have recently shown[6] that resetting of the carotid sinus reflex is identical in patients with renovascular hypertension and in patients with essential hypertension. Occurrence of secondary resetting does not rule out, however, that there might also be a primary component, and indeed there is some evidence[7] that primary baroreceptor resetting might occur in spontaneous hypertensive rats.

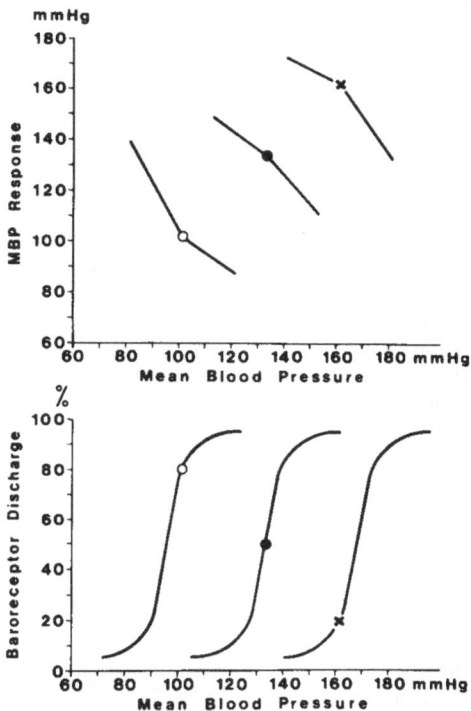

Fig. 1. Above: changes in mean arterial pressure responses
(ordinates) to changes in carotid sinus transmural pressure
in normotensives (hollow circle), moderate hypertensives
(filled circle) and severe hypertensives (cross). Below:
schematic drawing of the stimulus-response curves relating
arterial blood pressure with carotid baroreceptor firing.
The set-point of the reflex (i.e., the point corresponding
to the stimulus provided by the existing blood pressure)
may be located nearby baroreceptor saturation in normotensive subjects (line to the left) and migrate progressively to the baroreceptor threshold in moderate and severe
hypertension (modified from Mancia et al.[4]).

Plasma Catecholamines in Hypertension

The knowledge that plasma noradrenaline represents the spill-
over of transmitter released by postganglionic sympathetic endings
has suggested its use as a marker of sympathetic activity, and as
a test of the hypothesis that essential hypertension may be maintained by enhanced sympathetic activity. Goldstein[8] has recently
reviewed 32 studies comparing plasma noradrenaline concentrations

in hypertensive and normotensive groups (Figure 2). Pooling all the
data together, relating to 1085 normotensives and 1496 hypertensives,
there is a slight but statistically significant difference in plasma
noradrenaline between normotensives and hypertensives, the average
concentration being somewhat higher in hypertensives (285 vs 231
pg/ml). In the whole, 28 out of 32 studies have found a higher
noradrenaline concentration in hypertensives, but in only 13 studies
the hypertensive-normotensive difference was statistically significant. Furthermore, there are reasonable doubts that plasma noradrenaline, being only an indirect reflection of transmitter released
by sympathetic endings, is a sufficiently sensitive index of that
mild increase in tonic sympathetic activity which might occur in
essential hypertension, or in a few hypertensive subjects. For
instance, we have shown[9] that the increase and decrease in blood
pressure (and sympathetic activity) which follow baroreflex deactivation and stimulation by the neck pressure chamber is accompanied
by negligible changes in plasma noradrenaline. Plasma noradrenaline
might also be a poor marker of sympathetic overactivity in hypertension as there is evidence that plasma noradrenaline correlates
with sympathetic activity to muscle blood vessels[10] while there is
no excessive muscle vasoconstriction in hypertension[11]. Plasma
adrenaline might perhaps represent a better marker of enhanced
splanchnic sympathetic activity, and it is interesting that there
are reports[12,13] of increased plasma adrenaline concentration in
essential hypertension. Interest to this direction is added by
recent evidence[14] that adrenaline can enhance noradrenergic sympathetic transmission by a positive feedback action on pre-junctional
beta-adrenergic receptors.

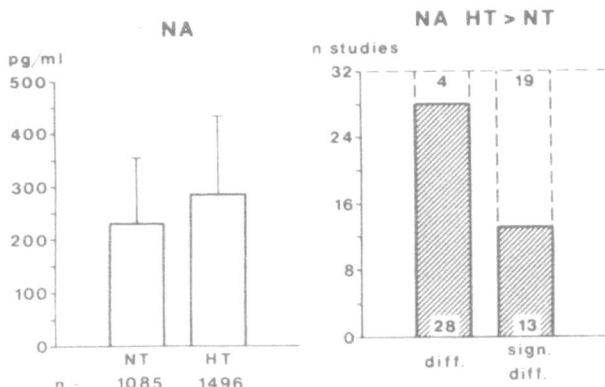

Fig. 2.   Left: means and SEM of plasma noradrenaline (NA) in 1085
          normotensive (NT) subjects and 1495 hypertensive (HT)
          subjects in 32 different studies. Right: number of studies
          in which NA was greater in HT than in NT, and number of
          studies in which this difference was statistically signi-
          ficant (from data of Golstein[8]).

ABNORMAL ION TRANSPORT ACROSS CELL MEMBRANES

The greatest interest has recently concentrated on abnormal ion transport across cell membranes[15,16] as a possible marker of essential hypertension and, even more importantly, of genetic predisposition to hypertension. Abnormal transport of sodium and/or potassium ions across membranes of erythrocytes[17-20], leucocytes[21] and lymphocytes[22] have been described in essential hypertensives and in normotensive children of hypertensive parents, and the hypothesis has been advanced that reduced cellular sodium extrusion might lead to hypertension, in the presence of excessive sodium intake, by increasing intracellular sodium and calcium concentration.

Several considerations do not yet allow us to use membrane abnormalities as safe markers of hypertension or of predisposition to hypertension. Firstly, there is no general agreement about which of the abnormalities described by the various investigators (of the ouabain-sensitive sodium-potassium pump[21], of the furosemide-sensitive sodium-potassium co-transport[23,24], and of the sodium-sodium (or sodium-lithium) counter-transport[20]) is the physiopathologic important marker. Secondly, the initial report[23,24] that some of these abnormalities would occur only in essential hypertension and in children of hypertensive parents, has not been confirmed by other investigators[25,26], who have found a considerable overlap between the distribution of these abnormalities in essential hypertensives, in normotensives with a family history of hypertension, and in normotensives without a family history of hypertension. Thirdly, there is no general agreement as to whether these abnormalities actually lead to increased intracellular concentrations of sodium[15], and, fourthly, it is largely unknown whether the abnormalities found in blood cells also occur elsewhere, and whether they might lead to hypertension by increasing vascular smooth muscle contractility, or by increasing peripheral or central excitability or rather by interfering with renal sodium excretion. Finally, it has recently been maintained[27] that these ion flux abnormalities would not be primary markers of a diffuse genetic membrane alteration, but would rather be secondary consequences of the action of a so-called natriuretic hormone, the secretion of which would be the consequence of a primary impairment of renal sodium excretion.

THE RENIN-ANGIOTENSION SYSTEM AND BODY FLUID VOLUMES

Plasma Renin Activity in Hypertension

It is agreed that plasma renin activity can vary widely under physiological conditions, and that patients with arterial hypertension may have different renin levels and can be classified as having low, normal and high renin hypertension[28]. The meaning of the classification of hypertensive patients in separate groups

according to the renin/sodium index is still the object of considerable debate, however. The Glasgow group[29] has made the point that
both in normotensives and in hypertensives renin values are distributed as a single uninterrupted frequency distribution curve.
It has also been remarked by several authors[29,30] that low renin
essential hypertension cannot be taken as an invariable marker of
increased volume. For the time being, plasma renin is a useful
diagnostic index for secondary hypertension, but its use as a marker
of subtypes of essential hypertension is of quite dubious significance.

Body Fluid Volumes in Hypertension

Plasma volume, extracellular fluid volume, exchangeable sodium
have been measured in hypertensive subjects by several authors, all
of whom have failed to identify any group of volume expanded patients
in essential hypertension. Recently, Beretta-Piccoli et al.[31] have
further explored the problem providing data of considerable interest.
Subnormal exchangeable sodium and the absence of a relation of exchangeable sodium and blood pressure in younger hypertensive patients
suggests that excess sodium intake or excessive fluid volume are not
particularly important as pathogenetic mechanisms in the early
stages of essential hypertension, although a positive relation
between exchangeable sodium and blood pressure in older hypertensives suggest that sodium and expanded body fluid volumes might
play a greater role in hypertension with advancing age.

MARKERS OF HYPERTENSION AS GUIDELINES TO TREATMENT AND PREVENTION

Plasma Renin Activity and Treatment of Hypertension

Plasma renin activity has been the most popular marker and
guideline for predicting the success of either beta-blockers or
diuretics according to a well-known theory expounded by John Laragh
and his group[32] who suggested that beta-blockers were particularly
effective in high and normal renin hypertensives, and diuretics in
low renin hypertensives. However, the various arguments discussed
above should caution against an indiscriminate use of these indices
as a sufficiently precise profile of the hypertensive patient and
as an approach to the pharmacologic management of hypertension[30,33].
Several of the inferences that have been made in recent years have
not resisted criticism, but caution should also be used against
translating sound criticism into an uncritical and generalized
denial. It is certainly true that recent research[30,33] has not
supported the opinion that hypotension induced by beta-blockers
results solely or mainly from renin suppression, and that the renin/
sodium index can effectively screen patients responsive from those
unresponsive to beta-blocking therapy. This does not mean, however,

that the renin-suppressive activity of beta-blockers is always and necessarily free of hypotensive consequences. There is evidence that renin may play some pressor role in a number of cases of hypertension, especially in those patients whose renin is stimulated by treatment with diuretics and vasodilators. Figure 3 shows that in those patients in whom an exaggerated increase in renin due to diuretic therapy blunted the hypotensive action of the diuretic, addition of either an angiotensin II-antagonist, saralasin, or of a beta-blocker can remove the counteraction of excessive renin and produce a hypotensive effect.

Membrane Abnormalities and Prevention of Hypertension

The discovery of membrane abnormalities in the cells of hypertensives and of normotensives with family history of hypertension has suggested that these abnormalities could be used to identify the subjects genetically prone to the development of hypertension if exposed to excessive dietary salt intake. Several investigators are preaching to drastically reduce dietary salt, and are waving the attractive image of the bon sauvage, the simple savage, who does not eat salt and is free from hypertension[34]. I have listed above the

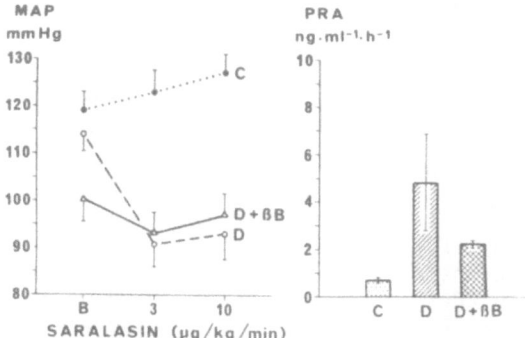

Fig. 3.   Effects of associating the beta-blocker, propranolol (βB) 160 mg/day for 1 week with the diuretic, chlorthalidone (D), in 12 patients whose plasma renin activity rose above 2.0 nmol.$^{-1}$.h^{-1} after administration of the diuretic alone. Left: effects on mean arterial pressure (MAP) of saralasin infusion starting from a sitting baseline (B) in control untreated conditions (C, filled circles and dotted line), after two week's diuretic therapy (D, hollow circles and interrupted line) and after one week's combined therapy with diuretic and beta-blocker (βB, hollow triangles and continuous line). Right: effects on supine plasma renin activity (PRA) (from Zanchetti et al.[33]).

many unanswered questions about the nature and the meaning of membrane abnormalities related to hypertension, and I would like to end by stressing that clinical and preventive application of these concepts must wait until an answer is provided to the many questions unsolved. Until more is learnt of the physiopathology of hypertension, extrapolation of hypotheses to the practice of medicine and, particularly to preventive medicine, is likely to bring about more disadvantages than benefits[35].

REFERENCES

1. A. L. Mark and R. E. Kerber, Augmentation of cardiopulmonary baroreflex control of forearm vascular resistance in borderline hypertension, Hypertension, 4:39 (1982).
2. P. Sleight, Reflex control of the heart rate, Am. J. Cardiol., 44:889 (1979).
3. G. Mancia, A. Ferrari, L. Gregorini, R. Valentini, J. Ludbrook and A. Zanchetti, Circulatory reflexes from carotid and extra-carotid baroreceptor areas in man, Circ. Res., 41:309 (1977).
4. G. Mancia, J. Ludbrook, A. Ferrari, L. Gregorini and A. Zanchetti, Baroreceptor reflexes in human hypertension, Circ. Res., 43:170 (1978).
5. A. Zanchetti, Overview of cardiovascular reflexes in hypertension, Am. J. Cardiol., 44:912 (1979).
6. G. Mancia, A. Ferrari, G. Leonetti, G. Pomidossi and A. Zanchetti, Carotid sinus baroreceptor control of arterial pressure in renovascular hypertension subjects, Hypertension, 4:47 (1982).
7. M. C. Andresen, J. M. Krauhs and A. M. Brown, Relationship of aortic walls and baroreceptor properties during development in normotensive and spontaneously hypertensive rats, Circ. Res., 43:728 (1978).
8. D. S. Goldstein, Plasma norepinephrine in essential hypertension. A study of the studies, Hypertension, 3:48 (1981).
9. G. Mancia, G. Leonetti, G. B. Picotti, A. Ferrari, M. D. Galva, L. Gregorini, G. Parati, G. Pomidossi, C. Ravazzani, C. Sala and A. Zanchetti, Plasma catecholamines and blood pressure responses to the carotid baroreceptor reflex in essential hypertension, Clin. Sci., 57, Suppl. 5:156 (1979).
10. B. G. Wallin, G. Sundlöf, B. M. Eriksson, P. Dominiak, H. Grobecker and L. E. Lindblad, Plasma noradrenaline correlates to sympathetic muscle nerve activity in normotensive man, Acta Physiol. Scand., 111:69 (1981).
11. J. Brod, Essential hypertension. Haemodynamic observations with a bearing on its pathogenesis, Lancet, 1:733 (1960).
12. R. Franco-Morselli, J. L. Elghozi, E. Joly, S. Di Giulio and P. Meyer, Increased plasma adrenaline concentrations in benign essential hypertension, Brit. Med. J., 2:1251 (1977).
13. O. Bertel, F. R. Bühler, W. Kiowski and B. E. Lütold, Decreased beta-adrenoceptor responsiveness as related to age, blood

pressure and plasma catecholamines in patients with essential
hypertension, Hypertension, 2:130 (1980).

14. L. H. Tung, M. J. Rand and H. Majewski, Adrenaline-induced
    hypertension in rats, Clin. Sci., 61, Suppl. 7:191 (1981).

15. D. C. Tosteson, N. Adragna, I. Bize, H. Solomon and M. Canessa,
    Membranes, ions and hypertension, Clin. Sci., 61, Suppl. 7:5
    (1981).

16. Y. Postnov and S. Orlov, Alterations of cell membranes in
    primary hypertension, Proc. IX World Congress of Cardiology,
    in press.

17. F. Wessels, G. Junge-Hulsing and H. Losse, Untersuchungen zur
    Natriumpermeabilität der Erythrozyten bei Hypertonikern und
    Normotonikern mit familiarer Hochdruckbelastung, Z. Kreislauf-
    forsch., 56:374 (1967).

18. Y. Postnov, S. Orlov, A. Shevchenko and A. Adler, Altered sodium
    permeability, calcium binding and Na^+, K^+-ATPase activity in the
    red blood cell membrane in essential hypertension, Pflügers
    Arch., 371:263 (1977).

19. R. P. Garay and P. Meyer, A new test showing abnormal net Na^+
    and K^+ fluxes in erythrocytes of essential hypertensive patients,
    Lancet, 1:349 (1979).

20. M. Canessa, M. Adragna, H. S. Solomon, T. M. Connolly and D. C.
    Tosteson, Increased sodium, lithium countertransport in red
    cells of patients with essential hypertension, New Engl. J. Med.,
    302:772 (1980).

21. R. P. S. Edmonsom, R. D. Thomas, P. J. Hilton, J. Patrick and
    N. F. Jones, Abnormal leucocyte composition and sodium transport
    in essential hypertension, Lancet, 1:1003 (1975).

22. E. Ambrosioni, L. Tartagni, L. Montebugnoli and B. Magnani,
    Intralymphocytic sodium in hypertensive patients: a significant
    correlation, Clin. Sci., 57, Suppl. 5:325 (1979).

23. R. P. Garay, G. Dagher, M. G. Pernollet, M. A. Devynck and P.
    Meyer, Inherited defect in Na^+, K^+ co-transport system in
    erythrocytes from essential hypertensive patients, Nature,
    284:281 (1980).

24. R. P. Garay, J. L. Elghozi, G. Dagher and P. Meyer, Laboratory
    distinction between essential and secondary hypertension by
    measurement of erythrocyte cation fluxes, New Engl. J. Med.,
    382:769 (1980).

25. M. Canali, L. Borghi, E. Sani, A. Curti, A. Montanari, A.
    Novarini and A. Borghetti, Increased erythrocyte lithium-sodium
    countertransport in essential hypertension: its relationship
    to family history of hypertension, Clin. Sci., 61, Suppl. 7:13
    (1981).

26. D. Cusi, C. Barlassina, M. Ferrandi, P. Palazzi, E. Celega and
    G. Bianchi, Relationship between altered Na^+-K^+ co-transport
    and Na^+-Li^+ countertransport in the erythrocytes of essential
    hypertensive patients, Clin. Sci., 61, Suppl. 7:33 (1981).

27. H. E. de Wardener and G. A. MacGregor, Dahl's hypothesis that
    a saluretic substance may be responsible for a sustained rise

in arterial pressure: its possible role in essential hypertension, Kidney Intern., 18:1 (1980).

28. J. H. Laragh, Vasoconstriction-volume analysis for understanding and treating hypertension. The use of renin and aldosterone profiles, Am. J. Med., 55:261 (1973).

29. P. L. Padfield, D. G. Beevers, J. J. Brown, D. L. Davies, R. Fraser, A. F. Lever, J. I. S. Robertson, M. A. D. H. Schalekamp, G. Kolsters and W. H. Birkenhäger, Low renin hypertension: a diagnostic entity attributable to mineralocorticoid excess?, in: "Hypertension - its nature and treatment", D. M. Burley, G. F. B. Birwood, J. M. Fryer, S. H. Taylor, eds., p. 135, Ciba, Horsham (1975).

30. A. Zanchetti, A. Stella, G. Leonetti, A. Morganti and L. Terzoli, Control of renin release: experimental evidence and clinical implications, in: "Topics in hypertension", J. H. Laragh, ed., chapter 7, Yorke Medical Books, New York (1980).

31. C. Beretta-Piccoli, D. L. Davies, K. Boddy, J. J. Brown, A. M. M. Cumming, B. W. East, R. Fraser, A. F. Lever, P. L. Padfield, P. F. Semple, J. I. S. Robertson, P. Weidmann and E. D. Williams, Relation of arterial pressure with body sodium, body potassium and plasma potassium in essential hypertension, Clin. Sci., 63:257 (1982).

32. F. R. Bühler, J. H. Laragh, E. D. Vaughan Jr., H. R. Brunner, H. Gavras and L. Baer, Antihypertensive action of propranolol. Specific antirenin responses in high and normal renin forms of essential, renal, renovascular and malignant hypertension, Am. J. Cardiol., 32:511 (1973).

33. A. Zanchetti, G. Leonetti, L. Terzoli and C. Sala, Beta-blockers and renin, in: "Beta Blockade in the 1980s", in publication.

34. E. D. Freis, Salt, volume and the prevention of hypertension, Circulation, 53:589 (1979).

35. A. Zanchetti, Essential hypertension today and tomorrow, in: "Blood pressure measurement and systemic hypertension", A. C. Arntzenius, A. J. Dunning, H. A. Snellen, eds., p. 261, Medical World Press, Breda (1981).

CONTROL AND TREATMENT OF ARTERIAL HYPERTENSION

F. Gross

Department of Pharmacology, University of Heidelberg
Im Neuenheimer Feld 366
D-6900 Heidelberg

Control of hypertension can be interpreted in two ways. According to the WHO Technical Report "Arterial Hypertension" (1978),
"the term 'hypertension control' includes all measures for health
protection and promotion related to high blood pressure", and "control programs" refer to public health actions aimed at hypertension
control. The other meaning applies to the efficacy of therapy in
the sense that high blood pressure of the patient should be kept
under control. In other words, aspects of community programs of
hypertension and of individual antihypertensive treatment have to be
considered when we speak of hypertension control. This lecture will
mainly deal with effective drug treatment of high blood pressure.
However, in view of the large number of subjects who have elevated
blood-pressure levels and the possible public health and economic
consequences that may arise if drug therapy is generally recommended,
it is advisable to discuss, at the beginning, some of the large controlled studies in which the significance of effective blood-pressure
control for the community was investigated.

The first reliable data on the effectiveness of antihypertensive
drugs in reducing morbidity and mortality caused by high blood pressure have been presented in the Veterans Administration Cooperative
Study (1967, 1970). It was demonstrated that in patients suffering
from severe hypertension, with diastolic pressures between 115 and
129 mm Hg, and in those with moderate hypertension, having an average
diastolic pressure of between 105 and 114 mm Hg, complications of
hypertension, such as cerebrovascular events and congestive heart
failure, were definitely reduced, whereas statistical significance
was not reached for the diminution of myocardial infarction. In subjects with diastolic pressures ranging from 90 to 104 mm Hg, no statistically significant reduction in morbidity and mortality due to

13

cardiovascular events was obtained in the treated group as compared
with the placebo control group (1970). Since then, various controlled
trials of the treatment of mild hypertension have been undertaken
and, with the exception of that organised by the British Medical
Research Council (1981), been finished and evaluated.

An interim analysis of the four completed trials has recently
been published (WHO/ISH Mild Hypertension Liaison Committee, 1982)
which compares the design of the projects and their results. It also
refers to the trials which are still in course, mainly that of the
Medical Research Council (MRC) in Britain and that of the European
Working Party on High Blood Pressure in the Elderly (EWPHE) (Amery
and De Schaepdryver, 1981). The results of the various studies differ: the positive outcome of the Australian National Blood Pressure
Study (ANBPS) (1980) and of the American Hypertension Detection and
Follow-up Program (HDFP) (1979) has not been confirmed in the US
Public Health Service Study (USPHS) (McFate Smith et al., 1979) and
the Oslo Study (Helgeland 1980) (Table 1). The reason for these dis-
crepancies is mainly the insufficient sample size in the two latter
trials, which failed to reveal a positive effect of treatment on the
frequency of cardiovascular events. However, care is also indicated
with respect to the interpretation of the two positive studies, of
which the American HDFP was not a placebo-controlled trial, but a
comparison between two ways of treatment - either in special clinics
(stepped care) or with the usual medical care in the community (referred care).

From the available data it is obvious that the annual risk in
individuals with mild hypertension is small. In the untreated control groups, mortality of all causes (not only cardiovascular) was
0.5% in the Australian Study, the Oslo Study, and the MRC trial.
It was higher in the HDFP Study, in which patients with mild hypertension had a 1.1% mortality rate per year under referred care, but
only 0.7% per year under the stepped-care management (WHO/ISH Mild
Hypertension Liaison Committee, 1982). In the ANBPS, fatal ischaemic
heart disease was less frequent in the treated group than in the
placebo group, but the absolute numbers were small (2 vs 8 patients),
and for non-fatal myocardial infarction no similar difference was
observed (18 vs 17 patients). In addition, the follow-up of the
placebo group revealed that, after the three years of the study, the
blood pressure fell further in 48% and rose in 12%, whereas it remained in the mild hypertension range in 32% (Report by the Management Committee of the Australian Therapeutic Trial in Mild Hypertension, 1982). From these data it may be concluded that a considerable
percentage of subjects with mild hypertension does not need drug
treatment, but that it suffices to observe them closely and to watch
the course of their blood pressure. Nevertheless, it has to be kept
in mind that, in a population control study of middle-aged male civil
servants in London, a blood-pressure dependent rise in mortality has
been calculated, the cause of death being either coronary heart disease or stroke (Rose, 1981).

Table 1.   Crude Mortality Rates (per 1000 person-years) in Treated Subjects and Controls* in A.N.B.P.S., H.D.F.P., (Stratum I), and the Oslo Trial, and in Controls in the M.R.C.Trial

Trial	Diastolic blood-pressure (mm Hg)	Age range (yr)	Person years	Mortality									
				All causes		All cardiovascular		All cerebrovascular		Coronary heart disease		cardiovascular	
				No.	Rate	No.	Rate	No.	Rate	No.	Rate	No.	Rate
A.N.B.P.S.													
Treated	} 95–109	30–69	6991	25	3.6	8	1.1	3	0.4	5	0.7	17	2.4
Controls			6868	35	5.1	18	2.6	6	0.9	11	1.6	17	2.5
H.D.F.P.													
Stepped care	} 90–104	30–69	19115	231	12.1	122	6.4	17	0.9	86	4.5	109	5.7
Referred care			19063	291	15.3	165	8.7	31	1.6	107	5.6	126	6.6
Oslo													
Treated	} <110	40–49	2233	10	4.5	7	3.1	0	0.0	6	2.7	3	1.3
Controls			2088	9	4.3	6	2.9	2	1.0	2	1.0	3	1.4
M.R.C.													
Controls	90–109	35–64	16415	83	5.1	46	2.8	7	0.4	35	2.1	37	2.3

*Stepped care and referred care for H.D.F.P.

So far, no indicators are available that would predict whether
a patient will benefit from drug treatment of mild hypertension.
In the ANBPS, analysis of the placebo controls revealed that one
fourth of the subjects who had a diastolic blood pressure below 95
mm Hg on the first three visits would be hypertensive three years
later, if they were left without treatment, whereas the remaining
75% would still have pressures below 95 mm Hg (Report by the Management Committee of the Australian Therapeutic Trial in Mild Hypertension, 1982). This, however, means that a substantial group would
receive unnecessary treatment, if antihypertensive drugs were automatically prescribed to subjects with mild hypertension. Hence, the
decision to treat mild hypertension should not only be based on the
values of diastolic blood pressure, but has to take into account
other factors as well that are characteristic for the individual,
such as age, sex, body weight, and possible risk factors - for instance high serum lipids, cigarette smoking, and others - which may
be of greater significance for the manifestation of cardiovascular
complications, especially ischaemic heart disease, than a slight
elevation in blood pressure (Bauer and Hunyor, 1978).

In connection with the observations made in the HDFP Study and
the demonstration that stepped care in special clinics may produce
better results - not only with respect to cardiovascular complications
of blood pressure - it should be mentioned that, also in uncontrolled
studies, care of hypertensive patients was somewhat more effective
in hospital out-patient departments than in general practice. However, after hospital treatment, discharge back to general practitioners may result in a satisfactory control (Bulpitt et al., 1982).

The fact that it is possible to lower the risk of fatal and
non-fatal myocardial infarction by the treatment of mild hypertension
should not let us forget that the number of those who benefit from
preventive treatment is only a fraction of those who are treated.
The mass approach to preventing complications of mild hypertension
means little benefit for the individual, or, as has been stated recently: "A measure that brings large benefits to the community offers
little to each participating individual" (Rose, 1982). There is the
danger that, on the basis of positive findings in epidemiological
studies, generalizing recommendations will be made to apply drug
treatment to all individuals with mild hypertension instead of making
a more careful selection considering additional criteria. Our efforts
should aim at singling out those who are at a higher risk than at
undifferentiated mass treatment. Keeping this in mind, we may now
turn to the various possibilities of effective treatment.

GENERAL MEASURES

At the beginning of active treatment, especially in patients
with mild to moderate hypertension, general therapeutic measures

are advisable. These include weight reduction by means of appropriate
dietary regimens, restriction of salt intake to 4-6 g daily, cessation
of cigarette smoking, and moderation in alcohol consumption. The
modest reduction in salt intake is generally recommended, but few
reliable data are available so far showing that it really affects
high blood pressure (Morgan et al., 1979). Further controlled studies
on the effect of a limited dietary salt restriction are necessary,
particularly in comparison with the administration of low doses of
diuretics. Physical activity has been claimed to diminish high blood
pressure, but there is little evidence to support such a statement;
there is at least no indication that physical inactivity enhances
the risk of developing high blood pressure. Psychological stress is
said to contribute to chronic blood-pressure elevation, but here
again no convincing data are in hand, and for this reason the ill-
defined term and the corresponding claim should be avoided. Similarly, various behavioral procedures have been said to be effective in
lowering high blood pressure such as biofeedback methods, yoga, relaxation, transcendental meditation, and psychotherapy (Patel, 1975a,
b). All these practices take a long time, are expensive, and may at
best bring transitory relief - they are certainly not suitable for
use on a large scale (Andrews et al., 1982). Hence, taken together,
the effects of general measures on high blood pressure remain limited
and will in most cases assist drug treatment rather than replace it.

ANTIHYPERTENSIVE DRUGS - THE PRESENT SITUATION

Today, an abundance of active drugs is available for the treatment of hypertension, and practising physicians are often confused
about the various pharmacological possibilities of interfering with
the regulation of blood pressure. The drugs differ with respect to
their pharmacodynamic profiles, their mechanisms of action, their
efficacy and potency, their pharmacokinetics and unwanted effects.
To a certain degree, this holds also true for the various representatives within a class of drugs, and, consequently, not all diuretics,
all β-blockers, or all vasodilators have identical profiles of activity
and are interchangeable. Admittedly, minor differences are occasionally overstated, mainly for promotional reasons, although they are
of little, if any practical significance. On the other hand, by far
not all the diversities are trivial, and quite a few make it possible
to adjust treatment better to the needs of the individual patient.

According to their mode of action, four large groups of antihypertensive agents can be distinguished (Table 2). Among the drugs
which act on the efferent sympathetic system, a further differentiation is possible between those which act on centrally located
adrenergic receptors and those which act preferentially in the
periphery, mainly on the heart and the resistance vessels.

Table 2. Antihypertensive Agents Grouped According to
          their Mode of Action

---

1. Drugs that interfere with the efferent sympathetic
   system, including the α- and β-adrenoceptors
2. Drugs acting directly on arteriolar smooth muscle
   (vasodilators)
3. Drugs affecting electrolyte–water balance, and,
   secondarily, total peripheral resistance
4. Drugs that interfere with the renin-angiotensin
   system

Monotherapy

According to the recommendations in the WHO Technical Report on
Arterial Hypertension (1978), treatment should usually start with
one drug in the form of monotherapy, either with a β-adrenoceptor
blocker or with a diuretic (Table 3). Only subsequently, if no
satisfactory response has been achieved with a single drug, combinations of various types of drug should be given. This principle has
been accepted by national organisations, such as the national societies or leagues against hypertension, but it is obvious that not
in all countries, for instance the Federal Republic of Germany, this
suggestion is observed. Many physicians here prefer the use of fixed
combinations right from the beginning instead of trying to achieve
a satisfactory result with the minimum of drugs. In favor of such
a policy it is often argued that the simultaneous administration of
various drugs makes it possible to reduce the dosages of the individual components, which have not only an additive, but often also
a synergistic action. Consequently, besides a more marked blood-
pressure lowering effect, the incidence and severity of side effects
and adverse reactions may be diminished. However, there is also the
danger to introduce unwanted effects together with an additional
drug, and therefore the principal requirement - to administer as few
drugs as possible - remains valid.

The debate about the criteria for the first choice in monotherapy still goes on (Withworth and Kincaid-Smith, 1982). It has
been claimed that in younger patients β-adrenoceptor blocking drugs
are preferable, and that in older patients or in those in whom the
blood pressure has been elevated for a long time the treatment may
start with a diuretic. However, it is difficult to draw a dividing
line between older and younger individuals, and there are also quite
a few exemptions from such a generalizing rule. Some years ago, the
activity of the renin-angiotensin system was also suggested as selection criterion, patients with high or normal plasma renin activity
being candidates for β-blocker therapy and those with suppressed
activity for a diuretic (Bühler et al., 1972); but also here, too

Table 3. Drugs to be used for Monotherapy

Standard drugs:
  β-adrenoceptor blockers

  relatively cardioselective ($\beta_1 > \beta_2$),
  non-selective ($\beta_1 - \beta_2$)

  or

  diuretics:

  thiazides, indapamide
  thiazides + potassium-sparing drugs

Possible alternatives:
  α-adrenoceptor blocker: prazosin (indoramin)
  α- and β-adrenoceptor blocking: labetalol
  converting enzyme inhibitor: captopril

---

many exceptions from the rule have been found besides the inherent
difficulties of the test method (Report on Round Table, 1975, Morgan,
1976). The assessment of the haemodynamic situation may provide
more helpful guidance but in many cases the trial-and-error principle
has to be applied, and the choice is left to the personal experience
and preference of the doctor (Waal-Manning, 1976; Gross, 1982a).
This holds also true for the selection of one of the numerous representatives that are in hand in the two classes of drugs. All the
available evidence indicates that the blood-pressure lowering potential of all β-adrenoceptro blockers is similar, provided they
are given in the correct dosage, and the same holds true for the
thiazides and related diuretics (Gross, 1982b).

β-Adrenoceptor blockers as well as diuretics cause only a moderate fall in blood pressure, which rarely exceeds 25 mm Hg systolic
and 15 mm Hg diastolic, the maximum response being generally achieved
after one or a few weeks of treatment. A positive correlation has
been found between the height of diastolic pressure at the beginning
of diuretic therapy and the reduction of pressure obtained after
several weeks (Turner, 1977). Whereas diuretics are usually prescribed in relatively small doses, corresponding to 25 or, at the
most, 50 mg of hydrochlorothiazide per day, the β-adrenoceptor blockers are, as a rule, given in higher doses than for the treatment of
angina or tachyarrhythmias. A slow increase in dosage may result in
a better response of blood pressure, but the dosage range is variable,
and the dose-response curve for the blood-pressure lowering effect
is shallow and does not follow closely that for antagonizing the
effects of isoprenaline on the blood pressure. This holds also true
for the delayed onset and for the duration of action, which exceeds
that derived from measuring plasma concentrations.

Various arguments have been brought forward in favor of using relatively cardioselective β-adrenoceptor blockers in the treatment of hypertension. However, no convincing data have been presented which support a better efficacy or tolerability of drugs which act preferentially on β_1-adrenoceptors. The attempt to distinguish between various generations of β-adrenoceptor blocking drugs is a promotional gag rather than a scientific reasoning. The intrinsic sympathetic activity and the duration of action may be of greater significance for the selection of the drug, the former being rather unwanted in the treatment of high blood pressure, the latter such that it permits the administration of one dose every 24 hours. Recently, it has been shown that blockade of β-adrenoceptors may be responsible for changes in plasma lipid concentrations, an increase in total and very low-density lipoprotein (VLDL) triglycerides, and a decrease in high-density lipoprotein (HDL) cholesterol and free fatty acid concentrations (Waal-Manning, 1976; Day et al., 1982; Leren et al., 1980). These changes in plasma lipid concentrations are ascribed to a marked stimulation of α-adrenoceptors, which results in an inhibition of lipoprotein lipase and a subsequent rise in plasma triglycerides. Excessive α-adrenoceptor stimulation has also been claimed to impair the production of HDL cholesterol in patients who had already a low HDL cholesterol concentration before the administration of β-adrenoceptor blockers (Day et al., 1982). However, it has not been proven that these changes in plasma lipids are of clinical significance, even if they are maintained for some time.

Special mentioning merit β-adrenoceptor blocking drugs such as labetalol, which, besides its affinity to β_1- and β_2-adrenoceptors, has an affinity to α_1-adrenoceptors, the ratio of β- to α-blocking activity being about 4:1. The lower affinity to α_1-adrenoceptors, however, suffices to induce a more marked blood-pressure lowering effect than is achieved with exclusive blockade of β-adrenoceptors and which may even result in occasional overshooting orthostatism (Prichard and Richards, 1982). So far, labetalol is the only marketed representative of drugs which bind to both types of adrenoceptors, but others may be expected which have more favorable pharmacokinetics and a longer duration of action than labetalol. In any case, this type of adrenoceptor blocking drug is suitable for monotherapy and may be administered at the beginning of treatment.

In this context, the question arises whether a selective α_1-adrenoceptor blocking drug, such as prazosin, is suitable for monotherapy. The drug has continuously gained acceptance after problems of orthostatic responses, produced by the first administration, had been overcome by the lowering of the initial dose (Brogden et al., 1977). Although prazosin may be used alone, it is preferably given together with a diuretic to keep the dosage down also during prolonged treatment and to avoid sodium fluid retention (Bolli et al., 1980). The lack of tachycardic response as well as the reduction in cardiac preload are haemodynamic advantages of prazosin, but the

danger of initial orthostatic reactions, the frequently observed
development of tolerance, and the subsequent increase in dose, necessary to obtain a reliable reduction in blood pressure, make it advisable to use the drug carefully. Hence, it is not suitable for
initial monotherapy.

Among the diuretics, it is especially hydrochlorothiazide, ben-
drofluazide, and the long-acting chlorthalidone, which are the standard drugs in this kind of monotherapy. The question arises whether
they should be given routinely together with potassium supplements,
as is widely done in the USA and the UK, or whether it would be
preferable to add a potassium-retaining diuretic to them. In general,
potassium loss is limited, and serum potassium concentrations rarely
fall below 3.5 mEq/l, provided the doses remain in the low range,
corresponding to 25 mg hydrochlorothiazide or even less of chlorthalidone. The fact that supplements of potassium chloride are much
more frequently administered in the USA than in Germany or other
European countries may be explained by the generally higher doses of
the diuretics that are given in America as compared to Europe. It
has, however, to be kept in mind that potassium chloride, administered
together with a diuretic, is excreted rapidly and does not cause a
rise in the serum concentration of potassium (Lowe et al., 1979).
In the majority of cases, there is no need for potassium supplements,
provided that dietary potassium supplementation is adequate. The
same holds true for the combination of two diuretics, a thiazide
derivative or a related drug together with a potassium-conserving
drug such as triamterene or amiloride. The occurrence of hypokalaemia
may be reduced by such a combination, but it has also been demonstrated that, in aequi-effective antihypertensive doses, the addition
of a potassium-conserving drug may have no special effect on serum
potassium concentration (Anavekar et al., 1979).

Indapamide merits special mentioning, since it differs chemically
from the thiazides and has in addition peculiar pharmacokinetic features, which are responsible for a prolonged duration of action.
Besides the diuretic activity, a vasodilatory effect is claimed for
indapamide, which may be demonstrable in low doses affecting electrolyte and water excretion little (Anavekar et al., 1979; Passeron et
al., 1981). Hence, the request to give low doses of diuretics in
the treatment of hypertension may be more easily realized with indapamide than with other diuretics owing to its vasodilatory component, its high lipophilicity, and its slow excretion (Wheeley et
al., 1982).

Like the β-adrenoceptor blockers, also the diuretics may be
responsible for slight changes in the lipoprotein pattern of the
plasma. A mild increase in VLDL lipoproteins has been shown simultaneously with a reduction in HDL cholesterol, but it remains doubtful
whether any clinical significance may be attributed to these variations. The diuretics have now been established in the treatment of

hypertension for 25 years and may be considered one of the best-
tolerated groups of drugs, being nearly free from severe adverse
reactions.

In the future, a third group of drugs may be more widely used
in the monotherapy of hypertension, namely the vasodilators which
act by interfering with calcium transport in the smooth-muscle cells
of the arterioles (Leonetti et al., 1981; Muiesan et al., 1981).
These drugs, also called calcium antagonists, have been widely used
in the symptomatic treatment of angina, but they also lower total
peripheral resistance. Usually, they cause an increase in heart rate
by stimulating the baroreceptors. An exception is verapamil, which
reduces heart rate by direct action on the atrioventricular conduc-
tivity. Besides verapamil, nifedipine and diltiazem have been used
in the treatment of hypertension, but further derivatives, with possibly a longer duration of action, may be expected soon (Hulthén,
U.L. et al., 1982; Krebs et al., 1982; Bühler et al., 1982 in press).
As long as reflex tachycardia will be marked, the calcium-channel
blockers will probably not be used in monotherapy, but only together
with β-adrenoceptor blocking drugs. However, as soon as derivatives
will arrive which do not increase heart rate or only transitorily so,
these drugs may find a place in the initial treatment of high blood
pressure.

Combined Treatment

In the step-wise treatment of hypertension, monotherapy is succeeded by the simultaneous administration of two or more drugs which
act by different mechanisms on the regulation of blood pressure.
The most obvious combination is that of β-adrenoceptor blockers and
diuretics, which have a partly additive effect on blood pressure
and in most cases cause a more pronounced lowering than either drug
alone. However, since treatment has usually been started with either
a β-blocker or a diuretic, it could also be that the response to the
added component is more marked, and that this second drug might be
more suitable for monotherapy than the drug used primarily. To make
sure that it is really necessary to give two drugs, the other component would have to be tested alone, before being joined to the drug
first used. In countries where drug combinations are preferred to
single drugs, such as in the Federal Republic of Germany, already
numerous fixed-ratio combinations of diuretics and β-adrenoceptor
blockers are available; in other countries, such as Sweden, there is
none so far, and the two types of drug have to be administered separately, with the advantage that they can be dosed individually allowing a greater flexibility.

The large number of available antihypertensive agents allows
numerous combinations, but it has to be requested that the two or
more drugs given together should not only differ with respect to

their mechanisms of action, but also act synergistically and correspond to one another with regard to their duration of action. In
most cases, combination therapy includes a diuretic in low dose,
which generally enhances the action of the other component(s). Recently, there has been the tendency to add a combination of two
diuretics, including a potassium-conserving one, but in most cases
this is unnecessary, especially in fixed-ratio combinations of antihypertensives, provided the diuretic dosage is kept low.

Not all the available and possible combinations can be mentioned,
but only a few examples shall be given. If the simultaneous administration of a diuretic and a ß-blocker results in an unsatisfactory
lowering of blood pressure, a vasodilator may be added - either one
of the hydralazine type, or a blocker of the slow calcium-channels,
or an α_1-adrenoceptor blocker (Table 4). Such a triple combination
has the advantage of a peripheral mechanism of action and, provided
the doses of the individual components may be varied, will allow
adequate control in 75 to 80% of the cases.

Further possibilities are drugs that stimulate centrally located
α_2-adrenoceptors, such as clonidine and α-methylnoradrenaline, the
active principle of α-methyldopa (Table 4). New interest has arisen
in clonidine, because it has been found to be active in smaller doses
than often recommended previously, i.e. in the order of 50 to 100 mcg,
and causes therefore fewer side effects. Guanfacine is very similar
to clonidine, and the same is the case with guanabenz. Guanethidine,
which, twenty years ago, was a definite progress in antihypertensive
therapy as the first specific peripheral adrenergic neurone blocker
is hardly used any more, since it is poorly absorbed, causes orthostatic reactions and other unwanted effects. All these drugs are
hardly given alone, but together with at least a diuretic and mostly
with a further drug in addition.

Quite recently, captopril, which interferes with the renin-
angiotensin system by inhibiting the angiotensin I converting enzyme,
responsible for the formation of the active octapeptide angiotensin
II, has been increasingly used in the treatment of severe hypertension, often in patients who had been resistant to other types of
drug treatment (Atkinson et al., 1980; White et al., 1980). The
mechanism by which captopril and other drugs, which inhibit the activity of the converting enzyme or kininase II similarly, interfere
with the blood-pressure regulation is not quite clear. The activity
of kininase II is not completely blocked by captopril, and some
angiotensin II is still present, but the main difficulty in understanding the antihypertensive action of the drug is the fact that
in essential hypertension the renin-angiotensin system is of little,
if any, pathogenic significance. Nevertheless, the success of captopril has stimulated research in this area, and similar drugs,
characterized as converting enzyme inhibitors, may be expected soon.
Of these, MK 421 or enalapril, which has a longer duration of action

Table 4.   Stepwise Treatment of Hypertension

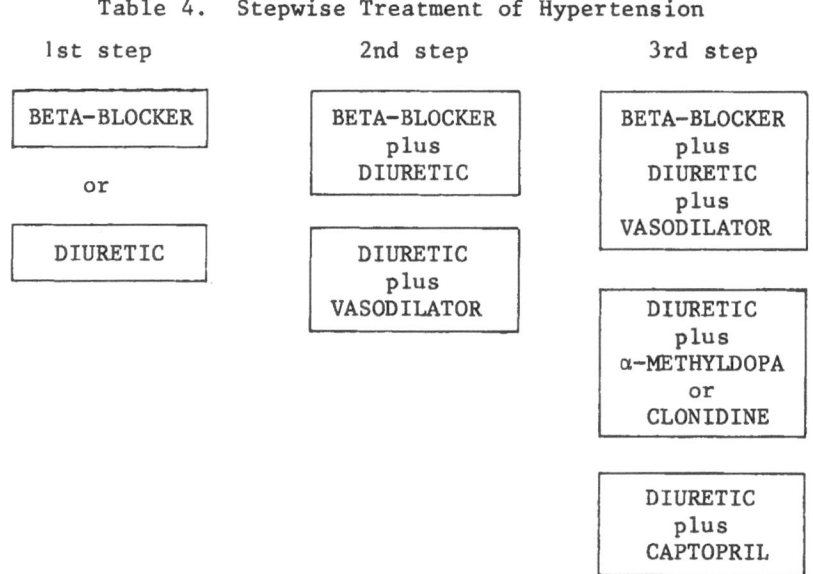

1st step   2nd step   3rd step

than captopril, is already quite advanced in clinical trials. Captopril itself and probably other converting enzyme inhibitors have
no marked antihypertensive activity, unless the renin-angiotensin
system is stimulated. By giving a diuretic simultaneously, preferably
a loop-diuretic, such as furosemide, the sensitivity to captopril is
enhanced, and this may be a suitable means to obtain a satisfactory
response. On the other hand, the combination of captopril with a
β-blocker does not enhance the blood-pressure lowering effect in
essential hypertension in a similar way as the addition of a diuretic
(MacGregor et al., 1982). This is a good example demonstrating that
combinations of antihypertensive drugs have to be selected carefully.
Even less clear than the antihypertensive mechanism is the beneficial
haemodynamic effect of captopril in congestive heart failure. Here,
not only afterload is reduced by a reduction in total peripheral resistance, but also preload, since the capacitance vessels are also
dilated under the influence of the drug. The onset of action is
quite prompt, and it seems that in most cases it is not necessary to
add a diuretic. It will, however, take some more time until the
place of this type of drug in the treatment of congestive heart failure is definitely established.

Treatment of Refractory Hypertension

     In the relatively small number of patients in whom the usual
stepped-care regimen (including a diuretic, a β-adrenoceptor blocker,

and a vasodilator) has not resulted in a satisfactory control of
blood-pressure, various drugs have been tried that have a more drastic
blood-pressure lowering effect. In a recent article, three of these
drugs - diazoxide, minoxidil, captopril - and a combination including
prazosin have been comparatively studied in the treatment of refractory hypertension (Swales et al., 1982). In such patients, care has
to be taken not to lower the blood pressure too abruptly, since
cerebral hypoxia with all its consequences or myocardial infarction
may occur, if the blood pressure falls suddenly to levels that are
far beyond those to which the perfusion of the tissues is adapted
(Ledingham and Rajagopalan, 1979). Minoxidil is certainly the most
powerful vasodilator, but it has to be given together with a diuretic
and a β-blocker (Figure 1) (Tenschert et al., 1980); captopril has
a lower efficacy, which, however, can be increased by the addition
of a diuretic. The quadruple therapy, which consists of the addition
of prazosin to the standard regimen of a diuretic, a β-blocker, and
hydralazine, is considered quite complex and may only be suitable in
the hospital, since problems of compliance may arise at home. Nevertheless, by suitable use of the drugs available today nearly all
hypertensives can be satisfactorily controlled and the progress of
cardiovascular complications stopped. Although such complex treatment regimens are anything but ideal and may include adverse reactions, one should keep in mind that, 25 years ago, these patients
would not have survived, but would have died of their disease within
a few months or years.

WHAT ARE THE PERSPECTIVES?

To come back to the beginning, one has to consider the prospects
for prevention and treatment of high blood pressure. Since we have
numerous active drugs in hand which enable the control of high blood
pressure - admittedly not ideally, but with a reasonable benefit/risk
as well as benefit/cost ratio - it would be more important to concentrate on developing preventive measures. However, prevention of
a chronic disease, of which the causes are unknown, is much more
difficult to realize than treatment and may be effective only if
substantial and continuous efforts are made which may not be feasible
economically. Furthermore, despite the fact that preventive interventions are generally suggested - such as weight control, reduced
salt intake, physical activity, behavioral education, and the avoid-
ance or elimination of adverse psychological and social factors -
hardly any convincing data are available which would justify definite
recommendations for the time being. Many more studies have to be
undertaken to answer at least part of the unsolved questions and to
provide a more solid basis for proposing changes in behavior, dietary
habits, or professional activities. We have to concede that there is
more belief than facts in supporting general measures as being effective in the control of high blood-pressure. This unsatisfactory
situation makes it urgent to start well planned long-term studies to
provide the urgently needed data.

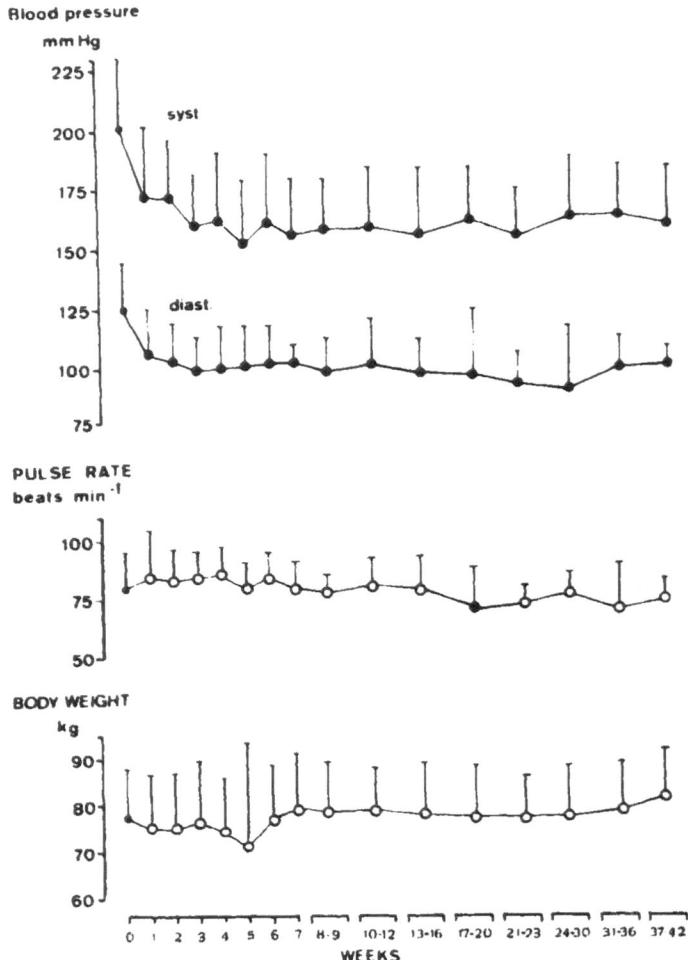

Fig. 1. Supine systolic and diastolic blood pressure, pulse rate
and body weight in 22 patients with severe hypertension.
Solid circles (●) indicate significant differences (p <0.05
- <0.001) to initial values, open circles (O) non-significant changes during the observed period of 42 weeks.

The easier way will be to develop further drugs for the treatment of hypertension, and here we shall see quite a few more come
up. Since most possibilities of interfering pharmacologically with
the regulation of blood pressure have already been extensively
studied and since corresponding drugs are in hand, it may hardly be
expected that there will be principally new types of antihypertensives. One of the new possibilities might be the interference with

the central serotoninergic system, and the development of ketanserin, a blocker of serotonin$_2$-receptors (5HT$_2$) could be a step in this direction. The drug is said to have a specific affinity to 5HT$_2$-receptors, but it has recently been demonstrated that it binds also to α_1-adrenoceptors (Van Nueten et al., 1981; Fozard, 1981). A blood-pressure lowering effect has been obtained in hypertensive patients (DeCree et al., 1981; Wenting et al., 1982) but it remains to be shown that it is due to blockade of 5HT$_2$ receptors and not mainly to blockade of α_1-adrenoceptors. Of course, continuous, more or less conspicuous improvements of already existing pharmacological principles will be made, with the result that the number of anti-hypertensive drugs will increase within the forthcoming years. This will not necessarily mean that the new drugs will be definitely better than those in hand today; they may have marginal advantages in one or the other direction, but it is hard to imagine that there will be a breakthrough comparable to that during the period from 1953 to 1962, when effective control of high blood pressure became possible for the first time.

If we consider the requirements for an ideal antihypertensive drug, as they have been defined many years ago (Table 5), we may say that most of them are satisfactorily met with the drugs available today. However, there still remains the request for improved tolerability, although we have to admit that quite a few of the drugs now in hand are remarkably well tolerated. We must also make it clear that there will be no ideal drug, and that all antihypertensives, those which are at our disposal and those to come, will have some unwanted effects and will have to be carefully studied in that direction.

The main problem to be settled is the control of mild hypertension, by far the most important from the community point of view. Should mild hypertension be treated in all subjects in whom it has been diagnosed, and should the elevated blood pressure be lowered by regular long-term intake of drugs? It is reassuring to know that effective treatment of severe and moderate hypertension is possible

Table 5. Requirements for an Antihypertensive Drug

1.	Decrease in blood pressure: slow onset, not too pronounced, similar in supine and standing positions
2.	Duration of action: 12 to 24 hours
3.	Active by mouth
4.	No negative inotropic effect on the heart, no tachycardia
5.	No tolerance
6.	No or only mild adverse reactions or side effects, no reduction of physical capacity and mental alertness
7.	Suitable for long-term treatment

today, and that cardiovascular complications may be prevented to a substantial degree. However, it is at least as important to avoid unnecessary treatment and not to expose all those who have a mild rise in blood pressure to drugs that may cause some risk without providing any benefit. More research is needed along these lines to improve further the control and treatment of hypertension.

In concluding, a few rules for the management and control of hypertension should be given (Table 6). It is not to be expected that there will be a change in these general rules in the future, and this holds true not only for the treatment with the drugs we have in hand, but also for the preparations that may be available tomorrow.

Table 6.   Management of Hypertension, General Rules for
           Drug Treatment

1. Gradual and slow lowering of blood pressure
2. Special care with old-age people; avoid abrupt changes, no strong-acting diuretics
3. Lowering of blood pressure to be achieved with minimum number of drugs
4. Application of the stepped-care program
5. One or two doses per day
6. Preference for peripherally acting drugs

REFERENCES

Amery, A., and De Schaepdryver, A., 1981, Antihypertensive therapy in patients above age 60. Fifth interim report of the European Working Party on High Blood Pressure in the Elderly (EWPHE). Current Concepts in Hypertension and Cardiovascular Disorders, 2:14-20.

Anavekar, S. N., Ludbrooke, A., Louis, W. J., and Doyle, A. E., 1979, Evaluation of indapamide in the treatment of hypertension, J.Cardiovasc.Pharmacol., 1:389-394.

Andrews, G., Macmahon, S. W., Austin, A., and Byrne, D. G., 1982 Hypertension: Comparison of drug and non-drug treatments, Brit.Med.J., 284:1523-26.

Atkinson, A. B., Lever, A. F., Brown, J. J., and Robertson, J. I. S., Combined treatment of severe intractable hypertension with captopril and diuretic, Lancet 1980/II, 105-107.

Australian National Blood Pressure Study Management Committee, The Australian therapeutic trial in mild hypertension, Lancet 1980/I, 1261-1267.

Bauer, G. E., and Hunyor, S. N., 1978, Mild hypertension: Is treatment worthwhile? Drugs, 15:80-86.

Bolli, P., Amann, F. W., and Bühler, F. R., 1980, Antihypertensive
    response to postsynaptic α-blockade with prazosin in low- and
    normal-renin hypertension, J.Cardiovasc.Pharmacol., 2:Suppl.3,
    399-405.
Brogden, R. N., Heel, R. C., Speight, T. M., and Avery, G. S., 1977,
    Prazosin: A review of its pharmacological properties and
    therapeutic efficacy in hypertension, Drugs, 14:163-197.
Bühler, F. R., Laragh, J. H., Baer, L., Vaughan, E. D., Jr., and
    Brunner, H. R., 1972, Propranolol inhibition of renin se-
    cretion. A specific approach to diagnosis and treatment of
    renin-dependent hypertensive diseases, New Engl.J.Med., 287:
    1209-1214.
Bühler, F. R., Hulthén, U. L., Kiowski, W., Müller, F., and Bolli, P.,
    1982, The place of the calcium antagonist verapamil in anti-
    hypertensive therapy, J.Cardiovasc.Pharmacol., 4:Suppl.3, in
    press.
Bulpitt, C. J., Daymond, M. J., and Dollery, C. T., 1982, Community
    care compared with hospital outpatient care for hypertensive
    patients, Brit.Med.J., 284:554-556.
DeCree, J., Verhaegen, H., and Symoens, J., Acute blood pressure
    lowering effect of ketanserin, Lancet 1981/I, 1161-1162.
Day, J. L., Metcalfe, J., and Simpson, C. N., 1982, Adrenergic mech-
    anisms in control of plasma lipid concentrations, Brit.Med.J.,
    284:1145-1148.
Fozard, J. R., The hypotensive effect of ketanserin in anaesthetized
    normotensive rats, Proc.Brit.Pharmacol.Soc., December 1981,
    Abstracts, P 63.
Gross, F., 1982a, Present concepts and perspectives of antihyperten-
    sive therapy, Clin.Exp.Hypertension, A4:1-25.
Gross, F., 1982b, The place of α-adrenoceptor and β-adrenoceptor
    blockade in the treatment of hypertension, Brit.J.Clin.Phar-
    macol., 13:Suppl.1, 5-11.
Helgeland, A., 1980, Treatment of mild hypertension: A five year
    controlled drug trial. The Oslo study, Am.J.Med., 69:725-732.
Hulthén, U. L., Bolli, P., Amann, S. W., Kiowski, W., and Bühler,
    F. R., 1982, Enhanced vasodilatation in essential hypertension
    by calcium-channel blockade with verapamil, Hypertension, 4:
    Suppl. , 26-31.
Hypertension Detection and Follow-up Program Cooperative Group, 1979,
    Five-year findings of the hypertension detection and follow-
    up program, I. Reduction in mortality of persons with high
    blood pressure, including mild hypertension, J.Am.Med.Assoc.,
    242:2562-2571.
Krebs, R., Graefe, K. -H., and Ziegler, R., 1982, Effects of calcium-
    entry antagonists in hypertension, Clin.Exp.Hypertension,
    A4:271-284.
Ledingham, J. G. G., and Rajagopalan, B., 1979, Cerebral complications
    in the treatment of accelerated hypertension, Quart.J.Med.,
    (N.S.) 48:25-41.

Leonetti, G., Pasotti, C., Ferrari, G. P., and Zanchetti, A., 1981,
    Double-blind comparison of the antihypertensive effects of
    verapamil and propranolol, in: "Calcium Antagonism in
    Cardiovascular Therapy." Internat. Symp. Florence, October
    1980 , A. Zanchetti and D. M. Krikler, eds., Excerpta Medica,
    Amsterdam-Oxford-Princeton, p. 260-267.

Leren, P., Foss, P. O., Helgeland, A., Hjermann, I., Holme, I., and
    Lund-Larsen, P. G., 1980, Effect of propranolol and Prazosin
    on blood lipids, Lancet 2:4-6.

Lowe, J., Gray, J., Henry, D. A., and Lawson, D. H., 1979, Adverse
    reactions to frusemide in hospital inpatients, Brit.Med.J.,
    2:360-362.

MacGregor, G. A., Markandu, N. D., Banks, R. A., Bayliss, J.,
    Roulston, J. E., and Jones, J. C., 1982, Captopril in essential
    hypertension: contrasting effects of adding hydrochloro-
    thiazide or propranolol, Brit.Med.J., 284:693-696.

McFate Smith, W., Edlavitch, S. A., and Krushar, W. M., 1979, U.S.
    Public Health Service hospitals intervention trial in mild
    hypertension, in: "Hypertension - Determinants, Complications
    and Intervention," G. Onesti and C. R. Klimt, eds., Grune and
    Stratton, New York, p. 381-399.

Morgan, T., 1976, Beta-adrenoceptor blocking drugs in the treatment
    of hypertension, Australia and New Zealand Journal of Medicine,
    6:612.

Morgan, T., Adam, W. R., Hodgson, M., and Myers, J., 1979, Duration
    of effect of different diuretics, Medical Journal of Australia,
    2:315-316.

M.R.C. Working Party on Mild to Moderate Hypertension, Adverse re-
    actions to bendrofluazide and propranolol used in the treat-
    ment of mild hypertension, Lancet 1981/II, 539-543.

Muiesan, G., Agabiti-Rosei, E., Alicandri, C., Beschi, M., Castellano,
    M., Corea, L., Fariello, R., Romanelli, G., Pasini, C., and
    Platto, L., 1981, Influence of verapamil on catecholamines,
    renin and aldosterone in essential hypertensive patients, in:
    "Calcium Antagonism in Cardiovascular Therapy," Internat.
    Symp. Florence, October 1980, A. Zanchetti and D. M. Krikler,
    eds., Excerpta Medica, Amsterdam-Oxford-Princeton, p. 238-249.

Van Nueten, J. M., Janssen, P. A. J., Van Beek, J., Xhonneur, R.,
    Verbeuren, T. J., and Vanhoutte, P. M., 1981, Vascular effects
    of R 41.468, a novel antagonist of 5-HT serotonergic receptors,
    J.Pharmacol.Exp.Ther., 218:217-230.

Passeron, J., Pauly, N., and Desprat, J., 1981, International multi-
    center study of indapamide in the treatment of essential
    arterial hypertension, Postgrad.Med.J., 57:Suppl.2, 57-59.

Patel, C., 1975a, Yoga and biofeedback in the management of 'stress'
    in hypertensive patients, Clin.Sci.Mol.Med., 48:Suppl.2, 171-
    174.

Patel, C., 12-month follow-up of yoga and bio-feedback in the manage-
    ment of hypertension, Lancet 1975b/I, 62-65.

Prichard, B. N. C., and Richards, D. A., 1982, Comparison of labetalol
    with other anti-hypertensive drugs, Brit.J.Clin.Pharmacol.,
    13:Suppl.1, 41-47.
Report on Round Table, 1975, on renin suppression and the hypotensive
    action of beta-adrenergic-blocking drugs, Clin.Sci.Mol.Med.,
    48:Suppl.2, 109-115.
Report of a WHO Expert Committee, 1978, Arterial Hypertension,
    Technical Report Series No.628, World Health Organization,
    Geneva.
Report by the Management Committee of the Australian Therapeutic
    Trial in Mild Hypertension, Untreated mild hypertension,
    Lancet 1982/I, 185-191.
Rose, G., 1981, Strategy of prevention: lessons from cardiovascular
    disease, Brit.Med.J., 282:1847-1851.
Swales, J. D., Bing, R. F., Heagerty, A., Pohl, J. E. F., Russell,
    G. I., and Thurston, H., Treatment of refractory hypertension,
    Lancet 1982/I, 894-896.
Tenschert, W., Studer, A., Záruba, K., Reuteler, H., Siebenschein,
    R., Siegenthaler, W., and Vetter, W., 1980, Minoxidil in
    hypertension, in: "Symposium: Clinical Pharmacology of Anti-
    hypertensive Agents." K. H. Rahn and H. A. J. Struyker-
    Boudier, eds., Arch. Int. Pharmacodyn. Ther., p.104-115.
Turner, P., Volans, N. G., and Rogers, H. J., 1977, Initial controlled
    evaluation of antihypertensive drugs: a study with indapamid,
    Curr.Med.Res.Opin., 5:Suppl.1, 124-128.
Veterans Administration Cooperative Study Group on Antihypertensive
    Agents, 1967, Effects of treatment on morbidity in hyper-
    tension: Results in patients with diastolic blood pressures
    averaging 115 through 129 mm Hg, J.Am.Med.Assoc., 202:1028-
    1034.
Veterans Administration Cooperative Study Group on Antihypertensive
    Agents, 1970, Effects of treatment on morbidity in hypertension
    II, Results in patients with diastolic blood pressure averaging
    90 through 114 mm Hg, J.Am.Med.Assoc., 213:1143-1152.
Waal-Manning, H. J., 1976, Hypertension: Which beta-blocker? Drugs
    12:412-441.
Wenting, G. J., Man in't Veld, A. J., Woittiez, A. J., Boomsma, F.,
    Schalekamp, M. A. D. H., 1982, Treatment of hypertension with
    ketanserin, a new selective 5-HT$_2$ receptor antagonist, Clin.
    Res., 284:537-539.
Wheeley, M. St. G., Bolton, J. C., and Campbell, D. B., 1982,
    Indapamide in hypertension: a study in general practice of
    new or previously poorly controlled patients, Pharmathera-
    peutica 2:143-152.
White, N. J., Yahaya, H., Rajagopalan, B., and Ledingham, J. G. G.,
    Captopril and frusemide in severe drug-resistant hypertension,
    Lancet 1980/II, 108-110.
Withworth, J. A., and Kincaid-Smith, P., 1982, Diuretics or β-blockers
    first for hypertension? Drugs 23:394-402.
W.H.O./I.S.H. Mild Hypertension Liaison Committee, Trials of the
    treatment of mild hypertension, An Interim Analysis, Lancet
    1982/I, 149-156.

BIOCHEMICAL MECHANISMS OF ALTERED METABOLISM IN ISCHEMIC HEART

Howard E. Morgan

Department of Physiology
The Milton S. Hershey Medical Center
The Pennsylvania State University
Hershey, Pennsylvania 17033

Oxygen deficiency in heart muscle is most commonly induced by reduction in coronary flow, referred to as ischemia. As contrasted to hypoxia or anoxia in which flow of blood with low or zero oxygen tension is maintained, ischemia leads to accumulation of metabolic products that further modify rates of biochemical reactions. After periods of severe ischemia ranging from 30 minutes to 1 hour or more, irreversible damage occurs.[1] Damage of this severity is characterized by disruption of the plasma membrane that is preceded by swelling of both the cell and mitochondria. Concurrently, the myofibrils and intercellular junctions are disrupted, and there is margination of nuclear chromatin. Reperfusion of an irreversibly-injured cell leads to accumulation of Ca^{++} within the mitochondria and failure to recover contractile activity.

In discussing the biochemical events leading to ischemic damage, attention will be directed to two aspects of cell metabolism. The first of these is energy metabolism. In oxygen-deficient muscle, formation of high-energy phosphates depends upon efficient utilization of the oxygen that remains by mitochondrial oxidative phosphorylation, and upon generation of ATP via the glycolytic pathway. As will be discussed, generation of high-energy phosphates by both of these pathways may be impaired by accumulation of metabolites. The second aspect of deranged metabolism in ischemic muscle to be discussed will be destruction of cellular organelles by hydrolytic enzymes. Activation of the lysosomal system has been observed frequently in ischemic tissue, including muscle.[2-7] Lysosomal enzymes possess the potential to hydrolyze macromolecules, such as proteins, nucleic acids and polysaccharides, and small molecular weight substances, such as phospholipids and metabolic intermediates. The possibility that

accumulation of metabolites may modify the hydrolytic activity of
lysosomal enzymes and that a link may exist between depletion of high-
energy phosphates and accelerated hydrolysis of cell constituents by
lysosomal enzymes will be discussed.

Energy Metabolism of Ischemic Muscle. Metabolism of Glucose in Ischemic Hearts

In aerobic cells supplied with normal plasma levels of glucose
and fatty acids, glycolysis makes a small contribution to generation
of ATP. Approximately 20% of myocardial oxygen consumption is accounted for by oxidation of glucose; about 1% of ATP synthesis occurs
in the passage of these glucose residues through the glycolytic pathway.[8] The steps restricting glycolysis in aerobic and ischemic
muscle are shown in Table 1. The major steps restraining glycolysis
in aerobic muscle are glucose transport, hexokinase, phosphofructokinase, and pyruvate dehydrogenase. The major oxidative substrate
of heart muscle is free fatty acid. Oxidation of free fatty acid
results in restraint of glycolysis at the transport, phosphofructokinase, and pyruvate dehydrogenase steps. The mechanism of the inhibition of transport is unknown, while phosphofructokinase is restrained by accumulation of citrate. Pyruvate dehydrogenase is inhibited by higher tissue levels of CoA and NADH, and by conversion
of the enzyme to the inactive phosphorylated form. Inhibition of
these steps accounts for preferential utilization of fatty acids
by heart muscle.

Addition of insulin accelerates glucose transport as much as
30-fold, and shifts the major restraint on glycolytic rate to glucose
phosphorylation. In aerobic hearts supplied only glucose, phosphofructokinase is the major reaction limiting glycolytic rate. Addition
of fatty acids inhibits this reaction, as well as pyruvate dehydrogenase, and restrains glycolytic rate despite the presence of insulin.

So long as coronary flow is maintained, oxygen deficiency accelerates glycolysis, as a result of faster rates of glucose transport, hexokinase, and phosphofructokinase. The mechanism of ac-
cleration of glucose transport is poorly understood, but appears to
involve greater sensitivity of the transport process to stimulation
by insulin, and perhaps a more direct effect, resulting from the fall
in energy levels. Acceleration of hexokinase results from a reduction in tissue levels of glucose-6-P, a potent product inhibitor
of the enzyme, and an increased tissue level of P_i, an activator.
The fall in glucose-6-P is a consequence of an acceleration of phosphofructokinase due to decreased tissue levels of ATP, an inhibitor
of the enzyme, and increased levels of AMP and P_i, activators of
phosphofructokinase. In anoxic hearts, glycolytic rate is limited
by flux through the glyceraldehyde-3-P dehydrogenase reaction.
Activity of the enzyme is increased by the higher levels of the substrates, glyceraldehyde-3-P and Pi, but restrained by higher tissue
concentrations of the product, NADH. NADH produced by glycolysis

Table 1. Rate-controlling reactions in glycolysis

Reaction	Effector	Direction of change
Glucose transport: extracellular glucose -------- intracellular glucose	insulin anoxia pressure development fatty acid	increase increase increase decrease
Hexokinase: glucose + Mg ATP→ glucose-6-P + MgADP	ATP, ADP, P_i glucose-6-P	increase decrease
Phosphofructokinase: fructose-6-P + MgATP → fructose-1,6 diP + MgADP	acid pH fructose-6-P ATP, citrate P_i, AMP. ADP fructose-1, 6-diP	decrease increase decrease increase increase
Glyceraldehyde-3-P dehydrogenase: glyceraldyhyde-3-P + NAD$^+$ + P_i--------1,3-diP glycerate + NADH + H$^+$	NADH 1,3-diP-glycerate	decrease decrease
Pyruvate dehydrogenase: pyruvate + CoA + NAD$^+$ → acetyl CoA + NADH + H$^+$ + CO$_2$	phosphorylation acetyl CoA, NADH	decrease decrease

must be oxidized either by transport of reducing equivalents into the mitochondria via the malate-aspartate shuttle[9] or by conversion of pyruvate to lactate. When glycolysis is increased, production of NADH by glyceraldehyde-3-P dehydrogenase accelerates. Oxidation of this extra NADH by either conversion of oxaloacetate to malate or pyruvate to lactate requires increased levels of NADH to accelerate these reactions. The level of NADH thus increases in proportion to glycolytic rate and eventually reaches a concentration that is inhibitory to glyceraldehyde-3-P dehydrogenase.[10] Although ATP production via glycolysis may be increased 10-fold, inhibition of oxidative phosphorylation leads to as much as a 90% inhibition of overall ATP production. In association, contractile activity of anoxic hearts is severely impaired, as are the enzymatic reactions dependent upon the availability of ATP and other high-energy compounds.

In ischemic heart, energy depletion is complicated by accumulation of metabolites, particularly lactate and hydrogen ions. Glycolysis is inhibited, as compared to anoxic hearts. Rates of glucose transport, hexokinase, and phosphofructokinase are sufficiently rapid to provide saturating levels of substrate for glyceraldehyde-

3-P dehydrogenase. Flux through this enzyme is reduced however, by a fall in intracellular pH together with higher levels of NADH.[11] The pH optimum of glyceraldehyde-3-P dehydrogenase is above pH 8. In ischemic muscle, the average intracellular pH was about 6.8 as compared to a pH of 7.0 in aerobic hearts.[12] Accumulation of lactate interferes with oxidation of NADH, causing the nucleotide to accumulate and glyceraldehyde-3-P dehydrogenase to be inhibited. These observations emphasize the importance of the accumulation of metabolites in producing the biochemical defects in glycolytic regulation found in ischemic hearts and indicate that low rates of flux through glyceraldehyde-3-P dehydrogenase in ischemic hearts are due to higher tissue levels of NADH and hydrogen ions.

Metabolism of Free Fatty Acids in Ischemic Hearts

Plasma levels of free fatty acids (FFA) are frequently elevated in the first 1 or 2 hours following a myocardial infarction and this increase has been implicated in frequency of serious ventricular arrythmias.[13] The free acid is the principal form that is utilized by heart muscle (for review[14]). The majority of serum FFA is bound to albumin. The amount of acid that is free in solution is small and is determined by the FFA/albumin molar ratio. The unbound pool of FFA is in equilibrium with a tissue pool of FFA (Fig. 1). The nature of the tissue pool is unknown, but it may be composed of FFA in the cytoplasm as well as FFA bound to intracellular membranes and soluble proteins. The first step in the cellular metabolism of fatty acids is their conversion to long-chain fatty acyl-CoA esters (FACoA). This process, referred to as activation, is catalyzed by long-chain acyl-CoA synthetases that are located on the outer mitochondrial membrane. The tissue levels of fatty acid and ATP are normally well above the K_m of the synthetases for these substrates. However, the concentration of free CoA (CoASH) in the cytosol is unknown, due to the fact that only 5-10% of total CoA is in the cytosol and is distributed among fatty acyl-CoA, acetyl-CoA and free CoA. The activity of the synthetases is inhibited by the products of the reaction, fatty acyl-CoA, AMP and PP_i.

After fatty acyl-CoA is formed, the fatty acyl moiety undergoes reactions which function to move the acyl group from the site of activation on the outer mitochondrial membrane to the mitochondrial matrix where it is oxidized. The first reaction is the transfer of the acyl group from CoA to carnitine (Carn). The second reaction(s) is transport of the acyl moiety across the inner mitochondrial membrane. The transport of acyl-carnitine (FACarn) involves an exchange reaction in which acyl-carnitine moves across the mitochondrial membrane in exchange for carnitine. This appears to be a 1:1 exchange which would mean that the content of carnitine on both sides of the membrane would remain constant under physiological conditions. The third reaction in this segment is the transfer of the acyl group from carnitine to matrix CoA, forming fatty acyl-CoA that can be used for β-oxidation. Heart muscle has a high carnitine/CoA ratio in the cytosol, about 175, which would favor transfer of acyl units to carnitine, maintain low levels of fatty acyl-CoA in the cytosol, and direct acyl units away from lipid synthesis toward oxidation.

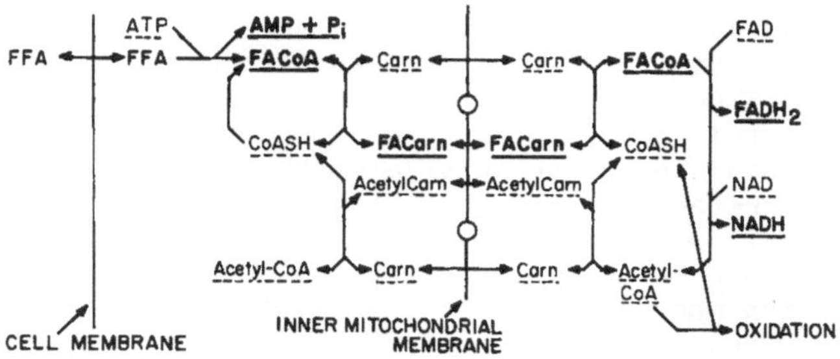

Fig. 1. Pathway for fatty acid oxidation in heart muscle illustrating intermediates that are elevated during ischemia in hearts perfused in the presence of fatty acid. This figure illustrates the two transferase systems for acyl units, each located on the inner and outer surfaces of the inner mitochondrial membrane. It includes compartmentation of CoA in two non-exchangeable pools (cytosolic and mitochondrial matrix); carnitine translocase is shown on the inner mitochondrial membrane between the two transferase systems. Metabolites that increase in ischemic hearts are shown with dark letters and are under-lined with a solid line; those that decrease are shown with light letters and are underscored with a broken line.

Following production of fatty acyl-CoA in the matrix, the next major sequence of reactions involves the β-oxidation system. Four separate enzymes are involved, and the overall reaction results in conversion of a two-carbon unit of fatty acyl-CoA to acetyl-CoA along with the reduction of NAD and FAD (1 mole each) to NADH and $FADH_2$. In order for the rate of β-oxidation to be sustained, the reduced nucleotides must be oxidized by electron transport, while acetyl-CoA is oxidized by the citric acid cycle.

In heart muscle, acetyl-CoA produced by β-oxidation can be used at appreciable rates only for oxidation by the citric acid cycle. Flux through the citric acid cycle is geared to the rate of oxidative phosphorylation through feedback control by changes in the levels of high energy phosphates and NADH. The only alternative route for the disposal of mitochondrial acetyl-CoA is transfer of the acetyl unit across the mitochondrial membrane to cytosolic carnitine where it is stored as acetyl-carnitine and provides a buffer against large changes in mitochondrial acetyl-CoA.

Under oxygen-deficient conditions such as ischemia or anoxia, the amount of oxygen available to support oxidation by the citric acid cycle is reduced (Figure 1). The levels of $FADH_2$ and NADH increase, and β-oxidation becomes inhibited. Levels of acetyl-CoA fall while the long-chain acyl derivatives of CoA and carnitine increase to very high levels. Since 95% of the total CoA is mitochondrial, most of the increase in acyl CoA must occur in this organelle. On the other hand, 95% of the total carnitine is cytosolic and most of the acyl carnitine must accumulate on the outside of the inner mitochondrial membrane. The uptake and activation of fatty acid is reduced. High levels of fatty acyl-CoA have been shown to inhibit the acyl-CoA synthetases[15-18] and adenine nucleotide translocase[19-20] in a specific manner, and many other enzymes in a non-specific way.[21] Free fatty acids[20] and long-chain acyl-carnitine,[23] in addition to having a detergent effect at high concentration, have been shown to inhibit Na^+-K^+ ATPase. Myocardial ischemia, therefore, in addition to resulting in a reduced capacity for ATP synthesis results in accumulation of compounds which are potentially detrimental to myocardial function and metabolism.

The Lysosomal System and Protein Turnover in Ischemic Hearts

As noted in the introduction to this paper, there is biochemical and morphological evidence of activation of the lysosomal system in ischemic hearts. Release of lysosomal enzymes into the cytoplasm or accelerated formation of autophagic vacuoles could lead to damage of cellular constituents, including the plasma membrane, sarcoplasmic reticulum and mitochondria, and lead to irreversible injury. Proteins, nucleic acids and phospholipids could be attacked by the appropriate hydrolases. At present, only the effects of ischemia on protein turnover have been investigated in detail.

If protein synthesis were inhibited more markedly than proteolysis in oxygen-deficient muscle, proteins with rapid rates of turnover could be lost, and marked metabolic derangements would ensue. Both synthesis and degradation of protein are energy-dependent processes[7,24-26] but these processes are modified to varying degrees by anoxia or ischemia.

In anoxic as compared to ischemic hearts, nitrogen balance was more negative in the absence of insulin (Figure 2). Protein degradation was more severely inhibited in ischemic than anoxic hearts, both in the presence and absence of insulin. Factors that may account for the more profound inhibition of protein degradation in

ischemic muscle include accumulation of lactate and hydrogen ions.[7]
In this regard, addition of a high concentration of lactate (50mM)
or a reduction in perfusate pH to 6.8 reduced proteolysis in aerobic
hearts by about 25%. When both lactate was added and pH reduced,
proteolysis was inhibited about 50%. These findings indicate that
inhibition of proteolysis in energy-poor muscle is due both to a
fall in high energy phosphate stores and to accumulation of metabolites.

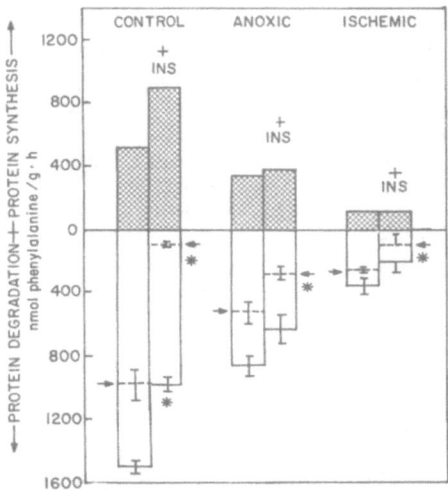

Fig. 2. Effects of ischemia and anoxia on protein synthesis, protein
degradation and nitrogen balance. Protein degradation (plotted downward from the zero line) was calculated by measuring
release of phenylalanine in the presence of cycloheximide -
nitrogen balance was measured by assessing phenylalanine release in the absence of cycloheximide (shown by the broken
lines and arrow heads). Protein synthesis was calculated by
subtracting nitrogen balance from protein degradation (plotted upward from zero line; cross-hatched bars). Six hearts
were perfused in each group with buffer containing 15mM
glucose, normal plasma levels of 19 amino acids and 0.01mM
phenylalanine. Insulin (25 mu/ml) was added as indicated.
Data represent the mean ± S.E. *p<0.05 versus no insulin.

Changes in the size of lysosomes or in the total activity of
lysosomal enzymes have been found to accompany a number of physiological and pathological modifications in the myocardium.[27] An increase in protein degradation in aerobic hearts perfused in the
absence of insulin was associated with a decrease in the latency of
cathepsin D.[28] These changes were associated with an increase

in the size of autophagic vacuoles within myocardial muscle cells.[29]
When insulin was present, rates of proteolysis were reduced by 50%,
and latency of lysosomal enzymes was increased.

Although accelerated rates of proteolysis was associated with decreased latency of lysosomal enzymes and appearance of autophagic
vacuoles in aerobic hearts, this correlation was lost in oxygen-
deficient tissue. As found in studies of liver lysosomes[2] activities
of cathepsin-D were higher in homogenates of anoxic and ischemic
hearts, even though the rate of protein degradation was inhibited.[7]
The effects of anoxia and ischemia on enzyme activity are thought to
reflect the greater fragility of autophagic vacuoles found within
ischemic hearts.[6] Although ultrastructural changes suggest that
tissue damage involved hydrolysis of cellular components by lysosomal
enzymes, proteolysis was not accelerated. The latter finding indicates that the energy requirement involves initial steps in the proteolytic pathway and that anoxia and ischemia do not lead to accumulation
of the products of proteolysis, peptides and free amino acids, within
the heart.[7,30] These findings indicate that protein breakdown is
inhibited in ischemic muscle, and that damage to this cellular component is unlikely to account for irreversible injury.

Concluding Remarks

In concluding this description of metabolism in the ischemic
heart, an overview of the changes will be presented in an attempt to
suggest common features and possible mechanisms of damage. Decreased coronary flow impairs oxygen delivery and removal of metabolic
products. As a result, ATP is converted to ADP and AMP. Loss of
total adenine nucleotide ensues, presumably due to hydrolysis of AMP
by 5'-nucleotidase. Decreased levels of ATP interfere with ion
pumping, Ca^{++} sequestration, and many other energy-dependent reactions. Reperfusion of ischemic hearts results in rapid resynthesis
of creatine phosphate, but ATP levels remain depressed. Irreversible
damage may result when ATP levels are too low to support critical
cellular functions such as contraction, volume control and substrate
activation. Metabolic intermediates in the pathways of glycolysis
and fatty acid oxidation accumulate and inhibit further flux of
substrate through these pathways. Inhibition of glycolysis impairs
even further the capacity for ATP generation, while accumulation of
fatty acyl-carnitine blocks the activity of Na^+ -K^+ ATPase and contributes to the difficulty in regulation of cell volume. The decrease in intracellular pH probably accounts for the initial fall
in contractility through interference with the calcium cycle, and
contributes to the fall in glycolytic rate. In some, as yet unknown
manner, the lysosomal system is activated and may be involved in disruption of sarcolemmal, mitochondrial, and other membrane systems.

This damage does not involve destruction of cellular proteins. The fall in intracellular pH and accumulation of compounds with detergent activity may enhance membrane damage. Future work could profitably be focussed on determining the nature of the damage that results from lysosomal activation and in identifying the link between energy-depletion and activation of this system.

REFERENCES

1. R. B. Jennings, and C. E. Ganote, Mitochondrial structure and function in acute myocardial ischemic injury, Circ. Res. 38: Suppl 1:180-191 (1976).

2. C. deDuve, and H. Beaufay, Tissue fractionation studies,Influence of ischemia on the state of some bound enzymes in rat liver, Biochem. J. 73: 610-616 (1959).

3. E. G. Leighty, C.D. Stoner, M. M. Ressallat, G. T. Passananti, and H. D. Sirak, Effects of acute asphyxia and deep hypothermia on the state of binding of lysosomal acid hydrolases in canine cardiac muscle, Circ. Res. 21: 59-64 (1967).

4. M. A. Riccuitti, Lysosomes and myocardial cellular injury. Am J. Cardio. 30: 498-502 (1972).

5. S. Hoffstein, G. Weissman, and A. C. Fox, Lysosomes in myocardial infarction: Studies by means of cytochemistry and subcellular fractionation with observations on the effects of methylprednisolone, Circulation 53: Suppl 1:134-140 (1976).

6. L. P. McAllister, B. L. Munger, and J. R. Neely, Electron microscopic observations and acid phosphatase activity in the ischemic rat heart, J. Mol. Cell. Cardiol 9: 353-364 (1977).

7. B. Chua, R. L. Kao, D. E. Rannels, and H. E. Morgan, Inhibition of protein degradation by anoxia and ischemia in perfused rat hearts, J. Biol. Chem. 254: 6617-6623 (1979).

8. J. R. Neely, and H. E. Morgan, Relationship between carbohydrate and lipid metabolism and the energy balance of heart muscle. Ann. Rev. Physiol. 36: 413-459 (1974).

9. K. F. LaNoue, and A. C. Schoolwerth, Metabolite transport in mitochondria, Ann. Rev. Biochem. 48:871-922 (1979).

10. S. Mochizuki, and J. R. Neely, Control of glyceraldehyde-3-P dehydrogenase in cardiac muscle, J. Mol. Cell Cardiol. 11: 221-236 (1979).

11. M. J. Rovetto, W. F. Lamberton, and J. R. Neely, Mechanisms of glycolytic inhibition in ischemic rat hearts, Circ. Res. 37: 742-751 (1975).

12. J. R. Neely, J. T. Whitmer, and M. J. Rovetto, Effect of coronary blood flow on glycolytic flux and intracellular pH in isolated rat hearts, Circ. Res. 37: 733-741 (1975).

13. M. F. Oliver, V. A. Kurien, and T. W. Greenwood, Relation between serum-free fatty acids and arrhythmias and death after acute myocardial infarction, Lancet 1: 710-714 (1968).

14. J. A. Idell-Wenger, and J. R. Neely, Regulation of uptake and metabolism of fatty acids by muscle, in: "Disturbances in Lipid and Lipoprotein Metabolism," J. M. Dietschy, A. M. Gotto, Jr., and J. A. Ontko, eds., American Physiological Society, Bethesda, pp 269-284 (1978).

15. J. W. DeJong, and W. C. Hulsman, A comparative study of palmitoyl CoA synthetase activity in rat liver, heart and gut mitochondrial and microsomal preparation, Biochem Biophys Acta 197: 127-135 (1970).

16. J. W. DeJong, and W. C. Hulsman, Effects of Nagarse, adenosine and hexokinase on palmitate activation and oxidation, Biochem. Biophys. Acta 210: 499-501 (1970).

17. S. V. Pande, Reversal by CoA of palmityl-CoA inhibition of long chain acyl-CoA synthetase activity, Biochem Biophys. Acta 306: 15-20 (1973).

18. J. F. Oram, J. I. Wenger, and J. R. Neely, Regulation of long chain fatty acid activation in heart muscle, J. Biol. Chem. 250: 73-78 (1975).

19. H. H. Chong, and S. V. Pande, On the specificity of the inhibition of adenine nucleotide translocase by long chain acyl-coenzyme A esters, Biochem. Biophys. Acta 369:86-94 (1974).

20. B. Chua, and E. Shrago, Reversible inhibition of adenine nucleotide translocation by long chain acyl CoA esters in bovine heart mitochondria and inverted submitochondrial particles, J. Biol. Chem. 252:6711-6714 (1977).

21. F. Morel, G. Lauquin, J. Lunardi, J. Duszynski, and P. V. Vignais An appraisal of the functional significance of the inhibitory effect of long chain acyl-CoAs on mitochondrial transports, FEBS Lett.39:133-138 (1974).

22. J. M. J. Lamers, and W. C. Hulsmann, Inhibition of $(Na^+ + Ka^+)$-stimulated ATPase of heart by fatty acids, J. Mol. Cell. Card. 9: 343-346 (1977).

23. J. M. Wood, B. Bush, B. J. R. Pitts, and A. Schwartz, Inhibition of bovine heart Na^+, K^+ - ATPase by palmitylcarnitine and palmityl-CoA, Biochem. Biophys. Res. Commun. 74:677-684 (1977).

24. R. Kao, D. E. Rannels, and H. E. Morgan, Effects of anoxia and ischemia on protein synthesis in perfused rat hearts, Circ. Res. 38: Suppl 1: 124-130 (1976).

25. H. E. Morgan, D. E. Rannels, and E. E. McKee, Protein metabolism of the heart, in: "Handbook of Physiology - The Cardiovascular System," R. M. Berne, ed., American Physiological Society, Bethesa, pp 845-871 (1979).

26. H. E. Morgan, B. Chua, and C. J. Beinlich, Regulation of protein degradation in heart, in: "Degradative Processes in Heart and Skeletal Muscle," K. Wildenthal, ed., North Holland Biomedical Press, Amsterdam, pp 87-112 (1980).

27. K. Wildenthal, Lysosomes and lysosomal enzymes in the heart, in: "Lysosomes in Biology and Pathology," J. T. Dingle and R. T. Deans, eds., Elsevier Publishing Company, Inc., New York, pp 167-190 (1975).

28. D. E. Rannels, R. Kao, and H. E. Morgan, Effect of insulin on
     protein turnover in heart muscle, J. Biol. Chem. 250: 1694-
     1701 (1975).
29. L. S. Jefferson, D. E. Rannels, B.L. Munger, and H. E. Morgan,
     Insulin in the regulation of protein turnover in heart and
     skeletal muscle, Fed. Proc. 33: 1098-1104 (1974).
30. E. H. Williams, R. L. Kao, and H. E. Morgan, Protein degradation
     and synthesis during recovery from myocardial ischemia, Am. J.
     Physiol. (Endocrinol. Metab. 3) 240: E268-E273 (1981).

.

CALCIUM AND CARDIOVASCULAR DISEASE

L. H. Opie

MRC Ischaemic Heart Research Unit
Department of Medicine
Groote Schuur Hospital and University of Cape Town
South Africa

INTRODUCTION

When the calcium-antagonist agents were initially used by Fleckenstein's group, it was found that beta-adrenoceptor agonists opposed the specific action of high dose verapamil (10^{-5}M) in inhibiting myocardial contractility (Figure 3 and 7 in Fleckenstein, 1971). The restorative effect of isoproterenol was very similar to that of an increased extracellular calcium (Figure 6 in Fleckenstein, 1971). Thus early thinking saw calcium-antagonists and beta-antagonists as having opposite effects on trans-sarcolemmal calcium flux. Some even argued that the calcium-antagonists had beta-blocking qualities, an argument that was laid to rest when it was found that verapamil was unable to inhibit an isoproterenol-induced tachycardia or inotropic response (Nayler et al, 1968). The explanation was that verapamil could not prevent catecholamine-induced increases in the tissue level of cyclic AMP nor the beta-mediated activation of adenyl cyclase; rather, verapamil blocked the trans-sarcolemmal calcium influx provoked in K^+ depolarized hearts by either catecholamines or by an increased external calcium (Watanabe et al, 1974).

This paper reviews the properties of calcium antagonist agents and evaluates a new hypothesis that trans-sarcolemmal calcium fluxes may play a role in provoking ventricular fibrillation (Thandroyen, 1982). This hypothesis is tested by examining the effects of calcium-antagonists on an isolated rat heart model. Previous data have suggested that beta-adrenergic stimulation can decrease ventricular fibrillation threshold in models of myocardial infarction (Lubbe et al, 1978).

45

Before evaluating this hypothesis, it is relevant to examine current concepts of the cellular modes of action of the beta-adrenoceptor antagonists and calcium-antagonists.

CONTRASTING PROPERTIES OF BETA-ADRENOCEPTOR BLOCKERS
CALCIUM-ANTAGONISTS

Mode of action of beta-adrenoceptor antagonists

A beta-adrenoceptor antagonist is an agent that interacts with the beta-receptor to provoke a characteristic series of events which include, in the case of the myocardium, a positive chronotropic and inotropic stimulation. Many of the effects of beta-stimulation are thought to be mediated by cyclic AMP. Hence because beta-adrenoceptor antagonists competitively interfere with the binding between the beta-antagonist and its receptor, beta-antagonists should decrease the tissue cyclic AMP response to beta-antagonists.

Mode of action of calcium-antagonists

In contrast to this rather clear sequence of events, the definition of a calcium-antagonist is somewhat obscure. It is best to go back to the original descriptions by Fleckenstein (Fleckenstein, 1971). In his basic experiment, acute contractile failure of the guinea-pig heart was produced by a large over-dose (1 mg/kg) of verapamil. There was an abrupt rise in the venous pressure and fall in the arterial pressure which was reversed by the injection of calcium chloride. Thus the first property of the calcium-antagonist drugs is that they selectively abolish "the contractile response of the guinea-pig papillary muscle in a low concentration without any significant change in the single fiber action potentials". This effect is antagonized by the calcium ions (Fleckenstein, 1971). Each molecule of verapamil antagonizes approximately 200 calcium ions whereas in the case of other antagonists such as the compound D-600 or nifedipine, 1 molecule antagonizes up to several thousand calcium ions. The second quality of the calcium-antagonists is that although they appear to affect the action potential in no significant way, when voltage clamp studies are undertaken, they can be shown to "block the transmembrane calcium influx into the excited heart muscle fibers but do not affect the simultaneous sodium movements which are connected with the action potential" (Fleckenstein, 1971). This inhibitory effect of calcium antagonists on the calcium slow inward current is also opposed by the addition of excess external calcium.

Properties of calcium channel

To control the vast difference in the concentration between calcium in the extracellular fluid and the cytosol (a concentration gradient of about 10^3) requires regulation of the calcium transmission across the sarcolemma. There are several possible modes of calcium entry. First, calcium can enter via the calcium channel or calcium channels (which have not been characterized). The sodium channel has been the subject of numerous models, including recent modifications of the classical Hodgkin-Huxley concept of the three "m" activation gates and the single "h" inactivation gate (Weld et al, 1982). Such data and models are not available for the calcium channel although a similar pattern of interaction is sometimes postulated.

Therefore, at the moment, the understanding of the calcium channel is largely descriptive. Some of the properties of calcium channels are:

1. They are "opened" by a voltage stimulus as the resting potential depolarizes to about -40 mV (Noble, 1979).
2. They "close" as calcium influx ceases and potassium efflux is enhanced (Bassingthwaighte et al, 1976).
3. They "open" in the presence of sodium and calcium ions externally (Schneider et al, 1975).
4. They can be "opened" by beta-stimulation (Reuter, 1974; Reuter & Scholtz, 1977). It is not sure in the case of the myocardium whether these receptor-operated channels are the same as the channels which respond to the influx of sodium ions. In the case of vascular smooth muscle clear arguments have been made (Bolton, 1979; Towart, 1981; Van Breemen et al, 1982) for the differentiation between DOC (depolarization operated channels) and ROC (receptor operated channels). In the case of the myocardium, K^+-depolarization inhibits the sodium channel so that an increased voltage stimulation plus beta-stimulation may be required to "open" the calcium channel (Schneider et al, 1975); hence the concept of DOC's for the myocardium seem invalid.
5. The channels are "closed" or "blocked" by calcium-antagonist group of drugs which include verapamil, nifedipine and diltiazem. It is not clear whether these drugs have similar or different modes of action on the calcium channel. It is also not clear whether these drugs act predominantly on the outside of the sarcolemma, as suggested in the case of verapamil (Langer et al, 1975); more recent evidence proposes that verapamil is concentrated many-fold within the heart (Lullman et al, 1979) cell and may act deeply in the membrane or on the inner surface of the sarcolemma (Payet et al, 1980).

This emphasis of the effects of calcium-antagonists on the trans-sarcolemma should not obscure the growing evidence that there is also an intracellular site of action, for example on calmodulin (Boström et al, 1981; Hidaka et al, 1979).

Functionally different calcium channels

Not only is the nature of the calcium channel not clear, but there are apparent differences between the calcium channels in various tissues. Although an increased extracellular calcium concentration antagonizes the effect of high-dose verapamil in depressing myocardial contractility (Hamm et al, 1982), calcium has no such effect when it comes to the inhibitory action of verapamil on the sinus node; in that case externally added calcium does not "antagonize" verapamil but rather leaves unchanged its effect in inhibition of conduction (Hariman et al, 1979). That difference provides a valuable practical approach to the problem of depressed myocardial function sometimes encountered when patients are given verapamil intravenously - injected calcium salts should restore myocardial contractility without impairing the therapeutic effect of verapamil on the atrioventricular node.

There is also very recent evidence that the calcium channel of vascular smooth muscle is stimulated by alpha-2 antagonists such as clonidine and inhibited by alpha-2 antagonists such as yohimbine (Van Meel et al, 1981). Hence the postjunctional alpha-2 receptors appear to be intimately linked to calcium transport in vascular smooth muscle. No such data exist for the myocardium.

Thus, from the practical point of view, the calcium channels in nodal tissue, in myocardial tissue and in vascular smooth muscle, all appear to have somewhat different characteristics although they share the property of being the site of action of the calcium-antagonist agents.

Ca^{2+}-ANTAGONISTS AND VENTRICULAR FIBRILLATION

We have proposed the hypothesis that calcium ions are involved in the genesis of ventricular fibrillation (Thandroyen, 1982). The first step in the evolution of the hypothesis was the recognition that elevation of tissue cyclic AMP in ischemic tissue could be linked to the onset of ventricular fibrillation (Lubbe et al, 1978; Opie et al, 1979; Opie et al, 1980). Calcium was seen as the further "messenger" of cyclic AMP (Opie et al, 1982). Recent data emphasize the role of calcium rather than of cyclic AMP. We tested the hypothesis by examining whether the three first generation Ca^{2+}-antagonist agents (verapamil, nifedipine, diltiazem) could inhibit ventricular fibrillation in the isolated rat heart model with coronary ligation (Thandoryen, 1982). All the agents were used in doses just below those causing atrioventricular block, and all elevated the ventricular fibrillation threshold of the isolated coronary ligated perfused rat heart. The antifibrillatory effects of the Ca^{2+}-antagonists were considerably greater than those of dℓ-propranolol (Opie et al, 1982). All the Ca^{2+}-antagonists tended to reduce cyclic AMP, although again not to the same extent as high-dose dℓ-propranolol. This "antifibrillatory" effect of the calcium-antagonist agents could be a non-specific phenomenon, as in the case of dℓ-propranolol (Lubbe et al, 1981).

Thus the effect of verapamil (1.5×10^{-7}M) is no more specific for the
Ca^{2+}-antagonist than for any Na^{+}-antagonist effects of verapamil, because the ℓ-isomer has a similar effect to the d-isomer. Hence, in
an isolated heart not subject to external catecholamine stimulation,
both sodium and calcium channels are involved in ventricular fibrillation. Our recent data show that in conditions of adrenaline-stimu-
lation (adrenaline 5×10^{-7}M) ℓ-verapamil caused a marked fall in
fibrillation threshold whereas d-verapamil had virtually no effect.
In theory, the ℓ-isomer inhibits the slow calcium channel (Bayer et
al, 1975) whereas the d-isomer inhibits the fast sodium channel
(Kohlhardt et al, 1978), hence the dℓ-isomer has local anesthetic
properties (Bondi, 1978). Consequently, the inhibition of adrenaline-
mediated effects by ℓ-verapamil rather than by d-verapamil favours
the view that the calcium antagonist effects of verapamil are involved
in these conditions of stimulation by external catecholamine. These
data suggest that calcium ions are involved in the production of increased sensitivity to stimulated ventricular fibrillation occurring
after the combination of coronary ligation and added beta-stimulation.

SUMMARY

    The properties of calcium-channel antagonist agents are described.
Because these agents render the isolated heart less sensitive to ventricular fibrillation a role for calcium ions in the genesis of ventricular fibrillation is proposed. The data obtained with verapamil
isomers in isolated hearts with coronary ligation suggest (i) a role
for both calcium and sodium ions in the fall of the fibrillation
threshold following coronary artery ligation, and (ii) a role only
for calcium ions when coronary ligation is combined with catecholamine
stimulation.

REFERENCES

Bassingthwaighte, J. B., Fry, C. H., McGuigan, J. A. S., 1976. Re-
    lationship between internal calcium and outward current in
    mammalian ventricular muscle: a mechanism for the control of
    the action potential duration? J. Physiol. 262: 15-37.
Bayer, R., Kalusche, D., Kaufmann, R., Mannhold, R., 1975. Inotropic
    and electrophysiological actions of verapamil and D600 in mam-
    malian myocardium. 111. Effects of the optical isomers on
    transmembrane action potentials. Naunyn-Schmied. Arch. Pharm.
    290: 81-97.
Bolton, T. B., 1979. Mechanisms of action of transmitters and other
    substances on smooth muscle. Physiol. Rev. 59: 606-718.
Bondi, A. Y., 1978. Effects of verapamil on excitation-contraction
    coupling in frog sartorius muscle. J. Pharmacol. Expt. Therap.
    205: 49-57.

Boström, S.L., Ljung, B., Mardh, S., Forsen, S., Thulin, E., 1981.
    Interaction of the antihypertensive drug felodipine with
    calmodulin. Nature 292: 777-778.
Fleckenstein, A., 1971. Specific inhibitors and promoters of calcium
    action in the excitation-contraction coupling of heart muscle
    and their role in the prevention or production of myocardial
    lesions. Harris, P., Opie, L.H. eds. In "Calcium and the Heart"
    London: Academic Press; 135-188
Hamm, C. W., Thandroyen, F. T., Opie, L. H., 1982. Protective effects
    on isolated hearts with developing infarction: slow channel
    blockade by diltiazem versus beta-adrenoceptor antagonism by
    metoprolol. Am. J. Cardiol. in press
Hariman, R. J., Mangiardi, L. M., McAllister, R. G., Surawicz, B.,
    Shabetai, R., Kishida, H., 1979. Reversal of the cardiovascular
    effects of verapamil by calcium and sodium: differences between
    electrophysiologic and hemodynamic responses. Circulation 59:
    797-804.
Hidaka, H., Yamaki, T., Naka, M., Tanaka, T., Hayashi, H., Kobayashi,
    R., 1979. Calcium-regulated modulator protein interacting
    agents inhibit smooth muscle calcium-stimulated protein kinase
    and ATPase. Mol. Pharmacol. 17: 66-72.
Kolhardt, M., Mnich, Z., 1978. Studies on the inhibitory effect of
    verapamil on the slow inward current in mammalian ventricular
    myocardium. J. Molec. Cell Cardiol. 10: 1037-1052.
Langer, G. A., Serena, S. D., Nubb, L. M., 1975. Localization of con-
    tractile-dependent Ca: comparison of Mn and verapamil in car-
    diac and skeletal muscle. Am. J. Physiol. 229: 1003-1007.
Lubbe, W. F., Muller, C. A., Worthington, M. G., McFadyen, L., Opie,
    L. H., 1981. Influence of propranolol isomers and atenolol on
    myocardial cyclic AMP, high energy phosphates and vulnerability
    to fibrillation after coronary artery ligation in the isolated
    rat heart. Cardiovasc. Res. 15: 690-699.
Lubbe, W. F., Podzuweit, T., Daries, P. S., Opie, L. H., 1978. The
    role of cyclic adenosine monophosphate in adrenergic effects
    on vulnerability to fibrillation in the isolated perfused rat
    heart. J. Clin. Invest. 61: 1260-1269.
Lullman, H., Timmermans, P. B. Ziegler, A., 1979, Accumulation of
    drugs by resting or beating cardiac tissue. Europ. J. Pharmacol
    60: 277-285.
Nayler, W. G., McInnes, I., Swann, J. B., Price, J. M., Carson, V.,
    Race, C., Lowe, T. E., 1968. Some effects of iproveratril
    (Isoptin) on the cardiovascular system. J. Pharmacol. Expt.
    Therap. 161: 247-261.
Opie, L. H., Muller, C., Nathan, D., Daries, P., Lubbe, W. F., 1980.
    Evidence for role of cyclic AMP as second messenger of arrhyth-
    mogenic effects of beta-stimulation. Adv. Cycl. Nucl. Res.
    12: 63-69.
Opie, L. H., Thandroyen, F. T., Hamm, C. W., 1982. Beta-blockade:
    metabolic and antiarrhythmic effects in myocardial infarction.
    Calcium as third messenger. In: Advances in beta-blocker
    therapy 11. Excerpta Medica; Amsterdam, pp. 40-64.

Opie. L. H., Thandroyen. F. T., Muller. C., Bricknell. O. L., 1979. Adrenaline-induced "oxygen-wastage" and enzyme release from working rat heart. Effects of calcium antagonism, β-blockade, nicotinic acid and coronary artery ligation. J. Molec. Cell. Cardiol. 11: 1073-1094.

Payet, M. D., Schanne, O. F., Ruiz-Ceretti, E., Demers, J. M., 1980. Inhibitory action of blockers of the slow inward current in rat myocardium, a study in steady state and rate of action. J. Molec. Cell Cardiol. 12: 187-200.

Reuter, H., 1974. Localization of beta-adrenergic receptors, and effects of noradrenaline and cyclic nucleotides on action potentials, ionic currents and tension in mammalian cardiac muscle. J. Physiol. 242: 429-451.

Reuter, H., Scholtz, 1977. The regulation of the calcium conductance of cardiac muscle by adrenaline. J. Physiol. 264: 49-62.

Schneider, J. A., Sperelakis, N., 1975. Slow Ca^{2+} and Na^+ responses induced by isoproterenol and methylxanthines in isolated perfused guinea pig hearts exposed to elevated K^+. J. Molec. Cell Cardiol. 7: 249-273.

Thandroyen, F. T., 1982. Protective action of calcium channel antagonist agents against ventricular fibrillation in the isolated perfused rat heart. J. Molec. Cell. Cardiol. 14: 21-32.

Towart, R., 1981. The selective inhibition of serotonin-induced contractions of rabbit cerebral vascular smooth muscle by calcium-antagonistic dihydropyridines. An investigation of the mechanism of action of nimodipine. Circ. Res. 48: 650-657.

Van Breemen, C., Mangel, A., Fahim, M., Meisheri, K., 1982. Selectivity of calcium antagonist action in vascular smooth muscle. Am. J. Cardiol. 49: 507-510.

Van Meel, J. C. A., de Jonge, A., Kalkman, H. D., Wilffert, B., Timmermans, B. M. W. M., van Zwieten, P. A., 1981. Vascular smooth muscle contraction initiated by postsynaptic α_2-adrenoceptor activation is induced by an influx of extracellular calcium. Europ. J. Pharmacol. 69: 205-208.

Watanabe, A. M., Besch, H. R. Jnr., 1974. Subcellular myocardial effects of verapamil and D600: comparison with propranolol. J. Pharmacol. Expt. Therap. 191: 241-251.

Weld, F. M., Coromilas, J., Rottman, J. N., Bigger, J. T. Jnr., 1982. Mechanisms of quinidine-induced depression of maximum upstroke velocity in ovine cardiac Purkinje fibers. Circ. Res. 50: 369-376.

CELLULAR AND MOLECULAR MECHANISMS OF ATHEROSCLEROSIS

E.I. Chazov

USSR Cardiology Research Center
Moscow

INTRODUCTION

The progress of science and technology, the development of fundamental studies in cardiology during the last decade have opened new frontiers for the exploration of mechanisms of cardiovascular diseases. Today the major thrust in atherosclerosis research is aimed at developing a molecular-cellular theory, which would explain molecular and cellular processes that give rise to morphological and clinical manifestations of the disease. The essence of the research boils down to the integral assessment of factors in pathogenesis of atherosclerosis. From the general to the particular and from the particular to the general - that is the way of scientific research. It is especially important to abide by this principle when studying such complex diseases as atherosclerosis.

Complexity of the disease is mainly manifested by dislipoproteinemia. The mechanism of lipid metabolism disorders during the atherosclerosis has been lately specified. In most cases the disorders proved to be localized in the system of transport, targeted delivery and removal of cholesterol, its esters, and phospholipids. Plasma lipoproteins play a key role in the system. Now it is becoming clear what defects lipoprotein synthesis, processing and catabolism lead to dislipoproteinemia in man.

STRUCTURE OF LIPOPROTEIN AND ATHEROSCLEROSIS

In this field the main effort is concentrated on deciphering the mechanism responsible for cholesterol and phospholipids donor-acceptor functions of plasma lipoproteins. This direction seems to

be promising for investigation of atherosclerosis since in the course
of epidemiological studies a negative correlation was found between
HDL cholesterol level and the incidence of ischemic heart disease in
men after 40 years of age.

On the other hand, the experiments on cell cultures and a perfused vessel demonstrated that HDL, particularly HDL_3, are capable
of uptaking cholesterol from cellular membranes and the vessel
wall.[1,2] The population of particles with HDL_2 density transports
cholesterol into the liver for excretion from the organism. It is
HDL_2 level that is reduced in IHD patients. That is why we took
interest in the characteristics of chemical composition of HDL and
their main subfractions (HDL_2 and HDL_3) in patients with documented
coronary atherosclerosis. (Figure 1).

It is assumed that the main acceptor characteristics of HDL are
determined by the phospholipid layer of lipoproteins. HDL phospholipids of healthy subjects consist of 70% lecithin and 12% sphingomyelin. It was shown in model systems that a lecithin increase in
HDL enhances their cholesterol acceptor capability and vice versa.[3]

These data served as a requisite for elucidation of the role of
HDL phospholipid composition in realization of their antiatherogenic
properties in patients suffering from coronary atherosclerosis.

Firstly, we were interested whether in patients with different
manifestation of coronary atherosclerosis: 1) lecithin/sphingomyelin
ratio of plasma HDL_2 and HDL_3 is changed, and if so, to what extent;
2) apo B/apo A ratio is changed at different lipoprotein spectrum,
assuming that cholesterol is transported into the vessel wall via
LDL and removed via HDL.

Two of these indices were studied in the plasma of patients with
different manifestations of coronary atherosclerosis by selective
angiography data. The area of total atherosclerotic lesion was calculated in arbitrary units according to a special formula, which took
into account the extent of occlusion, localization and spread of the
lesion.

At normal lipoprotein spectrum the area of atherosclerotic
lesion in CHD patients is smaller than that at dyslipoproteinemia-
hyperlipoproteinemia or at a low HDL cholesterol level. Apo B/apo
A_1 ratio in all CHD patients, even those with normal lipoprotein
spectrum, was higher than in the control group. The highest (Figure
2) values of such ratio were observed at low HDL cholesterol. We
assume that an increase of this ratio above one showed that cholesterol inflow to the arterial wall exceeded its outflow. It was still
unclear what accounted for the reduction of cholesterol outflow from
the arterial wall; a decrease in number of HDL particles, alterations
of their characteristics, or both.

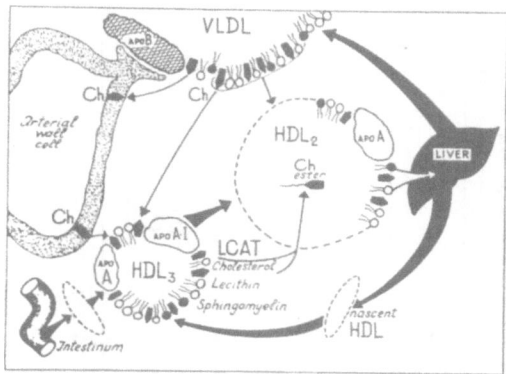

Fig. 1. Schematic representation of metabolism of VLDL and HDL.
VLDL—very high density lipoprotein. HDL—high density
lipoprotein. LCAT—lecithincholesterolacyltransferase.

To elucidate the question phospholipid composition and molar
ratio of lecithin to sphingomyelin have been studied in HDL_2 and
HDL_3. This ratio to a considerable degree determines the fluidity
of surface monolayer and cholesterol—acceptor function of these
particles.

A decrease of lecithin/sphingomyelin ratio was observed both in
HDL_2 and HDL_3 of patients with coronary atherosclerosis in comparison
with the control group. The greatest decrease was found in patients
with low HDL cholesterol (Figure 3).

These facts indirectly prove the assumption that relative lecithin content largely determines the fluidity and cholesterol—acceptor
function of HDL phospholipids. In our experiment a reduction of
lecithin/sphingomyelin ratio in HDL_3 resulted in the decrease of
biolayer fluidity and ability to accept cholesterol from cellular
membranes or VLDL.

It is also quite probable that a possibility of LCAT (lecithin-
cholesterolacyltransferase)—mediated transformation into HDL_2 is
somewhat limited for HDL_3 with a low lecithin level. Under normal
conditions this enzyme catalyzes cholesterol esters formation from
free lecithin and cholesterol. While esterifying, cholesterol moves
from biolayer into a hydrophobic "core". Lecithin is a substrate
for this reaction. The decrease of LCAT—reaction leads to a re-

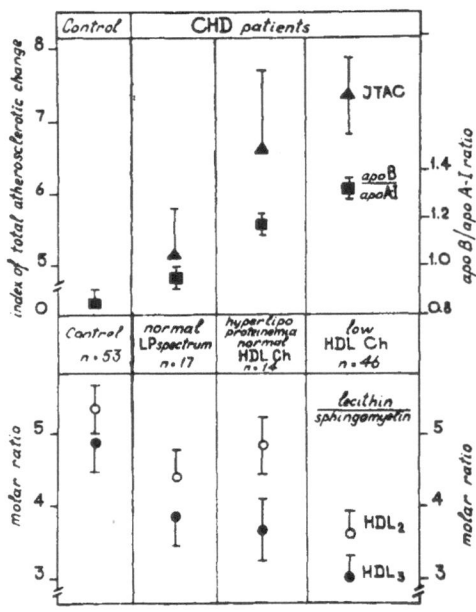

Fig. 2. HDL phospholipid composition and apo-B/apo-A ratio in healthy group and CHD patients. The left top ordinate-the degree of morphological involvement according to selective angiographic data. The right top ordinate- apo-B/apo-A ratio. The bottom ordinate- lecithin/sphingomyelin ratio. O- for HDL$_2$. O- for HDL$_3$.

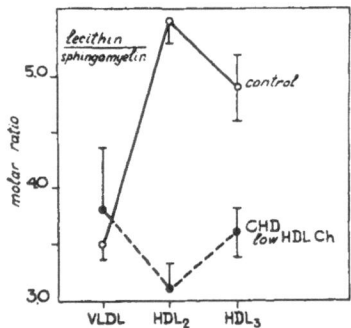

Fig. 3. VLDL,HDL$_2$ and HDL$_3$ phospholipid composition in healthy group and CHD patients with low HDL.

duction of cholesterol esters formation and thus decreases the formation from HDL_3 particles of HDL_2 which transport cholesterol to the liver for excretion.

Thus, the decrease of lecithin/sphingomyelin ratio in the phospholipid monolayer of lipoproteins of this class in patients with coronary atherosclerosis results both in lowering of the ability to accept cholesterol from membranes and expel it from the body.

The data on the lecithin/sphingomyelin ratio in three groups of particles, namely, VLDL, HDL_2 and HDL_3 are important with respect to investigation of mechanisms of atherosclerosis. Cholesterol inflow to and outflow from the membranes and its excretion from the organism are closely connected with cholesterol exchange between these particles. It was found that lecithin/sphingomyelin ratio in HDL_2 and HDL_3 of the control group was higher than in very low density lipoproteins. Naturally, that facilitates cholesterol inflow from VLDL to HDL_3 and HDL_2 in the control group of subjects. On the contrary, in patients with coronary atherosclerosis lecithin/sphingomyelin ratio did not exceed the values observed in VLDL. Naturally, under these conditions adequate amounts of cholesterol are not transferred from VLDL to HDL_3 and HDL_2. Thus, it is accumulated in these lipoproteins and together with them is transported into the vessel wall in larger quantities (Figure 3).

To confirm this assumption cholesterol content was calculated per a weight unit of apo B and apo A_1. In the group of patients with coronary atherosclerosis cholesterol share per a weight unit of apo B in VLDL was increased in comparison with the control group (Figure 4).

All these data indicate the decrease in cholesterol-acceptor and cholesterol-transport functions of HDL during coronary atherosclerosis which, in our view, is a possible mechanism of a tissue lipoidosis. We particularly stress the importance of changes in the molecular organization of HDL surface monolayer for this process. The obtained data lay the foundation not only for profound investigation of molecular basis of atherosclerotic process but, taking into account a possibility of changing antiatherosclerotic lipoprotein properties by affecting its phospholipid monolayer, open new prospects for the development of prevention techniques.

Along with lipoprotein structure the particles behavior in the organism is conditioned by a whole hierarchy of factors, which manifest themselves at different levels - from a single cell to the whole organism.

Surely, dislipoproteinemia is the most important sign of atherosclerosis. However, cells from different parts of the vascular system react quite differently to this metabolic disorder. Segmented

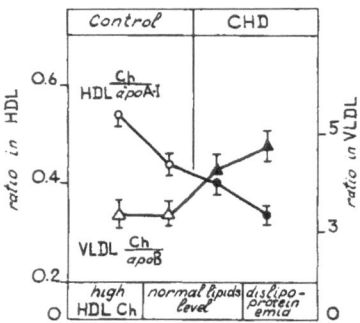

Fig. 4. Cho/apo-B ratio in plasma HDL and VLDL of control group
        and CHD patients.

character of atherosclerotic lesions in arteries and existence of
"predilected sites" for plaque formation prove that the intrinsic
characteristics of the vessel wall are really important for lesion
development. This is why we think it equally important to study
along with lipoproteins the structural and functional characteristics
of vessel wall cells.

VESSEL WALL IN CULTURE AND ATHEROSCLEROSIS

     At present most of the studies are concentrated on cellular
manifestations of atherosclerosis at early and late stages: functional and morphological endothelial injuries, migration and proliferation of intimal cells; dedifferentiation and redifferentiation
of medial smooth muscle cells; formation of foam cells and lipid-
laden cells; production of extracellular matrix components by the
endothelium and SMC. Cell-cell interactions are being intensively
studied: endothelial cells - SMC, blood born cells - intimal cells.
Special attention is paid to the adhesion of platelets and monocytes
(macrophages) in zones of endothelial damage. The latter event
plays a key role both in atherogenesis and thrombogenesis.

     Cellular aspects of human atherosclerosis mostly remain obscure.
The bulk of information on the problem has been öbtained on the basis
of histological analysis of autopsy material which does not allow to
precisely evaluate cellular dynamics in atherosclerotic lesion zones.
Only recently the methods of cellular biology, specifically a technique of culturing human vascular cells open new possibilities for
the study of human atherosclerosis.

     Nowadays cell culture may be figuratively called a "highway"
in the investigation of human atherosclerosis. Actually, so far
this is the only possible kind of experiment on man. It is of im-

portance that for a certain period of time cells in primary culture retain their intrinsic <u>in situ</u> properties.[4],[5] Main manifestations of atherosclerosis at a cellular level (endothelial monolayer damage and repair, SMS proliferation, lipoidosis, connective tissue matrix formation) can be reproduced in culture; the same simple chemical conditions make it possible to reproduce the early stages of thrombi formation: adhesion, platelet spreading and formation of aggregates and thrombi of platelets. Finally, the primary culture makes it possible to study the effect of different drugs on cellular manifestations of human atherosclerosis.

Therefore, the experiments on cell cultures performed in our Center are rather multipurpose.

The Center was the first to develop original techniques of obtaining endothelial and SMC cultures both from uninvolved and atherosclerotic areas of human aorta. We obtained a significantly high cell yield from tissue (50-90%), while 90% of cells retained viability and attached to the substrate. Thus, the cultures rather adequately reflected the cellular composition of various parts of human aorta.

Endothelial cells of human atherosclerotic aorta in primary culture are heterogenous: 5-20% of the population are made up by giant multinuclear cells. They have all signs of endothelial cells (VIII factor of coagulation, Weibel-Palade bodies). Similar cells were found on the luminal surface of the <u>in situ</u> human aorta by scanning electron microscopy. In the vessel affected by atherosclerosis giant endothelial cells are mainly concentrated in the region of fatty streaks and plaques. 40-50% of all the lesion area in these zones is covered with such atypical monolayer (Figure 5). That gave us reason to assume that giant endothelial cells are lesion zone "markers" on the luminal surface. Morphological heterogeneity of endothelium is most prominent in fatty streak and plague regions. Therefore, the study of endothelial polymorphism in culture, specifically of the mechanism responsible for giant multinuclear cells formation, seems to be a promising direction of research. It cannot be ruled out that these cells are the "hot spots" of lipoprotein metabolism-endocytosis, transendothelial transport etc.

Primary cultures of human aortic intimal cells also proved to be morphologically heterogenous. Four main types can be distinguished among them: 1) elongated, 2) polygonal, 3) asymmetric, and 4) stellate cells (Figure 6).

Judging by morphological criteria, cells of the <u>in situ</u> intimal aortic layer too are heterogenous (Figure 7). To study the morphology of vascular cells <u>in situ</u> the vessel was prefixed with formaldehyde and placed into alcoholic-alkaline solution till complete dissociation of collagen-elastic matrix. Thus, four morphologically

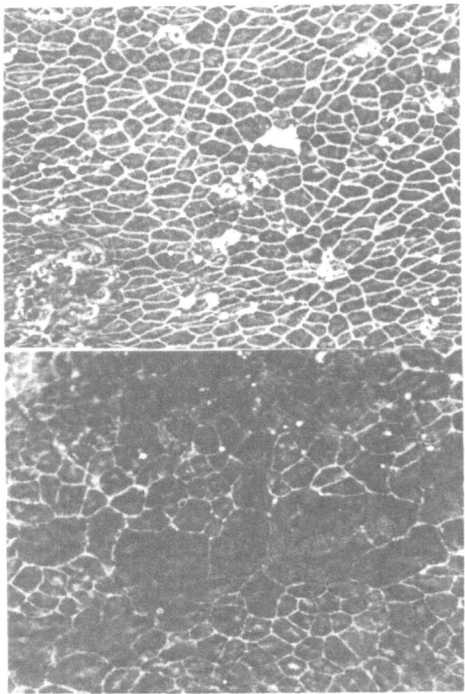

Fig. 5. Scanning electron microscopy of human aortic endothelium
         in situ. Vessel wall was silver stained and fixed under
         phisiological pressure. The upper part- homogenous endo-
         thelial surface of child aorta. The bottom part- the field
         of heterogenous endothelial lining of adult aorta. (x220)

different types of cells have been identified: 1) elongated, 2)
elongated with side processes, 3) flattened cells of irregular shape
and, 4) stellate cells. We have not yet identified the cell types
found in culture with their prototypes in the vessel, but hope to
do so in the nearest future. However, we already have reasons to
think that polymorphism of intimal cells in culture at least in part
reflects the morphological heterogeneity of the intimal layer of
human aorta.

     It stands to reason that the investigation of metabolic and
functional characteristics of cells in primary culture is a prerequisite for the understanding of the role of each cell type in
cellular manifestations of atherosclerosis. We have studied the
parameters that have bearing on atherosclerosis at the cellular
level: proliferation, lipoidosis and fibrosis.

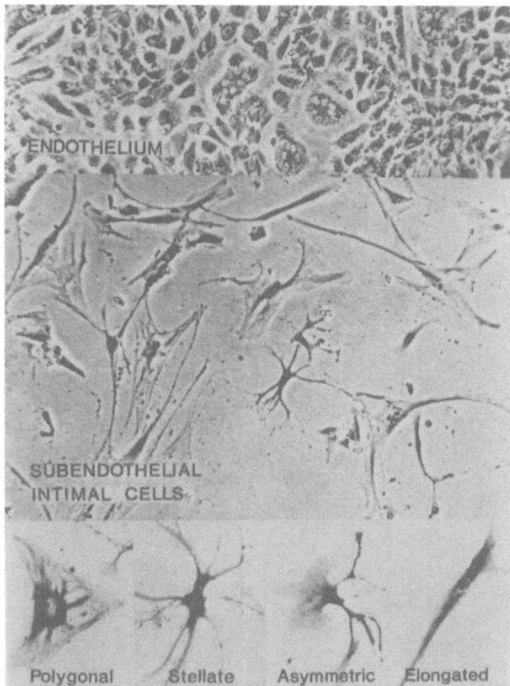

Fig. 6.   Phase-contrast microscopy of primary aortic endothelial
          and intimal cell culture. Upper section-confluent mono-
          layer with giant multinuclear endothelial cells. Medium
          section- primary intimal cell culture on the 7th day after
          seeding, general view. Bottom section- four main morpho-
          logical types of intimal cell in culture: polygonal,
          stellate, asymmetric and elongated cells.

     Intimal cells isolated from a normal region, fatty streak and
the plaque of one aorta differ as to their proliferative activity.
In cultures obtained from the zones of primary fatty infiltration
the thymidine index on average exceeded the normal value by 4-fold.
Cells from fatty streak divided more intensively as compared with
plaque cells (Figure 8). Our results contrast with the data obtained
on animals for we have not registrated intensive cell proliferation
in zones of advanced atherosclerotic lesions. The loci of proliferation are mainly associated with morphologically unchanged segments
of the vessel wall with minimal lipid infiltration.

     A lot of cells isolated from atherosclerotic lesions retain in
culture their main morphological feature - the lipid inclusions.[6,7]
In appearance they resemble the so-called "foam" cells. It is

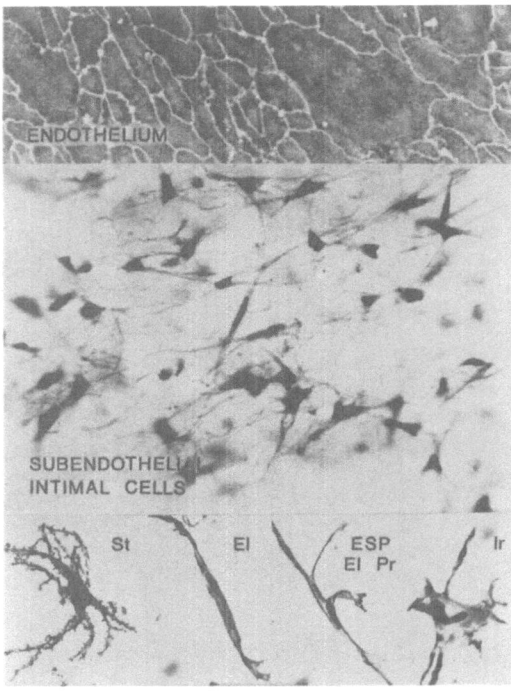

Fig. 7. Human aortic cell polymorphism in situ. The upper section-
         scanning electron microscopy of human aorta endothelial
         lining with small, medium-sized, large and giant endo-
         thelial cells. The medium section- population of intimal
         cell, isolated from prefixed vessel by alcoholic-alkaline
         dissociation, general view. The bottom section- four main
         morphological types of intimal cells in situ: St-stellate
         cells, El-elongated cells, ESP-elongated cells with side
         processes, Ir-flatten cells of irregular shape.

assumed that a part of foam cells may be formed from the smooth
muscle cells of intima; another part of foam cells is formed of
macrophages. The reasons for such a transformation are still unknown. We suppose that there are 2 possible ways of conversion into
a "foam" cell. Firstly, the accumulation of lipids inside the cell
may result from a dysfunction of intracellular lipid metabolism.
Secondly, it can be a consequence of the excessive uptake of LDL
circulating in the plasma. We have studied both possibilities.

     Cells of normal and atherosclerotic aorta were compared as to
their ability to synthesize lipids. For this purpose, radioactive
acetate was added into culture. The newly synthesized lipids became

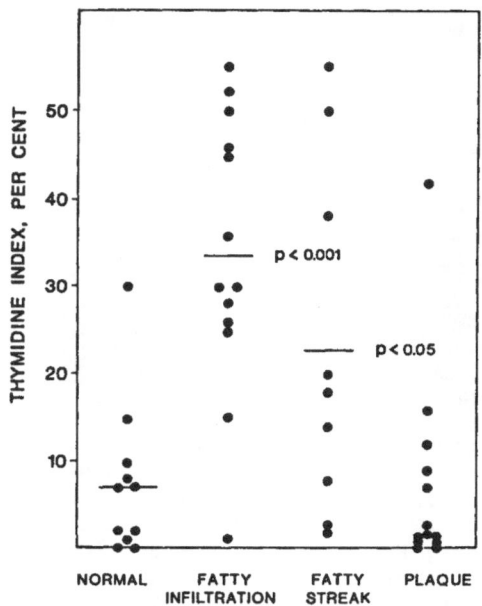

Fig. 8. ³H-Thymidine incorporation into cultured intimal cells.
The proliferation response of intimal cells in primary
culture isolated from non-involved area and lesions.
Ordinate- thymidine index in culture on the 7th day of
cultivation. -- mean value for a set of measurement. On
the absciss-results with primary intimal cell culture, obtained from normal, nonaffected region, fatty infiltration
area, fatty streak and plaque.

labeled; they were extracted, fractionated, and radioactivity was
measured in each fraction. It was shown that cells isolated from
atherosclerotic lesions include more label into the fraction of
phospholipids and cholesterol esters in comparison with the cells
isolated from uninvolved areas. In case of cholesterol esters
fraction the difference is nearly 10-fold. Since cholesterol esters
are the main class of lipids accumulated in the plaque, one can assume that accumulation of cholesterol esters results a shift in intracellular metabolism towards enhanced synthesis of these lipids
(Figure 9).

Another possible way of accumulation of cholesterol esters in
aortic cells is the uptake of LDL circulating in blood, which contain these lipids. We have studied LDL uptake by cells of normal
and atherosclerotic aorta, using fluorescence labeled lipoproteins.[8]
Protein part of LDL molecule was covalently bound with rhodamine

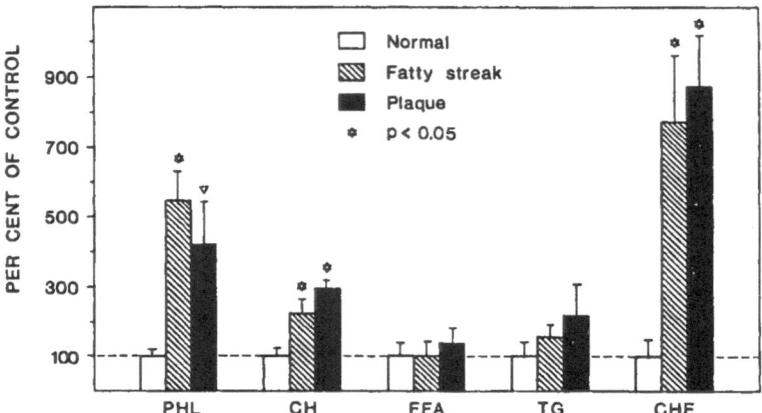

Fig. 9.   Incorporation of ^{3}H-Acetate into lipid fractions of cultured
intimal cells. Ordinate- mean value of radioactivity incorporation in per cent to control. Absciss-the main classes
of lipids. PHL-phospholipids, CH-cholesterol, CHE-choles-
teryl esters, FFA-free fatty acids, TG-triglycerides. White
columns-cells of healthy regions, shaded columns-cells of
fatty streaks, black columns-cells of plaques.

isothiocyanate. Fluorescence was excited, measured and recorded in
a FASC-II flow cytofluorimeter. We judged of LDL uptake into aortic
cells by the intensity of fluorescence. It was found that LDL uptake by atherosclerotic plaque cells exceeds that of the cells from
uninvolved areas of the same vessel by 1.5-2-fold and by 4-fold in
terms of LDL uptake per a surface unit. It is of interest that endo-
cytotic activity of plaque cells also exceeds the normal values.
Phagocytic activity was evaluated by the uptake of RITC-labeled
E.coli bacteria. The number of bacteria internalized by a cell was
measured in the flow cytofluorimeter. We have found a direct correlation between the effectiveness of LDL uptake by the plaque cells
and their phagocytic activity. We assume that plaque cells have a
higher level of specific and non-specific endocytosis.

It was demonstrated by cytofluorometry that the population of
plaque cells falls into two subpopulations differing in the effectiveness of non-specific LDL uptake. Under the indicated conditions
subpopulation A uptakes LDL several times more effectively than subpopulation B. Cells of both populations were sorted out, and it was
found that they have considerable morphological differences. Cells
of subpopulation A, which effectively incorporate LDL via non-specific
endocytosis, have numerous lipid inclusions; many of them are typical
"foam" cells. At the same time, cells of subpopulation B have low
effectiveness of LDL uptake under these conditions and no lipid in-

clusions. It can be assumed that lipid transformation of plaque
cells is, at least in part, a consequence of enhanced ability to uptake LDL via non-specific pathway (Figure 10).

As is known, high density lipoproteins (HDL) can discharge cells
overloaded with lipid inclusions. We decided to find out whether
HDL can completely discharge a human intimal cells of lipid inclusions. HDL were added into primary intimal cell culture, and in
24h the number of cells with inclusions was measured. Cultures not
treated with HDL served as a control. In cultures isolated from

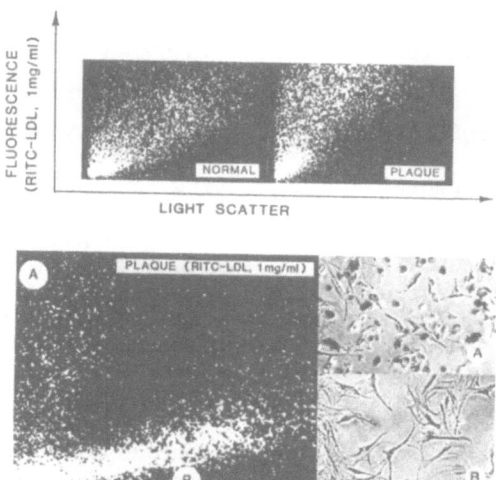

Fig. 10.   Features of fluorescently-labeled LDL interaction with
           human aortic intimal cells in the primary culture. Scat-
           tering diagram, obtained with fluorescence activated cell
           sorter FACS-II is presented on the upper part of this
           figure. Ordinate-the level of fluorescence of single cells
           in arbitrary units. Absciss-light scatter. Left population
           of normal intimal cell from noninvolved part of aorta. The
           level of fluorescence is proportional to the average size
           of cells. Right-population of intimal cells from plaque.
           It is seen that plaque cells has a higher level of fluor-
           escence. Bottom left: scattering diagram for intimal
           aortic cells from the plaque, incubated with RITC-LDL plus
           excess of non-labeled LDL. A-population with nonregulated
           high rate of RITC-LDL uptake. The top right part-phase-
           contrast microscopy of A-population of intimal cell sorted
           out and seeded on the plastic. B-population of intimal
           cell with down LDL control of RITC-LDL uptake. These cells
           were presented under phase microscopy to the right under A.

early atherosclerotic lesions HDL can decrease the number of cells
with lipid inclusions by 1.5-2-fold. HDL did not have such an effect
on cultures obtained from the plaque. Thus, the intimal cells of
human plaque have the following metabolic characteristics: 1) they
poorly proliferate in culture; 2) contain a lot of cholesterol esters;
and 3) their intracellular lipid metabolism is shifted towards accumulation of cholesterol esters. The intimal cells isolated from
fatty streaks and primary fatty infiltration have different characteristics: 1) they can actively proliferate in culture; 2) homogenous
with respect to the ability to uptake LDL; 3) HDL can completely free
these cells from lipid inclusions.

The differences found in the characteristics of cells localized
in the plaque and fatty streak may help to explain the mosaic pattern
of atherosclerotic lesion development in human aorta.

PLATELETS AND ATHEROSCLEROSIS

Along with lipoproteins, circulating in blood, platelets can
also play an important role in lipid infiltration of the vessel wall.
The mechanism of platelet participation in the plaque formation in
case of primary endothelial injury and following thrombus formation
is commonly known. In the experiments on animals platelet growth
factor, which stimulates the proliferation of smooth muscle in the
injury zone, has been found. It was also shown that lipid metabolism
and LDL incorporation into the wall is activated in the zone of endothelial repair.

Now, the plurality of platelet functions in the regulation of
lipid metabolism in the vessel wall becomes more and more evident.[9]

Thus, it was found in the in vivo experiments that platelets
exhibit specific reversible LDL binding and, when activated, can
chemically modify LDL apoprotein in such a way that specific endocytosis of the particles by macrophages is stimulated. So, in zones
of endothelial injury the inflow of LDL into the wall can be accelerated due to the directed LDL transport by platelets and via the stimulation of specific endocytosis. The interaction of LDL with vessel
wall cells and platelets in situ is more complex.

As is known, LDL of hypercholesterolemic animals increase
platelet "sensitivity" to aggregation inducers and have an expressed
cytotoxic effect on endothelial cells in culture. The initial phases
of endothelial cell injury are accompanied by the loss of athrombo-
geneity and an increase of platelet adhesion to the endothelium.
Such platelets can locally bind and modify LDL on the endothelial
surface and stimulate lipid accumulation via specific uptake.[9]

It is common knowledge that non-damaged endothelial sheet

in situ and in culture serves as a barrier limiting the inflow of LDL.
Vast de-endothelialization (denudation) of the vessel results in
sharp stimulation of LDL accumulation by the wall. Unregulated accumulation of LDL takes place in the de-endothelialized zone.

It was demonstrated in our experiments with a perfused artery
that HDL partially inhibited the uptake of LDL in the undamaged vessel
wall area, but did not change LDL uptake in the denuded zone. One
can conclude from these experiments that an integrate sheet of endothelial cells is the site of "antiatherogenic" HDL action (Figure 11).

Finally I would like to say a few words about our attempts at
correcting the manifestations of atherosclerosis at a cellular and
molecular level. We have seen that morphological features, metabolic
characteristics and main functions of cells of normal and atherosclerotic aorta are retained in primary culture. Cells in culture
are polymorphic like cells in vivo. The cells isolated from the
zones of early atherosclerotic lesions have enhanced proliferative
activity as compared with "normal" cells. Metabolism of lipids and
lipoproteins in plaque cells is shifted toward accumulation of cholesterol esters. These facts make it possible for us to regard the
primary cell culture as a suitable experimental model to testify some
antiatherogenic drugs.

Intimal cells in primary culture of atherosclerotic aorta were
treated with dibutiryl cAMP to decrease their proliferative activity

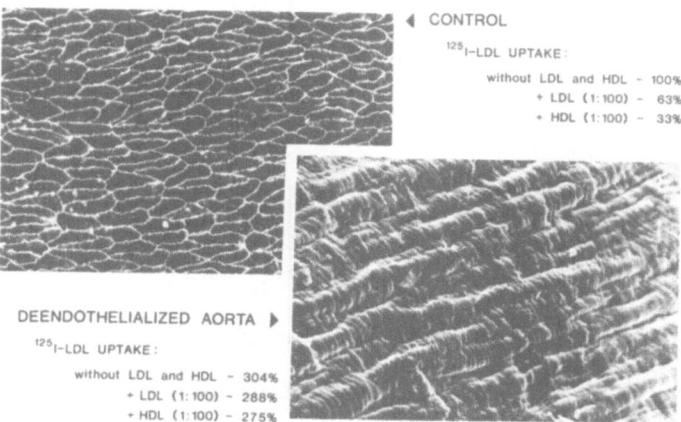

◄ CONTROL

^{125}I-LDL UPTAKE:

without LDL and HDL - 100%
+ LDL (1:100) - 63%
+ HDL (1:100) - 33%

DEENDOTHELIALIZED AORTA ►

^{125}I-LDL UPTAKE:

without LDL and HDL - 304%
+ LDL (1:100) - 288%
+ HDL (1:100) - 275%

Fig. 11. Effect of HDL on LDL uptake into intact and deendothelial-
          ized rabbit aorta. HDL regulates LDL uptake into non-
          damaged but not into deendothelialized area of rabbit
          aorta. Scanning electron microscopy of normal endothelial
          surface (left picture) and denuded surface (right).

and the level of cholesterol esters. As is known, cAMP inhibits
proliferation of many cells. Besides, this intracellular regulator
activates lipolysis and controls other pathways of lipid metabolism.
In our cultures dibutiryl cAMP significantly decreased the incorporation of thymidine into the cells of both normal and atherosclerotic
aorta (Figure 12).

The incubation with dibutiryl cAMP resulted in a reduction of
cholesterol esters level in cells isolated from the lesions of all
types, but did not change their content in the cells obtained from
the uninvolved intima. Thus, dibutiryl cAMP can be regarded as an
agent of double effect, which normalizes at least two cellular dys-
functions: enhanced proliferative activity and high level of cholesterol esters.

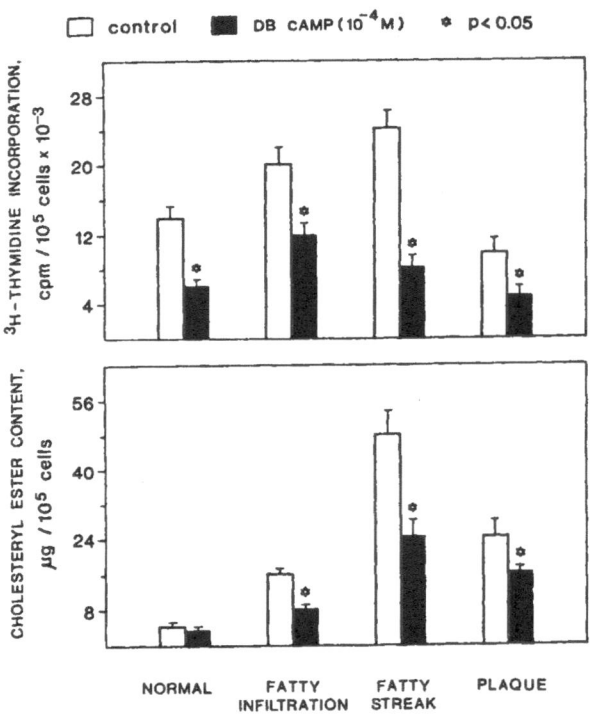

Fig. 12.   Effect of dibutyryl cyclicAMP on ^{3}H-thymidine incorporation
           and cholesteryl ester content in cultured intimal cells.
           White column-cells of normal region, lesions in standard
           media. Black column-the same cells with db-c AMP.

Finally, I would like to emphasize the close links between the fundamental studies of atherosclerosis carried out in the USSR Cardiology Research Center and the needs of practical medicine, and primarily of cardiology.

Thus, the studies of three-dimensional spatial HDL organization are aimed at investigation of the defects in the structure and packing of particles in various types of hypercholesterolemia and in CHD patients. This can lead to the engineering of artificial HDL-like particles with "improved" antiatherogenic characteristics.

The plurality of platelet functions in the control of athero-genesis and thrombi formation makes us regard the platelet as the key target for directed pharmacological action. In the light of the data we have obtained, it is of special interest to find out the mechanisms of LDL transportation and modification in the zone of thrombi formation. We assume that platelets stuffed with antithrom-bogenic and antiatherogenic drugs can be used as a container targeted to the zone of the vessel wall damage.

Our studies on primary cultures of normal and atherosclerotic human arteries have shown that polymorphism, functional and metabolic heterogeneity of endothelial and intimal cells are the prerequisites for emergence of atherogenesis. It is remarkable that cellular mani-festations of atherosclerosis (lipid infiltration of cells, prolifer-ation) can be corrected using a number of pharmacological prep-arations. These preliminary data make it possible to hope that the primary culture of cells of atherosclerotic vessels may be useful for the screening of drugs with pronounced antiatherogenic effect.

REFERENCES

1. Y. Stein and O. Stein, Metabolism of plasma lipoproteins, in: "Atherosclerosis V," A. M. Gotto, L. C. Smith, and B. Allen, eds., Springer Verlag, Heidelberg, Berlin, New York, p.653-65 (1979).
2. Y. Stein and O. Stein, Interaction between serum lipoproteins and cellular components of the arterial wall, in: "The Biochemistry of Atherosclerosis," A. M. Scanu, and R. W. Wissler, eds., Marcel Dekker Inc., New York-Basel, pp.313-340 (1979).
3. J. A. Glomset, Lecithin Cholesterol acyltransferase, in: "Bio-chemistry of Atherosclerosis," ibid, p.247-274.
4. G. R. Campbell and J. H. Chamley-Campbell, The cellular patho-biology of atherosclerosis, Pathology, 13:423-40 (1981).
5. E. I. Chasov, Advances and Perspectives of Thrombo- and Athero-genesis studies in the USSR, in: "Vessel Wall in Athero- and Thrombogenesis," E. I. Chasov and V. N. Smirnov, eds., Springer Verlag, Berlin, Heidelberg, New York, pp. 216-224 (1982).

6. J. C. Geer and D. M. Haust, Smooth muscle cells in atheroscler-
    osis, O. J. Pollak, H. S. Simms, and J. E. Kirk, eds., Karger,
    Basel, <u>Monogr.Atheroscler</u>., 2 (1972).
7. C. W. M. Adams, Local factors in atherogenesis: an introduction,
    <u>in</u>: "Atherosclerosis," R. J. Jones, ed., Springer, New York,
    p.28-34.
8. S. N. Preobrazhensky, A. S. Antonov, and V. A. Kosykh, Inter-
    action of fluorescently-labeled low density lipoproteins with
    human aortic cells in the primary culture, <u>in</u>: "Vessel Wall
    in Athero- and Thrombogenesis," E. I. Chasov and V. N. Smirnov,
    eds., Springer Verlag, Berlin, Heidelberg, New York, pp.151-160
    (1982).
9. Platelets: a multidisciplinary approach, G. deGaetano and S.
    Garratini, eds., Raven Press, New York, (1977).

CORONARY ARTERY DISEASE IN CHILDREN

Henry N. Neufeld and
Adam Schneeweiss

Heart Institute, Chaim Sheba Medical Center
Tel Hashomer, Sackler School of Medicine
Tel Aviv University, Tel Aviv, Israel

Because coronary disease is such a prevalent condition and is responsible for such a large number of fatalities, it is usually associated with age. However, recent documented evidence of the existence of coronary heart disease in the young, indicates that youth does not rule out the possibility of this condition. Even myocardial infarction and/or sudden death, which are the culmination of coronary arteriosclerosis, are encountered in the young.

The natural history of the development of coronary heart disease can be divided into three stages: (1) an incubation period (ab ova), which may start in foetal life and continue into infancy, childhood, and adolescence; (2) a latent period, which is asymptomatic but in which pathological changes can already be present in young age; and (3) a clinical period, in which signs and symptoms first appear.

Autopsy examinations of young adults who died of noncardiac causes (mostly of injuries sustained in war) first drew attention to the presence of atherosclerosis in young adults, a process which must have started in childhood. These findings triggered research which resulted in the description of several histologic coronary arterial changes in infancy and childhood which were directly correlated with the extent of coronary atherosclerosis in adults[1-7]. In addition some of the risk factors associated with coronary atherosclerosis such as hypertension and hypercholesterolemia, may be present in childhood[8,9].

In addition to the factors which affect large groups of the population, various relatively rare pediatric diseases are associated

71

with advanced coronary atherosclerosis or other types of coronary
narrowing in infancy. Among these are progeria[10]; congenital heart
diseases causing elevated pressure in the ascending aorta and coronary hypertension[11,12]; and inherited disorders of metabolism[13-17].

On the basis of the data collected on these subjects it is now
widely accepted that coronary atherosclerosis is a problem starting
in childhood, mainly in its pathogenic and preventive aspects, and
rarely also in its clinical presentation. The unusual finding of
myocardial infarction in infancy and childhood may also result from
many other systemic diseases and exogenous factors not associated
with atherosclerosis or other forms of gradual narrowing of the
arterial lumen.

Histologic Changes in the Coronary Arterial Wall in Infancy and Childhood

The coronary arterial walls undergo continuous changes throughout infancy and childhood. Since these changes have been proven to
be related to atherosclerosis, only coronary arteries of foetuses
may be considered completely normal. On this assumption a histologic study of coronary arteries of foetuses up to the age of 34
weeks was undertaken.

The normal foetal coronary arterial wall consists of (1) the
intima, a single layer of endothelial cells; (2) the internal elastic
membrane which consists of homogeneous elastic material surrounding
the intima as a continuous tube with longitudinal corrugations;
(3) the media, a few layers of smooth muscle cells and some elastic
fibers; and (4) the adventitia, an external layer of loose connective
tissue. The effect of risk factors influencing the foetal circulation was demonstrated[18].

After the 34 week gestation, the structure of the coronary
arterial wall becomes more complex. A musculoelastic layer develops
between the media and the intima where foci of fibrous thickening
appear. The musculoelastic layer is formed by a series of degenerative and proliferative processes, mainly splitting of the internal
elastic membrane, proliferation of smooth muscle cell within the
split areas, and increase in the amount of the elastic fibers within
the media[19]. The intimal changes include formation of intimal
cushions composed of fibroblasts, elastic fibers and droplets of
acid mucopolysaccharides.

In studies from our Institute, as well as from other centers,
it was demonstrated that the extent of the intimal and medial
changes is greater in males than in females. This sex difference
was more prominent in population groups with a high prevalence and
incidence of coronary heart disease in adult life[5,19].

The musculoelastic layer and the intimal thickening were prominent in ethnic groups with a high incidence of coronary artery disease such as Ashkenazy Jews, the population of the eastern part of Finland[5], and American Caucasians and Blacks[20,21]. On the other hand, the changes were minimal or absent in ethnic groups with a low prevalence and incidence of coronary heart disease such as Yemenite Jews, Bedouins from Negev Israel[7], the population of the western part of Finland[5] and Haitian Blacks[20]. These findings suggest that the coronary arterial morphologic changes in infancy and childhood underlie coronary atherosclerosis in adults. This would indicate that a genetic factor may be responsible for the structure of the coronary arteries we are born with, and partially responsible for the development of coronary atherosclerosis.

The combined results of these findings suggest that the presence of coronary atherosclerosis in adults is closely associated with the coronary arterial morphologic changes in infancy and childhood. In view of this, the presence of a genetic factor responsible for the structure of the coronary arteries we are born with is certainly indicated, and is also perhaps partially responsible for coronary atherosclerotic development in later life. The genetic disposition is probably combined with environmental factors.

Risk Factors for Coronary Atherosclerosis in Infancy and Childhood

<u>Hyperlipidemia</u>. Elevated levels of serum cholesterol are associated with an increased risk of coronary disease. However, only one type of hyperlipidemia associated with premature coronary heart disease presents a major risk factor in early childhood; this is hypercholesterolemia with xanthomatosis Fredrickson's type II, which is a genetically determined dominant trait with an incidence of 0.5-2%. It was shown that young people with hypercholesterolemia are more than 30 times susceptible to premature myocardial infarction than normocholesteremics of the same age group. Moreover, it has been shown that most young males sustaining myocardial infarction had hypercholesterolemia in youth. Although patients in the homozygote state are mainly affected, the heterozygote state is associated with increased incidence of coronary heart disease in patients over 30 years[22].

It is today an accepted policy in most medical centers that if a child from a high risk family has two elevated serum cholesterol measurements, lipoprotein fractions are measured to determine the distribution of total cholesterol among the lipid fractions. This information may be useful as more is learned about factors affecting cholesterol distribution among the lipoprotein fractions. Marked changes in the concentration of serum lipids and lipoproteins occur during the first year of life; a dramatic increase of serum total cholesterol, LDL and HDL begins around puberty; children tend to have higher HDL than do adults.

Recent epidemiologic investigations indicate that high levels of high density lipoprotein (HDL) cholesterol act as a protective factor against coronary artery disease and, conversely, that persons with subnormal levels of HDL cholesterol have a significantly increased risk of having arteriosclerosis.

It is premature to give prognostic significance to elevated HDL cholesterol levels in children: for the present, attention should be directed toward total serum cholesterol level and LDL cholesterol[8]. Mean HDL-C tends to be high at the areas with high mean total cholesterol, even in childhood. The mean HDL-C level could thus be a response of the metabolism to the total level, so as to assume a satisfactory HDL total level. We do know, however, that the latter varies greatly within adult populations and is inversely and strongly related to coronary risk. The relationship between dietary cholesterol and serum cholesterol is further complicated by genetic characteristics.

In spite of detailed descriptions in the literature and the fact that they are the most common known genetic diseases affecting man, the inherited hyperlipoproteinemias comprise only a small percentage of cases of hypercholesterolemia. The majority of hypercholesterolemic individuals are affected by environmental influences, dietary cholesterol intake has gained major attention and interest because it can potentially be controlled[8,23-29].

Hypertension. Hypertension has been established as a major risk factor for coronary atherosclerosis in adults[22]. It alone has been proven to produce atherosclerosis even in the absence of other risk factors[31]. The direct effect of hypertension on the coronary arteries was demonstrated by the finding of obliterative intimal hyperplasmia and medial thickening revealed by light microscopy studies performed in our Institute, and by others in patients with coarctation of the aorta or supraventricular aortic stenosis in experimental coarctation in a subhuman primate model[32].

In a recent electron microscopic study of coronary microcirculation in patients with coarctation of the aorta in our Institute[33], morphologic changes were also found in the small arterioles. These changes were more severe and widespread in young adults than in children and were directly related to age. A possible mechanism in which hypertension aggravates atherosclerosis is the stretching of the arterial wall, which increases its permeability to cholesterol and lipoproteins.

In recent years primary hypertension in children has been recognized as a public health problem[34]. Better recognition of the extent of the problem was achieved by blood pressure measurements in routine physical examination and better determination of the effect of age on blood pressure[35]. The study by Graham et al.[36]

and Londe's[37-40] studies demonstrated the importance of not using
the adult standards to define hypertension in children. The incidence of persistent hypertension in children is now estimated to be
1-4%. Until recent years primary hypertension in children was considered unusual. Londe et al.[37-40], however, demonstrated that
essential hypertension was much more common than previously thought.
Various studies have shown that blood pressure is continuously
rising from infancy, with acceleration in adolescence. On the
other hand, a hypertensive child may become a normotensive adult in
35% of the cases. Multiple determinations should be performed
before a child be considered hypertensive. Hypertension was found
to be more frequent in siblings of hypertensive individuals than in
those of normotensive individuals.

On initial evaluation (single determinations), Heyden et al.[35]
in the Evans County (Georgia) Study found that 11% of 435 adolescents
were hypertensive. Repeat evaluation carried out 7 years later on
30 of these 435 patients from the hypertensive group, revealed 11 to
have persistent high blood pressure, while 6 had some form of vascular complication during their early adulthood, including two
deaths. This indicates that not only do these children face an
increased risk of CHD later in life, but they also suffer significant
early morbidity and mortality.

Tobacco Smoking. The Joint Report of the Study Group on Smoking
and Health in 1957 [28] proved unequivocally that tobacco smoking is
a major contributing factor to the pathogenesis of atherosclerosis.
These findings were confirmed by epidemiologic studies which found
a direct relationship between smoking and coronary heart disease.
Further data on coronary arteriography studies proved a direct
relationship between the degree of cigarette consumption and the
severity of coronary atherosclerosis[42-47].

The incidence of hypertension and coronary heart disease is
highest and its onset earliest in those who began smoking at less
than 20 years of age. Because of this the increasing trend in
childhood smoking is particularly disturbing.

Inherited Disorders of Metabolism Associated with Coronary Obstructive Lesions in Infancy and Childhood

Disorders of Lipid Metabolism. In Sandhof's disease[14] there
is a neural accumulation of GM_2 ganglioside and neural visceral
accumulation of globoside due to deficient activity of hexosaminidase
A and B. Onset occurs in the first two months of life and the
clinical features include development retardation and cherry-red
macula. Two cases of Sandhof's disease with luminal narrowing of
the coronary arteries due to intimal proliferation of fibroblasts
have been reported[14].

In Fabry's disease[13] ceramide trihexoside accumulates in the walls of small blood vessels, due to a deficiency of ceramide tri- hexosidase. Coronary involvement is frequent and the clinical features include anginal pain, cardiac enlargement, congestive heart failure, and myocardial infarction. GM_1 gangliosidosis is a condition in which galactosidase deficiency causes neural and vis- ceral accumulation of GM_1 ganglioside. Cardiac lesions have been found in about 30% of the cases, but coronary atheromatous plaques containing balloon cells of foamy periodic-acid-Schniff-negative cytoplasma were reported in only one case[15].

Amino Acid Metabolism, Mucopolysaccharidoses
Disorders of Protein Metabolism

Homocystinuria. Homocystinuria is a defect in serine and homo- cystine metabolism, presenting clinically with ocular abnormalities, long extremities, scoliosis, osteoporosis, mental retardation, and thrombotic vascular disease, including coronary occlusion[17].

Alkaptonuria. In this condition homogentisic acid is accumu- lated and excreted in the urine, due to a deficiency of homogentisic oxidase. The clinical features include dark urine, pigmentation of cartilage, arthritis, and mitral and aortic valvulitis. Blue-black pigmented coronary atheromatous plaques cause myocardial infarction, which is a common cause of death in this condition[16].

Mucopolysaccharidoses. The coronary arteries are affected in two of the six mucopolysaccharidoses in which the heart is involved, namely Hurler's and Hunter's syndromes. The coronary arteries are narrowed by plaques containing mucopolysaccharides. Such cells also invade the myocardium[13].

Protein Metabolism. In primary hyperoxaluria there is excessive synthesis of oxalic acid with calcium oxalate accumulation in various organs, including the coronary arteries[13]. Tangier disease is an inborn error of metabolism characterized by deficiency of high density lipoprotein in plasma and storage of cholesterol esters in many tissues, including the heart. Patients with Tangier disease and coronary heart disease due to coronary deposition of cholesterol esters have been described[13].

Congenital Heart Anomalies with Coronary Obstructive Lesions

Conditions associated with elevated pressure in the ascending aorta and coronary arteries. Coarctation of the aorta and supra- ventricular aortic stenosis cause elevated pressure in the ascending aorta which affects the coronary arteries[11,12]. Light microscopy studies in these patients revealed coronary luminal narrowing due

to thickening of the media, proliferation of fibroblasts in the
intima, and degenerative and proliferative changes of elastic fibers.
The mortality rate from cardiovascular causes in patients undergoing
operative correction of coarctation of the aorta over the age of 35
years is ten times greater than the rate in patients between 15 and
34 years of age who were operated upon. This has been attributed
to the coronary arterial changes which develop with age[44].

In a recent electron microscopic study in our Institute[33], age-
related changes were found in the coronary microcirculation of
patients with coarctation of the aorta. These changes included
destruction of the normal wall of the small coronary arteries and
coronary arterioles with collagenous transformation. The precapillary sphincters, metarterioles capillaries and venules were
normal.

Single coronary artery. Single coronary artery is a congenital
anomaly which may be isolated or associated with other congenital
cardiac lesions. The incidence of coronary atherosclerosis in this
anomaly is not increased, but the patients are more susceptible to
its consequences[7].

Short main left coronary artery. It has been suggested that
patients with congenitally short main left coronary artery have an
increased incidence of atherosclerosis in the left coronary system[45].

Miscellaneous Conditions Associated with Coronary Obstructive Lesions in Infancy and Childhood

Progeria. Hutchinson-Gilford syndrome is a disease of extremely
accelerated aging, starting in infancy and developing throughout
childhood. The disease is characterized by thinning and atrophy of
the skin, loss of subcutaneous fat, growth failure, osteoporosis,
joint stiffness, and alopecia. Atherosclerosis begins in infancy
and presents clinically in the first decade of life as angina
pectoris, hypertension, congestive heart failure, and myocardial
infarction. The latter is rarely present in the first year of life,
but the basic disorder in the syndrome is dysplasia of mesenchymal
tissue of unknown etiology[10].

Werner's syndrome. Werner's syndrome is a condition of premature aging with retardation of development, hair loss or greying,
hyperkeratosis of skin, cataracts, hypogonadism and osteoporosis.
Atherosclerosis and arterial thrombosis are frequent[46].

Trisomy 18. A single case of trisomy 18 with arterial changes
including degeneration of the internal elastic membrane, thickening
of the intima by fibroblastic proliferation, and calcification of
the media has been reported[47].

Pseudoxanthoma elasticum. Pseudoxanthoma elasticum is an autosomal recessive condition in which calcification and fragmentation of elastic fibers occur in the eyes, skin and blood vessels, including the coronary arteries. Cardiovascular manifestations include anginal pain, congestive heart failure and hypertension[48].

Coronary Arteritis

Until recently the problem of coronary arteritis was limited to isolated cases of infantile periarteritis nodosa. In the last decade, however, increasing numbers of cases with Kawasaki's disease (mucocutaneous lymph node syndrome)[45] have been reported, mainly in Japan, but also in Europe and the United States. Kawasaki's disease is an acute febrile disease presenting in early childhood with conjunctical congestion, indurative edema, erythema, and desquamation of the palms and feet, strawberry tongue, dry red fissured lips, and exanthema of the trunk. Electrocardiographic changes and coronary periarteritis are frequent. In the chronic stage coronary aneurysms and myocardial infarction occur in an as yet undetermined number of the patients. The etiology of this condition is unknown. Some of the patients had aorta coronary bypass grafting. In most cases, however, the aneurysms disappear after one year and the coronary arteries are thin, with isolated obstructive lesions[49,50].

REFERENCES

1. H. D. Moon, Coronary arteries in fetuses, infants and juveniles, Circulation, 10:263 (1957).
2. H. E. Schornagel, Intimal thickening in coronary arteries in infants, AMA Arch. Pathol., 62:427 (1956).
3. H. N. Neufeld, C. A. Wagenvoort, and J. E. Edwards, Coronary arteries in fetuses, infants, juveniles and young adults, Lab. Invest. II, 837 (1962).
4. Z. Vlodaver, and H. N. Neufeld, The coronary arteries in coarctation of the aorta, Circulation, 37:449 (1968).
5. E. Pesonen, R. Norio, and S. Sarna, Thickenings in the coronary arteries in infancy as an indication of genetic factors in coronary heart disease, Circulation 51 and 52:218 (1975).
6. Z. Vlodaver, H. A. Kahn, and H. N. Neufeld, The coronary arteries in early life in three different ethnic groups, Circulation, 29:541 (1964).
7. Z. Vlodaver, H. N. Neufeld, and J. E. Edwards, "Coronary Artery Variations in Normal Heart and in Congenital Heart Disease", Academic Press, New York (1975) p.1.
8. H. N. Neufeld, and A. Schneeweiss, Etiology and prevention of coronary obstructive lesions in infancy and childhood, Clin. Cardiol., 4:217 (1981).

9. R. D. Voller, and W. B. Strong, Pediatric aspects of athero-
    sclerosis, Curriculum in Cardiology, 12:815 (1981).
10. W. L. Reichel, and R. Garcia-Bunuel, Pathologic findings in
    progeria: Myocardial fibrosis and lipofuscin pigment, Am.
    J. Clin. Path., 53:243 (1970).
11. H. N. Neufeld, C. A. Wagenvoort, P. A. Ongley, and J. E.
    Edwards, Hypoplasia in ascending aorta. An unusual form of
    supra valvular aortic stenosis with special reference to
    localized coronary arterial hypertension, Am. J. Cardiol.,
    10:746 (1962).
12. R. E. Schmidt, E. F. Gilbert, T. C. Ameno, C. R. Chamberlain
    and R. V. Lucas, Generalized arterial fibro-muscular
    dysplasia and myocardial infarction in familial supra-
    valvular aortic stenosis syndrome, Pediatrics, 74:576 (1969).
13. L. C. Blieden, and J. H. Moller, Cardiac involvement in
    inherited disorders of metabolism, Prog. Cardiovasc. Dis.,
    10:615 (1974).
14. L. C. Blieden, R. Desnick, and J. Carter, Cardiac involvement
    in Sandhof's disease: An inborn error of glyco-sphenogolipid
    metabolism, Am. J. Cardiol., 34:83 (1974).
15. R. N. Hadley, and J. W. Hagstrom, Cardiac lesions in a patient
    with familial neurovisceral lipidoses (generalized ganglio-
    sides), Am. J. Clin. Pathol., 55:237 (1971).
16. H. P. Smith, and H. P. Smith Jr., Ochronosis: report of two
    cases, Ann. Intern. Med., 42:171 (1955).
17. V. A. McKusick, R. N. Schmike, and A. D. Huang Pollaak,
    Thrombotic vascular disease in homocystinuria, a newly
    recognized inborn error of metabolism stimulating Marfan's
    syndrome, Circulation, 32 (suppl. II):149 (1965).
18. I. Asmussen, Fetal cardiovascular system as influenced by
    maternal smoking, Clin. Cardiol., 2:246 (1979).
19. H. N. Neufeld and Z. Vlodaver, Structural changes of coronary
    arteries in young age groups, Intl. Cardiol., Vol. 2 of
    Cardiovascular Clinic Series, (A. N. Brest and P. D. White,
    eds.,) F. A. Davies, Philadelphia (1977) p. 55.
20. D. Groon, E. E. Mckee, W. Adkins, V. Pean, and E. Hudicourt,
    Developmental patterns of coronary and aortic athero-
    sclerosis in young Negroes of Haiti and the United States,
    Ann. Intern. Med., 61:900 (1964).
21. H. C. McGill, "The Geographic Pathology of Atherosclerosis",
    Williams and Wilkins, Baltimore (1968).
22. W. B. Strong, "Atherosclerosis: Its Pediatric Aspects", Grune
    & Stratton, New York (1978) p. 1.
23. D. P. Barr, E. M. Russ, and H. A. Eder, Protein-lipid relation-
    ships in human plasma II, in: Atherosclerosis and Related
    Conditions, Am. J. Med., II:480 (1961).
24. J. W. Gofman, O. Delalla, and F. Glazier, The serum lipoprotein
    transport system in health, metabolic disorders, athero-
    sclerosis and coronary heart disease, Plasma, 2:413 (1954).

25. D. S. Fredrickson, R. I. Levy, and R. S. Lees, Fat transport
     in lipoproteins. Integrated approach to mechanisms and dis-
     orders, N. Engl. J. Med., 276:34, 94, 215, 273 (1967).
26. W. P. Castelli, J. T. Doyle, and T. Gordon, Cholesterol and
     other lipids in coronary heart disease, Circulation, 55:767
     (1977).
27. S. Bluementhal and M. J. Jesse, Risk factors for coronary heart
     disease in children of affected families, J. Pediatr., 87:
     1187 (1975).
28. W. B. Kannel, W. P. Castelli, T. Gordon, and P. M. McNamara,
     Serum cholesterol, lipoproteins, and the risk of coronary
     heart disease: The Framingham Study, Ann. Intern. Med.,
     74:1 (1971).
29. A. W. Voors, L. S. Webber, and G. S. Berenson, Time course
     studies of blood pressure in children - The Bogalusa Study,
     Am. J. Epidemiol., 109:320 (1979).
30. R. W. Wissler, and J. C. Geer, "The Pathogenesis of Athero-
     sclerosis", William & Wilkins, Baltimore (1972) p. 62.
31. E. D. Frees, Hypertension and atherosclerosis, Am. J. Med.,
     46:735 (1969).
32. D. I. Mininoshvili, G. O. Makakian, and G. I. Kokaia, Hyper-
     tension and coronary insufficiency in monkeys, in: "Theo-
     retical and Practical Problems of Medicine and Biology in
     Experiments on Monkeys", I. A. Utkin, ed., Pergamon Press,
     London (1960) p. 103.
33. A. Schneeweiss, E. Lehrer, L. Sherf, Y. Liberman, and H. N.
     Neufeld, Segmental study of the terminal coronary vessels
     in coarctation of the aorta: A natural model for study of
     the effect of coronary hypertension on human coronary
     circulation, Am. J. Cardiol., (in press, June 1982?).
34. D. E. Fixler, Epidemiology of childhood hypertension, in:
     "Atherosclerosis: Its Pediatric Aspects", W. B. Strong, ed.,
     Grune & Stratton, New York (1978) p. 177.
35. S. Heyden, A. G. Bartel, J. R. McDonough, and C. G. Hames,
     Elevated blood pressure levels in adolescents, Evans County,
     Georgia: Seven year follow-up of 30 patients and 30 controls,
     JAMA, 209:1683 (1969).
36. A. W. Graham, E.A. Hines, and R. P. Gage, Blood pressure in
     children between the ages of 5 and 16 years, Am. J. Dis.
     Child., 69:203 (1945).
37. S. Londe, Blood pressure in children as determined under office
     conditions, Clin. Pediat., 5:71 (1966).
38. S. Londe, Blood pressure standards for normal children as
     determined under office conditions, Clin. Pediat., 7:400
     (1968).
39. S. Londe, and D. Goldring, High blood pressure in children:
     Problems and guidelines for evaluation and treatment, Am. J.
     Cardiol., 37:650 (1976).
40. S. Londe, J. T. Bourgoingnine, A. M. Robson, and D. Goldring,
     Hypertension in apparently normal children, J. Pediat.,
     78:569 (1971).

41. Joint Report of the Study Group on Smoking and Health, Science, 125:1129 (1957).
42. J. T. Doyle, T. R. Dawber, W. B. Kannel, A. S. Heclin, and A. H. Kahn, Cigarette smoking and coronary heart disease. Combined experience of the Albany and Framingham studies, N. Engl. J. Med., 266:796 (1972).
43. W. B. Kannel, T. R. Dawber and P. M. McNamara, Detection of the coronary prone adult: The Framingham Study, J. Iowa Med. Soc., 56:26 (1966).
44. O. Paul, M. H. Lepper, W. H. Phelon, G. W. Dupertius, A. MacMillan, H. McKean and H. Park, A longitudinal study of coronary heart disease, Circulation, 28:20 (1963).
45. N. Gazetopoulos, P. J. Joannidis, C. Karydis, C. Lolas, K. Kiriakou, and C. Tountas, Short left coronary artery trunk as a risk factor in the development of coronary atherosclerosis: Pathologic study, Br. Heart J., 38:1160 (1976).
46. S. Goldstein and S. Niewiarowski, Increased procoagulant activity in cultured fibroblasts from progeria and Werner's syndrome of premature aging, Nature, 7:711 (1976).
47. R. L. Rosenfield, S. Breibart, H. Issacs Jr, and H. D. Kleoit, Trisomy of chromosomes 13-15 and 17-18, its association with infantile arteriosclerosis, Am. J. Med. Sci., 244:763 (1962).
48. Z. Schochner, and D. Young, Pseudoxanthoma elasticum with severe cardiovascular disease in childhood, Am. J. Dis. Child., 127:571 (1974).
49. T. Kawasaki, F. Kosaki, S. Okawa, J. Shigematsu and H. Yanagawa, A new infantile acute febrile mucocutaneous lymph node syndrome (MLNS) prevailing in Japan, Pediat., 54:271 (1974).
50. H. N. Neufeld, and A. Schneeweiss, "Coronary artery anomalies in infancy and childhood", Lea and Febiger, Washington (1981).

CARDIOMYOPATHIES: PATHOLOGY AND INFECTIOUS IMMUNE MECHANISMS

E. G. J. Olsen

National Heart Hospital
Westmoreland Street
London W.1.

Much confusion of defining and classifying cardiomyopathies has existed in the past. As a result of the work by the Task Force set up by the World Health Organization and the International Society and Federation of Cardiology[1], this has been clarified. Cardiomyopathies are now defined as "heart muscle diseases of unknown cause" and classified into three major types: dilated, hypertrophic and restrictive. For each type characteristic morphologic features exist.

Dilated cardiomyopathy

At necropsy all chambers of the overweight hearts are usually severely dilated, the endocardium is thickened, intercavitary thrombus frequent, and coronary arteries are normal[2]. Histologically, normal arrangement of myocardial fibers is found and if dilatation has been severe, disproportion of nuclear changes – which reflect hypertrophy – and myocardial fibers which may show normal diameters, reflecting dilatation, are seen[3]. Smooth muscle hypertrophy and hyperplasia in the endocardium confirm dilatation. An increase in interstitial fibrous tissue, limited to the inner rim of the myocardial wall, may be present. The intramyocardial vessels are usually normal.

Histochemical analysis undertaken on biopsy material obtained by bioptome[4] show no distinctive patterns and merely reflect the degree of hypertrophy and to some extent duration of heart failure. Thus the various enzyme components may be increased, normal or decreased.

Ultrastructural changes are those of hypertrophy[5] often with degenerative changes, particularly in long standing cases[6].

It has been argued that in view of the fact that no specific morphologic features exist that diagnosis can only be established with certainty at necropsy. This, of course, applies to every disease affecting the human body but diagnosis of dilated cardiomyopathy can be achieved during life clinically, aided by non-invasive techniques. Cardiac and extra-cardiac causes can be excluded with certainty in a large number of cases. There is, however, a significant number of patients in whom invasive techniques have to be undertaken, foremost among which is examination of endomyocardial tissue obtained by bioptome. By this means possible involvement of the myocardium by myocarditis, sarcoidosis or infiltrative diseases can be assessed[7].

Hypertrophic cardiomyopathy

Despite the denial of the existence of this type of cardiomyopathy as a distinct entity by some workers in the past, there is abundant evidence of sufficient highly characteristic features, not only clinically but also morphologically that hypertrophic cardiomyopathy is a separate, recognizable entity[8]. Macroscopically, asymmetric hypertrophy is often a striking characteristic feature. Echocardiographically, it has been shown that if the ratio of the ventricular septum to the posterior left ventricular free wall exceeds 1.3, hypertrophic cardiomyopathy is likely to be present[9]. Subsequently it has been established that minor degrees of asymmetric hypertrophy of the septum can be present in many other conditions and histologic confirmation needs to be undertaken in such instances [10]. Frequently however, if the ratio of the free ventricular wall with the septum is calculated[11], the ratio exceeds 3 (even in the severest form of other types of hypertrophy the ratio remains unity). If such severe disproportion is found, then asymmetric hypertrophy alone permits a diagnosis of hypertrophic cardiomyopathy to be made. The bulging of the septum displaces the anterior papillary muscle which contributes to the malfunction of the mitral valve apparatus, resulting in mitral insufficiency[12]. An impression of the anterior mitral valve leaflet may be found in the form of endocardial thickening in the outflow tract of the left ventricle[13]. The coronary arteries, as in dilated cardiomyopathy, are usually normal.

The characteristic histologic features include disarray of extremely hypertrophied myocardial fibers, bizarre shaped nuclei, often surrounded by a clear zone, the so-called perinuclear halo and varying degrees of often cellular fibrous tissue. Several years ago an index assessing semiquantitatively each of the histologic features was devised[14] and if the value exceeds 50%, then hypertrophic cardiomyopathy is present. Disarray, its distribution and severity has also been more recently undertaken[15] confirming and extending the findings previously reported[14].

Histochemical examination often shows severe accumulation of glycogen which has diagnostic importance. Other enzyme systems merely reflect severe hypertrophy[14].

Ultrastructurally, disarray of myocardial fibrils is often widespread and striking but is not diagnostically helpful[14]. Furthermore, abnormal intercellular junctions are also frequently found, at one time considered pathognomic[16], but previously and subsequently discounted[8]. Despite the overlap of ultrastructural changes with "ordinary" hypertrophy it can be concluded that if the changes of disorganization are widespread they characterize the condition and act as an adjunct to histologic and macroscopic diagnosis. The various histologic features considered in <u>combination</u> and the accumulation of glycogen permit a firm diagnosis[8].

Though previously the presence or absence of a systolic gradient has been emphasized, it has subsequently been established that it does not influence the natural history of the disease[17]. Similarly, at morphologic levels it has previously been found that if obstruction had been present, the abnormal features were principally concentrated in the asymmetrically thickened septum. If no obstruction was clinically present the same histologic and ultrastructural changes were seen but were widely distributed focally throughout the myocardium[18]. This distribution is, however, not always found[19].

Restrictive cardiomyopathy

Two hitherto considered separate entities are included under this heading, endomyocardial fibrosis, morphologically first described by Davies[20] and considered to be a disease limited to the tropics and Löffler's endocarditis parietalis fibroplastica (Löffler's endomyocardial disease)[21] considered to be confined to temperate zones. It has however been shown that both conditions belong to the same disease spectrum[22]. In this condition, irrespective of geographical origin, left, right or both ventricles, may be involved. The endocardium which is often several millimeters thick, is the characteristic feature. Inflow and partly outflow tract of the left ventricle, and the apex and the area beneath the tricuspid valve in the right ventricle, are the typical sites, but endocardial changes may be seen elsewhere in the ventricle as well as in the atria[23]. Thrombus is frequently superimposed, forming the obliterative "phase" of this disease.

Histologically, the endocardium is arranged in layers: superficially, beneath the thrombus a zone of loose and dense connective

tissue is present beneath which the so-called granulation tissue
layer is found. This consists of numerous dilated blood vessels,
embedded in loose connective tissue. Inflammatory cells including
occasionally eosinophils may be found. From this zone fine septae
extend into the underlying myocardium[24]. Histochemical and ultrastructural changes are those of hypertrophy.

By definition the etiology or etiologies for each of the types
of cardiomyopathy is unknown. Many suggestions have been made in
the past and these have been summarized previously[25].

Increasing evidence is accumulating that infectious immune
mechanisms may be responsible for some types of cardiomyopathy.
These will now be discussed. Before the various studies that have
been undertaken are detailed, it is perhaps relevant to summarize
some general remarks regarding infectious immune mechanisms. An
immunological reaction is defined as a specific combination of
antigens with humoral antibody or sensitized cells. An immunologic
event can be defined as tissue damage resulting from the initiation
of immune reactions[26]. These reactions have been classified into
four major types: I immediate hypersensitivity, involving reaginic
antibody; II other cytotoxic effects of antibody; III dependence on
immune complexes and IV dependence on delayed cell-mediated immune
reaction[27]. Modification of this classification has been suggested
[26], firstly immune disorders are rarely caused by a single mechanism
but involve interactions of several mechanisms and secondly it is
difficult to distinguish clearly between immunologic and inflammatory events, particularly in chronic disorders.

The possible infectious immune mechanisms or immune mechanisms
in the various types of cardiomyopathies will now be considered.

Dilated cardiomyopathy

By definition the etiology is unknown. The disease is often
heralded by an upper respiratory infection and increasing neutralizing antibody titres against Coxsackie B$_3$ Echo and Herpes virus
have been found in patients with this type of cardiomyopathy[28].
Significantly higher titres to B virus infections, particularly
with a history lasting less than one year have also been shown in
a significant number of patients when compared with an equal number
of age and sex matched normal individuals[29]. The linkage between
active viral infection and dilated cardiomyopathy is not yet well
established, though several clinical reports testify to such
relationship[30]. Heart-reactive antibodies have been demonstrated
correlating with the severity of symptoms and duration of disease[31].
Studies of cell mediated immunity have also been undertaken[32] and
defective T suppressor cell function in dilated cardiomyopathy have
also been demonstrated[33]. In the patients investigated with high

neutralizing antibody titres against Coxsackie virus[29], endomyocardial biopsies failed to show any evidence of present or past
myocarditis. The significance of the various reports is as yet
unclear but the possible pathogenetic mechanisms have been summarized[30]. A significant number of patients show evidence of an
immune disturbance and react in an unusual manner to common virus
infection. The progressive illness, punctuated by recurrences, may
be due to immune mechanisms. Virus infection may trigger production
of antibodies directed at suppressor cells. These antibodies may
inactivate or possibly coat the T cell receptors in such a manner
that their normal regulatory role in modulating T cell function is
impaired. This may result in heightened B cell activity with production of antibodies directed to self. Similarly T suppressor
cell dysfunction may also affect cell-mediated immunity. Further
work in these concepts is clearly indicated.

Hypertrophic cardiomyopathy

This type of cardiomyopathy has shown a human leukocyte antigen
(HLA) linkage. These antigens are closely associated with the gene
governing immune response (located on the sixth chromosome). It
has been shown that the differences between white and black races
exists (B12 and B5 antigens) and these patients were normotensive;
whereas patients without these antigens, sporadic cases, were hypertensive[34].

Restrictive cardiomyopathy

The possible association of infection such as filariasis[35] has
long been debated. Hypersensitivity response to streptococcal
infection[36], abnormal immunologic reaction, and immunologic factors
have also been previously reported[37,38]. The suggestion that endomyocardial fibrosis and Löffler's endomyocardial disease belong to
the same disease spectrum, the origin of which can be traced back
to the presence of eosinophils has been suggested several years
ago[39]. More recently, it has been shown that eosinophils when
associated with endomyocardial disease demonstrate certain abnormalities; these consist of degranulation. It has furthermore been
shown that eosinophilia may result from a variety of infectious
(and non-infectious) causes and it has been demonstrated that the
binding capacity for complexed IgG and increased phagocytosis of
eosinophils exists, with unmasking of Fc receptors. Degranulation
occurs as a result of binding of IgG or C3b coated particles or
parasites[40]. Electron microscopically it has been shown that the
granules are in appearance consistent with cationic proteins. These
proteins and possibly with combination of peroxidases result in the
changes that lead to endomyocardial disease.

It can, therefore, be concluded that a variety of infectious immune mechanisms may be operative in the various types of cardiomyopathy but much work needs still to be undertaken. Examination of fresh endomyocardial tissue obtained by bioptome[4] has demonstrated several important findings, for example in dilated cardiomyopathy IgG is preferentially bound to myocardial tissue, whereas if a virus infection had been the cause IgM is positive in many patients using direct fluorescent techniques[31]. The value of endomyocardial biopsies, particularly in cardiomyopathies is without doubt[41]. In patients with unsuspected myocarditis evidence is now accumulating that sequential biopsies of patients under treatment helps to monitor therapy[42]. This invasive form of investigation is also contributing greatly in elucidating pathogenic mechanisms of cardiomyopathy.

REFERENCES

1. Report of the WHO/ISFC Task Force on the Definition and Classification of Cardiomyopathies, Brit. Heart J., 44 No. 6:672 (1980).

2. E. G. J. Olsen, Cardiomyopathies, Cardiovasc. Clin., 4 No. 2: 239 (1972).

3. E. G. J. Olsen, Pathological recognition of cardiomyopathy, Postgrad. Med. J., 51:277 (1975).

4. E. G. J. Olsen, Postmortem findings and histologic, histochemical, and electron microscopic findings of myocardial biopsies, in: "Cardiomyopathy and myocardial biopsy", M. Kaltenbach, F. Loogen and E. G. J. Olsen, eds., Springer Verlag, Berlin (1978).

5. E. G. J. Olsen, "The Pathology of the Heart", 2nd edition, p.41 Macmillan Press, Basingstoke and London (1980).

6. H. Kuhn, G. Breithardt, H. J. Knieriem, F. Loogen, A. Both, W. A. K. Schmidt, R. Stroobandt and U. Gleichmann, Die Bedeutung der endomyokardialen Katheterbiopsie für die Diagnostik und die Beurteilung der Prognose der kongestiven Kardiomyopathie, Dtsch. Med. Wochenschr., 100:717 (1975).

7. E. G. J. Olsen, Edomyocardial biopsy, Brit. Heart J., 40:95 (1978).

8. E. G. J. Olsen, The pathology of idiopathic hypertrophic subaortic stenosis (hypertrophic cardiomyopathy). A critical review, Am. Heart J., 100 No. 4:553 (1980).

9. W. L. Henry, C. E. Clark and S. E. Epstein, Asymmetric septal hypertrophy (ASH): Echocardiographic identification of the pathognomonic anatomic abnormality of IHSS, Circulation, 47:225 (1973).

10. B. J. Maron, J. E. Edwards, V. J. Ferrans, C. E. Clark, E. A. Lebowitz, W. L. Henry and S. E. Epstein, Congenital heart malformations associated with disproportionate ventricular septal thickening, Circulation, 52:926 (1975).

11. J. H. Menges, R. D. Brandenburg and A. L. Brown Jr., The
     clinical, hemodynamic and pathologic diagnosis of muscular
     subvalvular aortic stenosis, Circulation, 24:1126 (1961).
12. E. G. J. Olsen,"Pathology of hypertrophic obstructive cardio-
     myopathy. Recent advances in studies of cardiac structural
     metabolism, Vol. 2 - Cardiomyopathies", E. Bajusz and G. Rona,
     eds., University Park Press, Baltimore, London, Tokyo (1973).
13. M. J. Davies, A. Pomerance and R. D. Teare, Pathological
     features of hypertrophic obstructive cardiomyopathy, J. Clin.
     Pathol., 27:529 (1974).
14. S. Van Noorden, E. G. J. Olsen and A. G. E. Pearse, Hypertrophic
     obstructive cardiomyopathy. A histological, histochemical
     and ultrastructural study of biopsy material, Cardiovasc.
     Res., V:118 (1971).
15. B. J. Maron and W. C. Roberts, Quantitative analysis of cardiac
     muscle cell disorganization in the ventricular septum of
     patients with hypertrophic cardiomyopathy, Circulation,
     59:689 (1979).
16. V. J. Ferrans, A. G. Morrow and W. C. Roberts, Myocardial
     ultrastructure in idiopathic hypertrophic subaortic stenosis.
     A study of operatively excised left ventricular outflow
     tract muscle in 14 patients, Circulation, 45:769 (1972).
17. J. F. Goodwin, Congestive and hypertrophic cardiomyopathies.
     A decade of study, Lancet, i:731 (1970).
18. E. G. J. Olsen,"The Pathology of the Heart",2nd edition, p. 323,
     Macmillan Press, Basingstoke and London (1980).
19. W. D. Edwards, R. Zakheim and L. Mattioli, Asymmetric septal
     hypertrophy in childhood. Unreliability of histologic
     criteria for differentiation of obstructive and nonobstructive
     forms, Human Pathol., 8:277 (1977).
20. J. N. P. Davies, Endocardial fibrosis in Africans, E. Afr.
     Med. J., 25:10 (1948).
21. W. Löffler, Endocarditis parietalis fibroplastica mit Blut-
     eosinophilie ein eigenartiges Krankheitsbild, Schweiz Med.
     Wochenschr., 17:817 (1936).
22. I. F. Brockington and E. G. J. Olsen, Löffler's endocarditis
     and Davies' endomyocardial fibrosis, Am. Heart J., 85:308
     (1973).
23. A. G. Shaper, M. S. R. Hutt and R. M. Coles, Necropsy studies
     of endomyocardial fibrosis and rheumatic heart disease in
     Uganda, Brit. Heart J., 30:391 (1968).
24. E. G. J. Olsen,"The Pathology of the Heart",2nd edition, p. 329,
     Macmillan Press, Basingstoke and London (1980).
25. E. G. J. Olsen,"The Pathology of the Heart",2nd edition, p. 317,
     Macmillan Press, Basingstoke and London (1980).
26. A. M. Denman, Immunological mechanisms and cardiovascular
     disease, in: "Immunology of Cardiovascular Disease", M. H.
     Lessof, ed., Marcel Dekker Inc., New York and Basel, (1981).
27. P. G. H. Gell, R. R. A. Coombs and P. Lachmann, eds.,"Clinical
     Aspects of Immunology",3rd ed., Blackwell Sci. Pub., Oxford
     England (1974).

28. C. Kawai and T. Takatsu, Clinical and experimental studies on cardiomyopathy, N. Engl. J. Med., 293:592 (1975).
29. G. Cambridge, C. G. C. MacArthur, A. P. Waterson, J. F. Goodwin and C. M. Oakley, Antibodies to Coxsackie B viruses in congestive cardiomyopathy, Brit. Heart J., 41:692 (1979).
30. S. K. Das, L. D. Stein, R. T. Reynolds, P. Thebert and J. T. Cassidy, Immunologic studies in cardiomyopathy and pathophysiologic implications, in: "Congestive Cardiomyopathy, Kiruna Sweden 1980", J. F. Goodwin, A. Hjalmarson and E. G. J. Olsen, eds., AB Hässle, Mölndal Sweden (1981).
31. H. D. Bolte and P. Schultheiss, Immunological results in myocardial diseases, Postgrad. Med. J., 54:500 (1978).
32. S. K. Das, R. E. Petty, W. L. Mengs and D. G. Tubergen, Cell mediated immunity in cardiomyopathy, Circulation, 53/54 suppl. 2:II-22 (1976).
33. R. E. Fowles, C. P. Bieber and E. B. Stinson, Defective in vitro suppressor cell function in idiopathic congestive cardiomyopathy, Circulation, 59:483 (1979).
34. J. R. Darsee, S. B. Heymsfield and D. O. Nutter, Hypertrophic cardiomyopathy and HLA linkage, N. Engl. J. Med., 300:877 (1979).
35. F. A. Ive and I. F. Brockington, Endomyocardial fibrosis and filariasis (letter), Lancet, 1:212 (1966).
36. A. G. Shaper, Endomyocardial fibrosis and rheumatic heart disease, Lancet, 1:639 (1966).
37. E. H. O. Parry and D. G. Abrahams, The natural history of endomyocardial fibrosis, Q. J. Med., 34:383 (1965).
38. A. G. Shaper, The geographical distribution of endomyocardial fibrosis, Pathol. Mecrobiol., 35:26 (1970).
39. E. G. J. Olsen and C. J. S. Spry, The pathogenesis of Löffler's endomyocardial disease, and its relationship to endomyocardial fibrosis, in: "Progress in Cardiology, 8", P. N. Yu and J. F. Goodwin, eds., Lea & Febiger, Philadelphia (1979).
40. D. J. McLaren, F. J. Ramalho-Pinto and S. R. Smithers, Ultrastructural evidence for complement and antibody-dependent damage to schistosomula of Schistosoma mansoni by rat eosinophils in vitro, Parasitology, 77:313 (1978).
41. E. G. J. Olsen, Diagnostic value of the endomyocardial bioptome (Annotation), Am. Heart J., 91:398 (1976).
42. K. Daly, P. J. Richardson, E. G. J. Olsen, J. Pattison, G. Jackson and D. E. Jewitt, Immunosuppressive therapy in acute inflammatory myocarditis, Circulation, 64 suppl. 4:IV-27 (1981).

TREATMENT OF CARDIOMYOPATHIES

J. F. Goodwin

Royal Postgraduate Medical School
Du Cane Road
London W12 OHS

In order to advise rational treatment it is necessary to define
and to classify the conditions known as cardiomyopathies. Cardiomyopathies are defined as "Heart Muscle Diseases of Unknown Causes"
to distinguish them from myocardial diseases due to disorders of
other systems; the "Specific Heart Muscle Diseases". This lecture
is concerned with the treatment of cardiomyopathies so defined.

Cardiomyopathies are classified into three main types according
to their disorders of structure and function:

1.   Hypertrophic; with and without systolic pressure gradients.
2.   Dilated (congestive).
3.   Restrictive/Obliterative.
(Goodwin and Oakley 1972; Goodwin 1974; 1979; 1981).

The report of the WHO/ISFC Task Force 1980 has confirmed this
earlier classification with only very minor modifications.

Hypertrophic Cardiomyopathy

This condition is characterized by massive hypertrophy of the
ventricular septum and free wall of the left ventricle and sometimes
of the right ventricle also. The systolic volume of the left ventricle is reduced; contraction is powerful, rapid and incoordinated.
Ejection fractions are in the region of 90%. The shape of the left
ventricle is grossly distorted. Diastolic function is seriously
impaired in a very complex way resulting in abnormal resistance to
filling and relaxation. The condition is familial; death is sudden
and unexpected in 50% of the patients, some families having a very

91

high incidence of sudden death (Malignant Hypertrophic Cardiomyopathy) (Maron et al., 1978[a]).

Treatment

Treatment aims at preventing sudden death, at improving hemodynamics, at reducing symptoms and at limiting progression of the
disease.

Sudden Death

Sudden death is most likely to be due to arrhythmia (Goodwin
and Krikler, 1976) for there is a significant relation between
sudden death and ventricular tachycardia (McKenna et al., 1981[a,b];
Goodwin and Krikler, 1976), but other factors such as impediment
to filling of the left ventricle and acute reduction in ventricular
volume also play a part. There is no relation between sudden death
and the presence or severity of systolic gradient.

Prevention of sudden death centers mainly around effective
antiarrhythmic therapy. Neither beta adrenergic blocking agents nor
calcium blocking agents have been shown by our group to reduce the
incidence of arrhythmias (McKenna et al., 1980; McKenna et al.,
1981[b]). Episodes of ventricular tachycardia detected by ambulatory
monitoring correlate inversely with prognosis. Amiodarone which
prolongs the action potential and increases the refractory period
has been shown to be effective in reducing the number and frequency
of ectopic rhythms and of ventricular tachycardia (McKenna et al.,
1981[c]).

All patients with hypertrophic cardiomyopathy should have
ambulatory ECG monitoring. If there are episodes of repeated multi-
focal ventricular premature contractions or runs of ventricular
tachycardia then Amiodarone should be started. The dosage should
be 200 mg three times daily for one week, then 200 mg twice daily;
the dose may be further reduced later, if necessary by discontinuing
the drug on one or two days of the week. There is a latent period
of one to two weeks before the drug begins to act. Since Amiodarone
affects thyroid function and can produce both hypo and hyperthyroidism, thyroid function tests should be performed before and during
treatment. The effects of calcium-blocking agents may be potentiated
by Amiodarone and thus Amiodarone and Verapamil should not be used
together. The effects of digitalis and anticoagulants are also
potentiated by Amiodarone. The action of Amiodarone persists for
many months after the drug has been stopped in patients who have
been taking it for long periods.

Complications of Amiodarone

Unfortunately, Amiodarone has a number of side effects. These include peripheral neuropathy, photosensitivity, headache, nausea, vertigo, but are usually mild and reversible. Vomiting may occur during the initial phase of treatment with the loading dose. Micro deposits on the cornea are regularly seen by slit lamp examination. They do not affect visual acuity though may impart a faint bluish tinge to the vision. Regular ophthalmic examination is important however. Amiodarone is rarely contraindicated in hypertrophic cardiomyopathy, but care should be taken to exclude patients with atrioventricular block or troublesome bradycardia unless a pacemaker has previously been inserted. Pulmonary fibrosis is a rare complication of Amiodarone treatment and usually reversible when the drug is stopped.

Measures to Prevent Sudden Death from Mechanical Causes

Attempts to prevent sudden death from resistance to ventricular filling center around measures to improve compliance, reduce resistance to filling and aid relaxation. Events which reduce ventricular volume add to the possibility of sudden death, and thus hypotension and hypovolemia should be avoided.

The effects of beta adrenergic blocking agents on ventricular filling and compliance are variable. In acute studies both Practolol (Webb Peploe et al., 1971) and Propranolol (Swanton et al., 1977) reduce diastolic filling pressure and increase diastolic volume. The effect of chronic oral treatment with beta adrenergic blocking agents is less consistent, but in most patients the active suction period of diastole (between the opening of the mitral valve and 0 point of the impulse cardiogram) when most of ventricular filling occurs is significantly prolonged. Filling of the left ventricle at the moment when left ventricular pressures are still falling is increased. This indicates improvement in relaxation, an effect that is independent of heart rate (Alvares, 1980). In theory, by these effects, and by slowing of heart rate, especially on effort, and by allowing more time for ventricular filling, beta blockade should help to reduce the risk of sudden death. Unfortunately, the available data apart from the series of Frank et al. 1978 who used very large doses of Propranolol, do not indicate that this is so.

Although Verapamil has been reported to improve diastolic function there is, as yet, no evidence of prolonation of life; indeed, Verapamil may shorten life because sudden death has occurred after starting Verapamil and pulmonary edema has been documented, both in our own experience and in that of Rosing et al. 1981.

However, it is encouraging that Nifedipine has been shown to improve diastolic compliance in acute studies (Lorell et al., 1982) though a disadvantage of Nifedipine would be its vasodilator effect which might reduce ventricular volume and so predispose to elimination of the cavity and arrest of blood flow.

There is no definite evidence that surgical treatment prevents sudden death, by an effect on ventricular function, except possibly by reduction in systolic pressure gradients and improvement in ventricular volume.

Treatment to Improve Hemodynamics

Hypertrophic cardiomyopathy is essentially a disease of impaired ventricular diastolic function: diastole is grossly disorganized (Alvares, 1980), relaxation and the rate of filling are impaired, both regionally and globally (Sanderson et al., 1978; Goodwin, 1982).. The massive ventricular hypertrophy, the reduced ventricular volume in systole and powerful contraction of the ventricle which expels all the contents in the first half of systole combine with the abnormalities of filling to offer serious impediment to effective left ventricular function. It is the powerful contraction of the massive left ventricular muscle that brings about apposition of the septum to the mitral valve apparatus and causes pressure gradients to develop in systole. Reduction of ventricular volume by impaired inflow and by reduced afterload both contribute to the elimination of the ventricular cavity. True obstruction does not occur (Criley et al., 1965; Goodwin, 1979; Murgo et al., 1980).

Systolic pressure gradients can be modified by beta blockade given acutely but there is no evidence that chronic beta blocking treatment is beneficial in this way. Verapamil has been reported to reduce pressure gradients (Rosing et al., 1979[a]). Reduction in the force of ventricular contraction may help to reduce cavity elimination but the most important area of impaired hemodynamics is diastole, and it is in this phase of the cycle that beta blocking agents exert their most important action. Chronic beta adrenergic blockade usually prolongs the active suction phase of diastole and improves relaxation independent of heart failure, the negative chronotropic effects of beta blocking agents is important also, as the bradycardia allows more time for filling of the ventricles.

Nifedipine improves diastolic filling acutely (Lorell, 1982) but may be disadvantageous chronically by reducing ventricular volume by vaso-dilatation and reduction of afterload.

Verapamil may improve diastolic function without vaso-dilatation. In my department the effect of Verapamil on systolic function has been studied in 18 patients with hypertrophic cardiomyopathy by

systolic time intervals. Verapamil was found to have negative
inotropic effects when left ventricular systolic function was normal
before treatment, but to have peripheral vaso-dilator effects when
left ventricular function was impaired before treatment. Two
patients in the study developed pulmonary edema (Herr, K. to be
published).

The effect of Amiodarone on hemodynamics has not yet been fully
worked out. Its beta blocking action may be of some value.

Surgical treatment reduces or abolishes gradients and reduces
left ventricular end diastolic pressure.

Thus, to improve hemodynamics beta blockade therapy is the
first line of treatment. In patients who do not respond, Verapamil
may be tried but atrioventricular conduction defects or high left
atrial pressures are contra-indications (Rosing et al., 1982).
Treatment with Verapamil should always be started in hospital.

At present Amiodarone is not indicated for hemodynamic reasons
but it may be combined with Propranolol to combine improvement in
hemodynamics relief of symptoms and control of arrhythmias.

Verapamil and Amiodarone should not be given together.

Symptomatic Treatment

The principle symptom is dyspnea on exertion, due to the high
left atrial pressure resulting from the stiff left ventricle and
the high left ventricular end diastolic pressure which rises on
effort. Angina is common, usually occurring on effort but prolonged
cardiac ischemic pain can occur at rest and myocardial infarction
(with normal coronary arteries) has been reported (Maron et al.,
1979). The exact reasons for the angina are not known; massive
oxygen demand by greatly hypertrophied muscle, impaired diastolic
coronary flow in diastole due to the abnormal relaxation of the
stiff left ventricle, and a metabolic fault leading to oxygen
deprivation may all be considered as possibilities. Dizziness,
syncope and palpitations, can all be ascribed to arrhythmia, but
syncope may be due to "mechanical" factors; sudden fall in cardiac
output due to reduction of left ventricular volume and resistance
of the left ventricle to filling. It is doubtful if the outflow
tract gradients alone contribute to syncope; they are produced by
the hypertrophied walls of the left ventricle collapsing inwards
when the ventricle is not distended with blood. When ventricular
volume is seriously reduced the cavity of the ventricle may be
virtually eliminated by the powerfully contracting hypertrophied
muscle and in this way gradients are created.

The treatment of dyspnea is by beta adrenergic blocking agents or calcium blocking agents. Propranolol improves dyspnea in around 70% of patients, probably by reducing the stiffness of the left ventricle, improving relaxation and increasing the time available for filling (Webb Peploe et al., 1971; Alvares, 1980; Goodwin, 1982). In my experience a non-selective beta adrenergic blocking agent gives better results than a selective one which has less effect on outflow tract gradients (Hubner et al., 1973). Large doses, up to 300 mg a day, of Propranolol, are needed but smaller doses (40 mg a day) should be used initially.

When arrhythmias have been detected and there are also symptoms of angina and dyspnea, Amiodarone and Propranolol may be tried. This combination may prove to be superior to Verapamil.

Beta blockade does not relieve symptoms in every patient, probably because, owing to the grossly global and regional irregular patterns of relaxation and filling (Sanderson et al., 1978; Alvares, 1980), the effects vary with the extent and severity of the mal-orientated myofibrillar lesions.

Verapamil has been reported to improve symptoms. Kaltenbach et al. (1979) reported reduction in symptoms and in left ventricular muscle mass in 22 patients. Rosing et al. (1979[b]) reported improvement in symptoms in 11 of 15 patients, with increase in exercise tolerance in 6.

Adverse effects included bradycardia, sinus arrest, pulmonary edema and systemic hypotension.

Personal experience indicates that while Verapamil may relieve symptoms in some patients, the incidence of side effects and complications may be higher than with beta adrenergic blockade. It has so far not been possible to identify precisely which patients with hypertrophic cardiomyopathy are most likely to benefit from Verapamil and which are most likely to sustain untoward effects.

The first line treatment for symptoms should be beta blockade and the agent of choice should be Propranolol. If beta adrenergic blockade fails, then Verapamil should be tried cautiously starting with a small dose (20 mg three times daily) and working up to 120 mg three times daily. Patients who have heart failure or conduction defects are unsuitable. On present evidence Verapamil and Propranolol should not be given together. It must be emphasized that more precise identification of the hemodynamics in individual patients and clearer identification of sub-groups of patients is required before the exact place of Verapamil can be determined. The place of other calcium blocking agents has not yet been studied in detail; Nifedipine may prove to be helpful but care should be taken to prevent undue vaso-dilatation and hypotension.

Attacks of severe and prolonged chest pain may be intractable and difficult to treat. Frequently they do not respond to Propranolol. Verapamil may be tried in such patients, while Amiodarone has occasionally been shown to have dramatic effects for reasons that are not fully understood but perhaps because of its weak beta adrenergic blocking action.

When atrial fibrillation occurs, the cardiac output usually falls dramatically and pulmonary edema or congestive heart failure may occur because of the loss of atrial drive and tachycardia; embolism may occur. The patient should immediately be given Heparin and cardioversion carried out. If this fails the ventricular rate must be slowed and digitalis may be cautiously given, together with diuretics. There is usually little risk of precipitating an outflow tract crisis in such patients. Amiodarone, which stabilizes atrial fibrillation, may convert it to sinus rhythm and should be started, but care is necessary since Amiodarone increases digitalis blood levels, and digitalis should be reduced when the Amiodarone starts to take effect in 3-10 days. Small doses of Propranolol to slow the ventricular rate may be used as an alternative to Amiodarone, but care is needed if heart failure threatens.

Infective Endocarditis

Treatment of infective endocarditis in hypertrophic cardiomyopathy does not differ from infective endocarditis complicating other forms of heart disease. Since the mitral valve is the most usually affected valve the need for mitral valve replacement should be remembered if hemodynamic reasons or failure to control infection dictate surgical treatment.

Congestive Heart Failure

Heart failure usually indicates a severe and late form of the disease. It should be treated cautiously with diuretics.

Digitalis in Hypertrophic Cardiomyopathy

The dire effects ascribed to digitalis in exacerbating gradients and causing sudden death have not been confirmed by subsequent experience. However, the positive inotropic effects of digitalis make it likely that it will further reduce ventricular volume and since there is no impairment of systolic function from the disease until it becomes far advanced, digitalis should be avoided except where atrial fibrillation or congestive heart failure are present. The inconstant effects reported for digitalis may be explained by the potentially adverse effects of the positive

inotropic action on the one hand and the potentially beneficial
effects of the negative chronotropic effect on the other.

Surgical Treatment

There is a small place for surgical treatment. There are two
operations available; septal resection or mitral valve replacement.
Septal resection is indicated in patients whose symptoms do not
respond to adequate medical treatment and who have appreciable
septal hypertrophy with a consistent systolic pressure gradient of
50 mmHg or more in the left ventricle. Results are excellent for
the relief of symptoms, and improvement in hemodynamics occurs
(Reitz et al., 1975; Kuhn et al., 1978; Maron et al., 1978). There
is no evidence that septal resection improves prognosis and the
operation is essentially for the relief of symptoms. The mortality
is not low (8% operative and 9% on late follow-up, making a total
of 17%) (Maron et al., 1978). Therefore, septal resection should
not be undertaken lightly.

Mitral valve replacement is indicated in patients in whom
mitral regurgitation is severe and intractable and requires surgical
relief in its own right. Such mitral regurgitation is usually the
result of secondary damage to the mitral valve as a result of calcification, turbulance or infection. In addition to relieving
mitral regurgitation, mitral valve replacement makes room in the
crowded ventricle by removal of the large papillary muscles. A low
profile disc type of mitral prosthesis must be used, as there is
usually insufficient room in the hypertrophied left ventricle for
a caged ball type of valve.

The presence of associated fixed outflow tract obstruction is
an important additional reason for operation.

Relief of Ventricular Hypertrophy and Modification of the Progress of the Disease

It has been postulated that beta adrenergic blockade by
relieving outflow tract gradients may lessen the stimulus to progressive hypertrophy but proof is lacking. Verapamil on the other
hand has been considered to reduce hypertrophy in one series
(Kaltenbach et al., 1979).

The possibility of retarding the progress of the disorder is
the most compelling reason for treating asymptomatic patients with
a good prognosis; that is, those with no family history of sudden
death and whose signs are of mild or moderate disease on clinical
and hemodynamic grounds, but the possible side effects of long term
treatment and the uncertainty of benefit tend to outweigh these

considerations. Regular ambulatory monitoring is advisable and if
arrhythmias are detected then treatment is needed, Amiodarone being
the drug of choice at the present time, quinidine being the next
best alternative.

Pacemaking Treatment

A pacemaker may be required occasionally to treat hypertrophic
cardiomyopathy. Patients who develop an unacceptable degree of
bradycardia on beta adrenergic blockade may require a pacemaker,
while those who have evidence of sinus node dysfunction with alternating tachycardia and bradycardia require a pacemaker in addition
to anti-arrhythmic drugs.

DILATED CONGESTIVE CARDIOMYOPATHY

The prognosis is usually poor, approximately 50% of patients
dying in the first two years after diagnosis and around 70% within
eight years. Just over 20% remain alive and have a reasonable
prognosis (Fuster et al., 1982). In our own experience of 146
patients followed for up to 20 years, prognosis was related mainly
to left ventricular function (MacArthur et al., 1982).

Treatment is essentially that for congestive cardiac failure
and no specific therapy is known. General measures include advice
against cigarette smoking and alcohol and prolonged reduction of
activity after the heart failure has been treated. Prolonged
inactivity has become a hallowed principle of treatment but there
is, in fact, little evidence or hard data to support this view.
Digitalis is indicated if there is atrial fibrillation but its use
in sinus rhythm has been questioned on the grounds that it may not
exert any effective action after the first few months of treatment.
Nevertheless if there is substantial cardiomegaly due to cardiac
dilatation, and heart failure in sinus rhythm, digitalis should be
given provided that there are no contra-indications. Careful
attention must be paid to avoid digitalis toxicity.

Recently treatment by new inotropic and vaso-dilator drugs
have been successful in the short term. Salbutamol given as an
intravenous infusion in severe heart failure improves cardiac function, mainly as a result of systemic vaso-dilatation but also
because of some positive inotropic effect (Sharma and Goodwin, 1978).
However, there are disadvantages, notably tachycardia, tachyphylaxis,
increase in blood sugar and fall in serum potassium. Vaso-dilator
therapy with Hydrallazine has been successful in reducing left
ventricular end diastolic pressure and pulmonary artery pressure,
and increasing cardiac output without a significant fall in blood
pressure or increase in heart rate. These effects are seen not

only when the drug is given intravenously, but also over a period
of weeks and months by mouth, in doses of up to 300 mg a day
(Fitchett et al., 1979). Patients who are slow acetylators may
experience side effects; headaches, flushing or lupus syndrome with
high doses. If possible acetylator status should be determined
before treatment is started as fast acetylators can probably be
given the larger doses with impunity.

As an alternative to Hydrallazine, Prazosyn may be used but
tachyphylaxis is common. In desperate situations, if the systolic
blood pressure is not below 90 mmHg, Nitroprusside may be cautiously
given intravenously and titrated against the blood pressure and
clinical response. Also, in desperate cases the positive inotropic
agents Dobutamine or Dopamine may be used, and in combination with
Nitroprusside may be life saving. Unfortunately, improvement after
such severe congestive cardiac failure is usually only temporary,
although a few patients make dramatic and unexpected recoveries,
so hope should not be abandoned lightly.

The angiotensin concerting enzyme inhibitor Captopril may
prove to be an effective agent for reducing afterload in chronic
heart failure (Sharp et al., 1980) and could be useful in congestive
cardiomyopathy.

Beta adrenergic Blockade in Congestive Dilated Cardiomyopathy

The use of beta adrenergic blocking agents in dilated congestive cardiomyopathy remains controversial and the indications
uncertain. The work of Hjalmarsson and his colleagues (Waagstein
et al., 1975) indicated improvement in cardiac function, on clinical
and hemodynamic evidence, after the use of graded oral doses of
Metoprolol, a cardioselective agent. Improvement in prognosis was
claimed also. The reason for the results are not understood. The
patients who are most suitable for treatment may be those with
disproportionate tachycardia who may have an excess of catecholamines
in the heart (Waagstein et al., 1979). Certainly judicious slowing
of the heart rate might be beneficial by allowing more time for
ventricular filling. Treatment with beta adrenergic blocking agents
should not be undertaken at random but should be part of a carefully
controlled clinical trial.

The treatment of complications or threatened complications of
dilated congestive cardiomyopathy is important. When there is
severe congestive heart failure, with low cardiac output and peripheral edema and the patient is immobilized, anti-coagulants are
advisable to protect against deep venous thrombosis and pulmonary
embolism. In patients with atrial fibrillation anti-coagulants
are indicated to avert systemic embolism.

The Implications of the Virus/Immune Theory of Causation on Treatment

The possibility that virus myocarditis or some infective agent might lead to dilated congestive cardiomyopathy either directly or by an auto immune mechanism was suggested a number of years ago (Kawii, 1971; Braimbridge et al., 1967). High titres to Coxsackie B viruses in the blood of patients with dilated congestive cardio-myopathy as compared to controls was reported by our group (Cambridge et al., 1979). In a number of patients endomyocardial biopsy did not show any evidence of myocarditis, and the possibility of a disturbance of cellular immunity resulting from the infection and causing progressive myocardial damage has been suggested. Work from Stanford University by Fowles et al. (1979) suggested a defect of suppressor cell function in dilated congestive cardiomyopathy, which might be explained in this way. However, the occasional finding of dilated congestive cardiomyopathy on a familial basis suggests that perhaps the opposite could sometimes be true; that is, that inherited defects in cellular immunity might predispose to virus infection. The matter is unsettled and the bearing on current treatment unclear. However, another recent report from Stanford by Mason et al. (1980) has therapeutic implications. These workers reported a small series of patients with a short history of congestive heart failure of unknown cause. Endomyocardial biopsy revealed evidence of myocarditis and treatment with immunosuppressive and steroid drugs caused improvement (as judged by clinical, hemo-dynamic and endomyocardial biopsy evidence) in the majority.

It is not clear whether these patients were suffering from myocarditis, or dilated congestive cardiomyopathy or that myo-carditis led to the latter, but the implications for treatment are clear. Patients who apparently have dilated congestive cardio-myopathy of recent onset should be investigated by endomyocardial biopsy if possible, and if evidence of myocarditis is found, treat-ment with immunosuppressive drugs and steroids should be considered.

In the terminal patient, for whom all methods of treatment have proved unavailing, cardiac transplantation may be considered provided that there are no contra-indications.

In patients with arrhythmic cardiomyopathies (Goodwin, 1979) Amiodarone may be of great value for it is effective in controlling arrhythmias without depressing myocardial function. Most anti-arrhythmic drugs have some negative effect on cardiac function, so Amiodarone is likely to be the drug of choice.

Restrictive/Obliterative Cardiomyopathy

Endomyocardial fibrosis is the usual cause of this type of cardiomyopathy. Since the hemodynamics and pathology are closely

similar in the tropical variety and in the temperate zone type
known as Löffler's endomyocardial disease, treatment is basically
the same and is in general unsatisfactory. The usual measures for
congestive heart failure are indicated and anti-coagulants should
be used because of the high risk of thrombosis in the ventricle.
In Löffler's disease the eosinophilia, which may affect other
organs, can be treated by cytotoxic drugs or steroids, but the
result is usually unsatisfactory except in relieving exacerbations.
The introduction of surgical means has improved prognosis. Resection
of endocardial fibrous plaques and replacement of atrioventricular
valves when severely involved in the disease has had considerable
success in the short term, but long term results are not yet available (Dubost et al., 1976; Davies et al., 1981; Spry and Tai, 1976).

Table 1. Suggested Plan of Management for Hypertrophic
          Cardiomyopathy

---

1. No family history, no symptoms, mild disease, no
    arrhythmia. Observe regularly. Holter monitoring.

2. Ventricular arrhythmia: Amiodarone.

3. Symptoms - no arrhythmia: beta blockade.

4. Symptoms - but unsuitable for beta blockade:
    Verapamil if no AV conduction defect and LA pressure
    not significantly elevated. Watch carefully.

5. Symptoms and arrhythmia: Propranolol, Amiodarone.

6. Symptoms - gradient at or greater than 50 mmHg, no
    response to medical treatment. Septal resection.

7. Severe complicated mitral regurgitation: mitral
    valve replacement with low profile mechanical
    prosthesis and excision of papillary muscle.

REFERENCES

Alvares, R., 1980, Diastolic function and prognosis in hypertrophic
      cardiomyopathy, PhD Thesis, University of London.
Braimbridge, M. V., Darracott, S., Chayen, J., Bitensby, L.,
      Poulter, L. W., 1967, Possibility of a new infective etiological
      agent in congestive cardiomyopathy, Lancet, 1:171-176.
Cambridge, G., MacArthur, C. G. C., Waterson, A. P., Goodwin, J. F.,
      Oakley, C. M., 1979, Antibodies to Coxsackie B virus in con-
      gestive cardiomyopathy, Brit. Heart J., 41:692.
Criley, J. M. et al., 1965, Pressure gradients without obstruction:
      a new concept of hypertrophic subaortic stenosis, Circulation,
      32:881.

Davies, J., Sapsford, R., Tai, P. C., Spry, C. J. F., Goodwin, J. F.,
    1981, Löffler's endomyocardial disease – cardiological and
    immunological study of nine patients with report of successful
    surgery in three patients, Brit. Heart J., 45:338 (P).
Dubost, C., Marine, P., Gerbaux, A., Bertrand, E., Rulliere, R.,
    Vial, F., Barrillon, A., Prigent, C., Carpenter, A., Soyer, R.,
    1976, Surgical treatment of constrictive fibrous endocarditis,
    Ann. Surg., 184:303-307.
Fitchett, D. H., Marin Neto J. A., Oakley, C. M., Goodwin, J. F.,
    1979, Hydrallazine in the assessment of left ventricular
    failure, Amer. J. Cardiol., 44:30.
Fowler, B. B., Bieber, C. P., Stinson, E. B., 1979, Defective in
    vitro suppressor cell dysfunction in idiopathic congestive
    cardiomyopathy, Circulation, 59:483.
Frank, M. J. et al., 1978, Long term medical management of hyper-
    trophic obstructive cardiomyopathy, Amer. J. Cardiol., 42:993.
Fuster, V. et al., 1982, Idiopathic dilated congestive cardio-
    myopathy – observations on the natural history, in: "Congestive
    Cardiomyopathy", eds., Goodwin, J. F., Hjalmarsson, A. and
    Olsen, E. G. J., Hessle, Molndal, Sweden, p. 208.
Goodwin, J. F., Oakley, C. M., 1972, The Cardiomyopathies, Brit.
    Heart J., 34:595.
Goodwin, J. F., 1974, International Lecture: Prospects and pre-
    dictions for the cardiomyopathies, Circulation, 50:210.
Goodwin, J. F., Krikler, D. M., 1976, Arrhythmia as a cause of
    sudden death in hypertrophic cardiomyopathy, Lancet, 2:937-940.
Goodwin, J. F., 1979, Cardiomyopathy: an interface between funda-
    mental and clinical cardiology, in: "Cardiology", ed., Hayase
    and Murao, Excerpta Medica Amsterdam, p. 103.
Goodwin, J. F., 1981, The frontiers of cardiomyopathy, Brit. Heart
    J., to be published.
Goodwin, J. F., 1982, The frontiers of cardiomyopathy, Brit. Heart
    J., in press.
Hubner, P. J. B., Ziady, G. M., Raine, G. K., Hardarson, T., Scales,
    B., Oakley, C. M., Goodwin, J. F., 1973, Double blind trial
    of Propranolol, and Practolol in hypertrophic cardiomyopathy,
    Brit. Heart J., 35:1116.
Kaltenbach, M., Hopf, R., Kober, G., Bussman, W.-D., Keller, M.,
    Peterson, Y., 1979, Treatment of hypertrophic obstructive
    cardiomyopathy with Verapamil, Brit. Heart J., 42:35-42.
Kawii, C., 1971, Idiopathic cardiomyopathy. A study on the infection/
    immune theory as a cause of the disease, Jap. Circ. J., 35:765.
Kuhn, H., Krelhaw, W., Bircks, W., Schulte, H. D., Loogen, F., 1978,
    Indication for surgical treatment in patients with hypertrophic
    obstructive cardiomyopathy, in: "Cardiomyopathy and myocardial
    biopsy",Eds., Kaltenbach, Loogen, Olsen, Springer Verlag,
    Berlin, p. 308.
Lorell, B. H., Poulus, Grossman, W., Fulton, M. A., Wynne, J.,
    Cohn, P. F., 1980, Improved diastolic compliance in hyper-
    trophic cardiomyopathy treated with Nifedipine, Circulation,
    3:62, 317.

MacArthur, C. G. C. et al., 1982, The effect of left ventricular
    function, arrhythmias and evidence of previous viral infection
    on the prognosis of congestive cardiomyopathy, in: "Congestive
    Cardiomyopathy", eds., Goodwin, J. F., Hjalmarsson, A. and
    Olsen, E. G. J., Hessle, Molndal, Sweden, p. 236.
McKenna, W. J., Chetty, S., Oakley, C. M., Goodwin, J. F., 1980,
    Arrhythmias in hypertrophic cardiomyopathy; exercise electro-
    cardiogram and 48 hour ambulatory electrocardiographic assess-
    ment with and without beta adrenergic blocking therapy, Amer.
    J. Cardiol., 45:1-5.
McKenna, W. J., England, D., Doi, Y. C., Deanfield, J. E., Oakley,
    C. M., Goodwin, J. F., 1981[a], Arrhythmias in hypertrophic
    cardiomyopathy: I, influence on prognosis, Brit. Heart J., in
    press.
McKenna, W., Deanfield, J., Faruqui, A., England, D., Oakley, C.,
    Goodwin, J. F., 1981[b], Prognosis in hypertrophic cardiomyopathy.
    Role of age and clinical electrocardiographic and hemodynamic
    features, Amer. J. Cardiol., 47:532.
McKenna, W. J., Harris, L., Perez, G., Krikler, D. M., Oakley, C.
    M., Goodwin, J. F., 1981[c], Arrhythmias in hypertrophic cardio-
    myopathy: II, comparison of Amiodarone and Verapamil in treat-
    ment, Brit. Heart J., in press.
Maron, B. J., Merrill, W. H., Freier, P. A., Kent, K. M., Epstein,
    S. E., Morrow, A. G., 1978, Long term clinical course and
    symptomatic status of patients after operative treatment for
    hypertrophic subaortic stenosis, Circulation, 57:1205.
Maron, B. J., Lipson, L. C., Roberts, W. C., Savage, D. D., Epstein,
    S. E., 1978[a], 'Malignant' hypertrophic cardiomyopathy, Amer.
    J. Cardiol., 41:1133-1140.
Maron, B. J., Epstein, S. E., Roberts, W. C., 1979, Hypertrophic
    cardiomyopathy and transmural myocardial infarction without
    significant atherosclerosis of the extramural coronary artery,
    Amer. J. Cardiol., 43:1086-1102.
Mason, J. W., Billingham, M. E., Ricci, D. R., 1980, Treatment of
    acute inflammatory myocarditis assisted by endomyocardial
    biopsy, Amer. J. Cardiol., 45:1037.
Murgo, J. P., et al., 1980, Dynamics of left ventricular ejection
    in obstructive and non-obstructive hypertrophic cardiomyopathy,
    Amer. J. Cardiol., 45:6.
Reitz, B. A., Epstein, S. E., Henry, W. L., Conkle, D. M., Iskoitz,
    S. B., Redwood, B. R., Morrow, A. G., 1975, Operative treat-
    ment in hypertrophic subaortic stenosis. Techniques and the
    results of pre and post operative assessment in 83 patients,
    Circulation, 52:88.
Report of the WHO/ISFC Task Force on the Definition and Classifi-
    cation of cardiomyopathies, Brit. Heart J., 1972, 34:545.
Rosing, D. R., Kent, K. M., Borer, J. S., Seides, S. F., Maron,
    B. J., Epstein, S. E., 1979[a], Verapamil therapy: A new approach
    to the pharmacological treatment of hypertrophic cardiomyopathy;
    I, hemodynamic effects, Circulation, 60:1201.

Rosing, D. R., Kent, K. M., Maron, B. J., Epstein, S. E., 1979[b],
    Verapamil therapy: A new approach to the pharmacological treat-
    ment of hypertrophic cardiomyopathy; II, effects on exercise
    capacity and symptomatic status, Circulation, 60:1208-1213.
Rosing, D. R. et al., 1981, Verapamil therapy: a new approach to
    the pharmacological treatment of hypertrophic cardiomyopathy;
    III, the effect of long term administration, Amer. J. Cardiol.,
    48:545.
Sanderson, J. E., Traill, T. A., Sutton, M. G. St.J., Brown, D. J.,
    Gibson, D. G., Goodwin, J. F., 1978, Left ventricular relax-
    ation and filling in hypertrophic cardiomyopathy. An echo-
    cardiographic study, Brit. Heart J., 40:596.
Sharma, B., Goodwin, J. F., 1978, Beneficial effects of Salbutamol
    on cardiac function in severe congestive cardiomyopathy.
    Effects on systolic and diastolic function of the left ven-
    tricle, Circulation, 58:449.
Sharpe, D. N. et al., 1980, Low dose Captopril in chronic heart
    failure: acute hemodynamic effect and long term treatment,
    Lancet, 2:1154.
Spry, C. J. F., Tai, P. C., 1976, Studies in blood eosinophils. II,
    patients with Löffler's cardiomyopathy, Clin. Exper. Immunol.,
    24:423.
Swanton, R. H. et al., 1977, Haemodynamic studies of beta blockade
    in hypertrophic cardiomyopathy, Europ. J. Cardiol., 5:327.
Waagstein, F., Hjalmasson, A., Vonrausker, E., Wolenkin, I., 1975,
    Effect of clinical beta adrenergic blockade in congestive
    cardiomyopathy, Brit. Heart J., 37:1022.
Webb-Peploe, M. M., Croxson, R. S., Oakley, C. M., Goodwin, J. F.,
    1971, Cardioselective beta adrenergic blockade in hypertrophic
    obstructive cardiomyopathy, Postgrad. Med. J., (suppl.),
    47:93-97.

HEART IN OUTER SPACE

Oleg G. Gazenko

Institute of Biomedical Problems
Moscow, USSR

During the 25 years that have elapsed since the first sputnik in space, space research has scored spectacular achievements. This follows from the simple fact that 109 men of the Earth have already made space flights and that men and lunar vehicles have left their traces on the Moon. Space probes have informed us about the environmental parameters on the planets of the solar system and in outer space.

Many investigations, particularly of recent years, give evidence that within the solar system the Earth appears to be the only place where life exists. This inference is fraught with very important consequences: 1) it points to the unique significance of the Earth biosphere in our solar system, 2) it attracts our attention to the very specific place man occupies in the "Earth biological envelope", to his historical responsibility for the preservation of the biosphere and the healthy development of the human society, and 3) it strictly confines hypotheses on the origin and evolution of planetary systems and the conditions required for the emergence, existence and evolution of life in the Universe.

A space environment as such is alien to life and, therefore, it can be penetrated if living creatures, man included, are protected against its harmful effects. This is why space cabin atmospheres are normally very close to those on the Earth. Space flights are characterized by the so-called free fall which gives rise to the state of dynamic weightlessness. Weightlessness or zero-g is of particular interest for biologists and medical people because the entire biological evolution, at least that which began with the emergence of the cell and ended with the appearance of man, developed under conditions of a constant gravity field.

Space flights greatly stimulated interest in the biological role of gravity. Today we have the right to speak about a new branch of biology, gravitational biology, the purpose of which is to study in great detail the effect of weightlessness on the structure and function of living organisms, including cardiovascular physiology. This is the subject of the present paper.

MAN IN SPACE

Man, as the prominent astronomer Shapley remarked, was born by stars and, therefore, it is not surprising that he tries to go back to them. But the wise men of ancient times who used to say that the road to the stars is hard were also correct. The problems man may encounter in space flight are of great diversity. Among them mention should be made of those that may influence the health state of man: weightlessness, cosmic radiation, abnormal environmental parameters, and factors causing nervous-emotional stress.

It is known that the sources of cosmic radiation are: galactic cosmic radiation from the depth of outer space, radiation of solar flares, and Earth radiation belts. Careful dosimetric measurements carried out in every space flight demonstrated that the absorbed radiation dose during lunar flights (whose trajectory crossed the Earth radiation belts) was about 0.5 rem and never exceeded 1.0 rem. During long-term orbital flights of about 6 months in duration the dose increased and reached 5.0 rem. However, this is still lower th the permissible dose which is taken of 15 rem per flight (in the US allowable dose is 25 rem).

Thus, the radiation factor is not very dramatic at least today and cannot be viewed as one influencing the cardiovascular function in space flight.

In flight crewmembers live and work in a specific environment which reflects tendencies of our technically advanced society. It is, first of all, characterized by the man-made environment. It is a classical example of a compromise between human requirements and technical feasibility. Then, a confined enclosure - a small living space which amounts to several cubic meters per man. This diminishes motor activity, enhances hypokinesia, stimulates cardio-vascular deconditioning.

At first sight, the physical and chemical parameters of the space cabin environment are stable. However, this is not quite the case, because the pressure, temperature, humidity and the concentration of the major constituents (O_2, N_2, CO_2) vary continuously; the content of trace contaminants, including anthro-pogenic, increases and the microbial composition changes. This gives rise to problems associated with the maintenance of the environmental parameters within normal limits because their marked deviations may affect the physiological functions of crewmembers.

     Of greater importance is a large group of various circumstances
and factors that may induce and maintain nervous-emotional stress.
As a matter of fact, flight starts still on the Earth and the
first critical state is the launch. Space crewmembers typically
show increased heart rate and a more or less increased blood
pressure as the launch time approaches. Immediately after launch
heart rate begins to go down, in spite of growing acceleration,
thus reflecting a typical "prelaunch" reaction of sympatho-adrenal
origin. The shock of novelty, great diversity of unexpected and
memorable impressions, heavy duties combined with expected and
actual complications and hazardous situations - these are
specific features of space missions which may bring about more or
less expressed reactions of the heart and the cardiovascular
system on the whole. Before considering the role óf zero-g, it is
appropriate to discuss general problems of gravitational biology.

BIOLOGICAL ROLE OF GRAVITY

     Gravity is a great and universal designer of the Universe -
the force of gravity has determined the emergence, structure and
environment of planets. Gravity is a constant and ubiquitous
phenomenon which generates a very weak field. Therefore, living
systems that have a different mass and spatial configuration show
different sensitivity to gravity effects. Large living organisms,
man included, distinctly react to gravity variations. Smaller
animals, e.g. insects, respond much more markedly to surface tension.
Microorganisms are indifferent to gravity and obey the laws of
viscosity and Brownian movement.

     In the course of evolution Nature has staged two important
experiments associated with gravity effect. The first took place
when living being moved from the ocean to the land, and the
second when our ancestors developed the ability of uprightness.
The success was due to the improvement of the structure and
function of the cardiovascular and musculoskeletal systems. The
development of two-leggedness, enlargement of the brain, ability
for conceptual thinking and the upright body position in the Earth
gravity field look like functionally ingenious achievements of
Nature. They have armed man with great advantages, including
social ones, and given rise to certain biological problems.

     Since man spends a considerable and most active part of his
life in the erect position, he has to maintain his body mass
center in unstable equilibrium, use his muscles constantly,
especially leg muscles in order to retain the posture. It is not
at all surprising that the leg mass is close to half of the total
body mass and the parameters characterizing motor activity are
important in the control of homeostatic reactions. In contrast
to man, very few mammals are capable to acquire the upright posture

and, if so, only for a short period of time. The fact that men do
that without any problems is a considerable evolutionary achievement,
because in this position the cardiovascular system actively counter-
acts gravity-induced blood redistribution. This ability is termed
orthostatic tolerance and realized via a concordant interaction of
the cardiovascular structure and regulatory mechanisms.

Concluding this Section, it should be emphasized again that
the force of gravity, at least in the limits faced on the Earth or
in space does not produce a direct effect at the molecular, subcellular or cellular levels. Its direct or indirect effect can be
seen in organisms weighing several grams and very clearly in us,
humans, who enjoy the privilege to view the world when standing.

The adaptation we have evolved is a philogenetic inherent
property. In our individual life we can improve it or we can
partially lose it. This normally occurs in aged or diseased
people. But it may also develop in young healthy men who are
travelling into outer space where weightlessness reigns.

WEIGHTLESSNESS

In the weightless state the body has no support, it is weightless and floats freely in the space cabin. On the Earth man can
face nothing of the kind. In the course of his evolutionary
development he was unable to acquire any specific mechanisms for
compensating the effects associated with the weightless state.
On the contrary, he developed the ability to counteract the
gravitational stress. What are his responses to weightlessness?

From the intellectual and emotional point of view - these are
more or less distinct disorders of spatial orientation, a wide
spectrum of emotional reactions of positive or negative nature.
With respect to autonomic functions these are equivalent physiological reactions which may arise on the ground when man drastically
reduces his motor activity (hypokinesia, hypodynamics), assumes a
horizontal position (bed rest) or goes down into the water (immersion).

Thus, weightlessness in space flight is a factor responsible
for changes in the self-regulation of an intact organism which
are aimed at establishing adequate relations with the lowered requirements of the environment. The exposure to zero-g is accompanied
by the phenomena of disuse or unloading and then atrophy from disuse
and deconditioning, which can be viewed as adaptive.

The functional changes that occur in weightlessness are primarily
produced by the following principal factors: changes in the afferent
compartment of the nervous system, withdrawal of the blood hydro-

static pressure, and the lack of weight load on the musculo-skeletal system. The responses to these changes develop at different time intervals. Besides, the physiological reactions have a characteristic time constant and may be modified by a simultaneous effect of other stress-factors of space flight. All this makes a very complicated picture of functional changes in response to the effects of weight-lessness.

INVESTIGATION OF CARDIOVASCULAR FUNCTION IN SPACE FLIGHT

Methods of Research

    After the historical flight of Yu. Gagarin in which ECG was recorded in one lead, a spectacular step forward was made in cardio-vascular research techniques. The spacecraft and especially space stations are well equipped with sophisticated biomedical equipment furnishing diagnostic and scientific information. Several generations of the biomedical equipment were used in succession and now the Salyut-7 station is supplied with devices to record electrocardiograms in 12 leads, to perform dynamic electrocardiography in one lead continuously during 24 hours, to perform rheography of the head, body and limbs, to measure blood pressure by means of Korotkoff sounds, to record sphygmo - and tachooscilograms, seismograms, kinetocardiograms, ballistocardiograms and, finally, echocardiograms using the ultrasound Doppler method. In addition, many other parameters necessary for interpreting cardiovascular data, e.g. variations in body mass, leg volume, hematocrit, can be measured.

    At first sight it looks as if space medicine has overcome the barrier of methodical problems. But this is not the case. The available methods enable one to get indirect and sometimes relatively inaccurate values of the main hemodynamic parameters, thus making difficult reliable evaluation of regulation mechanisms.

    Another characteristic feature of cardiovascular investigations is their discrete pattern. The crewmembers are to perform many duties associated with flight control, scientific and engineering experiments, etc. In short-term flights a comparatively small amount of biomedical information is transmitted to the Earth almost every day. In long-term space flights instrumented investigations are carried out approximately once every 10 days which appears adequate for the medical control but less than it is necessary to study the functional variations and the adaptation process.

    Without taking into account those who are aloft today and those who are on the verge of going into orbit there are 106 persons that have made space flights. Out of these 106 courageous space

travellers one (astronaut John Young) has made five flights, three
have made four flights, twelve have made three flights, twenty six
have made two flights and sixty four have made one flight, which is
in total 169 man-flights and about 8 years 105 days of life in
space.

When considering the scientific analysis of the accumulated
data, it should be borne in mind that in the 169 space studies
106 crewmembers participated, each having specific features of his
own. The scope of measurements in these flights varied substantially and each flight differed from another. All this makes it
difficult to compare and analyze the findings, to evaluate their
adequacy and to draw reliable conclusions concerning the effects to
which man is exposed.

However, this problem can be somehow resolved with the aid of
ground-based experiments simulating the physiological effects of
weightlessness which include: bed rest (hypokinesia) and its
modification - head-down tilt (antiorthostatic hypokinesia), and
water immersion (at neutral temperature).

A large number of studies of this kind have been conducted.
The results of ground-based studies and mathematical modeling
widely used at present are employed to elucidate physiological
reactions to weightlessness. This approach is undoubtedly well
justified because it allows the conduct of an unlimited number
of physiological experiments which can hardly be carried out onboard the spacecraft.

Primary and Delayed Cardiovascular Reactions

In weightlessness cosmonauts and astronauts experienced blood
run to the head and nasal congestion, then head heaviness and
pulsation. The level of these sensations varied. Sometimes they
reported that the sensations persisted for 10-15 days and then
disappeared. Sometimes they persisted throughout the flight
although were less distinct. When looking at his partner, the crewmembers noted face puffiness, eyelid swelling and sclera hyperemia.
Some of the symptoms augmented by the end of the working day or
weakened during exercise or LBNP (lower body negative pressure)
tests.

This is what happens after insertion into orbit when the hydrostatic pressure disappears and blood as well as the interstitial
fluid move headwards. Their major portions go to the intrathoracic
vessels, causing their enlargement. This also occurs in the cardiac
cavities. The remaining portion of the fluids accumulates in the
skin and in the subcutaneous tissue of the head and neck.

On the ground a similar situation occurs during the transition
from the vertical to the horizontal position. In this case fluid
redistribution is moderate; it is a normal physiological reaction
which does not manifest in the healthy man. Many experiments
carried out with the aid of different techniques yielded similar
results. The volume of this, so to say, mobile fluid is about
500-700 ml on the ground.

Today we have reliable data on the dynamics of blood filling of
different body compartments under various conditions and at a
different level of activity. The results of many ground-based
studies indicate that with respect to the effect of blood redistribution "laboratory models of weightlessness" can be ranked in a
certain order with the head-down tilt at -6^0 being the most accurate
simulation of what happens in real weightlessness. This is now
recognized by most researchers in the area.

Comparing a conservative number of indirect measurements in
space flights with solid data of ground-based studies, we can
evaluate the mobile fluid volume displaced from the lower body in
the cranial direction. It is estimated to be twice as much as
during the head-down tilt on the ground, i.e. about ±500ml.
Figuratively speaking, weightlessness turns the man upside-down.

The measurements during the Salyut and Skylab flights demonstrated that the leg volume decreased by 12-18%, lowering most
rapidly during the first days in weightlessness. An opposite
situation occurred upon return to Earth. In flight the body mass
center also shifted towards the head, being another indication of
the cephalad fluid displacement. Orthostatic tests have shown
that this reaction consists of two components: a rapid one
associated with blood movement along the vascular bed, and a slow
component induced by interstitial fluid accumulation.

It is obvious that the discussion of these primary, physically
meaningful processes developing in the vascular system should take
into consideration changes in the transcapillary fluid displacement.
The final volume of the displaced fluid may largely depend on the
contribution of the hydrostatic and osmo-oncotic pressure, as well
as on tissue distensibility. These problems have been poorly
studied. There are no data in the literature concerning the lymph
flow. Therefore, fluid regulation requires further study both on
Earth and in space.

It is believed that an increased blood inflow to the heart
causes reflex and humoral reactions which result in a decrease of
the plasma volume and, consequently, of the circulating blood
volume.

The scope and rate of the plasma volume decrease in weightlessness can be understood with the aid of immersion studies which
produce an effect that exceeds that of weightlessness. Following
an early increase, the blood and plasma volume declines, the reduction
being pronounced by the 2nd-3rd hour of the exposure. The greatest
changes are seen by the 6-8th hour, when the plasma volume decreases
by 8-15% (in some cases by 20%). Having reached this level, the
plasma volume remains practically unchanged till the end of the
exposure even if it lasts several days. This is easy to understand
because this is an adaptive reaction aimed at establishing equilibrium between the volume of the intravascular fluid and that of the
vascular bed.

This scheme gives a satisfactory explanation to the fluid
volume regulation at acute stages of different experiments and space
flights. However, as any other scheme, it disregards other possibilities and factors. It has been, for instance, shown that blood
redistribution during ortho- and antiorthostatic reactions are
noticeably affected by afferent somatic impulses that modify blood
redistribution between the cranial and caudal body parts.

Similar reactions can be elicited from the chemoreceptor zones
of the medulla oblongata ventral surface; this is of particular
importance in view of increased blood filling of the head. The
above hypothesis also ignores the role of hypothalamic osmo-
receptors which are assumed to regulate ADH secretion. It should
also be emphasized that in real life pathways of homeostatic
equalibrium are at least doubled, as in the case with redundant
spacecraft control systems. The actual reactions consist of
combinations of different elements which may be of greater or lesser
importance in different situations.

At the stage of acute adaptation when the circulating blood
volume and plasma volume diminish, crewmembers exhibit, as a rule,
losses of thirst and salt appetite, reduced water consumption and
sometimes they are requested to drink water or juice. Due to the
losses of plasma, the hematocrit level increases. These findings
were documented in flight and confirmed by ground-based investigations. So far it is still unclear in what way the normal relation
between the plasma volume and blood formed elements recovers, althougl
it is known that the production of red blood cells declines and they
have a tendency for microcytosis.

This essentially completes the early stage of adaptation to
weightlessness. A new homeostatic level of the cardiovascular
function is reached; it helps crewmembers maintain good health
condition. In flights ECG was recorded many times. No unusual or
abnormal changes in heart rate, rhythm (except for single cases of
ectopic beats and one case of higeminy), pattern or parameters
of ECG were observed.

Being very exacting, we can say that there was a difference
between heart rates at night and in the daytime. In very few cases
there were subjective complaints for discomfortable cardiac
sensations which were never supported by ECG or other objective
studies; there were no significant changes in blood pressure.

In a word, all the parameters measured and recorded at rest
demonstrate complete well-being of crewmembers. But as soon as
they increase their activity or start doing something difficult,
they show unstable or hypertrophic cardiovascular responses as
compared to those seen on the Earth. This was clearly seen during
bicycle ergometry and LBNP tests. Preflight data make it possible
to compare variations in their tolerance to exercises and orthostatic (LBNP) tests. As a rule, the tolerance declined, the reduction increasing as they diminished their exercises. However, the
time-course of these variations was not ascertained because in all
space flights of more than 2 weeks duration exercises were a
mandatory prophylactic measure.

On the whole, we can see a very curious picture. Following
the primary, acute phase of cardiovascular adaptation which completes
within the first hours or days in orbit, a new homeostatic level is
reached. This proceeds gradually and continuously for about a
month or sometimes a month and a half. This level may be termed
a relatively stable adaptation to weightlessness. Crewmembers adjust
to the new environment, feel well, develop habits and skills
necessary for their life and work in weightlessness, and face no
serious problems. It can be said that a man of the Earth has becom e
a man of space.

However, everyone who has made a space flight encounters certain,
sometimes significant problems upon return to Earth. This uneasy
and frequently difficult process of readaptation is the biological
price of the privilege to fly into space.

Unlike flight studies, pre- and postflight examinations are
wide, profound and less limited. However, the problem is that
postflight the investigator deals with a person who is not in
the weightless state but who was in zero-g but at the time of
examination is at 1 g. This, obviously, makes data analysis and
interpretation more difficult and speculative. Nevertheless, the
data accumulated are extensive and can be used not only to evaluate
readaptation reactions but also to take a glance into weightlessness
per se.

After touch-down physicians try to perform examinations as
soon as possible but sometimes fail to do that to a full extent.
Nevertheless, during the first hours after recovery the following
changes were demonstrated: losses of body mass, leg volume, and

circulating blood, increased heart rate, pulse variations, and trend
for hypotension. X-ray examination showed a decrease of the heart
shadow. Echocardiographic investigations suggested that the
decrease of the heart size may be induced partially or totally by
a reduction of the cardiac cavities rather than of the cardiac
muscle mass.

The application of quantitative electrocardiography (e.g.
according to Frank) and noninvasive methods to determine the phasic
structure of the cardiac cycle did not reveal any abnormalities but
indicated manifest individual variations. Biochemical and hormonal
parameters of blood varied substantially and often in different
directions. A consistent finding was a decrease of orthostatic
tolerance and exercise tolerance, as shown by bicycle ergometry.

The level of the variations was not always correlated with the
flight duration. It should be emphasized that a more active and
regular use of different countermeasures - bicycle ergometer, treadmill, bungee cords, LBNP box - combined with other measures (adequate
work-rest cycle, food and water consumption, water-salt supplementation) helped diminish the postflight reactions. In this context,
mention should be made of the long-duration space flights onboard
Salyut-6.

Nevertheless, we have to admit that our knowledge of cardiovascular reactions to weightlessness is still insufficient. In the
near future we have to clarify the effect of cephalad fluid shifts
and concomitant increased ventricular pressure on the morpho-
functional characteristics of the heart; we have to ascertain whether
a prolonged exposure to weightlessness may cause myocardial dysfunction; and we have to determine the role and importance of
general and local mechanisms of cardiovascular regulation in weightlessness. This can be done provided that the existing methods are
refined and the great achievements of modern cardiology are used
in the best way possible.

It is hoped that the progress achieved within a short period
of our space era will become more impressive. Many problems with
which we are concerned today will be resolved but they will be
replaced with new challenges which we will attempt to resolve with
similar enthusiasm and dedication.

PROGRESS IN RADIONUCLIDE METHODS

L. E. Feinendegen

Institute of Medicine
Nuclear Research Center Jülich GmbH
D-5170 Jülich, F.R.Germany

Radioisotopes are tools for observing the body at the molecular
level of organisation practically without discomfort and risk to the
patient. In this context, the method of imaging, for example, with
a fast gamma-camera, is not an end in itself, but a first step for
functional studies particularly at the molecular and cellular level
in small body volumes. Thus, radioisotopes have generally proved
useful for establishing diagnosis, for description and quantification
of findings involving metabolic reactions in the evolution of disease
and for control of therapy. Nuclear medicine has also become accepted in cardiology.

Radioisotopes are employed in cardiology mainly to study 1)
cardiac function, 2) myocardial perfusion, 3) myocardial metabolism.
This report emphasizes progress and covers these three topics.

1) CARDIAC FUNCTION

Cardiac function is essayed by measuring volumes, flow and wall
motion at rest, and exercise for defining cardiac reserve.

Multiple Blood Volume Analysis

A rather novel technique uses the simultaneous imaging of blood
pools of the heart, lung and liver.[1,2,3] Following equilibration of
the tracer such as 99m-Tc labelled erythrocytes within the circulation counting rates relate to blood volume and are simultaneously
measured over heart, lung and liver at frequent time intervals during
stepwise increase of exercise load. In normal individuals the cardiac

117

blood volume shows an initial adjustment at the lowest work load
level; then with increasing load it tends to decrease slowly. Over
the lung, there is initially little change, then with more than about
60 watt the blood volume increases. There is little initial change
in the liver blood volume and then a constant drop is seen. This
thus indicates in normals an exercise induced diminution of total
cardiac volume, an increase in pulmonary blood volume and a delayed
mobilization of liver blood pool.

The responses are quite different in patients with latent cardiac
insufficiency. There is an exercise induced increase in total cardiac
volume, an immediate rise in pulmonary blood volume and an immediately
induced mobilization of hepatic blood volume. The simplicity and
potential applicability of this multiple blood volume analysis is
obvious.

Cardiac Blood Pool Analysis

Cardiac function is most widely investigated by continuously
observing the left ventricular blood pool, as initiated by Hoffmann
and Kleine in 1965[4] and later adapted to the gamma-camera with ECG
triggering.[5,6] Following tracer equilibration in the blood, the left
ventricular blood pool is well recognized in the left anterior oblique
projection.

a) Beat by beat observation. Beat by beat analysis of the total
counting rate of the left ventricle is relatively simple by the
nuclear stethoscope[7] proposed by Wagner, or more recently by a mini-
probe with a sensitive solid state detector that may even be included
in a garment to observe the patient throughout his daily activities.[8]
These techniques permit continuous beat to beat analysis of left
ventricular function and thus are a radiocardiographic equivalent of
the continuous ECG monitoring.

b) Gated blood pool imaging. A commonly used mode permits the
collection of the total counting rates from the left ventricle from
at least 20 divisions of the cardiac cycle by ECG triggering, which
are then added up over about 400-500 cycles so that good counting
statistics for each cycle division are obtained. Thus, the counting
rates during a representative cardiac cycle present a volume curve
that lets one calculate left ventricular ejection fraction, filling-
time and -rate, and ejection-time and -rate, as shown in Figure 1.
The ejection fraction is given by the difference between enddiastolic
and endsystolic counting rates divided by the diastolic counting
rate after background substraction. Many investigators have shown
the ejection fraction to have a high prognostic value, especially
when the stress induced response is taken as major parameter.[9] A
stress induced reduction of the ejection fraction by more than 5%
indicates an about 60% incidence of a critical coronary artery
lesion.[10]

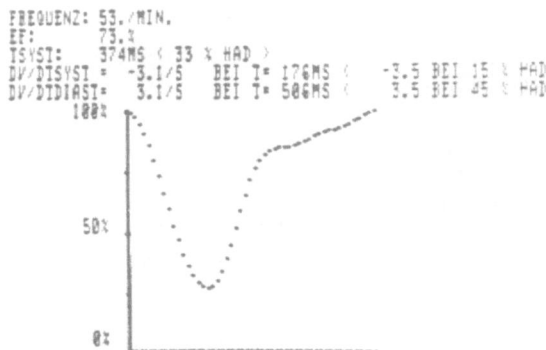

Fig. 1.   Left ventricular volume curve obtained from gated blood
          pool images. The curve permits the calculation of the
          ejection fraction, systolic time and diastolic time and
          the corresponding ejection and filling rates.

The left ventricular volume curve may also be obtained from
each individual image pixel and may be treated by Fourrier analysis,
as suggested by Adam.[11] Each curve from a pixel is adjusted to a
sinusoidal wave having a certain amplitude and phase. Whereas the
amplitude relates to the extent of wall motion, the phase emphasizes
the time at which contraction occurs. The values for phase and amplitude from each pixel may be displayed in colour for each individual pixel as shown in Figure 2. On the left there is a normal
display of pixel amplitudes with the maximum in the mid ventricular
region. On the right, the corresponding phase distribution image
is seen; the dark color throughout indicates a synchronous beginning
of ventricular contraction.

Figure 3 illustrates corresponding data from a patient with a
left ventricular aneurysm. The upper 2 images are the enddiastolic
and endsystolic unprocessed blood pool displays. After Fourrier
analysis for each pixel curve, the lower left gives the amplitude
image with a zero signal given in black in the mid ventricular region
where the aneurysm is located; on the right, the phase distribution
image shows an asynchronous contraction of the left ventricle with
initiation of contraction at the cardiac base in dark color and late
contraction in light color at the apical region.

Wall motion abnormalities are well correlated to the ejection
fraction. Stress induced abnormalities were found in 67% of cases
with 1 vessel disease, in 88% with 2 vessel disease and in about 75%
of the cases with 3 vessel disease.[12]

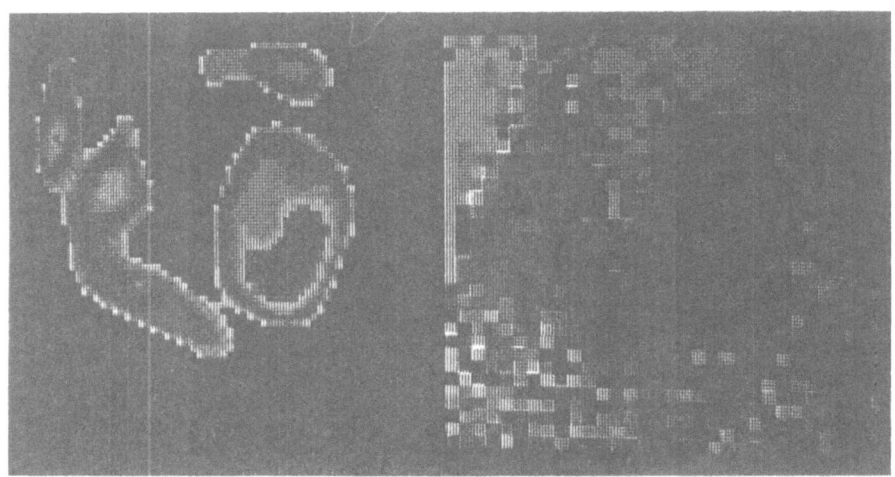

Fig. 2.   Parametric images of a normal left ventricle with respect
          to amplitude (left) and phase (right) of ventricular volume
          curves obtained for individual image pixels.

What is now easily achievable with the left ventricle, is in
most instances quite difficult with the right ventricle because of
overlapping of atrial and ventricular volumes.

Still, the right ventricular blood pool may be analysed, even
with difficulties, by the so-called first pass technique[13] and here
preferably with short lived radionuclides, such as 81m-Kr.[14]

The assessment of both ventricular volumes from the first pass
of an indicator bolus through the heart principally has the advantage
of speed, and short lived radionuclides are generally preferred, for
example 195-Gold.[15] Comparing right and left ventricular ejection
fractions may help to analyse valvular regurgitation.[16]

It is difficult to determine absolute volumes from the first
pass or from the gated blood pool technique.[17] A recent report by
Maurer et al.,[18] describes an easy measurement of the attenuation
of radiation coming from the ventricles. A gelatine capsule filled
with 99m-Tc is measured before the camera head and again on its
passage through the esophagus. The resulting attenuation coefficient

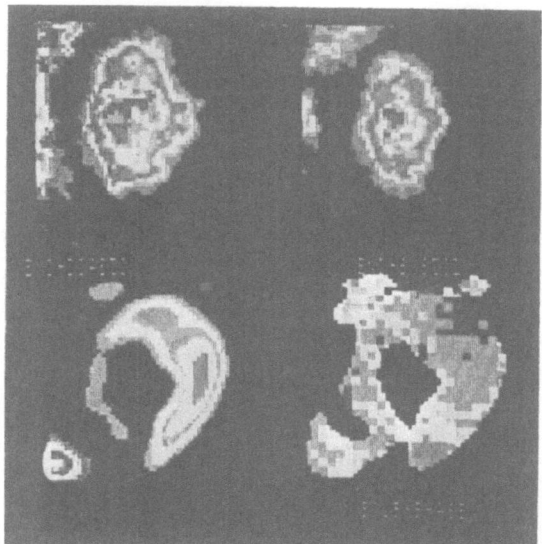

Fig. 3. Left ventricular aneurysm. The upper images show
          enddiastolic and endsystolic volume images. Below are
          the corresponding parametric images for amplitude and
          phase.

is then applied to a blood sample of the patient at the time of
ventricular counting; this quickly permits the conversion of left
ventricular counting rate into volume.

Flow Time, Minimal Transit Time

        Quantification of the entire first pass of a radioactive bolus
yields information on global function of all segments of the central
circulation. For this purpose the minimal transit times have proved
very useful, which my group began to measure in 1969.[19,20]

        Following injection of a radioactive bolus, for example of 99m-
Tc-pertechnetate, into an antecubital vein, the first pass is registered with the gamma-camera at a rate of at least 10 frames per
second. Subsequently, frames are summed up for image display of the
right and left side of the heart, as seen in Figure 4. Into these
images regions of interest are placed for covering the superior
caval vein, the right atrium, right ventricle, the pulmonary artery,

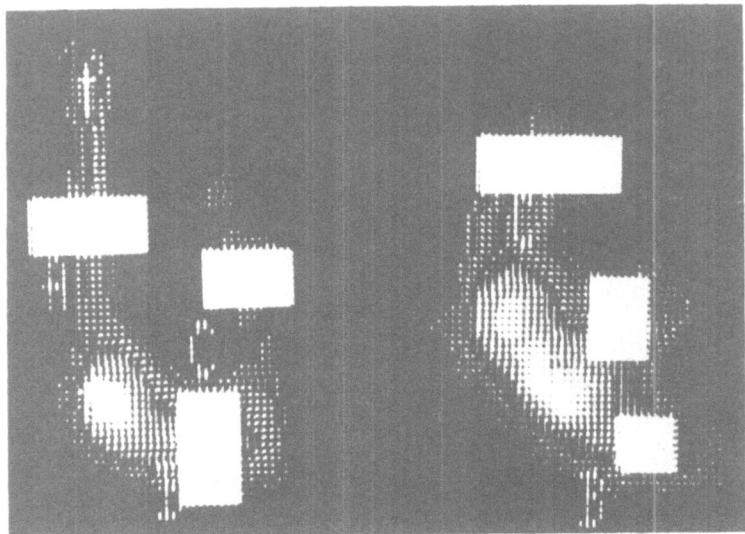

Fig. 4. The first pass of the indicator bolus through right and
         left heart may be quantified by measuring indicator arrival
         times at the indicated regions of interest for superior
         caval vein, right ventricle, pulmonary artery, left atrium,
         left ventricle and aortic arch.

the left atrium, left ventricle and the aortic root. It is not
necessary that these regions fully cover the anatomical site, yet
one must prevent the regions from extending into the intersegmental
boundaries. Time activity curves are then generated from each region,
as shown in Figure 5.

     The time activity curves are illustrated in Figure 5, from the
right atrium, right ventricle, pulmonary artery, left atrium, left
ventricle and aorta; they are smoothed in such a way that the arrival
of the tracer can be automatically detected.[21] The arrival of the
indicator in the various regions is here defined by vertical bars
on each corresponding curve. The time differences between consecutive arrivals are the fastest transport times or minimal transit
times. They are a function of the ratio of volume to flow and thus
are, in the absence of flow vortices, inversely proportional to the
ejection fraction and heart rate. At a heart rate of 80 per minute,
the total minimal transit time from the right atrium to the aorta
in normal individuals, supine position, is 6 seconds ± 5% standard

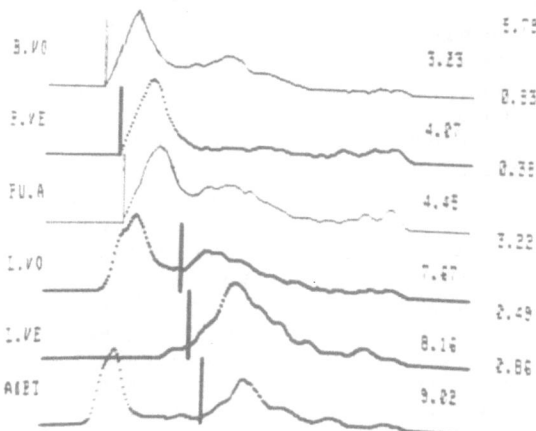

Fig. 5. Time activity curves from the regions of interest shown in
         Figure 4. The activity arrival is automatically recognized
         and is displayed here by vertical bars. The differences
         between consecutive arrival times are the fastest flow
         times or minimal transit times through the central circu-
         lation. These transit times are an expression of the ratio
         volume/flow.

deviation. The pulmonary minimal transit time is 3.2 seconds ± 8%
standard deviation, the individual segmental minimal transit times
through atria and ventricles vary between 0.5 and 1.0 second ± 15-
20% standard deviation.[19] The values are slightly different in
patients measured in the upright position.[22] It is thus relatively
easy to describe the global function in terms of volume to flow
ratio for each cardiac segment and the entire central circulation.
Also the right ventricle is easier accessible than with the gated
blood pool technique.

    I propose to combine quantification of the first pass by the
minimal transit times with the gated blood pool technique.[23]

    Whereas the gated blood pool technique gives detailed infor-
mation on left ventricular ejection fraction and wall motion, the
minimal transit times give global information on all cardiopulmonary
segments in terms of volume to flow ratios. The combined procedure
was tested in 65 patients with coronary artery disease, in supine
position. Thirty seven of the patients had a history of myocardial
infarction, of which 17 had developed left ventricular aneurysm.

Figure 6 shows the relationship between left ventricular ejection
fraction and cardiac minimal transit time, i.e. total transit time
minus pulmonary transit time; the patients with aneurysm are shown
by full dots. In patients without aneurysms, pathological minimal
transit times are about similarly frequent as are diminished left
ventricular ejection fractions. Patients with aneurysms have more
frequently a diminished left ventricular ejection fraction than a
pathological cardiac minimal transit time. It was interesting to
note that patients with a normal minimal transit time usually had a
better exercise tolerance than those with prolonged minimal transit
times. It is justified to speculate whether minimal transit time
readings may have prognostic value. A compact radiocardiograph was
designed for easily and specifically measuring simultaneously total
minimal transit time through the central circulation[24] and is now
also being used for simultaneously assaying left ventricular ejection
fraction, filling-time and -rate, and ejection-time and -rate.[24]

2) MYOCARDIAL PERFUSION

     Myocardial scintigraphy with 201-thallium has proven to be of
great diagnostic value in recognizing coronary artery disease with
a sensitivity ranging from about 75-90%.[25,26] This technique has
become the most widely used nuclear medical application in cardiology.

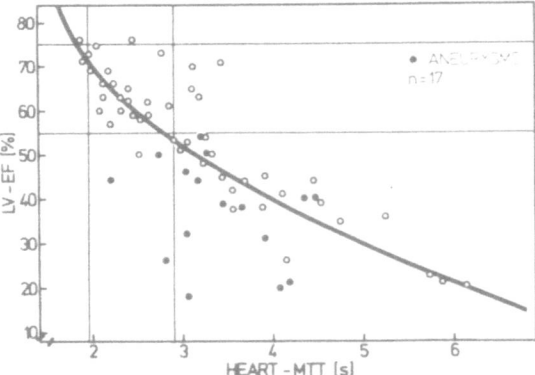

Fig. 6. Left ventricular ejection fraction, as measured by the
         gated blood pool technique, is correlated to the cardiac
         minimal transit time. Each individual sign relates to
         one patient. The solid dots relate to patients with left
         ventricular aneurysms.

It was tempting to check the potential diagnostic advantage of combining 201-thallium myocardial scintigraphy with the minimal transit time measurement and the gated blood pool analysis.

In a first study 33 patients with coronary artery disease including 9 with a history of myocardial infarction were investigated at rest and at peak exercise.

Figure 7 gives columns listing the number of patients with pathological findings either on the thallium-scan, upon gated blood pool analysis of ejection fraction and wall motion, or upon minimal transit time measurements, at rest and at exercise. A pathological score for minimal transit times was a significant prolongation; for the gated blood pool study it was a wall motion abnormality and/or a left ventricular ejection fraction below 55%; for the thallium-scan it was an accumulation defect. It is quite obvious that stress testing, of course, increases the sensitivity of all procedures. The highest sensitivity was obtained with the thallium-scan.

For evaluating the results of the 3 tests per individual at rest and exercise, the group of 33 patients with coronary artery disease was combined with additional 5 patients with the history of myocardial infarction but without obvious ischemia, 5 patients with cardiomyopathy and 10 normals, who, however, displayed some unspecific chest complaints. The 201-thallium-scan gave the highest sensitivity of 85% with a specificity of 60%. For the gated blood pool analysis

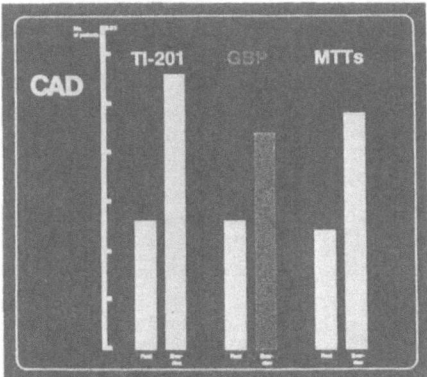

Fig. 7. Thirty three patients with coronary artery disease underwent examination for myocardial perfusion with 201-thallium, for cardiac function by the gated blood pool technique or by the minimal transit time measurement. The bars indicate the incidence of pathological findings at rest and exercise.

and the minimal transit time measurements about similar sensitivities
of about 70% were obtained with a highest specificity of 87% for the
gated blood pool study. When the values per patient were combined,
sensitivity and specificity was highest with 91 and 93% respectively.

Even if the thallium-scan gives the highest score, the low
gamma-energy, the relatively long half life of 75 hours, and the
price per examination is somewhat disadvantageous. Efforts are
being made to find 99m-Tc-labelled compounds that accumulate in the
myocardium as efficiently as does thallium. This search has apparently been successful in studies on primates, as it was reported by
Deutsch et al.,[27] for di-methyl-phosphino-ethane labelled with 99m-Tc.
This compound yields in the baboon high quality scans similar to
201-thallium.

3) MYOCARDIAL METABOLISM

In order to study metabolic reactions in vivo, it is necessary
to be aware of the principal metabolic pathways one wants to observe.
Moreover, attention must be paid to the proper tracer, the proper
substrate and the placement of the tracer on to the substrate so
that the reaction of interest may become observable. Also, one
should, whenever it is required, use counting techniques that permit
the distinction between the labelled substrate and its labelled cata-
bolite. Needless to say, the final choice for clinical use depends
on the diagnostic information obtained by the procedure.

Positron emission tomography has been elegantly used for analys-
ing uptake and turnover of various 11-C-labelled metabolites, especially fatty acids which are the main energy source of the myocardium in the fasting state.[28,29] Yet positron emission tomographs
are expensive and rare and should be close to a cyclotron that produces the short lived positron emitters. But planar, i.e. simple
gamma-camera imaging or single photon emission tomography is also
applicable to metabolic measurements and is therefore of wide interest
because of availability of the conventional imaging equipment.[30]

Prior to explaining the single photon imaging with labelled
fatty acids a short review of the principal pathways of fatty acids
in the myocardium is in order, as illustrated in Figure 8.

Free fatty acids are transported from the circulating blood
through the interstial space into the cell, obviously without need
of an active carrier system. Inside the muscle cell, there is a
pool of free fatty acids partially attached to myoglobin. The free
fatty acids are eventually bound to coenzyme-A on cytoplasmic membranes, and the coupling is a prerequisite for all further biochemical steps. There is evidence that some of the activated fatty acids
rapidly enter mitochondria by the carnitine shuttle. A large frac-

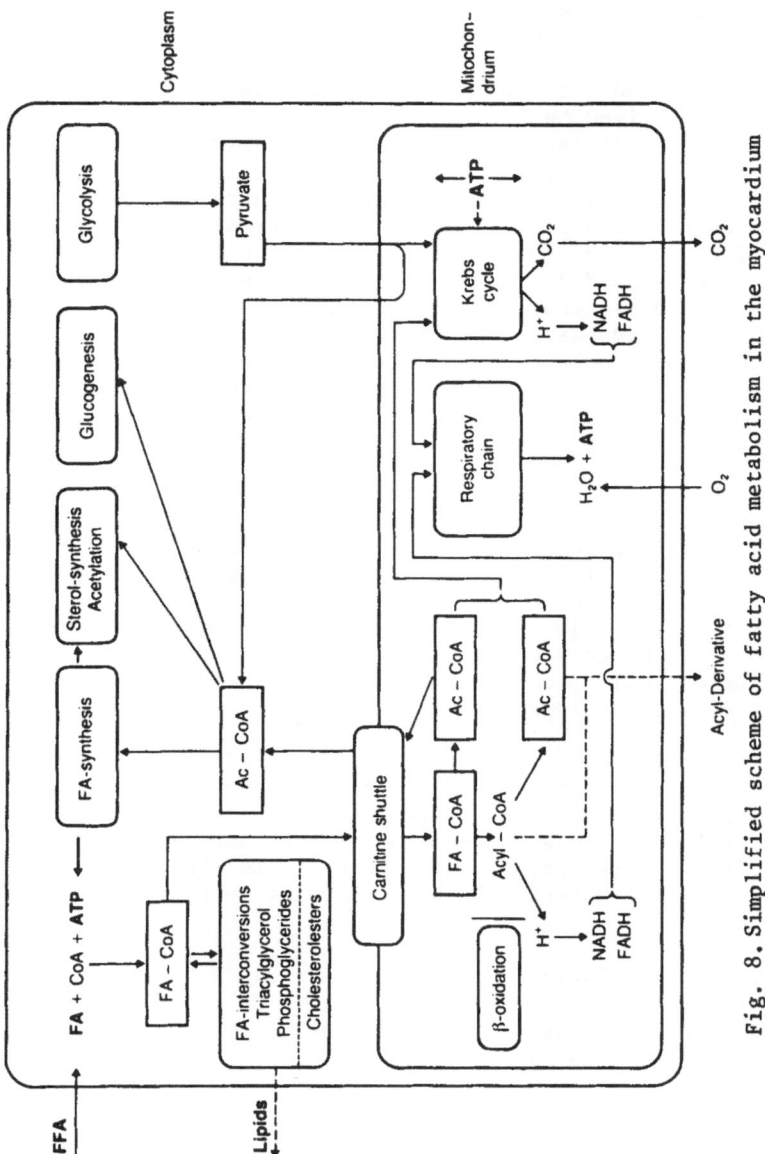

Fig. 8. Simplified scheme of fatty acid metabolism in the myocardium

tion of the fatty acid coenzyme-A is used for fatty acid intercon-
versions and for the synthesis of triglycerides and phospholipids,
also for cholesterol-esters. Mainly triglycerides and possibly
phospholipids may serve as fatty acid reservoirs from which varying
energy demands may be answered.

Having entered the mitochondria by the carnitine shuttle, fatty
acids are metabolized by beta-oxidation yielding acetyl-coenzyme-A
and protons. The latter are fed into the respiratory chain and the
acetyl-coenzyme-A either returns to the cytosol or is fed into the
Krebs cycle which produces CO_2 and protons which are again fed into
the respiratory chain for oxidative phosphorylation. It is to be
understood that acetyl-coenzyme-A in the cytosol is the central
source for fatty acid de-novo synthesis, various acetylation reactions
and sterol synthesis and also for glucogenesis. Thus, carbon fragments of fatty acids may be partially reutilized. Acetyl-coenzyme-A
is also the result of catabolism of glucose and aminoacids and enters
the Krebs cycle for generating protons for oxidative phosphorylation.
When glucose supply is large, there is a reduced demand for fatty
acid degradation.

Whereas fatty acid delivery to the cell largely depends on coronary flow and perfusion pressure, intracellular fatty acid degradation generally is governed by the energy demand and has been related
to ventricular work load, oxygen tension, pulse rate and action of
hormones. Metabolites, for example glucose, may partially substitute
for fatty acids as major source of energy. Answering energy demands
from any source depends on the integrity of the intracellular net
work of the metabolic reaction chains, especially on the integrity
of the mitochondrial apparatus.

It is clear that it is exceedingly difficult to measure by in
vivo nuclear medical techniques a specific reaction in the fatty
acid degradative system and relate this to a specific disorder.
What has thus far been shown possible is the distinction between the
accumulation of fatty acid inside the cell and the rate of release
of activity. The latter will be shown below to signal fatty acid
degradation.

Thus far, the fatty acids shown in Figure 9 have been employed
for myocardial scintigraphy. 11-C-labelled palmitic acid obviously
is a physiological substrate and has been successfully used with
positron emission tomography for measuring fatty acid metabolism.[28]

123-I-heptadecanoic acid is an analogue of stearic acid; the
final methyl-group is replaced by iodine.[31] Iodine labelled long
chain fatty acids were first used by Evans[32] and by Poe[33] and shown
to accumulate in the myocardium. 123-I-heptadecanoic acid was shown
to behave kinetically similar to palmitic acid and was employed for
measuring fatty acid utilization and turnover in the human myocardium.[34]

1 – ^{11}C	–	PALMITIC ACID
17 – ^{123}I	–	HEPTADECANOIC ACID
p – ^{123}I	–	PHENYLPENTADECANOIC ACID
22 – ^{123}I	–	ERUCIC ACID
17 – ^{131}I	–	IODO–9–TELLURA-HEPTADECANOIC ACID
9 – [^{123m}Te]	–	TELLURA-HEPTADECANOIC ACID
3 – [^{11}C]	–	METHYL-HEPTADECANOIC ACID

Fig. 9. Some fatty acids presently employed in order to measure myocardial metabolism.

123-I-phenyl-pentadecanoic acid is artifical.[35,36,37] It does not follow the pathway of natural fatty acid but tends to become trapped mainly in the triglyceride pool with a turnover in the cell slower than palmitic acid. A similar behavior was shown for the long chain erucic acid.[38]

Other fatty acids have been especially synthesized to prevent beta-oxidation, thus permitting the observation of substrate accumulation in the cell. There is the long chain fatty acid which carries tellurium in the carbon chain and may be labelled by radioiodine or by a suitable tellurium radioisotope.[39] Another fatty acid in this category is the 3-methyl-heptadecanoic acid that was shown to be metabolically trapped in beta-oxidation.[40]

Thus there are 3 groups of labelled fatty acids: 1) natural fatty acids and their metabolic analogues, 2) the "artificial" fatty acids that differ from natural fatty acids in that they get specifically and temporarily trapped in pools, 3) fatty acids that are engineered in order to accumulate in mitochondria by virtue of being trapped in beta-oxidation.

For the development of a diagnostically useful assay of myocardial metabolism by planar imaging mainly 123-I-heptadecanoic acid was chosen. It is also easily applied to single photon tomography.

Single Photon Imaging of Fatty Acid Metabolism

High quality images and turnover measurements with 123-I-heptadecanoic acid required the development of a correction procedure that eliminates signal contribution from fatty acids in circulation or from catabolites such as free 123-iodine.[34] Frequent imaging over the first 40 minutes after tracer injection and using this correction technique thus creates time activity curves showing tracer accumulation and wash out from the myocardium.

The half times of the first component of tracer release from the total left ventricular myocardium and for the individual myocardial segments varied around 24 ± 5 minutes at rest, and were somewhat yet statistically not significantly shorter at exercise.[34]

Examination of patients with coronary artery disease led to the conclusion: 1) heptadecanoic acid accumulation defects correlate with coronary artery stenosis or occlusion; 2) heptadecanoic acid elimination rate for the entire myocardium may be normal; 3) heptadecanoic acid uptake and elimination is normal and areas with normal perfusion; regions with accumulation defects have diminished, normal or at times even increased elimination rates.[41]

As shown by Dudczak et al.,[42] the first and second components of the elimination rate of heptadecanoic acid in normal individuals as in patients with coronary artery disease promptly respond to an infusion of insulin and glucose, in fact indistinguishable from the response reported for 11-C-palmitic acid.[29] This further supports the elimination rates to be an expression of myocardial metabolism.

Both measurements, that of accumulation and of turnover, were applied to investigate the effect of rehabilitation training in 8 patients after myocardial infarction. The elimination half times for various myocardial regions after 1 year of rehabilitation training following myocardial infarction improved in 5 of the 8 patients, and 3 patients showed no change or even a slight deterioration.[41]

Of special interest is the application of 123-I-heptadecanoic acid for noninvasively recognizing cardiomyopathies. The accumulation images of patients with early or advanced congestive cardiomyopathy show gross, spotty heterogeneous distribution of the tracer in the left ventricular wall, similar to images at times obtained with 201-thallium and often not clearly distinguishable from those of patients with coronary artery disease (Figure 10). We have assayed the relationship between accumulation and turnover of the tracer in groups of patients with advanced and early congestive cardiomyopathy.[43,44] In contrast to results in coronary artery diseases, the quality of regional tracer accumulation does not correlate with the elimination half time in that region. Thus, accumulation and turnover of fatty acid in the various myocardial regions were unrelated and discordant. Discordance between distribution of accumulation defects and of altered elimination rates was also seen in patients with early stage of congestive cardiomyopathy as illustrated in Table 1. This data lets one speculate whether a systematic analysis of fatty acid accumulation and elimination may considerably aid the diagnosis of cardiomyopathy, in distinction from coronary artery disease.

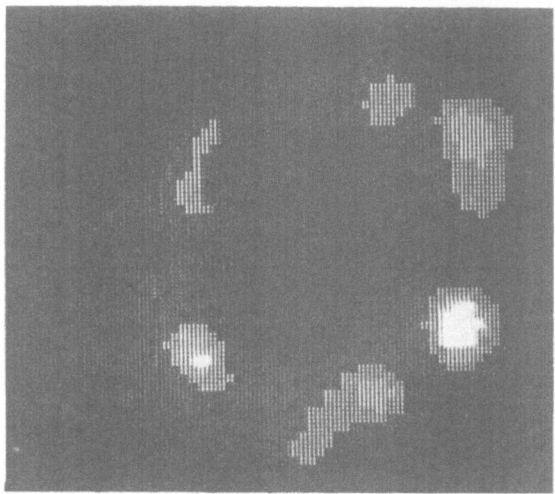

Fig. 10. Myocardial scintigram following the injection of 123-I-
          heptadecanoic acid in a patient with early stage of con-
          gestive cardiomyopathy.

Positron Emission Tomography

Metabolic measurements are the primary domain of positron emission tomography. This technique is presently limited to few institutions only.

A variety of 11-C-labelled substrates has thus far been employed
for measuring myocardial metabolism; just to list a few:

(a) 11-C-palmitic acid[28,29,31] served to measure myocardial fatty
     acid metabolism and 18-F-deoxyglucose[45,46] has been used for
     measuring local glucose utilization and was shown to increase
     in areas of myocardial ischemia, where fatty acid utilization
     was depressed.
(b) 11-c-acetate,[47] 13-N-glutamat[48] and 13-N-ammonia[49] were tried
     and data correlated with cardiac disease.
     Local perfusion may be measured with 15-O labelled CO_2.[50]

Table 1. Regional Myocardial Elimination Half Times (Min)
of 123-I-Heptadecanoic Acid in Patients with
Congestive Cardiomyopathy in Early Stage

PAT.	TOTAL HEART t 1/2	SEPTUM t 1/2 Acc	INFERIOR t 1/2 Acc	POSTERO-LATERAL t 1/2 Acc
M.W.	13.0	11.0 + 11.0 ++	9.4 −	12.8 + 12.4 +
K.H.	21.0	16.8 ++ 15.4 ++	16.5 +	31.4 + 19.6 ++
K.R.	46.5	47.6 + 35.0 +	38.8 ++	48.5 ++ 35.6 ++
B.M.	20.5	20.8 + 16.3 +	17.7 +	21.1 + 18.3 ++
F.B.	57.8	167.7 − 35.4 +	32.8 +	49.0 + 63.2 ++
R.A.	41.5	41.0 − 32.0 +	33.4 +	43.4 − 23.5 ++
D.R.	80.7	53.0 − 74.0 −	39.0 ++	344.0 − 277.0 ++
D.H.	30.4	28.8 + 26.6 ++	32.0 +	31.2 + 35.6 ++
R.A.	34.7	33.5 + 34.8 +	21.8 −	41.2 + 30.9 ++
M.G.	41.5	40.9 − 32.0 +	32.5 +	43.4 + 23.5 +

++ = Acc. normal, + = Acc. diminished, − = Acc. bad
a = basal part, b = distal part

I would like here to draw attention to the potential use of
75-Br amongst the newer positron emitting radionuclides.[51] This
isotope is certainly easily handled chemically, and has the advantage
of a long enough half life of 97 minutes for permitting transport
from the cyclotron to the site of medical application. Figure 11
shows a dog heart on the left in a transmission image, and on the
right is the ECG gated diastolic emission tomographic image of the
myocardium taken at the level on the AV valves, after intravenous
injection of 75-Br labelled phenyl-pentadecanoic acid. This approach
appears practical and eventually useful for clinical research.

A potentially useful compound is 11-C labelled methylglu-
cose.[52,53] This glucose analogue is transported like glucose across
the cellular membrane, but it is not metabolised. It is transported
back from the primary intracellular glucose pool into the circulation.
After a single injection of the tracer into a suitable vein, activity

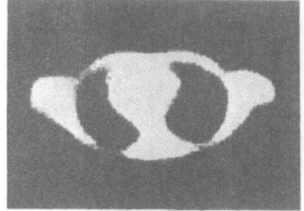 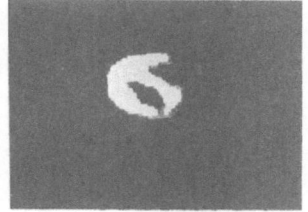

Transmission image   Emission image

Fig. 11.   ECG-gated diastolic image of the myocardium registered by
           positron emission transaxial tomography at the level of
           A-V valves, after intravenous injection of 15(p-75-Br-
           phenyl)-pentadecanoic acid in a normal dog. The trans-
           mission image is given for comparison on the left.

over tissue increases to a steady state between the concentration
in tissue and that in blood. The 2 values finally give a fixed ratio
for each tissue volume.

   - By taking the blood concentration as internal standard, the
     transport of methylglucose into tissue to equilibrium may be
     selectively and quantitatively measured and relates to the rate
     of activity of the sugar transporting enzyme.[54] At steady
     state, tissue accumulation is readily seen when correction is
     made for the blood pool, as shown in Figure 12 giving the ECG
     gated diastolic image of the human myocardium registered by
     emission tomography at mid ventricular level, after i.v. in-
     jection of about 5 mCi 11-C-methylglucose.

   - The dual analysis of blood and tissue concentration not only
     permits measuring glucose transport into the cell but also
     promises to yield local perfusion.[55] In normal myocardium
     local perfusion was 0.68 ml/min/g average; in the subendocardium
     local perfusion was 0.74 ml/min/g; and in the subepicardial
     region it was 0.67 ml/min/g.

   - After transient ischemia in subendocardial areas the local glu-
     cose transport rate was significantly reduced whereas the local
     perfusion rate returned to normal values.

Conclusion

     There has been an enormous advance over the past 10 years in
using radioisotopes in cardiology because of improvement of counting
and imaging devices, because of discovery of new useful radiopharma-
ceuticals, because of advancement of data processing techniques and
of new concepts of evaluation of data. Most important is the inter-

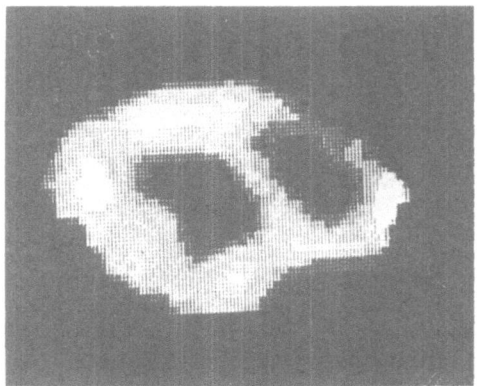

Fig. 12. ECG-gated diastolic image of a human myocardium obtained
          by positron emission transaxial tomography at mid ventricu-
          lar level, after intravenous injection of 3-0-11-C-methyl-
          D-glucose in a normal individual.

disciplinary awareness amongst cardiologists, nuclear medical special-
ists, physicists, nuclear chemists, engineers and mathematicians.
It is foreseeable that this broad approach continues to be rewarding
particularly emphasizing the elucidation of defined metabolic reaction
steps, i.e. biochemistry in vivo eventually with regard to many different enzyme reactions.

REFERENCES

1. R. D. Okada, G. M. Pohost, H. D. Kirshenbaum, F. G. Kushner,
    Ch. A. Boucher, P. C. Block, and H. W. Strauss, Radionuclide-
    determined change in pulmonary blood volume with exercise:
    improved sensitivity of multigated blood pool scanning in
    detecting coronary artery disease, N.Engl.J.Med., 301:569
    (1979).
2. A. Höck, P. Schürch, Ch. Freundlieb, K. Vyska, N. Kunz, L. E.
    Feinendegen, and W. Hollmann, Globale and regionale kardio-
    pulmonale Blutvolumen-Änderungen unter kontinuierlicher
    Belastung, Nucl.-Med., 19:166 (1980).
3. A. Höck, K. Vyska, Ch. Freundlieb, L. E. Feinendegen, H. P.
    Schürch, H. Breitbach, and W. Hollmann, Cardiac, pulmonary
    and hepatic blood volumes during exercise, in: "Nuklear-
    medizin," H. A. E. Schmidt and H. Rösler, eds., F. K.
    Schattauer Verlag, Stuttgart – New York (1982).
4. G. Hoffmann and N. Kleine, Eine neue Methode zur unblutigen
    Messung des Schlagvolumens am Menschen uber viele Tage mit
    Hilfe von radioaktiven Isotopen, Verhandl.Dtsch.Ges.
    Kreislaufforschg., 31:93 (1965).

5. W. E. Adam, F. Bitter, and W. J. Lorenz, Der Computer als
    Hilfsmittel zur Verbesserung der nuklearmedizinischen
    Funktionsdiagnostik, in: "Computers in Radiology," R. de
    Haene and A. Wambersie, eds., Karger, Basel (1970).
6. H. W. Strauss, B. L. Zaret, P. J. Hurley, T. K. Natarjan, and
    B. Pitt, A scintiphotographic method for measuring left
    ventricular ejection fraction in man without cardiac cath-
    eterization, Amer.J.Cardiol., 28:575 (1971).
7. H. N. Wagner, P. Rigo, R. H. Baxter, P. O. Alderson, K. H.
    Douglass, and D. F. Housholder, Monitoring ventricular
    function at rest and during exercise with a non-imaging
    nuclear detector, Amer.J.Cardiol., 43:975 (1979).
8. R. A. Wilson, P. J. Sullivan, R. H. Moore, J. S. Zielonka,
    N. Alpert, C. A. Boucher, K. A. McKusick, and H. W. Strauss,
    The vest – validation of a device for the ambulatory
    measurement of ejection fraction, J.Nucl.Med., 23:47 (1982).
9. J. H. Caldwell, G. W. Hamilton, S. G. Sorensen, J. L. Ritchie,
    D. L. Williams, and J. W. Kennedy, Detection of coronary
    artery disease with radionuclide techniques: comparison of
    rest-exercise thallium imaging and ejection fraction response,
    Circulation 61:610 (1980).
10. J. Borer, S. Bacharach, M. Green, P. Phillips, C. Hochreiter,
    and H. Goldberg, Uses and limitations of radionuclide cine-
    angiography in patients with coronary and valvular heart
    diseases, IX World Congress of Cardiology, Moscow (1982).
11. W. E. Adam, A. Tarkowska, F. Bitter, M. Stauch, and H. Geffers,
    Equilibrium (gated) radionuclide ventriculography, Cardio-
    vascular Radiology, 2:161 (1979).
12. W. Strauss, Nuclear cardiology: the challenge of the eighties,
    IX World Congress of Cardiology, Moscow (1982).
13. R. Slutsky, W. Hooper, K. Gerber, A. Battler, V. Froelicher,
    W. Ashburn, and J. Karliner, Assessment of right ventricular
    function at rest and during exercise in patients with coronary
    heart disease: a new approach using equilibrium radionuclide
    angiography, Am.J.Cardiol., 45:63 (1980).
14. T. J. Ruth, R. M. Lambrecht, and A. P. Wolf, Cyclotron isotopes
    and radiopharmaceuticals: XXX. aspects of production,
    elution, and automation of ^{81}Rb/^{81}Kr generators, Int.J.Appl.
    Radiat.Isot., 31:51 (1980).
15. D. S. Dymond, A. T. Elliott, W. Flatman, J. Caplin, R. Bett,
    J. G. Cuninghame, H. E. Sims, and H. H. Willis, First pass
    radionuclide angiography in man using gold-195m (T1/2 30.5
    seconds), J.Nucl.Med., 23:71 (1982).
16. P. Rigo, Ph. O. Alderson, R. M. Robertson, L. C. Becker, and
    H. N. Wagner, Jr., Measurement of aortic and mitral regurgi-
    tation by gated cardiac blood pool scans, Circulation,
    60:306 (1979).
17. R. Slutsky, J. Karliner, D. Ricci, R. Kaiser, M. Pfisterer,
    D. Gordon, K. Peterson, and W. Ashburn, Left ventricular
    volumes by gated equilibrium radionuclide angiography: a
    new method, Circulation 60:556 (1979).

18. A. H. Maurer, J. A. Siegel, B. Dennenberg, P. S. Robbins,
    B. Carabello, A. Gash, J. F. Spann, and L. S. Malmud,
    Absolute left ventricular volumes by a noninvasive in vivo
    esophageal transmission measurement, J.Nucl.Med., 23:70
    (1982).

19. L. E. Feinendegen, V. Becker, K. Vyska, H. Schicha, and L.
    Seipel, Minimal cardiac transit times - diagnostic radio-
    cardiography in heart disease, J.Nucl.Biol.Med., 16:211
    (1972).

20. L. E. Feinendegen, K. Vyska, H. Schicha, V. Becker, and Chr.
    Freundlieb, The minimal transit times, Der Nuklearmediziner
    Suppl.93 (1979).

21. P. Bosiljanoff, H. Herzog, A. Schmid, D. Sommer, K. Vyska, and
    L. E. Feinendegen, Automatisches Auswerte-programm fur die
    Bestimmung der minimalen cardialen Transitzeiten (MTTs),
    KFA-JUEL-Report, in press (1982).

22. H. Schicha, K. Vyska, V. Becker, and L. E. Feinendegen, Radio-
    cardiograph of minimal transit times. A useful diagnostic
    procedure, in: "Dynamic Studies with Radioisotopes in
    Medicine," IAEA Wien (1975).

23. P. Bosiljanoff, V. Becker, K. Vyska, and L. E. Feinendegen,
    Assessment of combined gated blood pool studies and minimal
    cardiac transit time measurement in nuclear cardiology, in:
    "Nuklearmedizin," H. A. E. Schmidt and H. Rösler, eds.,
    F. K. Schattauer Verlag, Stuttgart - New York (1982).

24. P. Bosiljanoff, V. Becker, K. Vyska, and L. E. Feinendegen,
    Development and testing of a compact radiocardiograph for
    measuring minimal cardiac transit times (MTT), in:
    "Nuklearmedizin," H. A. E. Schmidt, and G. Riccabona, eds.,
    F. K. Schattauer Verlag, Stuttgart - New York (1980).

25. J. L. Ritchie, G. W. Hamilton, and F. J. T. Wackers, "Thallium-
    201 myocardial imaging," Raven Press, New York (1978).

26. D. E. Johnstone, M. J. Sands, H. J. Berger, L. A. Reduto, A. B.
    Lachman, F. J. Wackers, L. S. Cohen, A. Gottschalk, and
    B. L. Zaret, Comparison of exercise radionuclide angiocardio-
    graphy and thallium-201 myocardial perfusion imaging in
    coronary artery disease, Am.J.Cardiol., 45:1113 (1980).

27. E. Deutsch, K. Libson, J. - L. Vanderheyden, D. L. Nosco, V. J.
    Sodd, and H. Nishiyama, Chemistry and preparation of the
    potential myocardial imaging agent $[^{99m}Tc(dmpe)_2Cl_2]^+$ (Tc-
    99m DMPE), J.Nucl.Med., 23:9 (1982).

28. R. A. Goldstein, M. S. Klein, M. J. Welch, and B. E. Sobel,
    External assessment of myocardial metabolism with ^{11}C-
    palmitate in vivo, J.Nucl.Med., 21:342 (1980).

29. E. Henze, R. G. Grossman, S. C. Huang, J. R. Barrio, M. E. Phelps
    and H. R. Schelbert, Myocardial uptake and clearance of C-11
    palmitic acid in man: effects of substrate availability and
    cardiac work, J.Nucl.Med., 23:12 (1982).

30. L. E. Feinendegen, K. Vyska, Chr. Freundlieb, H. J. Machulla, G. Kloster, and G. Stöcklin, Non-invasive analysis of metabolic reactions in body tissues, the case of myocardial fatty acids, Europ.J.Nucl.Med., 6:191 (1981).

31. H. - J. Machulla, G. Stöcklin, Ch. Kupfernagel, Chr. Freundlieb, A. Höck, K. Vyska, and L. E. Feinendegen, Comparative evaluation of fatty acids labeled with C-11, Cl-34m, Br-77, and I-123 for metabolic studies of the myocardium: concise communication, J.Nucl.Med., 19:298 (1978).

32. J. R. Evans, R. W. Gunton, R. G. Baker, D. S. Beanlands, and J. C. Spears, Use of radioiodinated fatty acids for photoscans of the heart, Circ.Res., 16:1 (1965).

33. N. D. Poe, G. E. Robinson, and N. S. MacDonald, Myocardial extraction of labeled long-chain fatty acid analogs, Proc.Soc. Exp.Biol.Med., 148:215 (1975).

34. Chr. Freundlieb, A. Höck, K. Vyska, L. E. Feinendegen, H. - J. Machulla, and G. Stöcklin, Myocardial imaging and metabolic studies with (17-123-I)iodoheptadecanoic acid, J.Nucl.Med., 21:1043 (1980).

35. H. J. Daus, S. N. Reske, K. Vyska, and L. E. Feinendegen, Pharmacokinetics of ω-(p-^{131}I-phenyl)-pentadecanoic acid in heart, in: "Nuklearmedizin," H. A. E. Schmidt, F. Wolf, and J. Mahlstedt, eds., F. K. Schattauer Verlag, Stuttgart - New York (1981).

36. S. N. Reske, H. J. Machulla, D. Aurich, H. J. Biersack, H. Simon, D. Koischwitz, R. Knopp, and C. Winkler, Myocardial turnover of p-^{123}I-phenylpentadecanoic acid (I-PPA) in patients with valvular heart and coronary artery disease, in: "Radioaktive Isotope in Klinik und Forschung," R. Höfer, H. Bergmann, eds., Verlag H. Egermann, Wien (1982).

37. R. Dudczak, R. Schmoliner, P. Angelberger, K. Kletter, and H. Frischauf, Myocardial studies with I-123p-phenylpentadecanoic acid (PPA) in patients with coronary artery disease (CAD) and cardiomyopathy (CMP), J.Nucl.Med., 23:35 (1982).

38. D. M. Solheim, ^{123}I-erucic acid: a promising substance for myocardial imaging, in: "Radioaktive Isotope in Klinik und Forschung," R. Höfer, H. Bergmann, eds., Verlag H. Egermann, Wien (1982).

39. F. F. Knapp, Jr., M. M. Goodman, G. W. Kabalka, K. A. R. Sastry, and A. P. Callahan, Synthesis and evaluation of I-125 (*I)-labeled 18-iodo-13-tellura-17-octadecenoic acid, J.Nucl.Med., 23:10 (1982).

40. E. Livni, D. R. Elmaleh, S. Levy, D. A. Varnum, G. L. Brownell, and H. J. Strauss, Carbon-11 labeled beta methyl fatty acids as potential tracers for myocardial metabolism, J.Nucl.Med., 23:9 (1982).

41. A. Höck, Ch. Freundlieb, K. Vyska, L. E. Feinendegen, R. Rost, P. M. Schürch, and W. Hollmann, The influence of physical training on fatty acid metabolism in patients with coronary artery disease, in: "Nuklearmedizin," H. A. E. Schmidt and

H. Rösler, eds., F. K. Schattauer Verlag, Stuttgart - New York (1982).

42. R. Dudczak, R. Schmoliner, D. K. Derfler, P. Angelberger, K. Kletter, U. Losert, and H. Frischauf, Effect of ischemia and pharmacological interventions on the myocardial elimination of I-123 heptadecanoic acid (HDA), J.Nucl.Med., 23:34 (1982).

43. A. Höck, Chr. Freundlieb, K. Vyska, L. E. Feinendegen, B. Lösse, and R. Erbel, Uptake and elimination rates of labelled fatty acids in patients with cardiomyopathy, in: "Nuklearmedizin," H. A. E. Schmidt, F. Wolf, J. Mahlstedt, eds., F. K. Schattauer Verlag, Stuttgart - New York (1981).

44. A. Höck, Chr. Freundlieb, K. Vyska, B. Lösse, R. Erbel, and L. E. Feinendegen, Myocardial imaging and metabolic studies with (17-^{123}I) iodoheptadecanoic acid in patients with idiopathic congestive cardiomyopathy, J.Nucl.Med., in press (1982).

45. R. C. Marshall, S. C. Huang, J. H. Tillisch, R. Carson, D. Plummer, H. R. Schelbert, and M. E. Phelps, Development of regional criteria to assess the significance of changes in 18-fluoro-deoxyglucose (F) and n-13-ammonia (N) activities evaluated with positron computed tomography (PCT), J.Nucl. Med., 23:33 (1982).

46. O. Ratib, M. E. Phelps, S. C. Huang, E. Henze, C. Selin, and H. R. Schelbert, Noninvasive measurement of the myocardial glucose metabolic rate with positron tomography and fluoro-18 deoxyglucose, in: "Nuklearmedizin," H. A. E. Schmidt, H. Rösler, eds., F. K. Schattauer Verlag, Stuttgart - New York (1982).

47. A. P. Selwyn, personal communication (1982).

48. A. S. Gelbard, R. S. Benua, R. E. Reiman, J. M. McDonald, J. J. Vomero, and J. S. Laughlin, Imaging of the human heart after administration of L-(N-13) Glutamate, J.Nucl.Med., 21:988 (1980).

49. P. V. Harper, K. A. Lathrop, H. Krizek, N. Lembares, V. Stark, and P. B. Hoffer, Clinical feasibility of myocardial imaging with ^{13}NH$_3$, J.Nucl.Med., 13:278 (1972).

50. S. C. Huang, M. Schwaiger, R. E. Carson, E. Henze, E. J. Hoffman, M. E. Phelps, and H. R. Schelbert, An 0-15 water clearance method for quantitative regional myocardial blood flow (rMBF) measurements, J.Nucl.Med., 23:69 (1982).

51. H. H. Coenen, M. - F. Harmand, G. Kloster, and G. Stöcklin, 15-(p-[^{75}Br]bromophenyl)pentadecanoic acid: Pharmacokinetics and potential as heart agent, J.Nucl.Med., 22:891 (1981).

52. G. Kloster, C. Müller-Platz, and P. Laufer, 3-(^{11}C)-methyl-D-glucose, a potential agent for regional cerebral glucose utilization studies, in: "Nuklearmedizin," H. A. E. Schmidt, G. Riccabona, eds., F. K. Schattauer Verlag, Stuttgart - New York (1980).

53. A. Höck, C. Freundlieb, K. Vyska, L. E. Feinendegen, G. Kloster, S. H. Qaim, and G. Stöcklin, 30-P-labelled phosphate and

11-C-labelled methyl D-glucose for metabolic studies, in: "Radioaktive Isotope in Klinik und Forschung," R. Höfer, H. Bergmann, eds., Verlag H. Egermann, Wien (1980).

54. K. Vyska, C. Freundlieb, A. Höck. V. Becker, L. E. Feinendegen, G. Kloster, G. Stöcklin, H. Traupe, and W. D. Heiss, The measurement of glucose transport across the blood brain barrier in man by use of 3-(C-11)-methyl-D-glucose, J.Cerebr. Blood Flow Met., Suppl.1, 1:42 (1981).

55. K. Vyska, C. Freundlieb, A. Höck, V. Becker, L. E. Feinendegen, F. J. Schuier, H. U. Thal, G. Kloster, G. Stöcklin, and W. D. Heiss, Simultaneous measurement of local perfusion rate (LPR) and glucose transport rate (LGTR) in brain and heart, with C-11-methylglucose (CMG) and dynamic positron-emission-tomography (dPET), J.Nucl.Med., 23:13 (1982).

CLINICAL TRIALS WITH ANTIAGGREGATING AGENTS IN THROMBOSIS

M. Verstraete

Center for Thrombosis and Vascular Research
Department of Medical Research
University of Leuven, Campus Gasthuisberg
Herestraat 49, B-3000 Leuven, Belgium

Many agents capable of interfering with normal platelet function in vitro have been described in recent years; most are nonsteroidal anti-inflammatory agents. Not all these compounds have been shown to affect platelet aggregation and adhesiveness in experimental animals, but since animals do not develop spontaneous thrombosis, the relevance of such experiments to clinical medicine is rather tenuous. The only drugs suppressing platelet function that have been evaluated in clinical trials are aspirin, sulfinpyrazone, dipyridamole, hydroxychoroquine, clofibrate, flurbiprofen, and lidocaine, all of which were originally used for other therapeutic purposes. Even today one still has a poor understanding of the relationship between some of their effects on platelets and a potential antithrombotic effect. It is even uncertain whether the latter property is due to their impact on platelets or to some other unknown mode of action.

Aspirin does not inhibit the adherence of platelets to collagen and subendothelium but is a clear inhibitor of platelet aggregation and release induced by mild stimuli in vitro and in ex vivo experiments. Aspirin has however unequivocal effects in experimental venous, arterial and foreign shunt thrombosis in animals and was even shown to enhance thrombosis at high doses. Aspirin is unable to normalize shortened platelet survival in man.

Dipyridamole is a weak inhibitor of aggregation in vitro and ex vivo but was shown to prevent experimental thrombosis in most animal models. Moreover, it normalizes shortened platelet survival in animals and man.

Sulfinpyrazone is a poor inhibitor of platelet function in
vivo and ex vivo although it has a protective effect against experimental thrombosis in animals. It also normalizes enhanced platelet
survival in man. There is meagre evidence that sulfinpyrazone may
be effective against the vessel wall.

PRIMARY PREVENTION OF MYOCARDIAL INFARCTION IN APPARENTLY
HEALTHY AND IN AGED INDIVIDUALS

In a prospective American trial in over 2,000 hyperlipemic men
(average age 42 years) free of coronary heart disease, treated with
clofibrate (2 g daily), a reduction in the incidence of angina
pectoris and non-fatal myocardial infarction but no statistically
significant reduction in overall mortality was obtained (Krasno et
al., 1972). However, major deficiencies in trial design and exe-
cution of the study prevent an unequivocal interpretation of the
data.

The World Health Organization (WHO) sponsored in Edinburgh,
Prague and Budapest a primary prevention, placebo-controlled trial
with clofibrate on the incidence of ischemic heart disease in
healthy men with a known cholesterol level (Report of the Committee
of Principal Investigators, 1980). In total 15,000 healthy blood
donors between 30 and 59 years were studied for an average of 5.3
years. The treatment group was given 1.6 g clofibrate per day.
The overall lowering of non-fatal ischemic heart disease was 20%
in the clofibrate group. However, the number of deaths and the
crude mortality rates from all causes in the clofibrate group were
significantly higher than those in the control group, the excess
being particularly due to a group of noncardiovascular diseases
including malignant neoplasms.

Evidence is also uncertain for aspirin. While the Boston
Collaborative Drug Surveillance Group (1974) and Jick et al. (1976)
had hinted a protective effect of aspirin in the prevention of
myocardial infarction, subsequent follow-up studies, some of which
involved very large numbers, showed no relationship between the
regular use of aspirin and fatal or non-fatal myocardial infarction
(Hammond et al., 1975; Hennekens et al., 1978).

Also in a prospective placebo-controlled trial carried out in
a municipal old age home involving 430 elderly people (82% were
females), there was no evidence of any prophylactic effect of
aspirin (1 g/day) on the incidence of fatal or non-fatal myocardial
infarction after 1 year follow-up observation (Heikinheimo, 1971).

A double-blind between-patient study was therefore carried out
over 4 years in 291 institutionalized elderly males allocated at
random to receive either sulfinpyrazone (0.6 g/day) or a placebo

(Blakely et al., 1975). At entry to the trial more than half of these elderly men had clinical signs of atherosclerosis (coronary, cerebral or peripheral arteries). No statistically significant reduction in mortality could be demonstrated in the sulfinpyrazone-treated patients.

The evidence available at present therefore does not allow the recommendation for use of clofibrate, aspirin or sulfinpyrazone for the primary prevention of myocardial infarction in apparently healthy men or in elderly individuals.

ANTIAGGREGATING AGENTS IN PREVENTION OF A FIRST MYOCARDIAL INFARCTION IN PATIENTS WITH ANGINA

In two Scottish trials 1.5 to 2 g clofibrate was given daily for 5 years to patients who had only angina when admitted to the trial (Research Committee of the Scottish Society of Physicians, 1971; Newcastle-upon-Tyne Physicians, 1971). There was a significant reduction in all cardiac deaths, sudden death and non-fatal death in the clofibrate-treated patients who had only angina when admitted to the trial.

While clofibrate looked promising in the prevention of a first myocardial infarction in patients with angina, this agent cannot - because of major side effects - be recommended for long term use (Committee of Principal Investigators, 1978, 1980).

PREVENTION OF RECURRENT MYOCARDIAL INFARCTION

The two Scottish trials discussed above and the Coronary Drug Project Research Group (1975) failed to show a significantly beneficial effect of clofibrate (1.8 g daily for 5 years) on cause-specific mortality or total mortality in patients who survived a previous myocardial infarct.

The first major double-blind trial of aspirin for the prevention of death after recovery from myocardial infarction was reported by Elwood et al. (1974). On the 1,239 males studied within 6 months after discharge from hospital, half were given a low dose of aspirin (0.3 g daily for 24 months) and half were given a placebo. After 12 months, the follow-up revealed that the treated group had a cumulative mortality of 12.2% and the control group of 18.5%; at no point during the study did this 24% reduction in mortality reach a level of statistical significance. One defect of this trial was that the 9% men who withdrew from treatment were not followed to ascertain death or survival.

Similar findings emerged from a second double-blind trial, also set up by Elwood et al. (1979) to evaluate the prophylactic effect of 300 g aspirin 3 times daily, started within 2 weeks after infarction. After 1 year the all-cause mortality was 12.3% in the aspirin-treated group and 14.8% in the control group, a not statistically significant difference of 17%. The major weakness of this trial is the high withdrawal rate from treatment (26%).

In the study of the Aspirin Myocardial Infarction Research Study Group (1980) 4,524 patients were randomly allocated to either aspirin (1 g/day) or placebo for three years. Endpoints determined before the beginning of the trial included total mortality, coronary incidence (that is the combination of coronary deaths plus proved non-fatal myocardial infarction) and fatal or non-fatal strokes. Entry was eight weeks to five years after myocardial infarction and analysis was by life tables and final outcome. As regards the three endpoints total mortality, coronary deaths combined with non-fatal myocardial infarction and fatal or non-fatal strokes, the results for aspirin and placebo were almost identical.

In a German-Austrian multicenter trial 946 survivors of a myocardial infarction were randomly allocated to aspirin, placebo or phenprocoumon and followed during 2 years (Breddin et al., 1980). There was little difference in total mortality among the three groups, but sudden death and non-fatal recurrent myocardial infarction combined were significantly lower in the aspirin group than in the placebo or phenprocoumon group.

In the "PARIS" Study (Persantine Aspirin Reinfarction Study Research Group, 1980) 2,026 patients were randomly allocated to three treatment groups; one group received 75 mg dipyridamole and 324 mg aspirin three times a day. The second group received the same dose of aspirin with a persantin placebo, and the third group (half the size of the two previous groups) placebo only. After 3 years of treatment, there was a trend in favor of aspirin and dipyridamole, and of aspirin as compared with placebo, but statistical significance was not achieved with regard to total mortality (respectively 10.7%, 10.5% and 12.8%), coronary deaths and coronary incidence. Life table analysis however showed that dipyridamole and aspirin were significantly better than placebo at 4, 8, 12, 16, 20 and 24 months, and aspirin was significantly better than placebo at 8 and 24 months. Subgroup analysis showed that the effects on the three primary endpoints were much more marked in patients who entered the study within six months of myocardial infarction.

Two major trials of sulfinpyrazone have been reported - the "ART" Study (carried out by the Anturane Reinfarction Trial Research Group (1978, 1980)) and the Anturane Reinfarction Italian Trial (1982). In the ART trial 1,629 patients who had suffered a myocardial infarction, were allocated at random to sulfinpyrazone

200 mg four times daily, or to placebo, for 12 to 24 months. Entry
to the trial was 25 to 35 days after myocardial infarction. 43
deaths were regarded as "non-analyzible" according to criteria
defined in the protocol. Deaths from all causes and cardiac deaths
were reduced at up to 24 months, although conventional levels of
significance were not achieved. Although deaths from myocardial
infarction were almost identical in the treatment and placebo groups,
there was a marked and significant reduction in sudden deaths (43%)
which took place almost entirely during the first six months of
treatment. An independent committee re-analyzed all deaths and
when the principles of a so-called clinical efficacy trial are
applied, their results are in general agreement with the original
report, although the levels of statistical significance are less
striking (The Anturane Reinfarction Trial Policy Committee, 1982).
If the data from the "ART" study are analyzed on an "intention-to-
treat" basis, including all patients and all deaths in the 24 months
follow-up, there were 74 deaths in the 813 sulfinpyrazone-treated
patients and 89 deaths in 816 placebo patients ($p > 0.05$) (McNicol,
1980).

     The results of a similar trial with the same daily dose of
sulfinpyrazone were recently published (Anturane Reinfarction Italian
Trial, 1982). There are some important differences between the
American and Italian sulfinpyrazone trials, eg., all patients who
had a myocardial infarction, a stroke or a transient ischemic attack,
withdrew from the Italian trial. The death rate during the first
6 months in Italian placebo-patients (cardiac death rate 4.4% and
sudden death rate 2.5%) was much lower than in the American placebo-
patients (cardiac death rate 10.3% and sudden death rate 7.0%),
which may be due to less patients with recurrent infarction and
heart failure in the Italian trial. Therefore it is not surprising
that in contrast to the American trial, the Italian study did not
demonstrate a reduction in either total mortality or sudden death
rate. However, it did reduce the incidence of reinfarction during
the entire 24 months observation period (75 in the sulfinpyrazone
group, 34 in the placebo group).

PREVENTION OF GRAFT OCCLUSION AFTER AORTOCORONARY BYPASS SURGERY

     Early occlusion of a coronary bypass is most often related to
the level of blood flow through the bypass which depends mainly
upon the size of the anastomosis and distal run-off. Late occlusion
is more related to the progression of the basic disease in which
platelet adherence to the graft wall could be an important factor.

     A preliminary nonrandomized trial suggested that all groups
of patients who received dipyridamole, aspirin or oral coumarin
anti-coagulant drugs experienced higher survival rates over a 4
year observation period than control groups who did not receive

one of these drugs (Hall et al., 1974). These findings were not
confirmed in a strictly randomized trial in which the protective
effect of aspirin (1 g daily), dipyridamole (0.225 g daily) and oral
anti-coagulants were compared to oral anti-coagulants. Six months
after coronary bypass surgery, the occlusion rate was similar in
the 4 treatment groups (Oblath et al., 1978). The treatment however
was started 3 days after surgery which may be too late to prevent
myo-intimal proliferation (Goldberg et al., 1979).

PREVENTION OF THROMBOEMBOLISM IN PATIENTS WITH PROSTHETIC
HEART VALVES

Newer materials employed in modern prosthetic valves are less
thrombogenic than the first artificial valves. Also the location
of the artificial valve is important, the mitral location being
associated with the highest thromboembolic risk. Oral anti-coagulants
provide a satisfactory protection provided the level of anti-coagu-
lation is effective, which requires frequent and accurate monitoring
of the prothrombin time. The risk of bleeding complications still
prevails and the potentially dysmorphogenic properties of oral anti-
coagulants in the first trimester of pregnancy constitutes a problem
in young women with cardiac valve replacement who wish to become
pregnant. These drawbacks explain the interest in the possible use
of antiaggregating agents, combined or not with oral anti-coagulants
in patients with synthetic heart valves.

The first double-blind trial demonstrated that <u>dipyridamole</u>
(0.4 g daily) given in addition to oral anti-coagulants resulted in
a greater protection (1.3% arterial emboli) than oral anti-coagulants
used alone (14.3% arterial emboli) (Sullivan et al., 1971). Several
other trials confirmed these findings although they all had a less
than satisfactory design (Arrants et al., 1970; Meyer et al., 1971;
Pell, 1975; Groupe de Recherche Pacte, 1978).

Two trials in which <u>aspirin</u> (0.5 g or 1 g daily) was given in
addition to oral anti-coagulants also had fewer thromboembolic
complications than patients receiving anti-coagulants alone (Altman
et al., 1976; Dale et al., 1977). Dipyridamole or aspirin prevention alone does not result in a satisfactory protection (Isom et
al., 1973; Dale et al., 1977; Sutton et al., 1978). While a combination of oral anti-coagulants and either dipyridamole or aspirin
results in a greater protection, one should not disregard the
incidence of bleeding induced by aspirin, which may be 7 to 15%
(Altman et al., 1976; Dale et al., 1977).

ANTIAGGREGATING AGENTS IN PATIENTS WITH OBLITERATIVE
DISEASE IN LIMB ARTERIES

The most common cause of obliterative arterial disease in the
legs is slowly progressive atherosclerosis which is eventually
superimposed by thrombosis. The danger of the condition is the
underlying disease, as most patients die from a cardiac or cerebral
complication of atherosclerosis. The increased mortality in claudi-
cating patients corresponds approximately to the mortality rate one
would expect in an overall population aged 10 years older. The
message is therefore very clear. A patient with claudication is to
be treated first for the underlying illness and medical risk factors,
and not for the presenting symptoms. Abstinence from smoking,
appropriate diet and physical exercise are therefore the first
treatment guidelines while percutaneous transluminal dilatation and
reconstructive surgery often relieve the most severe cases.

There is a widespread interest in the use of antiaggregating
agents in patients with atherosclerotic limb arteries as thrombosis
of a stenotic lesion is a rather frequent event. Damaged endothelium and other atherosclerotic lesions may activate platelets
which in turn accelerate the atherogenic obliterative process.
Inhibition of platelet deposition, aggregation and release would
then in the long run be beneficial in these patients.

There are very few well controlled trials demonstrating that
antiaggregating agents are clinically effective in patients with
intermittent claudication. A recent double-blind trial suggests
that ticlopidine (0.5 g daily) decreases the extent of cutaneous
lesions (Katsumara et al., 1980). This study has so far not been
confirmed.

Aspirin (1.5 g daily) has been used after arterial thrombo-
endarterectomy and found to increase the patency rate after 1 year
from 11.2% in the control group to 22% in the aspirin-treated
patients (Ehresmann et al., 1977). Similar findings were obtained
after a 2 year follow-up with either aspirin alone (1 g daily) or
in combination with dipyridamole (0.225 g daily) (Bollinger et al.,
1978, 1981). This beneficial effect of aspirin was obtained in
patients subjected to endarterectomy, not after venous bypass
operation. It should be noted that arterial endarterectomy is at
present an almost abandoned operation.

None of the published trials with sulfinpyrazone after peripheral arterial surgery resulted in a beneficial effect (Blakely
et al., 1977; Rodvian et al., 1978).

Several reports have appeared on the beneficial effects of
aspirin (0.3 to 1 g daily) in patients with thrombocytosis and
intermittent arterial ischemia. The painful "blue toe" syndrome is

the consequence of a blocked microcirculation due to platelet emboli
or spontaneously aggregating platelets. Aspirin immediately relieves
the pain; treatment of the underlying disorder will prevent further
ischemic attacks in toes or fingers (Vreeken et al., 1971; Bierme
et al., 1972; Preston et al., 1974). Similar symptoms can also
result from platelet emboli originating on ulcerated atherosclerotic
plaques.

PREVENTION OF TRANSIENT CEREBRAL ISCHEMIA

The most important warning symptoms of impending stroke are
Transient Ischemic Attacks (TIA's), which are focal cerebral dys-
functions, rapid in onset, variable in duration, lasting 2 to 15
minutes but no longer than 24 hours. Each attack leaves no persistent neurological deficit. In general, TIA's have a bad prognosis;
25 to 40% of patients with TIA's will eventually develop cerebral
infarction within 5 years. The risk of stroke in the first year
after TIA may be over 15%.

The origin of TIA's and stroke is multicausal and deals with
a variety of heart diseases, blood vessel disorders, hypertension
and blood disorders. Considering the multicausal origin of TIA's
and stroke and the uncertainty of the role of platelets in many of
them, it may be questioned whether administration of an antiaggregating agent may ever result in therapeutic large scale benefit in
such a mixed population. The effectiveness of antiaggregating
agents would certainly increase, could one predict which patients
have an increased risk for fibrin-platelet emboli as the specific
cause of their TIA.

A controlled clinical trial in America compared aspirin (1.3 g
daily) in patients with a history of TIA's. The endpoints were the
recurrence of TIA's, stroke and death. Aspirin did not reduce
significantly these endpoints at 24 months of follow-up. Subgroup-
analysis revealed that patients who had multiple TIA's before
entering the trial and those with angiographically demonstrated
lesions of the carotid artery had after 24 months a significant
reduction of the absolute endpoints death and stroke combined
(Fields et al., 1977, 1978).

The Canadian Cooperative Trial (1978) concerns patients who
had experienced at least 1 TIA in the 3 months before entry in the
trial. They were randomized for an average of 26 months to aspirin
(1.2 g daily), aspirin (1.2 g) plus sulfinpyrazone (800 mg), sulfinpyrazone alone (800 mg) or placebo. Aspirin reduced the risk
of continuing TIA's, stroke or death by 19% (p < 0.05) and also the
risk for the harder, more important events of stroke or death by
31% (p < 0.005). For sulfinpyrazone, no risk reduction of TIA was
observed and only a 10% (p > 0.05) reduction of stroke or death.

No overall synergism was observed between the 2 drugs. The aspirin effect was not observed in women and was less marked in patients with diabetes, hypertension or previous myocardial infarction.

In a more recent Swedish trial the combined effect of aspirin (1 g daily) and dipyridamole (0.15 g daily) appeared during the first year of follow-up to be in TIA patients as effective as oral anti-coagulants against stroke (Olsson et al., 1980).

One can therefore conclude that aspirin reduces significantly in the first 2 years the recurrence of TIA's, stroke or death in male patients with a recent transient ischemic attack. Many neurologists consider that patients with TIA's in whom arteriographic examination reveals a surgically accessible lesion, should be operated first and subsequently take aspirin. Considering the prominent role of hemodynamic processes which apparently are considerably more frequent than solely occlusive factors in the pathogenesis of TIA's in a general population (Herman et al., 1981), a complete clinical and technical examination of the patients is mandatory before any treatment is decided.

REFERENCES

Altman, R., Boullon, F., Rouvier, J., Raca, R., De la Fuente, L., and Favorolo, R., 1976, Aspirin and prophylaxis of thromboembolic complications in patients with substitute heart valves, J. Thorac. Card. Surg., 72:127.
Anturane Reinfarction Trial Research Group, 1978, Sulfinpyrazone in the prevention of cardiac death after myocardial infarction, N. Engl. J. Med., 298:289.
Anturane Reinfarction Trial Research Group, 1980, Sulfinpyrazone in the prevention of sudden death after myocardial infarction, N. Engl. J. Med., 302:250.
Anturane Reinfarction Trial Policy Committee, 1982, The Anturane reinfarction trial: reevaluation of outcome, N. Engl. J. Med., 306:1005.
Anturane Reinfarction Italian Study, 1982, Sulphinpyrazone in postmyocardial infarction, Lancet, i:237.
Arrants, J. E., Hairston, P., and Lee, W. H. Jr., 1970, Use of dipyridamole (Persantine) in preventing thromboembolism following valve replacement (Abstract), Chest, 58:275.
Aspirin Myocardial Infarction Study Research Group, 1980, A randomized controlled trial of aspirin in persons recovered from myocardial infarction, JAMA, 243:661.
Bierme, R., Boneu, B., Giraud, B., and Pris, J., 1972, Aspirin and recurrent painful toes and fingers in thrombocythaemia, Lancet, i:431.
Blakely, J. A., and Gent, M., 1975, Platelets, drugs and longevity in a geriatric population, in: "Platelets, Drugs and Thrombosis",

Hirsh, J., Cade, J. F., Gallus, A. S., and Schönbaum, E., eds.,
Karger, Basel, p. 284.

Blakely, J. A., and Pogoriler, G., 1977, A prospective trial of
sulfinpyrazone after peripheral vascular surgery, Proc. VIth
Congr. Int. Soc. Thrombosis and Hemostasis, Philadelphia, p. 238.

Bollinger, A., Fitschy, J., Torres, C., and Piquerez, M. J., 1978,
Thrombozytenaggregationshemmer nach offener oder halfoffener
Endarteriektomie; Vorläufige Resultate einer prospektiven
Studie, VASA, 7:82.

Boston Collaborative Drug Surveillance Group, 1974, Regular aspirin
intake and acute myocardial infarction, Brit. Med. J., 1:440.

Breddin, K., Loew, D., Lechner, K., Ueberla, K., and Walter, E.,
1980, Secondary prevention of myocardial infarction: a comparison of acetylsalicylic acid, placebo and phenprocoumon, Hemostasis, 9:325.

Canadian Cooperative Study Group, 1978, A randomized trial of
aspirin and sulfinpyrazone in threatened stroke, N. Engl. J.
Med., 299:53.

Committee of Principal Investigators, 1978, A cooperative trial on
the primary prevention of ischemic heart disease using clofibrate, Brit. Heart J., 40:1069.

Committee of Principal Investigators, 1980, WHO cooperative trial
on primary prevention of ischemic heart disease using clofibrate to lower serum cholesterol: mortality follow-up, Lancet,
ii:379.

Coronary Drug Project Research Group, 1975, Clofibrate and niacin
in coronary heart disease, JAMA, 27:360.

Dale, J., Myhre, E., Storstein, O., Stormorken, H., and Efskin,
D. L., 1977, Prevention of arterial thromboembolism with
acetylsalicylic acid. A controlled clinical study in patients
with aortic ball valves, Am. Heart J., 94:101.

Ehresmann, V., Alemany, J., and Loew, D., 1977, Prophylaxe von
Rezidivverschlussen nach Revascularisation - Eingriffen mit
Acetylsalicylsaure, Med. Welt., 28:1157.

Elwood, P. C., Cochrane, A. L., Burr, M. L., Sweetnam, P. M.,
Williams, G., Welsby, E., Hughes, S. J., and Renton, R., 1974,
A randomized controlled trial of acetylsalicylic acid in the
secondary prevention of mortality from myocardial infarction,
Brit. Med. J., 1:436.

Elwood, P. C., and Sweetnam, P. M., 1979, Aspirin and secondary
mortality after myocardial infarction, Lancet, i:1313.

Fields, W. S., Lemak, N. A., Frankowski, R. F., and Hardy, R. J.,
1977, 1978, Controlled trial of aspirin in cerebral ischemia,
Stroke, 8:301; 9:309.

Gent, A. E., Brook, C. G. D., Foley, T. H., and Miller, T. N., 1968,
Dipyridamole. A controlled trial of its effect in acute myocardial infarction, Brit. Med. J., 4:366.

Goldberg, I. D., Stemerman, M. B., and Schnipper, L. E., 1979,
Vascular smooth muscle cell kinetics: a new assay for studying
patterns of cellular proliferation in vivo, Science, 205:920.

Groupe de Recherce PACTE, 1978, Prévention des accidents thrombo-
    emboliques systémiques chez les porteurs de prothèses val-
    vulaires artificielles: essai coopératif contrôlé du dipyrida-
    mole, Coeur, 19:915.
Hall, R. J., Garcia, E., Al-Bassam, M. S., and Dawson, J. T., 1974,
    Aortocoronary bypass surgery 1969-1973; Review of 2,566
    patients, Cardiovasc. Dis. Bull., 1:74.
Hammond, E. C., and Garfinkel, L., 1975, Aspirin and coronary heart
    disease: findings of a prospective study, Brit. Med. J., 2:269.
Heikinheimo, R., and Jarvinen, K., 1971, Acetylsalicylic acid and
    arteriosclerotic thromboembolic diseases in the aged, J. Amer.
    Geriat. Soc., 19:403.
Hennekens, C. H., Karlson, L. K., and Rosner, B., 1978, A case-
    control study of regular aspirin use and coronary deaths,
    Circulation, 58:35.
Herman, B., de Waard, F., and Colette, H. J. A., 1981, Unexpected
    trends in the analysis of a questionnaire and interview pro-
    cedure to detect transient cerebral ischemic attack in a female
    population, Clin. Neurol. Neurosurg., 83:225.
Isom, O. W., Williams, C. D., Falk, E. A., Spencer, F. C., and
    Glassman, E., 1973, Evaluation of anti-coagulant therapy in
    cloth-covered prosthetic valves, Circulation, suppl. III:48.
Jick, H., and Miettinen, O. S., 1976, Regular aspirin use and myo-
    cardial infarction, Brit. Med. J., 1:1057.
Katsumara, T., Kusaba, A., Shionoya, S., Kamiya, K., Myaucchi, Y.,
    and Nishimura, A., 1980, Therapeutic effects of ticlopidine,
    a new inhibitor of platelet aggregation in chronic arterial
    occlusive disease, Blood Vessels, 11:152.
Krasno, L. R., and Kidera, G. J., 1972, Clofibrate in coronary
    heart disease, JAMA, 219:845.
McNicol, G. P., 1980, Anti-platelet drugs in the secondary preven-
    tion of myocardial infarction, Lancet, ii:736.
Meyer, J. S., Charney, J. Z., Rivera, V. M., and Mathew, N. J.,
    1971, Cerebral embolization: prospective clinical analysis of
    42 cases, Stroke, 2:541.
Mitchell, J. R. A., 1980, Secondary prevention of myocardial infarc-
    tion - the present state of the ART, Brit. Med. J., 280:1128.
Newcastle-upon-Tyne Physicians, 1971, Trial of clofibrate in the
    treatment of ischemic heart disease, Brit. Med. J., 4:767.
Oblath, R. W., Buckley, F. O., Green, R. M., Schwartz, S. E., and
    de Weese, J. A., 1978, Prevention of anastomic neointimal
    fibrous hyperplasia in femoral bypass by aspirin and dipyrida-
    mole, Surgery, 84:37.
Olsson, J. E., Brechter, C., Bäcklund, H., Krook, H., Müller, R.,
    Nitelius, E., Olsson, O., and Tornberg, A., 1980, Anticoagulant
    vs antiplatelet therapy as prophylactive cerebral infarction
    in transient ischemic attacks, Stroke, 2:4.
Pell, E., 1975, Essai clinique contrôlé du Dipyridamole dans le
    traitement préventif des accidents thromboemboliques chez les
    porteurs de prothèses valvulaires, Thèse, Lyon.

Persantine-Aspirin Reinfarction Study Research Group, 1980, Persan-
    tine and aspirin in coronary heart disease, Circulation, 62:449.
Preston, F. E., Emmanuel, I. G., Winfield, D. A., and Malia, R. G.,
    1974, Essential thrombocythemia and peripheral gangrene, Brit.
    Med. J., 3:548.
Research Committee of the Scottish Society of Physicians, 1971,
    Ischemic heart disease: a secondary prevention trial using
    clofibrate, Brit. Med. J., 4:775.
Rodvian, R., and Salzman, E. W., 1978, Thrombotic and hemorrhagic
    problems in surgery, Thrombos. Hemost., 39:254.
Sullivan, J. M., Harken, D. E., and Gorlin, R., 1971, Pharmacologic
    control of thromboembolic complications of cardiac valve
    replacement, N. Engl. J. Med., 284:1391.
Sutton, M. G., and John, S. T., 1978, Anticoagulation and Björk-
    Shiley prosthesis. Experience of 390 patients. Brit. Heart J.,
    40:558.
Vreeken, J., and van Aken, W. G., 1971, Spontaneous aggregation of
    blood platelets as a cause of idiopathic thrombosis and recurrent
    painful toes and fingers, Lancet, ii:1394.
Wilcox, R. G., Richardson, D., Hampton, J. R., Mitchell, J. R. A.,
    and Banks, D. C., 1980, Sulphinpyrazone in acute myocardial
    infarction: studies on cardiac rhythm and renal function,
    Brit. Med. J., 2:531.

ECHOCARDIOGRAPHY: PRESENT STATE OF THE ART

J. Roelandt

Thoraxcentre
Erasmus University and Academic Hospital
Dijkzigt
Rotterdam, The Netherlands

Among the new diagnostic methods in cardiology, echocardiography is certainly the most informative. The field has grown so rapidly in recent years that it is almost impossible to keep up with the new technical developments and their application in patient care. The principle of the method is based upon the detection of echoes produced by a beam of short ultrasound pulses transmitted into the heart. Ultrasound is harmless at the energy levels used. The examination can thus readily and repeatedly be used without untoward effects to the patient making it the ideal method for serial analysis and follow-up studies.

It is important to appreciate some distinct differences between echocardiography and X-ray imaging for a better understanding of its specific applications. With ultrasound local changes in acoustic impedance along the sound beam pathway are registered. X-ray techniques register cumulated attenuation of energy along the pathway so that cardiac structures are superimposed in depth and seen as shadows. As a result, the specific details of intracardiac anatomy and pathology such as the attachment and morphology of the atrioventricular valves, the interventricular septum, mass lesions, etc. are better documented with ultrasound that with X-ray techniques.

Since its introduction in 1954 by Edler and Hertz[1] to the mid 1970's, M-mode echocardiography has been exclusively used and its clinical value and limitations are well established.[2,3]

The ultrasound beam is aimed manually at selected cardiac structures and a "diagram" showing how the position of these structures change during the cardiac cycle is obtained (time-motion

display of B-mode or intensity-modulated echoes). The high sampling
rate (1,000 transmit-receive cycles/sec) permits recording of
rapidly occurring events (e.g. valve opening, closure and fluttering)
and facilitates measurement of cardiac dimensions and the analysis
of time relationships with other physiological parameters (e.g.
simultaneously recorded pulse and pressure tracings). The method
however, does not provide information on the spatial relationships
of different cardiac structures to each other. This can be
accomplished by rapidly and automatically moving the ultrasound beam
through a section of the heart to create a "tomographic image"
yielding instantaneous structure information and thus cardiac anatomy
in motion (Fig. 1).

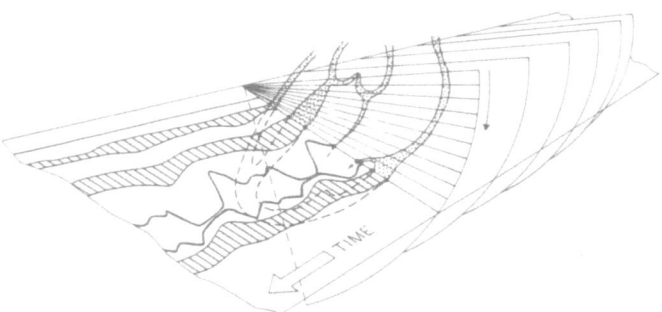

Fig. 1.   Diagram illustrating the relationship between the two-
          dimensional and the M-mode echocardiogram. The motion
          pattern of the small part of the mitral valve hit by the
          sound beam is accurately tracted (1,000 transmit-receive
          cycles/sec). However, no information on its anatomical
          relationships is obtained. This is available from the
          two dimensional images.

     The spatially oriented display of two-dimensional echocardi-
ography allows information to be appreciated and utilized which is
meaningless in the absence of such a spatial reference. This allows
a multitude of cardiac cross-sections to be imaged from several
chest wall transducer positions (parasternal, apical, subcostal and
suprasternal) providing a wealth of diagnostic information.[4]
Recently, the American Society of Echocardiography (ASE) has published recommendations for nomenclature and image orientation
standards.[5] Such standards obviously are needed to make studies
from different laboratories comparable. Building up a two-
dimensional image requires time limiting the frame rate which is

25 or 30 frames/sec. As a consequence, two-dimensional echocardiography is less suitable for analysis of functional abnormalities. The relative advantages of M-mode and two dimensional echocardiography are listed in Table 1.

Table 1.   Relative Advantages of M-Mode and Two-Dimensional Echocardiography

M-mode echocardiography
- Excellent time resolution
- Accurate dimensional measurements
- Timing of events against other parameters
- Easy storage and retrieval of data

Two-dimensional echocardiography
- Anatomical relationships
- Shape information
- Multiple tomographic views
- Complex motion patterns
- Easier to understand

It is obvious that both methods are complementary and best used in combination for a comprehensive analysis of cardiac conditions where anatomic and functional abnormalities overlap. Because the "ultrasonic windows" to the heart are limited by the ribs and lungs, all presently used two-dimensional imaging systems are of the sector type, either mechanical or electronic. Comparative advantages and limitations of each tupe of instrument are continually changing and their sophistication is increasing which makes differences between them less pronounced.[6]

Mechanical scanners use an oscillating or a rotating scan head. The principle of image formation in the oscillating systems relies on the rapid pivoting motion about a fixed axis of a single transducer by means of a magnetic deflection mechanism. In the rotating systems, several transducers are mounted on a spinning wheel inside a fluid-filled scanning head and are active when they pass over the heart. Signals from the scanning heads are used to steer the oscilloscope beam in the same manner as the ultrasound beam to create a tomographic image. Advantages of the mechanical scanners are their relative simplicity, the possibility to adapt them to existing M-mode units, and the retention of the straight-forward resolution characteristics of a single crystal.

Phased-array scanners make use of a small stationary transducer with multiple small elements. They are all utilized in producing each of the individual ultrasound beams which comprise the sector image. The ultrasound beam is steered electronically through the scan plane by firing them in an extremely rapid and precisely controlled sequence. These systems are very complicated and, hence, the most costly. Despite the necessary complexity, they offer the possibility for reducing the effective beam width by dynamic focusing, a feature not possible with mechanical scanners. Their major advantage is that they can simultaneously display the two-dimensional image while repeatedly sampling areas of the selected scan plane for M-mode recording. An alectronic cursor superimposed on the display is adjusted to the desired position and the appropriate B-mode lines are printed on a M-mode strip-chart recorder.

In order to document two-dimensional images we presently make use of digital scan converters which allow to change the image into a standard TV format. They comprise a matrix of memory cells (typically 512 x 512 elements, each called a "pixel"). When fully loaded, the memory matrix can be "read" in any desired sequence, e.g. as a series of horizontal lines to form a TV image for a video recorder, or as a series of vertical lines to enable it to be printed along with the M-mode on a strip-chart recorder. Digital stored images offer additional advantages since they can be manipulated in a number of ways. Alpha-numeric data (e.g. patient identification) can easily be added, various techniques can be employed to enhance the image quality, and measurements can be made directly from the displayed image using a light-pen or a joystick-controlled cursor and the results encoded in the image.

These capabilities allow accurate and reproducible measurements of the mitral valve orifice area from parasternal short axis views in patients with mitral valve stenosis.[7,8] They further enhance and simplify segmental wall motion analysis in patients with coronary artery disease.[9] Most of their attractiveness, however, lies in the measurement of left ventricular volume and quantitation of left ventricular function. The extreme accuracy reported in vitro and in animal studies proves that the models and formulas applied are satisfactory and suggest that quantitation is an obtainable goal.[10,11] The reported results in patients, however, are less convincing.[12,15] It seems that accurate measurement of left ventricular volumes in humans using two-dimensional echocardiography must await further instrument improvements and better display techniques.

Pulsed Doppler echocardiography is gaining increasing interest and currently undergoing intensive evaluation. The method uses the frequency shift of an ultrasound beam backscattered from the red blood cells and allows to detect the nature, direction and velocity of blood flow at one point (sample volume) within the heart and great vessels. Doppler echocardiography provides data

on the integrity of valve function and detection of septal defects
but this information is qualitative at its best.[16] Doppler evaluation should nevertheless be considered as part of a comprehensive
cardiac evaluation and is optimally used in conjunction with M-mode
or preferably two-dimensional echocardiography. Some newer units
offer these integrated capabilities, all information being obtained
from one and the same transducer (Fig. 2). Such a combination with
multigate, digital Doppler technique promises to obtain two-
dimensional images similar to cineangiocardiograms, in which
valvular regurgitation or shunting blood flow is translated directly
into an anatomic form of display.

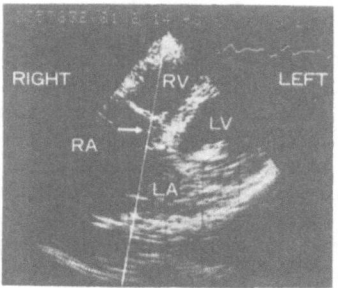

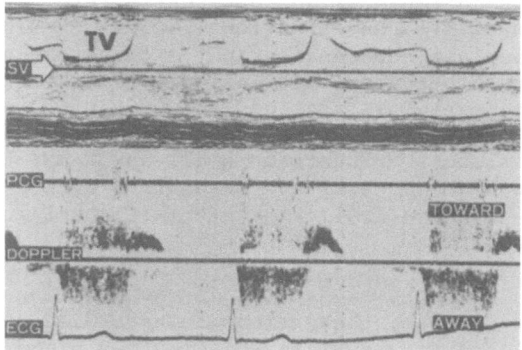

Fig. 2.   Phased array sector image of a patient with tricuspid
          regurgitation. The imaging plane is a foreshortened
          four chamber view. The cursor indicates the B-mode line
          from which the M-mode echocardiogram is obtained and
          passes through the tricuspid valve. The position on the
          B-mode line of the range gate from which the Doppler is
          sampled is indicated by the arrow. The M-mode echo-
          cardiogram is shown below and the position of the sample

volume (SV) is here indicated by the straight line on the
tracing. The Doppler shift indicating flow velocity and
its direction and the M-mode cardiogram are recorded
simultaneously. Laminar flow is represented by a narrow
band of dots and turbulence by a broad band of dots. By
convention, deflection of dots above the baseline indicates
an increase in flow velocity toward the transducer and flow
away from the transducer is indicated by the dots below the
baseline. Note the systolic flow away from the transducer indicating tricuspid regurgitation. ECG: electrocardiogram, PCG: phonocardiogram, TV: tricuspid valve.

With presently available single sample volume instruments,
accurate quantitation of volume flow is not possible and this
possibility should probably be awaited with cautious optimism.

Contrast echocardiography is the technique of injecting an
echoproducing biologically compatible solution into the blood-
stream and using M-mode and two-dimensional techniques, observing
the bloodflow patterns as revealed by the resulting cloud of
echoes. The method is increasingly used and makes it possible
to derive information that was heretofore available only from
cardiac catheterization and angiocardiography. The source of ultrasound contrast is microbubbles of air present in the injectate.[17]
Dextrose 5% in water, saline, and indocyanine green dye are the
most commonly used contrast agents. Right sided structures are
delineated by peripheral venous injections, and left sided structures
are opacified by injections performed directly into the left heart
chambers during cardiac catheterization (Fig. 3).[18] The clinical
applications of contrast echocardiography are indicated in Table 2.
Since echocardiographic contrast is entirely removed from the circulation by the pulmonary capillary bed, the appearance of contrast
in the left heart after a peripheral venous injection is diagnostic
for a right-to-left shunt. Shunts as small as 5% can be detected.[19]
The method thus provides a sensitive means to diagnose uncomplicated
atrial septal defects as a small right-to-left shunt is always
present in this condition.

The technique is extremely useful in complex congenital heart
disease helping to diagnose the various intracardiac connections
and communications and to visualize the shunting blood flow (Fig. 4).
The method is further helpful to diagnose tricuspid regurgitation.[20]
Normally contrast injected in an upper extremity flows from the
superior vena cava into the right atrium and right ventricle without
retrograde flow into the inferior vena cava. In patients with
tricuspid regurgitation, however, it can be detected in the inferior
vena cava and hepatic veins during the "v" wave on the right atrial
pressure tracing. Timing of its appearance is much easier from
M-mode than from two-dimensional studies. Kerber et al. were using
the technique during cardiac catheterization for the identification

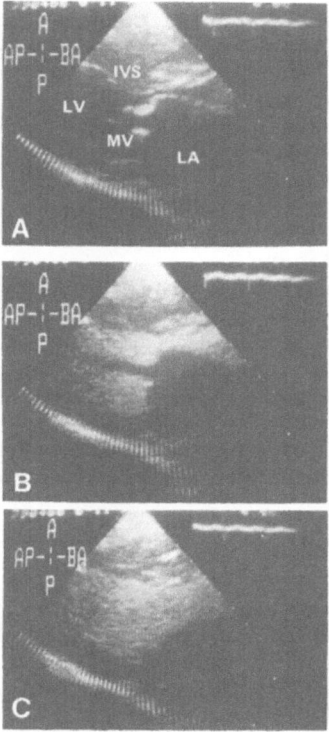

Fig. 3. Stop-frame photographs of parasternal long axis views of
         a patient with mitral valve stenosis before (panel A) and
         after injection of echo contrast via a catheter in the
         left ventricle. Panel B shows a frame recorded during
         diastole. The negative shadow caused by the noncontrast
         blood flowing from the left atrium into the ventricles
         visualizes the transmitral blood flow pattern. During
         systole (panel C), the echo contrast does not pass into
         the left atrium, excluding mitral incompetence. A:
         anterior; AP: apical; BA: basal; IVS: interventricular
         septum; LA: left atrium; LV: left ventricle; MV: mitral
         valve; P: posterior. (From Roelandt J et al: Contrast
         echocardiography of the left ventricle. In Rijsterborgh
         H (ed),"Echocardiology", M. Nijhoff, The Hague, 1981,
         p 219-232).

of valvular regurgitation and regurgitant volumes as small as 10%
of the forward stroke volume can be demonstrated.[21] Recent studies
have shown that injections in the pulmonary wedge position can cause
contrast to appear on the left side of the heart and may enable us

Table 2. Clinical Applications of Contrast Echocardiography

- Structure identification (M, 2-D)
- Diagnosis (or exclusion) of shunts
    Localization (2-D)
    Direction shunting blood flow (M, 2-D)
    Timing (M)
- Complex congenital heart disease (2-D)
- Valvular insufficiency
    Venous injections: tricuspid and pulmonic (M)
    Catheter injections: aortic and mitral (M, 2-D)
- Intracavitary and transvalvular flow patterns (2-D)
- Videodensitometric analysis of echo contrast
- Improved quantitation of left ventricle (2-D)

M, 2-D: indication for which points M-mode or two-dimensional echocardiography offer relative advantages.

---

to visualize left-to-right shunting.[22] There are several interesting additional future prospects for contrast echocardiography. Recent studies have suggested that quantitative videodensitometric techniques may allow to measure ejection fraction and cardiac output,[23] and to quantify intracardiac shunts[24] from two- dimensional contrast echocardiograms.

Exercise echocardiography is a recent experimental technique. Its important limitations at present are that successful exercise studies are technically difficult to perform and that there is a large proportion of patients in whom adequate study for analysis are unobtainable. Nevertheless there are some important advantages to this method. It allows to study cardiac physiology during exercise[25] and to detect left ventricular dysfunction in selected patients with coronary artery disease.[26] Because of the methodological difficulties, the method will probably not become a routine clinical screening method but may gain wider application in the investigation of normal and abnormal physiology in the future.

Summary

The combined use of two-dimensional and M-mode echocardiography complemented with contrast and Doppler techniques makes echocardiography an extremely accurate noninvasive method for the diagnosis of various cardiovascular diseases. It should be realized, however, that despite its apparent simplicity and safety, echocardiography is a difficult procedure to perform and that the interpretation of the results are subject to many pitfalls. It

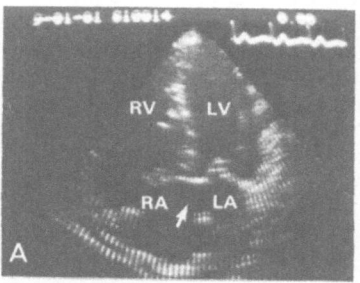

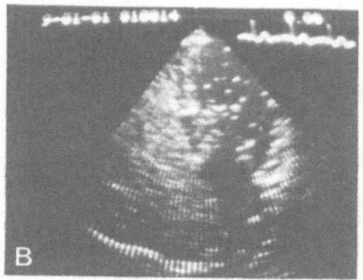

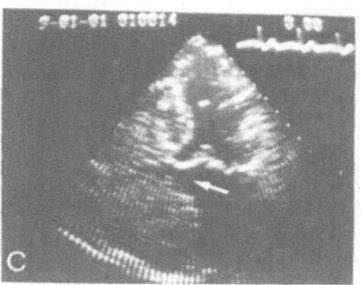

Fig. 4   Apical four chamber views obtained from a patient with an
          atrial septal defect of the primum type. The defect is
          indicated by the arrow on panel A. Panel B shows opaci-
          fication of the right-sided heart after peripheral venous
          injection of 5 ml of dextrose 5% in water. Echo contrast
          is seen in the left ventricle indicating right-to-left
          shunting. The negative contrast effect proving the atrial
          septal defect is seen on panel C (arrow) when noncontrast
          blood flows from the left atrium into the right atrium.
          A bidirectional shunt is demonstrated. AP: apex; BA:
          basal; L: left; R: right; LA and RA: right and left
          atrium; LV and RV: left and right ventricle. (From
          Roelandt J et al: Contrast echocardiography: clinical
          applications. Verh Dtsch Ges Herz u Kreislaufforschg
          47: 185-192, 1981)

appears that routine cardiac catheterization is presently being
displaced from its dominant role for the preoperative assessment
of patients with congenital and valvular heart disease.[27] Refinements of the technique will further increase its role in the
diagnosis and management of cardiac patients.

REFERENCES

1. I. Edler, Ch. Hertz, Use of ultrasonic reflectoscope for
    continuous recording of movements of heart walls. Kungl
    Fysiogr Sällsk Forhandl (Lund) 24: 5, 1954.
2. J. Roelandt, "Practical echocardiology". Research Studies
    Press, Forest Grove, (1977).
3. H. Feigenbaum, "Echocardiography". 3rd Edn, Lea & Febiger,
    Philadelphia, (1981).
4. A. J. Tajik, J. B. Seward, D. J. Hagler, D. D. Mair, J. T.
    Lie, Two-dimensional real time ultrasonic imaging of the
    heart and great vessels. Technique, Image Orientation,
    Structure identification and validation. Mayo Clin
    Proc 53: 271-303, (1978).
5. W. H. Henry, A. N. DeMaria, R. Gramiak, et al, Report of the
    American Society of Echocardiography Committee on
    Nomenclature and Standards in two-dimensional echocardi-
    ography. Circulation 60: 212-17, (1980).
6. J. W. Helak, T. Plappert, A. Muhammad, N. Reichek, Two
    dimensional echocardiographic imaging of the left ventricle:
    comparison of mechanical and phased array systems in vitro.
    Am J. Cardio 48: 728-35, (1981).
7. P. M. Nichol, B. W. Gilbert, J. A. Kisslo, Two-dimensional
    echocardiographic assessment of mitral stenosis.
    Circulation 55: 120, (1977).
8. L. S. Wann, A. E. Weyman, H. Feigenbaum, J. C. Dillon, K. W.
    Johnston, R. C. Eggleton, Determination of mitral valve
    area by cross-sectional echocardiography. Ann Intern Med
    88: 337, (1978).
9. L. W. Eaton, J. L. Weiss, B. H. Bulkley, J. B. Garrison, M. L.
    Weisfeldt, Regional cardiac dilatation after acute myo-
    cardial infarction: recognition by two-dimensional echo-
    cardiography. New Engl J. Med 300: 57-62, (1979).
10. H. L. Wyatt, M. K. Heng, S. Meerbaum, R. Davidson, E. Corday,
    Evaluation of models for quantifying ventricular size by
    two-dimensional echocardiography. Amer J. Cardiol 41: 369,
    (1978)(abstract).
11. L. W. Eaton, W. L. Maughan, A. A. Shoukas, J. L. Weiss,
    Accurate volume determination in the isolated ejecting
    canine left ventricle by two-dimensional echocardiography.
    Circulation 60: 320-26, (1979).

12. K. W. Carr, R. L. Engler, J. R. Forsythe, Measurement of left ventricular ejection fraction by mechanical cross sectional echocardiography. Circulation 59: 1196-1206, (1979).

13. W. Bommer, L. Weinert, A. Neumann, J. Neff, D. T. Mason, A. N. DeMaria, Determination of right atrial and right ventricular size by two-dimensional echocardiography. Circulation 60: 91-100, (1979).

14. N. B. Schiller, H. Acquatella, T. A. Ports, et al, Left ventricular volume from paired biplane two-dimensional echocardiography. Circulation 60: 547-555, (1979).

15. E. D. Folland, A. F. Parisi, P. F. Moynihan, D. R. Jones, C. L. Feldman, D. E. Tow, Assessment of left ventricular ejection fraction and volumes by real-time, two-dimensional echocardiography: a comparison of cineangiographic and radio-nuclide techniques. Circulation 60: 760-66 (1979).

16. A. S. Pearlman, J. G. Stevenson, D. W. Baker, Doppler echocardiography: applications, limitations and future directions. Amer J Cardiol 46: 1256-62, (1980).

17. R. S. Meltzer, E. G. Tickner, T. P. Sahines, R. L. Popp, The source of ultrasonic contrast effect. J. Clin Ultra-sound 8: 121-7, (1980).

18. J. Roelandt, R. S. Meltzer, P. W. Serruys, Contrast echo-cardiography of the left ventricle. In Meltzer R. S. and Roelandt J (editors), "Contrast Echocardiography", Martinus Nijhoff, The Hague, (1982), p. 72-85.

19. D. R. Pieroni, J. Varghese, R. M. Freedom, R. D. Rowe, The sensitivity of contrast echocardiography in detecting intra-cardiac shunts. Cathet Cardiovasc Diagn 5: 19, (1979).

20. R. S. Meltzer, D. Van Hoogenhuyze, P. W. Serruys, M. M. P. Haalebos, P. G. Hugenholtz, J. Roelandt, Diagnosis of tricuspid regurgitation by contrast echocardiography. Circulation 63: 1093-99, (1981).

21. R. E. Kerber, J. M. Kioschos, R. M. Lauer, Use of ultrasonic contrast method in the diagnosis of valvular regurgitation and intracardiac shunts. Am J Cardiol 34:722, (1974).

22. A. Reale, F. Pizzuto, P. A. Gioffré, A. Nigri, F. Romeo, E. Martuscelli, E. Mangier, G. Scibilia, Contrast echocardi-ography: transmission of echoes to the left heart across the pulmonary vascular bed. Europ Heart J 1: 101, (1980).

23. W. Bommer, J. Neef, A. Naumann, L. Weinert, G. Lee, D. T. Mason, A. N. DeMaria, Indicator-dilution curves obtained by photometric analysis of two-dimensional echocontrast studies. Am J Cardiol 41: 370, (1978) (abstract).

24. D. J. Hagler, A. J. Tajik, K. B. Seward, D. D. Mair, D. G. Ritter, E. L. Ritman, Videodensitometric quantitation of left-to-right shunts with contrast sector echocardiography. Circulation 57-58 (suppl 11): 11-70, (1978)(abstract).

25. J. L. Weiss, M. L. Weisfeldt, S. J. Mason, J. B. Garrison, S. V. Livengood, N. J. Fortuin, Evidence of Frank-Starling effect in man during severe semisupine exercise. Circulation 59: 655-661, (1979).

26. L. S. Wann, J. V. Paris, R. H. Childress, J. C. Dillon, A. E.
     Weyman, H. Feigenbaum, Exercise cross-sectional echo-
     cardiography in ischemic heart disease. Circulation 60:
     1300-8 (1979).
27. M. G. St John Sutton, M. St. John Sutton, P. Oldershaw, R.
     Sacchetti, M. Paneth, S. C. Lennox, R. V. Gibson, D. G.
     Gibson, Valve replacement without preoperative cardiac
     catheterization. New Engl J Med 305: 1233, (1982).
28. J. Roelandt, R. S. Meltzer, P. W. Serruys. Contrast echocardi-
     ography of the left ventricle. In Rijsterborgh H (ed),
     "Echocardiology", Martinus Nijhoff, The Hague, (1981), p. 219.

HIGH BLOOD CHOLESTEROL AND HIGH BLOOD PRESSURE:
STATE OF KNOWLEDGE TODAY AND IMPLICATIONS FOR PREVENTION
AND CONTROL OF EPIDEMIC ADULT CARDIOVASCULAR DISEASE

Jeremiah Stamler

Department of Community Health and Preventive Medicine
Northwestern University Medical School
Chicago, Illinois, U.S.A.

INTRODUCTION

This presentation aims to review the key data sets on the role
of elevated serum cholesterol and elevated blood pressure in the
production of mass premature coronary heart disease (CHD). Its purpose is to set down the information needed by the health professions
and the general public to act effectively in the growing effort to
control the contemporary CHD epidemic in the industrialized countries
and to prevent its emergence in the developing countries. To aid
in accomplishing this objective, a most useful document is the just
published report of the World Health Organization Expert Committee
on the Prevention of Coronary Heart Disease[1]. This document sum-
marizes current knowledge on these matters and on that basis presents
an effective strategy for the health services and the general public
for the effort to control this epidemic. (For an extensive review
of the research literature in this field - i.e., the scientific basis
of the preventive effort - see also the recently published Volume 2
of the Report of the Working Group on Arteriosclerosis of the U.S.
National Heart, Lung, and Blood Institute[2].

THE STRATEGIC·IMPORTANCE OF PRIMARY PREVENTION

First, a set of data dealing with the very important question
of why a strategy emphasizing primary prevention - the prevention
of the first CHD episode - is crucial for control of this disease
(Figure 1)[3,4]. These are data from five major long-term prospective
studies of populations in the United States, the Pooling Project
study, involving 7,545 men originally aged 30 to 59, free at baseline of evidence of definite CHD and followed for almost 10 years.

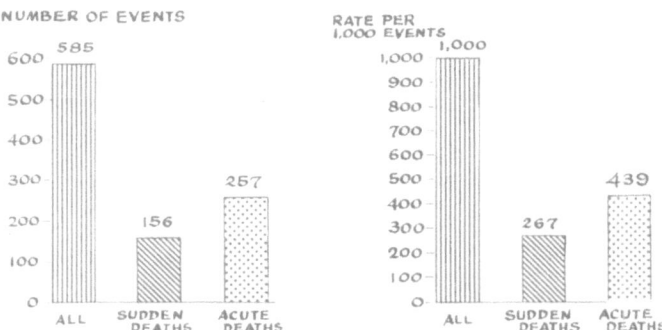

Fig. 1.   U.S. national cooperative Pooling Project; sudden death
          and acute mortality with first major coronary events, men
          age 30-59 at entry, pooled data from five studies, ex-
          perience over the first 10 years of follow-up; first major
          coronary events were definite non-fatal myocardial in-
          farction, sudden (≤3 hours) coronary death, non-sudden
          coronary death (>3 hours-1 month)[3,4].

There were 585 first major coronary events during that time, of
which more than a quarter (27%) were sudden deaths, and another 17%
were non-sudden deaths with this first episode. (Sudden death was
defined as observed death within 3 hours of onset of sickness in
people previously well and without a history of definite CHD). Al-
together, 44% of these first coronary episodes ended in death, in
these men originally age 30 to 59, a typical experience with this
disease all over the world[5]. About 70% of the deaths occur so rapidly that no medical care can be brought to bear and there is not
time for hospitalization. For the 56% surviving the first attack,
risk of dying in the next five years is increased about five times
compared to similar men without a history of such an event, with
most of the excess risk due to CHD, and with almost half the deaths
being sudden death.

     These data not only emphasize that this is a grim and difficult
disease. More relevant practically, they also make the point that
if we are to make major progress against a disease with this natural
history, the fundamental strategic emphasis must be on primary prevention. Note that this is also fully in keeping with the lessons
from past control of mass disease. The triumphs against infectious
disease and against under-nutritional disease were achieved first
and foremost by primary prevention, prevention of the disease from
ever developing, based on approaches from infancy on, often long
before people reached the stage of life when the mass occurrences of
the diseases take place.

The second point I want to make on this matter is an elaboration of the remarks made by Finn Monahan on the roots of epidemic disease. Over a hundred years ago, one of the great founders of modern medicine – Rudolph Virchow – pointed out that when disease occurs at very high epidemic rates, this is due to, "... disturbances of human culture"[6]. In the case of CHD and the other atherosclerotic diseases afflicting both the middle-aged and the elderly in the industrialized countries at epidemic rates, the disturbances of human culture are mainly the "rich" diets, the cigarette smoking habit, the sedentary life-style all so widely prevalent in these countries in the second half of the 20th century, for the first time in human history. The consequence is that the major atherosclerotic disease risk factors, including high blood cholesterol and high blood pressure, are present at very high levels throughout the population, assuring the mass occurrence of these diseases.

SERUM CHOLESTEROL

Extensive data on the relationship of serum cholesterol to CHD risk are available both from studies comparing different populations (inter- or cross-population studies) and within-population studies. Figure 2 is from the invaluable Seven Countries Study of 16 cohorts in northern Europe (Finland, Netherlands), southern Europe (Italy, Greece, Yugoslavia), Japan, and the U.S.A.[7]. Each cohort is a large group of men age 40-59 at baseline and free of evidence of definite CHD. Each circle in this Figure represents the population average for serum cholesterol, i.e., a group value, one for each of the 16 cohorts. As is evident, the northern European groups had high mean values of serum cholesterol (especially the East Finns – about 270 mg/dl), as did the Americans, and high CHD rates. In contrast, the southern European and especially the Japanese cohorts had much lower mean cholesterol values and lower CHD rates. The relationship between population mean serum cholesterol and risk of fatal CHD is strong and significant statistically.

Table 1 takes us from comparisons of populations, in which the only statistic is the average for a whole population, to the situation within populations. In this case, data are again from five studies of the Pooling Project in the U.S.A.[8,9]. Each of 8,247 middle-aged men is classified – based on his entry serum cholesterol – into one of five quintiles, the lowest 20%, the next 20%, etc. From the third quintile on, the higher the serum cholesterol level, the greater the risk of a first major coronary event before age 65. Compared to men in quintiles 1 and 2, those in quintiles 3, 4, and 5 had a progressive increase in risk, of 15%, 64%, and 99% respectively. Thus, 60% of the population was at greater risk compared to the two lowest quintiles, with serum cholesterol values under 220 mg/dl. This clearcut relationship was registered with only one measurement, with all its limitations because of fluctuations of

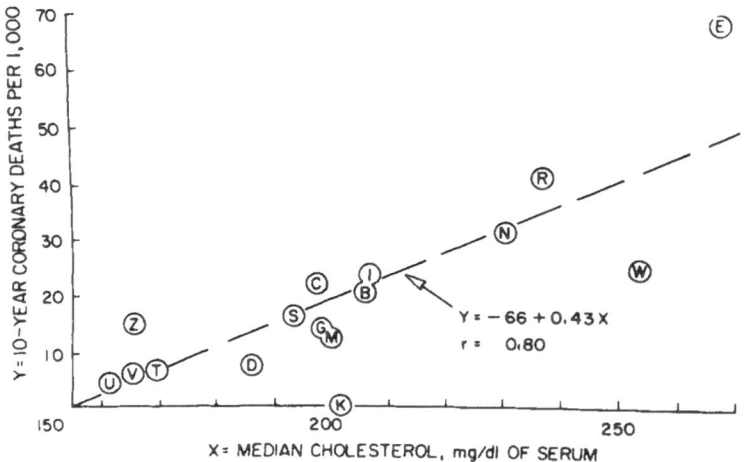

Fig. 2. Seven Countries Study; relationship between population
         cohort median serum cholesterol at entry and 10-year rate
         of coronary death; B is Belgrade faculty, Serbia, Yugoslavia;
         C is Crevalcore, Bologna Province, Italy; D is Dalmatia,
         Croatia, Yugoslavia; E is east Finland; G is Corfu, Greece;
         I is Rome-based Italian railroad workers; K is Crete, Greece;
         M is Montegiogio, Marche Region (near Ancona), Italy; N is
         Zutphen, The Netherlands; R is northwest U.S. railroad
         workers; S is Slavonia, Croatia, Yugoslavia; T is
         Tanushimaru (farming village), Kyushu, Japan; U is
         Ushibuka (fishing village), Kyushu, Japan; V is Velika
         Krsna, Serbia, Yugoslavia; W is west Finland; Z is
         Zrenjanin, Serbia, Yugoslavia[7].

individual levels and because of laboratory errors (even in research
laboratories!).

    Note the overall high risk of these American men in the 1950s
and 1960s - 221.4 chances per 1,000 of a first major coronary event
by age 65, almost 1 chance in 4, the epidemic onslaught of premature
CHD.

    Based on these data, it was possible to estimate the proportion
of all these coronary attacks attributable to hypercholesterolemia,
levels of about 220 mg/dl and above - about 25% of all attacks.

    What are key environmental factors that influence the serum
cholesterol level of populations and individuals? They are first and
foremost the components of the habitual diet, especially its fat
components. The higher the saturated fat and cholesterol in the
diet, the higher the serum cholesterol level (all else being equal),

Table 1. Serum Cholesterol and Risk of a First Major Coronary Event
Between Ages 40-64 (8,274 White Men, Pool 5, Pooling Project, Final Report)

Quintile of Level and Level (mg/dl)		Number of Events	Risk of An Event per 1,000	Relative Risk	Absolute Excess Risk per 1,000	Per Cent of all Excess
I+II	≤218	166	162.7	1.00	---	---
I	≤194	86	172.4	---	---	---
II	194-218	80	153.0	---	---	---
III	218-240	104	186.8	1.15	24.1	8.3%
IV	240-268	167	266.3	1.64	103.6	35.8%
V	>268	210	324.1	1.99	161.4	55.8%
ALL		647	222.4	---	---	---

$$\frac{QIII-QV \text{ Excess Events, } 3,000 \text{ Men}}{All \text{ Events, } 5,000 \text{ Men}} = \frac{289.1}{1,112.0} = 25.6\%,$$
of all events are excess events, attributable to
hypercholesterolemia.

as well illustrated in the data from the Seven Countries Study*
(Figure 3, upper)[7]. (In contrast, dietary polyunsaturated fat has
a modest serum cholesterol lowering effect). And the higher the
saturated fat and cholesterol in the diet of populations, the greater
their coronary risk (Figure 3, lower)[7]. This is true also for individuals within a population[10]. In addition, diets low in fiber, as
well as high in cholesterol and saturated fat, tend to be associated
with high serum cholesterol levels.

Correspondingly, changes in diet pattern - with sizeable decrease in saturated fat and cholesterol intake, moderate increase in
intake of polyunsaturated fat and fiber (particularly of the pectin
and gum types, from fruits and from legumes) - produces marked reduction in serum total cholesterol and its most atherogenic fraction
(LDL-cholesterol) and in serum triglycerides, with little change in

---

*Dietary cholesterol was not measured in the Seven Countries Study.
However, extensive data from other epidemiologic studies, from
controlled nutritional experiments in man, and from animal research,
indicate its important influence on serum cholesterol and risk of
atherosclerotic disease[2].

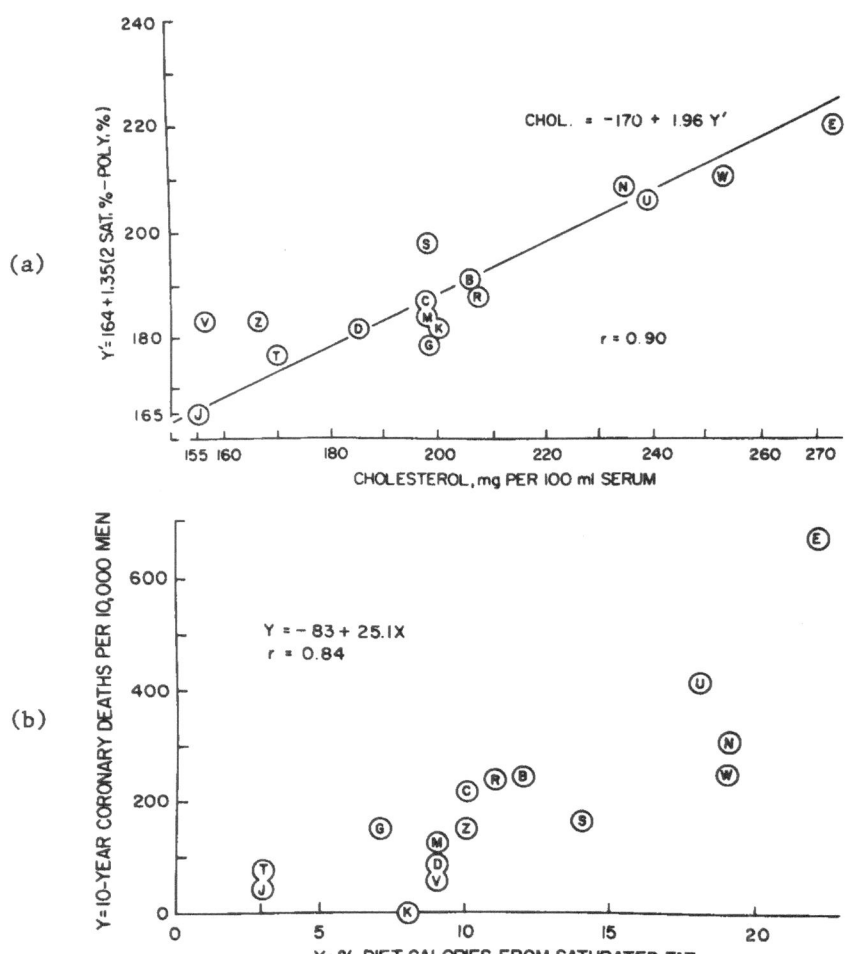

Fig. 3.   Seven Countries Study; upper graph: relationship between
          population cohort mean intake of dietary saturated fat and
          polyunsaturated fat as per cent of total calories, and
          median serum cholesterol level at entry; lower graph:
          relationship between population cohort mean per cent of
          total calories from saturated fat at entry and 10-year
          rate of coronary death; for identification of the cohorts[7],
          see legend for Figure 2.

the putatively protective fractions (HDL and HDL_2). These changes
are well illustrated by the findings with Diet C of the recent study
on Dutch monks (Table 2)[11]. Note that the fall in serum total

Table 2. Diet Composition and Change in Serum Lipids-Lipoproteins
          Controlled Experiment, 12 Healthy Dutch Monks

Nutrient	Reference Diet A	Fat-Modified Diet B	High-Fiber Fat-Modified Diet C
Protein-% Cal.	14	14	14
Vegetable Protein-% Protein	34	34	52
Fat-% Cal.	40	27	27
Polyunsaturates-% Cal.	5.2	8.5	8.7
Saturates-% Cal.	19.3	8.4	8.7
Cholesterol-mg/2,500 Cal.$^\Delta$	617	245	252
Available Carbohydrate-% Cal.[+]	46	59	59
Fiber-g/2,500 Cal.$^\Delta$	19	20	55
Pectin-g/2,500 Cal.$^\Delta$	1.2	1.8	6.3

Serum Lipid-Lipoprotein- Per Cent Change	Reference Diet A	Fat-Modified Diet B	High-Fiber Fat-Modified Diet C
Total Cholesterol	----	-21.6%	-29.2%
LDL Cholesterol	----	-26.5%	-34.5%
HDL Cholesterol	----	-12.0%	-10.6%
HDL$_2$ Cholesterol	----	-34.6%	-11.5%
Total Triglycerides	----	0.0%	-20.8%
VLDL Triglycerides	----	+ 4.8%	-19.0%
Ratios			
Total Chol./HDL Chol.	4.49	4.02	3.56
LDL Chol./HDL$_2$ Chol.	17.7	19.9	13.1

$^\Delta$Energy intake varied from 1,550 to 4,250 Cal/day.
[+]Mono- and di-saccharides contributed 18-20% of calories.

cholesterol was a substantial 29%; in LDL-cholesterol, 34%. Corresponding results were obtained in a Boston study of a population
group eating a predominantly vegetarian diet low in animal products
(Table 3)[12].

   Figure 4 illustrates - from the experience of the Framingham
population - the effect of caloric balance on serum cholesterol
(and glucose, uric acid, and blood pressure as well)[13]. Caloric

Table 3. Serum Cholesterol and Lipoprotein Levels in "Macrobiotic"
          Vegetarians and Controls in Boston

Group	Serum Cholesterol-mg/dl				Weight kg.
	Total	LDL	VLDL	HDL	
115 Controls	184±37	118±34	17.2±11.0	49±12	73±15
115 Vegetarians	126±30	73±24	11.8± 7.0	43±11	58± 9
Mean Difference	58±48***	45±44***	5.4±13.3***	6±15***	15±16***
% Difference	−31.5%	−38.1%	−31.4%	−12.2%	−20.5%
Mean Difference△	55±53***	39±46***	4.6±14.4*	9±17**	0± 9

△Weight matched pairs − N = 42.
*   p≤.05
** p≤.01
***p≤.001

balance is, of course, a resultant of both diet and physical activity.
With weight gain, especially on a diet high in saturated fat and
cholesterol, serum cholesterol rises; with weight loss on an ordinary or a fat-reduced diet, it falls. The changes can be sizeable,
even with modest changes in weight. The Multiple Risk Factor Intervention Trial demonstrated this in extenso in its large group of
free-living men[14]. For obese men, weight loss of 4 to 5+ kg. on its
diet − reduced in saturated fat and cholesterol, with a moderate increase in polyunsaturated fat − was associated with favorable changes
in all plasma lipid-lipoprotein components. Plasma total cholesterol,
LDL-cholesterol, VLDL-cholesterol, total triglycerides, VLDL-tri-
glycerides all fell sizeably, and HDL rose. The MRFIT progressive
eating pattern emphasized delectable fare based upon Mediterranean
and Far Eastern cuisine, with concomitant attention to dietary fat
composition and level, fiber intake from fruits and vegetables,
grains and legumes, and moderation in sodium intake.

    Is it possible by dietary means to influence the occurrence of
atherosclerotic disease, i.e., severe atherosclerosis of the coronary, cerebral, trunk, and peripheral arteries? In the first decade
of this century, Anitschkow working as a young man with colleagues
in Petrograd demonstrated in rabbits the relationship among dietary
lipid (dietary cholesterol in particular), serum cholesterol, and
the atherogenic process[15]. This was a major breakthrough in experimental medicine, the basis for the great acquisition of knowledge
by animal experimentation in this field over the last 70 years.
Anitschkow was probably the first scientist to demonstrate that with

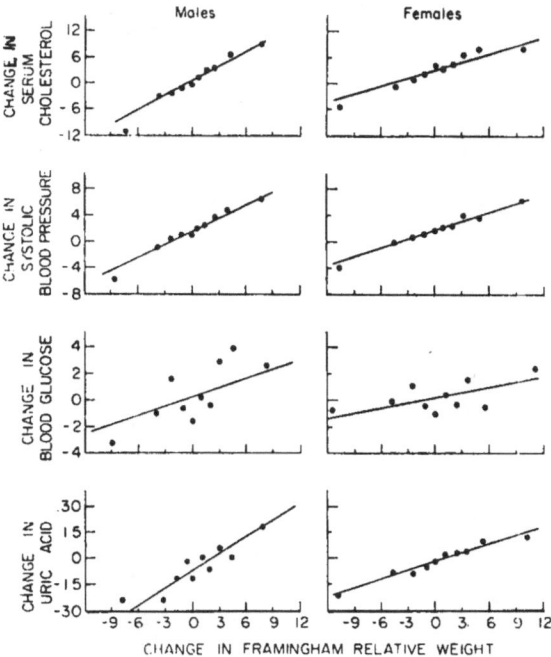

Fig. 4. Framingham Heart Study; relationship between change over time in relative weight and change in serum cholesterol, systolic blood pressure, blood glucose, serum uric acid[13].

cessation of cholesterol-fat feeding, and consequent restoration of low normal serum cholesterol in animals, atherosclerotic lesions regressed. Figure 5 illustrates this phenomenon, from a modern classic experiment in monkeys[16]. For 18 months a diet high in egg yolk (hence high in dietary cholesterol) was fed, and sustained hypercholesterolemia was thereby induced. One-third of the animals were sacrificed to study the resultant atherosclerosis and narrowing of the coronary arteries (upper 4 frames, Figure 5). The two-thirds of the animals remaining alive were then taken off this atherogenic diet and were maintained for 40 months on a diet low in saturated fat and free of cholesterol, so that the serum cholesterol was quickly restored to low normal levels. As is evident from the lower six frames of Figure 5, after these 40 months marked reversal of lesions took place and the coronary arteries opened up, with only minimal residual thickening of the arterial walls. Another study in monkeys, recently completed, showed that such regression of lesions can be achieved if the serum cholesterol is brought down to a level of about 200 mg/dl, but regression does not take place at 300 md/dl[17]. (Figure 6 and Table 4). Thus, the disease is not only preventable by nutritional means but is also within limits reversible.

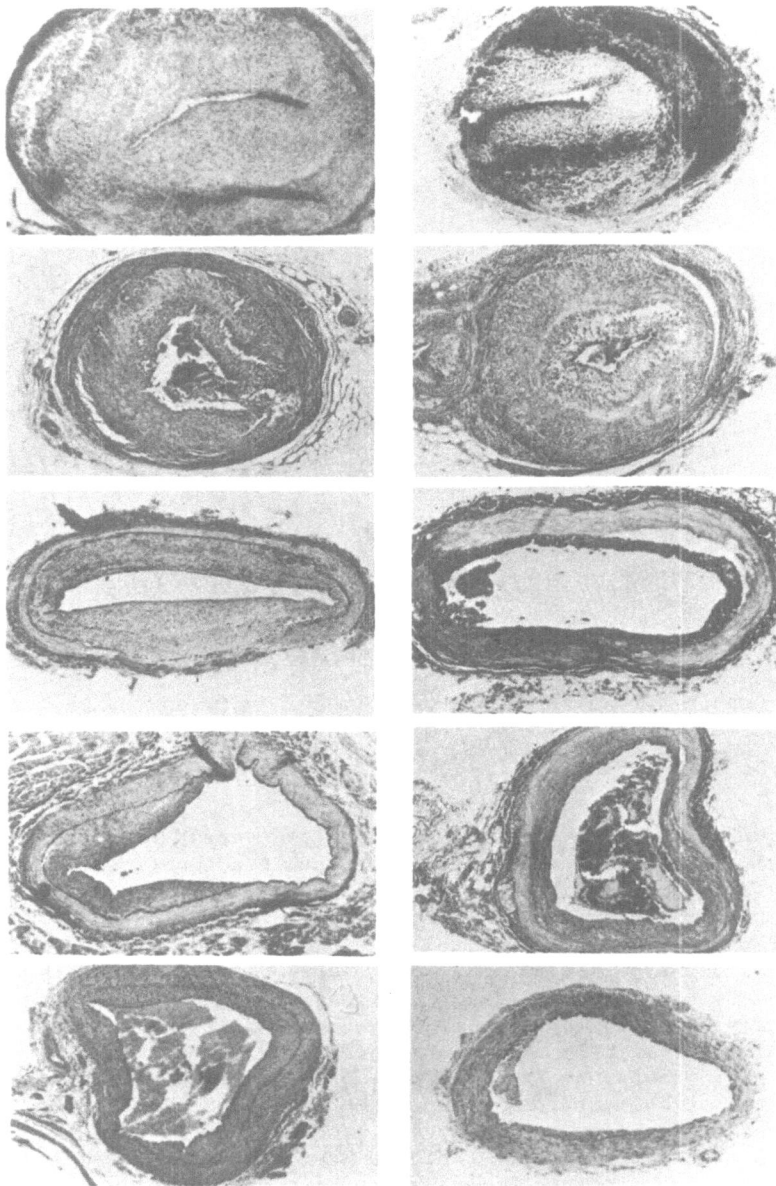

Fig. 5.   Experiment on regression of coronary atherosclerosis in
          male rhesus monkeys; upper 2 rows (4 figures) - coronary
          atherosclerosis after 18 months on a high-cholesterol diet
          from egg yolk; lower 3 rows (6 figures) - regression of
          atherosclerosis 40 months after cessation of feeding of the
          high-cholesterol diet[16].

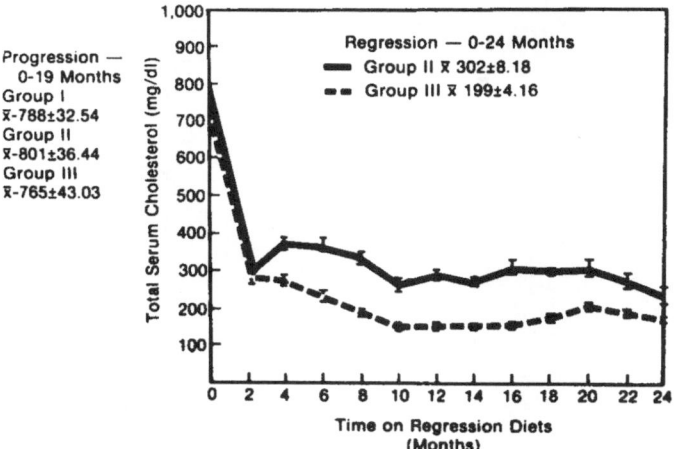

Fig. 6.   Experiment on regression of atherosclerosis in macaca
          mulatta monkeys; mean serum cholesterol concentration
          after 19 months of feeding an atherogenic diet high in
          cholesterol and fat, and over the next 24 months, for
          Groups II and III, fed diets to yield mean serum chol-
          esterol levels of approximately 300 mg/dl and 200 mg/dl
          respectively[17].

Table 4.   Primate Regression Study Coronary Atherosclerosis

Group	Stenosis %	Fat %	Medial Damage %	IEL Damage %
I	25±5.2	41±3.9	40±8.0	25±5.8
II (Chol 300)	35±4.7	20±2.9	37±5.3	22±3.5
III (Chol 200)	17±4.2	6±1	20±5.4	17±4.1

Data are available on the human species supporting this thesis,
although such data are much more difficult to obtain. Figure 7 illustrates such findings from an important study of 846 American men
in late middle-age, residing in a home for veterans in Los Angeles[18].
The data are on the incidence in 8.5 years of major atherosclerotic

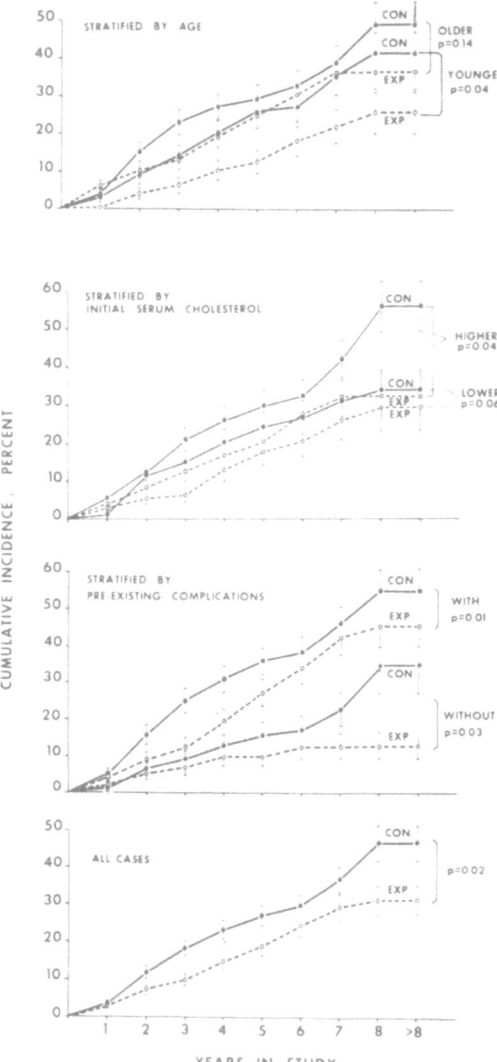

Fig. 7.   Los Angeles Veterans Administration Domiciliary Facility
          double blind trial on dietary fat modification to reduce
          serum cholesterol and atherosclerotic disease; cumulative
          incidence rates over 8.5 years in experimental and control
          groups overall (bottom graph), and stratified by entry age
          (top graph), entry serum cholesterol level (graph 2nd from
          top), and entry findings with respect to clinical evidence
          of atherosclerotic disease; the incidence end point was a
          combination of "hard" atherosclerotic disease events, in-
          cluding coronary death, definite non-fatal myocardial in-
          farction, definite cerebral infarction[18].

disease events, fatal and non-fatal, involving chiefly the heart and brain, in two groups – one eating a usual American diet, the other a fat-modified diet, reduced in cholesterol and saturated fat, increased in polyunsaturated fat, with a resultant reduction in serum cholesterol of about 10 to 15% over the years. Overall there was a statistically significant 34% reduction in the incidence of the major atherosclerotic diseases (lowest frame, Figure 7), even though these men were already rather elderly – median age 65.5 years – when the study began. Benefit was more clearcut and greater for the 50% of men under 65.5 years at entry (top frame, Figure 7) and for men hypercholesterolemic at entry (2nd frame, Figure 7). Both those without and with clinical evidence of atherosclerotic disease at entry benefitted, i.e., there was significant achievement in both primary and secondary prevention (although not in regard to all causes of mortality).

Table 5 presents similar positive findings from the primary prevention study in Oslo (Norway), for men age 40-49 at entry. This study involved both diet intervention for these markedly hypercholesterolemic (normotensive) men and an effort to achieve cessation of cigarette smoking[19]. Over the five years of the trial, the intervention group had a serum cholesterol level 42.6 mg/dl (13.0%) lower than the controls, and a greater degree of weight reduction by 3 kg. Of the intervention group, 31% quit smoking cigarettes; of the controls, 19%. No differences in blood pressure were recorded. Incidence of CHD and all cardiovascular diseases was markedly lower in the intervention group compared to the controls, by over 40%, and striking positive results were also obtained in regard to death rates[19]. (Table 5). Thus, as difficult as it is to acquire accurate information on ability to prevent atherosclerotic disease in man (properly designed and executed large-scale randomized controlled trials are very complex undertakings), meaningful results are indeed available, and they support all the other sets of data – from observational epidemiology, clinical medicine, autopsy studies, and animal experimentation – on the relationship among diet, serum cholesterol, and atherosclerotic disease.

BLOOD PRESSURE

Figure 8, again from the Seven Countries Study, shows the independent relationship of blood pressure, in addition to serum cholesterol, in contributing to differences across populations in risk of premature CHD[7]. Again, each population is treated as a single unit. The higher levels of both blood pressure and serum cholesterol at baseline for the northern European and U.S. population samples play a key role, in an additive way, in accounting for their much higher 10-year CHD death rates, compared to the Greek, Italian, Yugoslav, and Japanese cohorts. Measured only once at the outset of this prospective epidemiologic study, these two factors by themselves explain a good deal of the differences in CHD risk among the populations.

Table 5.   5-Year Intervention Results, Oslo Trial

End Point	Intervention Group-604 Men		Control Group 628 Men		% Difference*	p Value
Coronary heart disease incidence	19$^\Delta$	31.5°	36	57.3	-45.0%	.028
Cardiovascular disease incidence	22	36.4	39	62.1	-41.4%	.038
Sudden CHD mortality	3	5.0	11	17.5	-71.4%	.024
Coronary heart disease mortality	6	9.9	14	22.3	-55.6%	.086
All cardiovascular disease mortality	8	13.2	15	23.9	-44.8%	.168
Cancer mortality	5	8.3	8	12.7	-34.6%	---
All mortality	16	26.5	24	38.2	-30.6%	.246

$$*\frac{\text{Intervention group rate minus control group rate}}{\text{Control group rate}} \times 100$$

As to the effect of blood pressure on the risk of individuals within a population, Table 6 gives representative data, again from the national cooperative Pooling Project in the U.S.A., again with combined findings from five long-term studies, with the population divided into quintiles based on the entry diastolic pressure reading[8,9]. Again, there are the limitations of only one measurement. Nevertheless, diastolic pressure is highly related to long-term CHD risk (as is also systolic pressure). Even for men with diastolic readings in the 80 to 88 mm Hg range (quintile 3), usually regarded as normal for middle-aged men, there is already a 42% increase in risk of a first major coronary event by age 65. Given such findings, it seems wise to begin designating such levels as not simply normal, but at the very least, as what we are now calling high-normal. As one goes further up the scale of diastolic pressure, to 90 and over, risk increases progressively. Again, a simple calculation leads to the estimate that over 30% of all cases of heart attack in this middle-aged U.S. population of men in the 1950s and 1960s were attributable to levels of blood pressure above the optimal. Note that such elevated levels were recorded at baseline for 60% of the population (quintiles 3, 4, and 5). This is not a minority phenomenon. Almost 40% of these men had frankly elevated or hypertensive readings, based on the currently accepted medical standard of 90+ mm Hg diastolic.

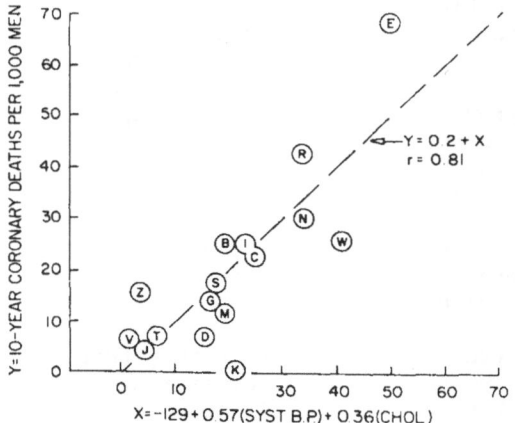

Fig. 8. Seven Countries Study; relationship between population
cohort average values for systolic blood pressure and
serum cholesterol at entry, and 10-year rate of coronary
death; for identification of the cohorts[7], see legend
for Figure 2.

Table 6. Diastolic Pressure and Risk of a First Major Coronary
Event between Ages 40-64 (8,381 White Men, Pool 5, Pooling
Project, Final Report)

Quintile of Level and Level (mmHg)	Number of Events	Risk of An Event Per 1,000	Relative Risk	Absolute Excess Risk Per 1,000	Per Cent of all Excess
1+11 ≤80	182	149.7	1.00	---	---
1 <76	91	162.6	---	---	---
11 76-80	91	136.7	---	---	---
111 80-88	126	212.4	1.42	62.7	18.1%
1V 88-94	142	239.7	1.60	90.0	26.0%
V ≥94	208	343.5	2.29	193.8	55.9%
ALL	658	223.0	---	---	---

$$\frac{\text{Q111-QV Excess Events, 3,000 Men}}{\text{All Events, 5,000 Men}} = \frac{346.5}{1,094.9} = 31.6\%$$

of all events are excess events, attributable to elevated
blood pressure.

What makes high blood pressure so common in our populations? Table 7 gives typical data on one important trait that has repeatedly been shown to be related to occurrence of elevated pressure, namely overweight[20,21]. This is the case for older and younger, men and women, all ethnic groups, persons with and without a positive family history of high blood pressure. Prospective studies - e.g., as illustrated in Figure 4 above[13] - confirm that overweight and weight gain are indeed associated with increased risk of developing high blood pressure, for persons originally normotensive. Thus, a major risk factor for high blood pressure is overweight, and one key strategic aspect of improving blood pressure levels of populations is the prevention and control of overweight.

Figure 9 illustrates the role of another trait influencing prevalence of high blood pressure in the population, i.e., level of sodium intake[22]. Again, this is a modifiable aspect of modern human eating habits.

Another trait that is a predictor of high blood pressure is a rapid heart rate[23]. This too is amenable to influence by regular frequent rhythmic (isotonic) exercise to improve cardiopulmonary fitness.

Another important trait related to prevalence and incidence of high blood pressure is heavy consumption of alcohol - 50 or 60 or more grams of alcohol per day (4, 5, or more drinks per day), irrespective of type (beer, wine, whiskey, vodka, etc.)[24]. (Table 8).

Table 7. Family History of Hypertension, Weight and Prevalence of Hypertension by Age, Chec Screening, One Million Americans, 1973-5

Weight	Family History	Age-Averaged Prevalence of Hypertension[Δ] per 1,000	
		Age 20-39	Age 40-64
Normal	Positive	82.8	309.4
	Negative	46.7	181.7
	P/N[†]	1.84	2.02
Overweight	Positive	182.4	443.5
	Negative	118.2	293.2
	P/N[†]	1.66	1.92

[Δ]DBP$\geq$95 mmHg or reported current use of antihypertensive medication.
[†]$P_1 (1,000.0 - P_2)/P_2(1,000.0 - P_1)$

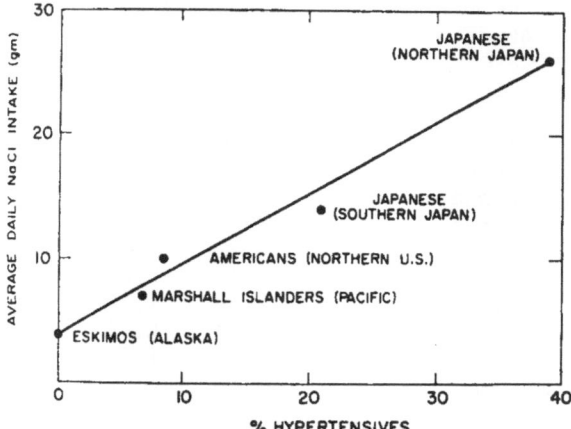

Fig. 9. Relationship between population average daily sodium
         chloride intake and prevalence of hypertension, based
         on data from 5 populations[22].

Finally, as illustrated in regard to serum cholesterol, so in
regard to high blood pressure, it is possible to control or prevent
the development of high blood pressure[25] (Table 9). This can be
achieved by safe nutritional-hygienic means - without drugs - in
many people with high-normal or already frankly elevated blood
pressure levels, by reduction of weight, moderation of sodium intake,
improvement of physical fitness by regular rhythmic exercise, and
control of alcohol intake. For many of those who are frankly hypertensive, of course, it may also be necessary to use modern pharmacologic treatment for the long-term control of high blood pressure.
And recent trials have shown that it is indeed possible to improve
prognosis in regard to death from all causes and from the major
cardiovascular diseases by such treatment, both for those with so-
called "mild" and for those with more marked hypertension[26-28].

In summary, there is a great deal of information available on
the contribution of hypercholesterolemia and hypertension to risk
of coronary heart disease and the other atherosclerotic diseases.
There is also much information available on the main aspects of life
style of populations that influence these two traits. There is also
now considerable information on the ability to apply all that knowledge to prevent these traits from developing in the first place,
or to control them if already present - and the utility of these
approaches for control of epidemic atherosclerotic disease. In a
number of countries this knowledge is being progressively applied.
There is good reason to believe that the favorable changes in life

Table 8. Per Cent with High Blood Pressure Among Problem
          Drinkers and Non-Problem Drinkers

Chicago Peoples Gas Company
1233 White Males Age 40-59 in 1958

Variable	Problem Drinkers N = 38	Non-Problem Drinkers N = 1195	t	Adjusted* t
SBP ≥ 140	55.3	33.1	2.85	2.92
SBP ≥ 160	18.4	10.7	1.50	1.68
DBP ≥ 90	34.2	20.4	2.06	2.66
DBP ≥ 95	15.8	9.1	1.39	1.95

Chicago Western Electric Company
1899 White Males Age 40-55 in 1957

Variable	Heavy Drinkers N = 117	Non-Heavy Drinkers N = 1782	t	Adjusted* t
SBP ≥ 140	59.0	36.9	4.75	4.30
SBP ≥ 160	28.2	11.7	5.18	4.66
DBP ≥ 90	64.1	42.1	4.65	4.27
DBP ≥ 95	40.2	20.4	5.02	4.75

*Adjusted by analysis of covariance for age, serum chol-
 esterol, pulse, relative weight, and cigarettes/day.

style and medical care that have resulted are related to recent declines in CHD and stroke mortality, and all causes mortality as well.
That is, the trail has been blazed indicating that prevention of
these diseases is possible in the population as a whole.

Acknowledgements

It is a pleasure to express thanks to research colleagues and
their publishers for permission to reproduce published findings here,
including M. L. Armstrong, T. B. Clarkson, S. Dayton, I. Hjermann,
A. Keys, B. Lewis, M. L. Pearce, and F. M. Sacks; colleagues of the
U.S. national cooperative Pooling Project, H. Blackburn, J. M.
Chapman, T. R. Dawber, J. T. Doyle, F. H. Epstein, W. B. Kannel,
A. Keys, F. E. Moore, O. Paul, and H. L. Taylor; American Heart
Association, American Heart Journal, Archives Internal Medicine,
Circulation, Circulation Research, Experimental and Molecular
Pathology, Harvard University Press, Journal of the American Medical

Table 9. Sequential Mean Changes in Weight, Relative Weight, Pulse Rate, Blood Pressure and Serum Cholesterol, Nondropouts, Not on Antihypertensive Drugs, Chicago Coronary Preventive Evaluation Program

Years in CPEP	No.of Men	ΔWeight lbs.°	ΔRelative Weight	ΔPulse Rate beats/min.	ΔSystolic Pressure mm Hg	ΔDiastolic Pressure mm Hg	ΔSerum Cholesterol mg/dl
Men with Last Baseline Diastolic Pressure ≥ 90 mm Hg							
1	115	-11.9***	-7.9***	-3.1***	-11.5***	-8.1***	-28.1***
3	99	-10.1***	-6.7***	-2.5*	-12.5***	-8.6***	-22.8***
5	96	-8.4***	-5.5***	-5.1***	-10.8***	-8.0***	-21.8***
7	65	-8.1***	-5.4***	-3.6*	-13.4***	-9.7***	-23.2***
9	35	-6.3***	-4.4***	-3.9	-11.8***	-12.6***	-25.3*
Baseline Value 115 Men	---	197.3	129.6	81.2	147.7	96.3	248.5
Men with Last Baseline Diastolic Pressure 80-89 mm Hg							
1	101	-10.6***	-7.1***	-2.3**	-7.9***	-4.4***	-22.4***
3	97	-9.8***	-6.5***	-3.5***	-7.3***	-4.0***	-14.7***
5	89	-7.7***	-5.1***	-3.2**	-7.0***	-3.3***	-12.8***
7	72	-6.7***	-4.4***	-2.7**	-2.8*	-3.1***	-13.7***
9	46	-8.4***	-5.5***	-3.5*	+0.1	-3.0*	-7.2
Baseline Value 101 Men	---	189.9	126.2	78.1	131.5	82.9	259.5

*p≤.05 **p≤.01 ***p≤.001   Δis "Change in". °Relative Weight is the ratio of observed weight to desirable weight for height and sex, from the 1959 actuarial data[6,18].

Association, Journal of Chronic Diseases, The Lancet, and New England Journal of Medicine. It is also a pleasure to acknowledge the contribution to the research reported here from our group of colleagues working with the author, particularly D. M. Berskon, A. Dyer, E. Farinaro, Y. Hall, M. H. Lepper, H. A. Lindberg, K. Liu, J. Marquardt, D. Moss, L. M. Mojonnier, R. B. Shekelle, R. Stamler, and E. Stevens. Many Chicago organizations have over the years given invaluable cooperation in the cited research efforts, particularly the Chicago Health Department, the Chicago Heart Association, Peoples Gas Light and Coke Company (Peoples Energy Company), Western Electric Company, American Oil Company, Arthur Andersen and Company, Armour and Company, Internal Revenue Service, International Harvester Company, Newspaper Division of the Field Enterprises.

The research of our group reported here was supported by the American Heart Association; Chicago Heart Association; National Heart, Lung, and Blood Institute; Best Foods Institute of Nutrition; Chicago Health Research Foundation; Ciba-Geigy Corporation; Standard Brands (Nabisco Brands); National Dairy Council; the Upjohn Company; the Wesson Company.

REFERENCES

1. WHO Expert Committee on the Prevention of Coronary Heart Disease. Prevention of Coronary Heart Disease - Report of a WHO Expert Committee, World Health Organization, Geneva, Switzerland, Technical Report Series 678 (1982).
2. Working Group on Arteriosclerosis of the National Heart, Lung, and Blood Institute, Report of the Working Group on Arteriosclerosis of the National Heart, Lung, and Blood Institute, Vol.2, U.S. Department of Health and Human Services, Public Health Service, National Institutes of Health, NIH Publication No. 81-2035, Bethesda, MD, September 1981.
3. Inter-Society Commission for Heart Disease Resources. Atherosclerosis Study Group and Epidemiology Study Group. Primary Prevention of the Atherosclerotic Diseases, Circulation, 42:A55-A95 (1970). Revised April 1972.
4. H. Blackburn, J. Chapman, T. R. Dawber, J. T. Doyle, F. H. Epstein, W. B. Kannel, A. Keys, F. Moore, O. Paul, J. Stamler, and H. L. Taylor, Revised Data for 1970 ICHD Report, Letter to the Editor, Amer.Heart J., 94:539-540 (1977).
5. WHO International Collaborative Group, WHO Regional Office for Europe, Myocardial Infarction Community Registers, Regional Office for Europe, World Health Organization, Copenhagen, Denmark (1977).
6. E. H. Ackerknecht, "Rudolf Virchow - Doctor, Statesman, Anthropologist," Madison, WI, University of Wisconsin Press (1953).
7. A. Keys, ed., "Seven Countries - A Multivariate Analysis of Death and Coronary Heart Disease," Cambridge, MA, Harvard University Press (1980).

8. Pooling Project Research Group: Relationship of blood pressure,
    serum cholesterol, smoking habit, relative weight and ECG
    abnormalities to incidence of major coronary events: Final
    report of the Pooling Project, J.Chron.Dis., 31:201-306
    (1978).

9. J. Stamler, Improved life styles: Their potential for the
    primary prevention of atherosclerosis and hypertension in
    childhood; the fat-modified diet: its nature, effectiveness,
    and safety; can an effective fat-modified diet be safely
    recommended after weaning for infants and children in general?
    "Childhood Prevention of Atherosclerosis and Hypertension,"
    Edited by R. M. Lauer and R. B. Shekelle, New York, Raven
    Press, pp 3-36, 387-403 and 407-410 (1980).

10. R. B. Shekelle, A. M. Shryock, O. Paul, M. Lepper, J. Stamler,
    S. Liu, and W. J. Raynor, Jr., Diet, serum cholesterol, and
    death from coronary heart disease - the Western Electric
    Study, N.Engl.J.Med., 304:65-70 (1981).

11. B. Lewis, M. Katan, I. Merkx, N. E. Miller, F. Hammett, R. M.
    Kay, A. Nobels, and A. V. Swan, Towards an improved lipid-
    lowering diet: additive effects of changes in nutrient in-
    take, Lancet, 2:1310-1313 (1981).

12. F. M. Sacks, W. P. Castelli, A. Donner, and E. H. Kass, Plasma
    lipids and lipoproteins in vegetarians and controls, N.Engl.
    J.Med., 292:1148-1151 (1975).

13. F. W. Ashley and W. B. Kannel, Relation of weight change to
    changes in atherogenic traits: The Framingham Study, J.Chron.
    Dis., 27:103-114 (1974).

14. A. W. Caggiula, G. Christakis, M. Farrand, S. B. Hulley, R.
    Johnson, N. Lasser, J. Stamler, and G. Widdowson, The Multiple
    Risk Factor Intervention Trial (MRFIT), IV. Intervention on
    blood lipids, Prev.Med., 10:443-475 (1981).

15. N. Anitschkow, Experimental arteriosclerosis in animals,
    "Arteriosclerosis," Edited by E. V. Cowdry, New York,
    Macmillan, pp 271-322 (1933).

16. M. L. Armstrong, E. D. Warner, and W. E. Connor, Regression of
    coronary atheromatosis in rhesus monkeys, Circ.Res., 27:
    59-67 (1970).

17. T. B. Clarkson, M. G. Bond, B. C. Bullock, and C.A. Marzetta,
    A study of atherosclerosis regression in macaca mulatta.
    IV. Changes in coronary arteries from animals with athero-
    sclerosis induced for 19 months and then regressed for 24
    or 48 months at plasma cholesterol concentrations of 300 or
    200 mg/dl, Exper.Molecular Path., 34:345-368 (1981).

18. S. Dayton, M. L. Pearce, S. Hashimoto, W. J. Dixon, and U.
    Tomiyasu, A controlled clinical trial of a diet high in un-
    saturated fat - In preventing complications of athero-
    sclerosis, Circulation, 39,40 (Suppl.2):1-63 (1969).

19. I. Hjermann, I. Holme, K. V. Byre, and P. Leren, Effect of diet
    and smoking intervention on the incidence of coronary heart
    disease, Report from the Oslo study group of a randomized
    trial in healthy men, Lancet, 2:1303-1310 (1981).

20. R. Stamler, J. Stamler, W. F. Riedlinger, G. Algera, and R. H. Roberts, Weight and blood pressure, Findings in hypertension screening of 1 million Americans, JAMA, 240:1607-1610 (1978).

21. R. Stamler, J. Stamler, W. F. Riedlinger, G. Algera, and R. H. Roberts, Family (Parental) history and prevalence of hypertension: results in a nationwide screening program, JAMA, 241:43-46 (1979).

22. L. K. Dahl, and R. A. Love, Evidence for relationship between sodium (chloride) intake and human essential hypertension, Arch.Intern.Med., 94:525-531 (1954).

23. J. Stamler, Hypertension: aspects of risk, J. C. Hunt, T. Cooper, E. D. Frohlich, R. W. Gifford Jr., N. M. Kaplan, J. H. Laragh, H. M. Maxwell, and C. G. Strong, eds., Hypertension Update: Mechanisms, Epidemiology, Evaluation, Management, Health Learning Systems, Inc., Bloomfield, N.J. pp.23-37 (1979).

24. A. R. Dyer, J. Stamler, O. Paul, D. M. Berkson, R. B. Shekelle, M. H. Lepper, H. McKean, H. A. Lindberg, D. Garside, and T. Tokich, Alcohol, cardiovascular risk factors and mortality: the Chicago experience, Circulation, 64(Suppl.III):III-20-III-27 (1981).

25. J. Stamler, E. Farinaro, L. M. Mojonnier, Y. Hall, D. Moss, and R. Stamler, Prevention and control of hypertension by nutritional-hygienic means - long-term experience of the Chicago Coronary Prevention Evaluation Program, JAMA, 243:1819-1823 (1980).

26. Hypertension Detection and Follow-Up Program Cooperative Group, Five-year findings of the Hypertension Detection and Follow-Up Program. I. Reduction in mortality of persons with high blood pressure, including mild hypertension, JAMA, 242:2562-2571 (1979).

27. Hypertension Detection and Follow-Up Program Cooperative Group, Five-year findings of the Hypertension Detection and Follow-Up Program. II. Mortality by race-sex and age, JAMA, 242:2572-2577 (1979).

28. Hypertension Detection and Follow-Up Program Cooperative Group, Five-year findings of the Hypertension Detection and Follow-Up Program. III. Reduction in stroke incidence among persons with high blood pressure, JAMA, 247:633-638 (1982).

DETECTION AND TREATMENT OF VENTRICULAR ARRHYTHMIAS

Donald C. Harrison and William G. Irwin

Stanford University School of Medicine
Stanford, California 94305, U.S.A.

INTRODUCTION

During the past 15 years the techniques available to detect
ventricular arrhythmias in hospitalized and ambulatory patients have
been developed to permit characterization and quantitation of the
ventricular arrhythmias.[1] These advances have permitted the assessment of ventricular arrhythmia in many cardiac disorders and determination of their importance in the natural history of each syndrome.[2]
Recently, a number of new antiarrhythmic drugs have been developed
to provide the cardiologist a number of highly effective therapeutic
agents for almost all ventricular arrhythmias.[3] However, each advance has raised new problems such as stratifying patients requiring
treatment, documenting the effects of treatment and assessing the
impact of treatment, on the natural history of the cardiac disorder.
The report focuses on the latest available information about the
detection and treatment of ventricular arrhythmias.

MAGNITUDE OF THE PROBLEM

In the USA there are more than 300,000 arrhythmic sudden deaths
annually. Almost 90% of these patients have coronary artery disease
(CAD), but other cardiac disorders are associated with ventricular
arrhythmias and sudden death (Table 1).

Since CAD is the largest single cause of ventricular arrhythmias
and is the area where sufficient studies have been performed to permit
conclusions, we focus our presentation on the early and late occurrences of ventricular arrhythmias in the CAD patients.

Table 1. CV Disease Associated with Arrhythmic Death

---

1. Coronary Artery Disease
   a) Post-myocardial infarction
   b) Unstable angina
   c) Stable angina
   d) "Sudden Cardiac Death Syndrome"
   e) Coronary spasm

2. Cardiomyopathy
   a) Dilated forms (advanced)
   b) Hypertrophic - obstructive and non-obstructive

3. Aortic Valve Disease

4. Prolapsed Mitral Valve

5. Congenital Disease
   a) Pre-excitation syndrome
   b) Repaired shunt lesions
   c) Conduction disease

6. Idiopathic

Early Post-Myocardial Infarction Ventricular Arrhythmias

Electrical inhomogeneities occur within seconds of coronary occlusion and ventricular arrhythmias are almost universal. The ventricular arrhythmias and sudden death rate decreases thereafter almost logarithmically with time. While the concept of "warning ventricular arrhythmias" occurring before ventricular fibrillation in the CCU was developed in the 1960's, it is now well documented that many patients have ventricular fibrillation with no or very short warning times. In addition, CCU's without computer monitoring do not detect many serious ventricular arrhythmias and there is marked delay or failure to commence therapy. For these reasons, I and others have advocated the prophylactic administration of lidocaine (or other agents) for all patients following acute infarction.[4,5,6] With new understanding of the pharmacokinetics of lidocaine, the ability to monitor plasma concentration and understanding the influence of disease on the disposition of the drug, it can be administered safely and effectively in most patients in the CCU for 36 to 48 hours.[7]

Late Post-Myocardial Ventricular Arrhythmias

After myocardial infarction late occurring ventricular arrhythmias are seen in from 52 to 88% of all patients depending on the duration of monitoring.[9,10] Many studies have documented a higher sudden cardiac death rate for 6 to 12 months after myocardial

infarction, but stratification of risk depends on quantitation of
ventricular arrhythmia and the association of decreases in ventricular function due to myocardial loss.

In patients with the "sudden death syndrome" almost 90% have
underlying severe CAD, but only approximately 16-25% experience
myocardial infarction at the time of ventricular fibrillation.
Untreated, these patients have 46-60% recurrence of ventricular
fibrillation in one year.

MONITORING AND INTERPRETATION OF VENTRICULAR ARRHYTHMIAS

A number of technologies permit monitoring of ambulatory
patients for ventricular arrhythmias. These include: telemetry
units in hospitals, analog (Holter) tape units, ambulatory event
recorders which activate when ventricular arrhythmias are detected
and record "snapshots" and telephone coupling transmission devices.
The greater the period of monitoring, the higher yield of detected
events.[2] However, the costs, complexity of analysis, the need for
a computer system for quantitation, and the inability of the patient
to keep electrodes functional for long periods limits recording
times.[2] Indications for ambulatory monitoring are outlined in
Table 2.

Table 2. Indications for Ambulatory Monitoring in CAD

---

1. Prognostic stratification of post-MI patients

2. Symptoms
    a) Palpitations
    b) Syncope or presyncope
    c) Stroke or cerebral ischemic attacks

3. To assess results of therapy

4. Post-resuscitation of sustained VT/VF

Interpretation of ventricular ectopic activity to determine its
prognostic value and when it should be treated remains controversial
although careful clinical studies permit tentative conclusions.[8,10]
Frequent and complex ventricular ectopic activities (VT, couplets,
R on T, and multiformed ventricular ectopic activities) are common:
greater than 10-20/hour in 7-26% of studies; complex forms in 27-
43% and VT in 1-14%, of reported studies in post-myocardial infarction groups. Spontaneous variability is considerable.[11,12] And
all types of ventricular ectopic activities are more common with
CHF,[10] reduced ejection fractions and ventricular aneurysm. However,

I conclude that frequent and complex ventricular ectopic activities have independent prognostic value.

TREATMENT OF VENTRICULAR ARRHYTHMIAS POST-MYOCARDIAL INFARCTION

A number of studies have documented that beta-blocking drugs reduce overall mortality and sudden deaths when given after myocardial infarction. They should be used when not contraindicated.

Studies do not definitively document that treatment of ventricular arrhythmias with Class 1 antiarrhythmic agents reduces mortality. However, existing studies have problems demonstrating that effective treatment has been given, that suppression of ventricular ectopic activities is required and that the observed reduction of ventricular ectopic activities is not just spontaneous variation.[11,12] For these reasons I recommend Class 1 antiarrhythmic agents when frequent and complex ventricular ectopic activities are detected (Table 3).

Table 3. Ventricular Ectopic Activity to Treat

---

1. When sustained VT occurs (greater than 20 beats

2. Greater than 20 VEA's/hour
   a) Nonsustained VT (less than 20 beats)
   b) Couplets
   c) R on T
   d) Multiformed VEA's

3. When 1 or 2 (above) occur with heart failure exceptional effort

---

Several methods have been developed to determine effectiveness of treatment. First, use plasma levels of antiarrhythmic drugs to be certain each patient is in therapeutic range and do not attempt ventricular ectopic activity monitoring.[7] Secondly, do two ambulatory monitorings before instituting treatment and 4 to 7 afterwards with probability statistical analysis.[13] Thirdly, two pretreatment quantitations with analysis of variance and confidence intervals established for judging one or more post-treatment monitoring results.[13] Fourthly, to require 90% suppression of all ventricular ectopic activities. Further studies are clearly needed.

Schema for Post Myocardial Infarction Management

Based on clinical studies, the new technologies available, and the potential for salvaging large numbers of patients, I offer a schema for post-myocardial management (Table 4).

Table 4. Schema for Post-MI Management

---

1. Beta-blocker to all with no CHF, exercise ECG ischemia or frequent or complex VEA's.

2. For angina, exercise ECG ischemia, and complex and frequent VEA's - coronary angiography and stratification for surgery or medical treatment.

3. For suitable patients - CABG based on symptoms and anatomy.

4. For suitable CABG patients - Class 1 antiarrhythmic treatment
    a) Vessel anatomy
    b) Ventricular function poor

5. If CABG not required - antiarrhythmic drugs based on electro-physiologic induction study.

While such an approach is experimental at this time, background suggestive supporting data are available for each new technology, for each new quantitative approach and for a larger group of safe and effective drugs.[14] The potential salvage of young patients with CAD makes it imperative to launch such approaches in the near future.

REFERENCES

1. D. C. Harrison, J. W. Fitzgerald, R. A. Winkle, Contribution of Ambulatory Electrocardiographic Monitoring to Anti-arrhythmic Management, Am. J. Cardiol. 41: 996-1004 (1978).
2. D. C. Harrison, J. W. Fitzgerald, R. A. Winkle, Ambulatory Electrocardiography for Diagnosis and Treatment of Cardiac Arrhythmias, New Eng. J. Med. 294: 373-380 (1976).
3. D. L. D. Keefe, R. E. Kates, D. C. Harrison, New Antiarrhythmic Drugs: Their Place in Therapy, Drugs 22: 363-400 (1981).
4. D. C. Harrison, L. E. Berte, Should Prophylactic Antiarrhythmic Drug Therapy Be Used in Acute Myocardial Infarction, Clin. Cardiol. 247: 2019-2021 (1982).
5. H.S. Ribner, E. S. Isaacs, W. H. Frishman, Lidocaine Prophylaxis Against Ventricular Fibrillation in Acute Myocardial Infarction, Prog. Cardiovasc. Dis. 21: 287-313 (1979).

6. M. G. Wyman, L. Hammersmith, Comprehensive Treatment Plan for the Prevention of Primary Ventricular Fibrillation in Acute Myocardial Infarction, Am. J. Cardiol. 33: 661-667 (1974).

7. D. C. Harrison, P. J. Meffin, R. A. Winkle, Clinical Pharmacokinetics of Antiarrhythmic Drugs, Prog. Cardiovasc. Dis. 20: 217-242 (1977).

8. R. A. Winkle, Indications for Ambulatory ECG Monitoring, in: "Cardiology Update," E. Rapaport, ed., (1981), Elsevier, New York.

9. J. T. Bigger, C. A. Heller, T. L. Wenger, F. M. Weld, Risk Stratification After Acute Myocardial Infarction, Am. J. Cardiol. 42: 202-210 (1978).

10. W. Ruberman, E. Weinblatt, J. Goldberg, C. W. Frank, S. Shapiro, Ventricular Premature Beats and Mortality After Myocardial Infarction, New Eng. J. Med. 297: 750-757 (1977).

11. R. A. Winkle, Antiarrhythmic Drug Effect Mimicked by Spontaneous Variability of Ventricular Ectopy. Circulation 57: 1116-1121 (1978).

12. J. Morganroth, E. L. Michelson, L. N. Horowitz, M. E. Josephson, A. S. Pearlman, W. B. Dunkman, Limitations of Routine Long-Term Electrocardiographic Monitoring to Assess Ventricular Ectopic Frequency, Circulation 58: 408-414 (1978).

13. M. Sami, H. Kraemer, D. C. Harrison, N. Houston, C. Shimaski, R. F. DeBusk, A New Method for Evaluating Antiarrhythmic Drug Efficacy, Circulation 62: 1172-1179 (1980).

14. Sudden Coronary Death, H. M. Greenberg and E. M. Dwyer, Jr., eds., Ann. New York Acad. Sci. 382: 1-483 (1982).

CLINICAL EFFICIENCY AND SIDE-EFFECTS OF OLD AND NEW ANTIARRHYTHMIC DRUGS

Erik Sandøe, Ellen Damgaard Andersen, Jens Damgaard
Andersen and Bjarne Sigurd

Medical Department B, Rigshospitalet
Copenhagen, Denmark

The number of antiarrhythmic drugs has increased greatly during the last three decades. From the triad of digitalis, quinidine and procainamide in 1951 to now a multitude of drugs. The purpose of the present paper is to assess the therapeutical potentials of this large armory of drugs. Focus will be on long-term prophylaxis of symptomatic paroxysmal tachycardia and fibrillation with a few comments on the treatment of ventricular extrasystole.

Drug Action Through Suppression of Arrhythmia Generating/Triggering Event (Calcium Channel Blockers and Beta Blockers).

In the more infrequent case, the mechanism of drug action is causal in that it suppresses the pathophysiological event underlying the arrhythmia, or protects a functionally unstable myocardium against the arrhythmia triggering influence of an increased adrenergic tone.

Calcium channel blockers, both those with effect on the AV nodal cells (verapamil and diltiazem) and the one without (nifedipine), act against arrhythmias related to Prinzmetal's variant angina.[1] By their vasodilatatory effect coronary artery spasm is prevented and with it attacks of chest pain and arrhythmia. While chest pain may be slight and not reported by the patient at the history taking, arrhythmia symptoms like fainting may prevail in the clinical picture. The ST elevation preceding the arrhythmia and signaling transmural myocardial injury may not be visible in the monitoring lead, or the ECG registration may first have been started after the onset of the arrhythmia. Thus, occasionally all signs of myocardial

ischemia may be missing and with them the clues for the choice of
the proper antiarrhythmic treatment.

By protecting the myocardium against adrenergic influence, beta-
blocking agents are capable of:

- suppressing attacks of torsade de pointes ventricular tachycardia in a substantial part of the patients with congenital
  long QT syndrome with or without associated hearing defect[2],
  and
- alleviating exercise/emotion induced attacks of ventricular
  tachycardia/fibrillation with fainting in the child or adolescent with normal ECG[3], or in the individual with mitral
  valve prolapse and T wave anomalies.[4] Exercise induced ventricular tachycardia/fibrillation related to coronary artery
  disease is best managed by coronary artery surgery.[42]

The therapeutical response is usually all to none with complete
alleviation of the attacks of tachycardia/fibrillation. The efficacy
of an initiated antiarrhythmic treatment can often be challenged by
provocation test: by hyperventilation or ergonovine test in Prinzmetal's variant angina[1], by abrupt awakening in the early morning in
a few of the patients with long QT syndrome[5,41], and by work load
on a bicycle ergometer or treadmill in the patient with exercise
induced fainting.[3] Particularly in the younger age groups, failure
to comply with regular medicine intake can result in recurrence of
the attacks of tachycardia and sometimes in sudden death.[3]

Drug Action Through Modification of Cardiac Cell Electrophysiological Properties (Quinidine, Mexiletine, Propranolol, Amiodarone and Verapamil

In the great majority of patients, drugs exert their effect directly on the cardiac cell by modifying its electrophysiological
properties. The mechanism of action can be that of a suppression of
enhanced ectopic activity; or the evening out of differences in myocardial refractoriness within a potential reentry circuit; or the
conversion of an unidirectional block in such a circuit to a bi-
directional one blocking for further impulse circling.

To create some form of order in the electrophysiological potentials of the multitude of antiarrhythmic drugs, they are usually
divided into four classes according to their dominant effect on the
action potential (Table 1). The digitalis glycosides form an additional fifth class of their own, being the only drugs which increase vagal heart tone on a chronic basis.[6] A clinically more valid
classification is a differentiation between "wide spectrum" antiarrhythmic drugs with action potential against both supraventricular
and ventricular arrhythmia and more "narrow spectrum" ones with
effect primarily on either supraventricular or ventricular arrhythmia
(Table 2).

Table 1.   Classification of anti-arrhythmic drugs from their dominant effect on the cellular action potential (AP). Class 1 drugs are divided in class 1 A drugs (quinidine-like drugs) which slightly prolong the duration of AP, and class 1 B drugs (lidocaine-like drugs) which shorten or do not affect the duration of AP. Modified after Vaughan Williams.[39]

Class 1		Class 11	Class 111	Class 1V
Depressors of max. rate of rise of AP		Beta-blocking agents	AP-prolongators	Calcium channel blockers
(Fast response inhibitors)		(Adrenergic tone inhibitors)	(Refractoriness prolongator)	(Slow response inhibitor)
A	B			
Quinidine	Lidocaine	Propranolol	Amiodarone	Verapamil
Ajmaline	Aprindine	Acebutolol	Sotalol	Diltiazem
Disopyramide	Encainide	Atenolol		
Procainamide	Ethmozin	Metoprolol		
Propafenone	Flecainide	Pindolol		
	Lorainide	Sotalol		
	Mexiletine	Timolol		
	Tocainide			

Table 2. Classification of antiarrhythmic drugs from their effect
          on supraventricular arrhythmia (SVA) and ventricular
          arrhythmia (VA)

Wide Spectrum Drugs for SVA and VA	Narrow Spectrum Drugs for	
	SVA	VA
Class 1 A drugs	Digitalis[a]	Class 1 B drugs
Beta-blocking agents	Verapamil	(Verapamil)[b]
Amiodarone		

[a] Digitalis should not be given to the adult patient with WPW.

[b] Verapamil is usually not effective in ventricular tachycardia
   but may be so in Gallavardin's repetitive ventricular tachycardia[40]

    Independent of arrhythmia type and mechanism sensitivity and
tolerance to various drugs varies greatly from one individual to
another. The optimal result of drug prophylaxis is usually restricted to a relative bettering of the arrhythmic status with a
reduction in rate, duration and/or severity of the arrhythmic events.
Complete elimination of the arrhythmias is the exception.

Selection of the Optimal Drug

    Within the framework of the statements in Table 2, selection of
the optimal drug is based on the cumbersome trial and error method.
An alternative approach in advanced cardiological centers is invasive electrophysiological investigation with programmed electrical
stimulation (PES).[7] PES is performed with the intention of deliberately provoking arrhythmia before and after drug administration
to challenge the antiarrhythmic efficacy of drug treatment. Prospects
of the method seem good for selecting the optimal drug and, particularly for excluding the dangerous one which may worsen the arrhythmia
and endanger the life of the patient.[8,9] However, long-term validity
of these optimistic preliminary results awaits corraboration by
large scale, well planned investigations. The resource demand of
the method will also have to be dramatically reduced before it can
significantly influence management of the average arrhythmia patient.
The method seems not equally applicable for the assessment of all
antiarrhythmic drugs. Thus, a poor correlation has been reported
between PES inducibility of the tachycardia and the often very impressive reduction in symptomatic events observed in the amiodarone
treated patient.[10]

Drug Prophylaxis in Chronic Ventricular Extrasystole

Individual patients with <u>chronic</u> ventricular extrasystole (VE)
often show large degrees of spontaneous variability. Repeated 24-
hour Holter monitoring was performed in an own series of 28 clinically stable patients - 11 with chronic coronary artery disease, 5
with cardiomyopathy and 12 without organic heart disease. The
selection criterion was an average VE count of 200/hour or more at
a previous 24-hour Holter monitoring. The spontaneous variations
from the first to the second investigation with 95% and 99% confidence limits are shown in Fig. 1. Through a further statistical
evaluation (regression analysis) it was found that in a clinical
trial a reduction of at least 80% in average number of VE/hour is
required to confirm drug efficacy. Figures of 65 - 83% have been
reported by former investigators.[11,12]

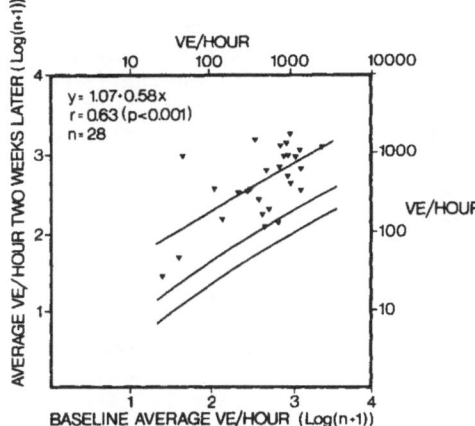

Fig. 1. Spontaneous variability in ventricular extrasystole (VE)
        frequency of 28 patients investigated with 24-hour monitoring
        at 14-day intervals. VE/hours at the first investigation
        is indicated along the abscissa, from the second investigation
        along the ordinate (log. scale). Linear regression analysis
        was used to describe the relationship between the two re-
        cordings and to establish 95% and 99% one-tailed confidence
        intervals for this relationship. To distinguish a true drug
        response from spontaneous variability at the 0.05 and 0.01
        level of significance, the coordinate corresponding to no-
        treatment/post-drug response must fall below the 95% or 99%
        confidence limits, respectively.

Judged by these criteria, several corss-over studies[14,15] convey
the impression that most antiarrhythmic drugs of class I A and B
possess a reasonable rate of success in the suppression of ventricular extrasystole. The individual sensitivity/tolerance varies
from patient to patient. No single agent seems to be out-standing
in efficacy over the other, but in the individual case the one may
work where the other has failed. Beta-blocking agents seem somewhat
less efficient in suppressing ventricular extrasystole than class I
drugs. When tried in an open series, the class III drug, amiodarone,
proved efficient in a substantial number of cases where other drugs
had failed.[16] Verapamil is usually non-effective.

Drug Prophylaxis in Symptomatic Paroxysmal Supraventricular Tachy-cardia

The episodic nature of the paroxysms and lengthiness of the required study period preclude the use of expensive Holter monitoring
in the evaluation of the patient with paroxysmal supraventricular
tachycardia. With all of its inbuilt shortcomings we have tried
to assess the problem by persuading a series of patients to keep a
diary of their attacks over periods extending from several months
to several years. At intervals, the accuracy of the diary keeping
has been checked by telemetric ECG monitoring during hospital admission. Irrespective of the type of supraventricular arrhythmia
and underlying heart disease, if any, arrhythmic activity was
usually erratic and highly unpredictable in appearance (Fig. 2).
The wide spontaneous variability in attack rate, duration and severity makes it obvious that any proper assessment of drug efficacy
in paroxysmal supraventricular tachycardia ought to build on the
outcome of controlled trials or preferably double-blind crossover studies extending over a period of at least several months.
The extent of such trials is extremely limited.[17,18] What we "know"
today about antiarrhythmic drug efficacy in paroxysmal supraventricular tachycardia is based primarily on the outcome of non-
controlled trials supported by evidence from electrophysiological
investigations in the cardiac laboratory with programmed electrical
stimulation (PES). The drugs presumed to be efficient are the ones
listed in the first two columns of Table 1. Each of the two class
I A drugs, quinidine and disopyramide, are often administered in
combination with digitalis to counteract their vagolytic effect,
which in the event of atrial fibrillation/flutter may otherwise
result in high ventricular rates. In infants with paroxysmal tachycardia digitalis is the drug of first choice. The main object of
digitalis in this context is to counteract heart failure, and it is
often given as the only drug.[19] As a general rule digitalis should
not be given to adult patients with Wolff-Parkinson-White syndrome
since it may decrease refractoriness in the accessory pathway
causing a very high ventricular rate in the event of atrial fibrillation with accompanying risk for development of ventricular fibril-

ation.[20] Due to possible side-effects, amiodarone, at least in the
hands of the authors, is used as the drug of second or third choice
although it will often prove effective in a substantial number of
cases where the other drugs will fail (see special section on
amiodarone).

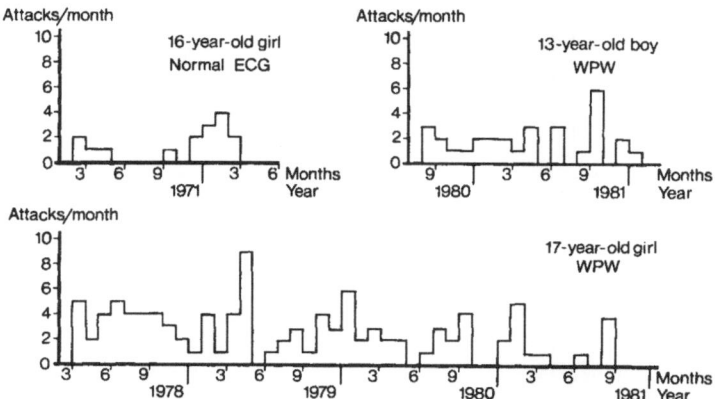

Fig. 2. Spontaneous variability in paroxysmal supraventricular tachy-
        cardia. Three adolescents without organic heart disease,
        two with, one without WPW. Diagrams based on patient diaries.

     With these limitations drugs are usually tested on a trial and
error basis with no universally accepted rank of order for the
testing. It is obvious from a view of Fig. 2 that spontaneous
variations in the attack rate of paroxysmal supraventricular tachycardia can mimic drug-induced bettering or worsening. To avoid this
fallacy it is recommendable to start out with a no-treatment or
placebo period establishing the individual "attack profile" as
baseline for drug efficacy in the subsequent periods of treatment
(fig. 3). After selection of the better drug for continued treatment it might be worthwhile to check the accuracy of the baseline
and the assumed antiarrhythmic efficacy of the selected drugs by
renewed account of attack rate/duration during another no-treatment
or placebo period. For various reasons it may be necessary to omit
the initial no-treatment or placebo period completely and instead
establish an attack profile from the case history in the knowledge
that this frequently will be inadequate.

Drug Prophylaxis in Symptomatic Paroxysmal Ventricular Tachycardia

     A great spontaneous variability is also seen in symptomatic parox-
ysmal ventricular tachycardia (Fig. 4). Judged from non-controlled

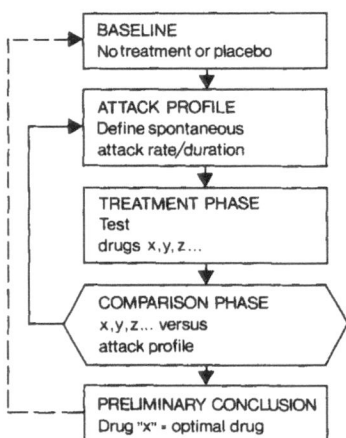

Fig. 3. A "trial and error" model for selecting the optimal drug
         treatment in paroxysmal supraventricular tachycardia.

series, class I antiarrhythmic drugs or beta-blocking agents given
alone or in combination will often reduce the attack rate. Again,
when tried, amiodarone often proves effective where other drugs have
failed (see special section on amiodarone).

Drug Prophylaxis in the Prevention of Sudden Death in Coronary Artery Disease.

It has been widely assumed that reducing ventricular extrasystole
in the patient with coronary artery disease is synonymous with reducing the risk of sudden death due to paroxysms of ventricular tachy-
cardia/fibrillation. An incredible number of Holter monitoring
hours have been spent in first finding the patient with a high incidence of ventricular extrasystole and next following the effect
of various antiarrhythmic drugs in reducing the frequency of ventricular extrasystole. However, for evaluating drug efficacy in
preventing sudden arrhythmic death, reduction in ventricular extrasystole appears to be a faulty substitution parameter. Thus, in
four large long-term controlled trials with various class I antiarrhythmic drugs in acute myocardial infarction survivors, all
drugs proved efficient in decreasing the frequency of ventricular
extrasystole. However, in no case was the reduction in ventricular
extrasystole followed by a significant lowering of sudden death
mortality.[21] In contrast, drug prophylaxis with beta-blocking agents
exerting less suppressive effect on ventricular extrasystole have
proved efficient in lowering both total mortality and mortality

related to sudden death, probably because they are able to protect
the myocardium against ischemic events and hereby intervene in the
disease process.[21]

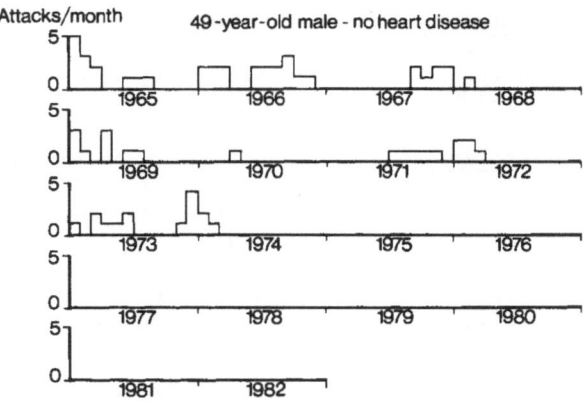

Fig. 4. Spontaneous cessation of paroxysmal ventricular tachycardia
        after repeated attacks over a period of 9 years. The patient
        is a 49-year-old male with normal ECG and no sign of heart
        disease (normal coronary arteriography and ventriculography).
        From 1965 to 1974 repeated attacks of sustained ventricular
        tachycardia lasting for hours to days which often had to be
        stopped by DC conversion. During the same period of time
        treated with many various drugs without definite benefit.
        Since 1974 and up to the last follow-up in 1982 - no treat-
        ment and no attacks. It appears that the start of a drug
        treatment in the last month of 1973 might have conveyed the
        impression of high efficacy with the recommendation that the
        treatment should be continued on a lifetime basis.

Side-Effects of Antiarrhythmic Drugs

    Side-effects, cardiac and non-cardiac side-effects, are common
in antiarrhythmic drug treatment. They can be due to high plasma
concentrations of the drug, but in a substantial number of cases
are not dose dependent and can occur at drug concentrations definitely within the therapeutical level. Interactions can occur. Thus,
quinidine[22], amiodarone[23], and to some extent verapamil[24], when given
combined with digoxin, will increase the plasma concentration of
digoxin increasing the risk of digoxin intoxication. Cardiac ar-
rhthmias are potential complications of any antiarrhythmic drug
regimen. They can take the form of

Worsening of the original arrhythmia which can occur in up to
10% of the patients deduced from electrophysiological studies using
programmed electrical stimulation (PES)[8,9] and a single clinical
series.[25]

Torsade de pointes ventricular tachycardia preceded by QT prolongation observed particularly during treatment with quinidine[26,27],
disopyramide[28], and aprindine[29], but occurring also with the beta-
blocking agent sotalol[30], and with amiodarone.[31]

Increase in ventricular rate in atrial fibrillation or flutter
related to the vagolytic effect of disopyramide and quinidine or in
WPW syndrome due to digitalis or more rarely verapamil, lowering the
refractory period in the accessory pathway.

SA block, AV block, bradycardia and/or asystole complications
developing primarily in patients with latent or manifest dysfunction
of the SA and AV conduction system.

In general, antiarrhythmic agents (except digitalis) have a
depressing effect on cardiac contractility. The depressant effect on
cardiac contraction is regarded as primarily true of disopyramide[32],
and is considered to be rare with amiodarone.[33] Among the many noncardiac side-effects attention will be called only to those of
amiodarone as listed below.

Amiodarone, the Better Drug and the Drug with the Unusual Side-Effects

Amiodarone is a drug of several virtues, thus-

- evidence from several open series states that it is effective
  in a substantial part of patients both with supraventricular
  and ventricular tachycardia where other drugs have failed,
  and that it more often than other drugs leads to total suppression of the attacks of tachycardia/fibrillation[16,33,34],
  results from own series of 50 patients support this view
  (Table 3);

- it is particularly effective in the prevention of tachycardia
  in WPW syndrome and is the drug of choice for slowing down
  the ventricular rate in WPW related attacks of atrial flutter/
  fibrillation.[35]

- its long halflife (1 month) ensures continued drug effectivity
  by a single daily oral dose, not endangered even by a few days'
  lapse in medicine intake.

Meanwhile, more general use of amiodarone is restricted due to
a number of unusual, worrisome side-effects including: thyrotoxicosis,
myxoedema, goitre, photosensitivity, pneumonitis and pulmonary

fibrosis.[10,34,36,37,38] Incidence of thyrotoxicosis in own series
(Table 4) was as high as 10%; much smaller percentages have been
reported by other investigators.[37] Corneal micro-deposits are observed in almost all patients receiving amiodarone, but these rarely
interfere with vision, are dose related and disappear after some time
when treatment is discontinued. Because of the thyroid complications,
monitoring of thyroid function is essential in all patients on long-
term therapy.

Table 3. Amiodarone in 50 patients with symptomatic
paroxysmal tachycardia resistant to treatment
with a variety of other antiarrhythmic drugs.
27 patients were without signs of organic
heart disease (4 with WPW); 11 had ischemic
heart disease; 3 congenital heart disease,
hereof 2 with WPW; 3 congestive cardiomyopathy; and 6 miscellaneous forms of heart
disease.

| Effect of Treatment · | Paroxysmal Tachycardia | |
	Supraventricular	Ventricular
No symptomatic events	8	7
Fewer attacks	15	–
Unchanged	12	7
Worsened	–	1[a]
Total no. of patients	35	15

[a] Repeated attacks of torsade de pointes ventricular tachycardia.

CONCLUSIONS

The state of the art of antiarrhythmic therapy continues to be
a difficult balancing between therapeutic and toxic effect of the
applied drugs. The expansion in recent years with the introduction
of a vast number of class I drugs has brought with it only limited
progress. It can be hoped for the future that:

- new drugs of the amiodarone type will be in the offing, but
  drugs without its unusual and worrisome side-effects and with
  simpler pharmacocinetics and easily measureable plasma concentration.

Table. 4. Side effects of amiodarone
in 50 patients (same series
as in Table 3). Treatment
duration 1 month to 5 years,
average 2½ years. Development
of thyrotoxicosis was observed
in 5 patients treated for periods varying from 16-29 months
in the two patients during
treatment and in the three patients 6-9 months after cessation
of treatment.[36]

Side-effect	No. of patients
Corneal micro-deposits	50
Thyrotoxicosis	5
Goitre,eumetabolic	3
Photosensitization	3
Aggravation of SA block	2
Torsade de pointes VT	1
Vasculitis	1

- electrophysiological testing will live up to its promise and
  evolve into a less resource demanding method.

- pacing and surgery may father better treatment alternatives
  for the many patients with arrhythmias who are presently poorly
  helped by medicine.

REFERENCES

1. R. Vilhelmsen, S. A. Mortensen, and E. Sandøe, Diagnostic fal-
    lacies and drug management in Prinzmetal's variant angina,
    in: "Myocardial Revascularization. Medical and Surgical Ad-
    vances in Coronary Disease," D. T. Mason, J. J. Collins, Jr.
    eds., Yorke Medical Books, New York, N.Y. (1981)
2. B. Sigurd, M. Suenson, A. Wennevold, and E. Sandøe, Means of
    management of the long Q-T syndrome, in "Management of
    Ventricular Tachycardia - Role of Mexiletine," E. Sandøe,
    D. G. Julian, and J. W. Bell, eds., Excerpta Medica, Amsterdam
    Oxford (1978).

3. A. Wennevold, and E. Sandøe, 6-14 years' beta-blockade in three
    children with paroxysmal ventricular fibrillation, in: "Manage-
    ment of Ventricular Tachycardia - Role of Mexiletine," E. Sandøe
    D. G. Julian, and J. W. Bell, eds., Excerpta Medica, Amerster-
    dam - Oxford (1978).

4. W. A. Pocock, and J. B. Barlow, Postexercise arrhythmias in the
    billowing posterior mitral leaflet syndrome, Am. Heart J.
    80:740 (1970)

5. E. Gymoese, E. Skovlund, and E. Sandøe, Paroxysms of ventricular
    tachycardia provoked by auditory stimuli in Romano-Wards
    syndrome, Abstract, Acta med. Scand., Suppl. 651:29 (1981).

6. R. Gillis, and J. A. Quest, The role of the nervous system in
    the cardiovascular effects of digitalis, Pharmacol. Rev.
    31:19 (1980).

7. B. Surawicz, Intracardiac extrastimulation studies: how to?
    where? by whom? - Editorial, Circulation 65:428(1982).

8. R. W. F. Campbell, M. R. Nicholson, and D. G. Julian, Ventricular
    tachycardia - management with encainide, Abstract, Europ.
    Heart J., (Suppl. A)2:185 (1981).

9. R. L. Rinkenberger, E. N. Prystowsky, W. M. Jackman, G. V.
    Naccarelli, J. J. Heger, and D. P. Zipes, Drug conversion of
    nonsustained ventricular tachycardia to sustained ventricular
    tachycardia during serial electrophysiologic studies: Ident-
    ification of drugs that exacerbate tachycardia and potential
    mechanisms, Am Heart J. 2:178 (1982).

10. J. J. Heger, E. N. Prystowsky, W. M. Jackman, G. V. Naccarelli,
    K. A. Warfel, R. L. Rinkenberger, and D. P. Zipes, Amiodarone:
    Clinical efficacy and electrophysiology during long-term
    therapy for recurrent ventricular tachycardia or ventricular
    fibrillation, New Engl. J. Med.10: 539 (1981).

11. J.Morganroth, E. L. Michelson, L. N. Horowitz, M. E. Josephson,
    A. S. Pearlman, and W. B. Dunkman, Limitations of routine long-
    term electrocardiographic monitoring to assess ventricular
    ectopic frequency, Circulation 3:408 (1978).

12. M. Sami, H. Kraemer, D. C. Harrison, N. Houston, C. Shimasaki,
    R. F. DeBusk, A new method for evaluating antiarrhythmic drug
    efficacy, Circulation 62:1172 (1980).

13. B. Sigurd, J. Fischer Hansen, K. Mellemgaard, and J. Damgaard
    Andersen, Comparative effects of tocainide and procainamide
    in the treatment of ventricular ectopic complexes, in:
    "Workshop on Tocainide - Conference Held in Copenhagen,
    November 1979," A. Pottage, and L. Tyden, eds., Hässle,
    Mölndal, Sweden (1981).

14. J. P. Van Durme, M. Bogaert, I. Bekaert, D. De Clercq, and
    E. Moerman, Comparison of the antidysrhythmic efficacy of
    atenolol, disopyramide, mexiletine and placebo, in: "Manage-
    ment of Ventricular Tachycardia - Role of Mexiletine," E.
    Sandøe, D. G. Julian, and J. W. Bell, eds., Excerpta Medica,
    Amsterdam - Oxford (1978).

15. M. A. Warnowicz, and P. Denes, Chronic ventricular arrhythmias:
    Comparative drug effectiveness and toxicity, Prog. Cardiovasc.
    Dis. 23:225 (1980).

16. M. B. Rosenbaum, P. A. Chiale, M. S. Halpern, G. J. Nau, J. Przybylski, R. J. Levi, J. O. Lazzari, M. V. Elizari, Clinical efficacy of amiodarone as an antiarrhythmic agent, Am. J. Cardiolog. 38:934 (1976).

17. M. W. Millar Craig, and E. B. Rafferty, A double-blind trial of disopyramide, procaineamide and digoxin in paroxysmal supraventricular tachycardia, Clin. Cardiol. 2:179 (1980).

18. K. Midtbφ, Verapamil in the prophylactic treatment of paroxysmal supraventricular tachycardia, Curr. Ther. Res. (1981).

19. E. Damgaard Andersen, J. Ramsφe Jacobsen, E. Sandφe, J. Videbæk, and A Wennevold, Paroxysmal tachycardia in infancy and childhood: A review and a long-term follow-up study, Acta Pædiat. Scand. 62:341 (1973).

20. T. D. Sellers, T. M. Bashore, and J. J. Gallagher, Digitalis in the pre-excitation syndrome, Circulation 56:260 (1977).

21. G. S. May, K. A. Eberlein, C. D. Furberg, E. R. Passamani, and D. L. DeMets, Secondary prevention after myocardial infarction: A review of long-term trials, Prog. Cardiovasc. Dis 24: (1982).

22. J. T. Bigger, Jr., The quinidine - digoxin interaction - Editorial review, Intnl. J. Cardiol. 1:109 (1981).

23. J. O. Moysey, N. S. V. Jaggarao, E. N. Grundy, D. A. Chamberlain, Amiodarone increases plasma digoxin concentration - short reports, Brit. Med. J. 282: 272 (1981).

24. K. E. Pedersen, A. Dorph-Pedersen. S. Hvidt, N. A. Klitgaard, and F. Nielsen-Kidsk, Digoxin-verapamil interaction, Clin. Pharmacol. Therap.30: 311 (1981).

25. V. Velebit, P. J. Podrid, I. B. Graboys, and B. Lown. Aggravation of ventricular arrhythmia by antiarrhythmic drugs - Abstract, Am. J. Cardiol. 43:359 (1979).

26. P. Denes, A. Gabster, and S. K. Huang, Clinical, electrocardiographic and follow-up observations in patients having ventricular fibrillation during Holter monitoring. Role of quinidine therapy, Am. J. Cardiol. 48:9 (1981).

27. R. W. Koster, H. J. J. Wellens, Quinidine-induced ventricular flutter and fibrillation without digitalis therapy, Am. J. Cardiol. 38:521 (1976).

28. G. Ellrodt, B. N. Singh, Adverse effects of disopyramide (Norpace) Toxic interactions with other antiarrhythmic agents, Clin Pharmacol. Critical Care 9:469 (1980).

29. D. Scagliotti, B. Strasberg, H. A. Hai, R. Kehoe, K. Rosen, Aprindine-induced pholymorphous ventricular tachycardia, Am. J. Cardiol.49:1297 (1982).

30. M. Laakso, P. J. Pentikäinen, K. Pyörälä, and P. J. Neuvonen, Prolongation of the QT interval caused by sotalol - possible association with ventricular tachyarrhythmias, Europ. Heart J. 2: 353 (1981).

31. J. M. McComb, K. R. Logan, M. M. Khan, J. S. Geddes, and A. A. J. Adgey, Amiodarone-induced ventricular fibrillation, Europ. J. Cardiol. 11:381 (1980).

32. P. J. Podrid, A. Schoeneberger, and B. Lown, Congestive heart failure caused by oral disopyramide, New Engl. J. Med. 302: 614 (1980).

33. K. Nademanee, J. A. Hendrickson, D. S. Cannom, B. N. Goldreyer, B. N. Singh, Control of refractory life-threatening ventricular tachyarrhythmias by amiodarone, Am. Heart J. 101:759 (1981).

34. W. J. McKenna, L. Harris, G. Perez, D. M. Krikler, C. Oakley, J. F. Goodwin, Arrhythmia in hypertrophic cardiomyopathy. II Comparison of amiodarone and verapamil in treatment, Brit. Heart J. 46:173 (1981).

35. M. B. Rosenbaum, P. A. Chiale, D. Ryba, M. V. Elizari, Control of tachyarrhythmias associated with Wolff-Parkinson-White syndrome by amiodarone hydrochloride - Reports on therapy, Am. J. Cardiol. 34:215 (1974).

36. E. Damgaard Andersen, Long-term antiarrhythmic therapy with amiodarone. High prevalence of thyrotoxicosis (11%), Abstract, Europ. Heart J., (Suppl. A) 2:199

37. M. H. Jonckheer, Amiodarone and the thyroid gland. A review, Cardiologica 36:199 (1981).

38. S. M. Sobol, and L. Rakita, Pneumonitis and pulmonary fibrosis associated with amiodarone treatment: A possible complication of a new antiarrhythmic drug, Circulation 65:819 (1982).

39. E. M. Vaughan Williams, Electrophysiological basis for a rational approach to antiarrhythmic drug therapy, Adv. Drug Res. 9:69 (1974).

40. P. Coumel, P. Attuel, and J. -F Leclercq, The role of calcium antagonists in ventricular arrhythmias, in: "Calcium Antagonism in Cardiovascular Therapy: Experience with Verapamil." Proceedings of International Symposium, Florence October 1980, A. Zanchetti, and D. M. Krikler eds., Excerpta Medica. Amsterdam (1981).

41. H. J. J. Wellens, A. Vermeulen, and D. Durrer, Ventricular fibrillation occurring on arousal from sleep by auditory stimuli, Circulation 46: 661 (1972).

42. J. L. Cox, Indications and results of surgery, in: "Proceedings of Symposium on Chronic Antiarrhythmic Therapy, Gent 1982," J. P. Van Durme, and M. G. Bogaert eds., Astra, Mölndal, Sweden (In press).

ACKNOWLEDGEMENT

The authors would like to acknowledge the assistance of Mrs. Susan Hebsgaard.

GENERAL AND LOCAL FACTORS IN ARTERIAL THROMBOSIS:

PLATELETS, PROSTAGLANDINS AND POSTULATES

J. P. Caen and J. Maclouf

U. 150 INSERM, LA 334 CNRS
Hôpital Lariboisière, 6, rue Guy Patin
75475, Paris   Cedex 10, France

The discovery by Moncada et al., (1976) that vessel fragments could convert prostaglandin endoperoxide G_2 in an unstable metabolite with a potent antiaggregating as well as vasodilating property appeared to be a major step in the understanding of arterial thrombosis. The fact that this substance was mainly produced in the endothelial cells of the vessel wall (Moncada et al., 1977) seemed to be an additional explanation to the non thrombogenicity of the endothelium. These discoveries were followed by the emergence of the concept of antagonistic substances, namely platelet thromboxane (TX) A_2 and vascular prostaglandin (PG) I_2 playing a key role in the thrombocyte-vessel wall interactions. According to this concept, a balance might exist between TXA_2 and PGI_2 for the homeostatic regulation of platelet-vessel wall interactions. This very tempting hypothesis has stimulated a tremendous effort in the cardiovascular field, aimed at the verification of this theory as a likely explanation of most thrombotic disorders. However, at the present time, it appears that the $TXA_2 - PGI_2$ axis may only be one part of the mediators that play a role in vascular disorders. Plasma factors, membrane components, blood cells other than platelets... may be involved in those processes. In this chapter, we will try to review some of these aspects.

DYSFUNCTION OF CYCLOOXYGENASE REGULATIONS IS SUPPOSED TO BE RESPONSIBLE FOR THROMBOTIC EVENTS

Let us consider some pathophysiological situations for which an alteration of the TXA_2/PGI_2 balance has been claimed to be the main explanation.

Non Steroidal Antiinflammatory Drugs as Antithrombotic Molecules

The finding that aspirin irreversibly acetylated platelet cyclo-oxygenase (Roth and Majerus, 1975) and therefore inhibited PGH_2 as well as TXA_2 production was a good justification to its use as an antithrombotic drug. However, although a lot of wide scale trials have been conducted in cardiovascular diseases, the best estimate of reduction in total mortality was just less than 10% (Sweetnam and Elwood, 1982). At the present time, it is not clear whether aspirin should be more active in some defined categories of patients nor why it is less effective in women in the prevention of strokes. Further, although the administration of aspirin to patients was intended to act as an antiplatelet drug it is known that platelet aggregation undergoes via several metabolic pathways. Actually, no one knows exactly which pathway of aggregation or which mediator predominates in many situations where aggregation seems to play an important role in the disease. Among the cyclooxygenase-independent pathways, PAF-acether has been claimed to aggregate platelets independently of TX formation. We have shown in in vitro studies that platelet activation (i.e. release reaction involving the liberation of vasoactive sub-stances such as 5-Hydroxy-tryptamine from the dense bodies or of products facilitating cell-cell interactions such as fibrinogen or fibronectin stored in the α granules) did not depend on TX synthesis but rather of the triggering of internal Ca^{2+} fluxes (Levy-Toledano et al., 1982). These facts emphasize the need for designing new drugs more adapted to antithrombotic functions than anti-inflammatory drugs.

Key Role of PGI_3 in the Diet

In 1978, Dyerberg et al., who were doing epidemiological studies on the Greenland eskimos mainly fed on fish diet observed a very prolonged bleeding time that they related to the rarity of atheros-clerosis. They hypothesized that the replacement of arachidonic acid by fish eicosapentaenoic acid in the membrane phospholipids of those individuals caused a synthesis of vascular PGI_3 (whose bio-logical activity was comparable to PGI_2) contrasting with an inactive platelet TXA_3. However biochemical regulations turned out to be more complex since Hornstra and collaborators (1981) showed that experi-mental animal diet with fish oil resulted in an equal decrease of TXA_2 and PGI_2 suggesting a competition of eicosapentaenoic acid with arachidonic acid at the cyclooxygenase level rather than conversion. Further it was also shown (Berlin et al., 1980) that dietary fat modification also altered the fluidity of platelet membranes leading rather to physical perturbations of the cell membrane reactivity rather than a modification of the TXA_2/PGI_2 balance.

Circulating PGI_2 as a Hormone

Since a number of years it was admitted that PG were autacoids rather than hormones. However in 1978, the report of the existence of circulating PGI_2 (Gryglevski et al., Moncada et al.,) in the peripheral blood brought the concept of prostacyclin playing a beneficial antiaggregating and vasodilator role as a circulating hormone which may be responsible for the resting state of platelets under normal conditions. Since then several groups could neither detect circulating PGI_2 nor the stable hydrolysis product, 6-Keto-$PGF_1 \alpha$ (Siess and Dray, 1982), by direct measurement and it is well accepted that there is no circulating prostacyclin.

PGI_2 as the major Cyclooxygenase product of Endothelial Cells

Isolated human endothelial cells from the umbilical cord have been shown to produce high amounts of PGI_2 contrasting with the small concentrations of $PGF_2 \alpha$ or PGE_2 (Weksler et al., 1977). However, although this situation seems the most frequent it has then been hypothesized that regional vascular differences may exist and that PGI_2 may not be the unique regulatory PG of vessel function. The findings that bovine endothelial cells in culture (Ingerman - Wojenski et al., 1981) or rabbit intrapulmonary arteries (Salzman et al., 1980) synthesize PGI_2 and TXA_2 may raise pathophysiological arguments concerning a possible heterogeneity of the vasculature.

PROSTANOID DERIVATIVES AS MODULATORS OF THE THROMBOTIC EVENTS

Modification of Platelet Adhesion to Collagen by PGI_2, PGD_2, and PGE_1

After a vascular lesion, adhesion to subendothelium is the primary step of platelets with the different macromolecules exposed to the blood. Several in vitro techniques have been designed to investigate platelet adhesion. The Baumgartner and Muggli technique (1976) using deendothelized rabbit aorta placed in a perfusion chamber through which the blood is passed at different shear rates allows a quantitative estimation of both adhering and subsequently aggregating platelets. Using this technique, we were able to show, in a joint work with the Wellcome group, that PGI_2 could inhibit platelet adhesion to subendothelium although this inhibition was much less potent than that observed on the subsequent formation of thrombi (Higgs et al., 1978). However the interference of plasmatic factors or biorheologic parameter may modify dramatically this primary step. Therefore a quantitative method was developed in our laboratory to estimate specifically the platelet adhesion to collagen without other interference (Legrand et al., 1979). In this situation we could show that inhibition of adhesion to collagent, by PGI_2, was

correlated to the enhancement of the intracellular cAMP level by
adenylate cyclase (Karniguian et al., 1982). These effects were
also found using PGD_2 and PGE_1 and they were potentiated by the
phosphodiesterase inhibitor, theophylline.

On another hand, structural and amino acid sequences have allowed the finding of a collagen-derived peptide which represents the
smallest part of the molecule that can interact with platelets, thus
providing an inhibitor of collagen-platelet reactions, independent
of PG modulation (Legrand et al., 1980). Such approach may be a
basis for a development of a novel strategy of antithrombotic drugs.

Platelets-Von Willebrand Factor Interactions in the Presence of PGI_2

It appears that the fixation and attachment of platelets to
damaged endothelial cells depends mainly on a complex molecule
present in the circulating plasma and platelets as well as in the
endothelium or in subendothelial regions, namely the von Willebrand
factor. Factor VIII/von Willebrand factor (F VIII/WF) is composed
of a pro-coagulant portion and of a ristocetin cofactor activity
necessary for the aggregation of normal platelets in the presence
of the antibiotic. It has been shown (Moake et al., 1981) that
PGI_2 could reverse ristocetin-induced platelet agglutination although it did not suppress the ristocetin induced binding of FVIII/WF
to platelets. From these data it was concluded that PGI_2 could
suppress platelet-platelet cohesion sites without suppressing the
binding of platelets to subendothelial FVIII/WF necessary for hemostasis.

IMPORTANCE OF OTHER BLOOD FACTORS IN THE INTERACTION WITH VASCULAR CELLS

Red Blood Cells

Diabetes mellitus is associated with a high prevalence of microvascular and atherosclerotic disease; it has also been observed that
whole-blood viscosity was increased and that the erythrocyte deformability was reduced. Recently, the adhesion of erythrocytes from
diabetic patients to endothelial cells was studied in our laboratory
(Wautier et al., 1981). After labeling of washed erythrocytes with
^{51}Cr, the cells were incubated with confluent endothelial cells
cultures from umbilical veins. After sequential washings, it was
found that the percentage of adhering red cells from diabetic
patients was higher than when they were from controls ($P<0.005$).
These results could be correlated to a vascular score which suggested
that in diabetes an intrinsic erythrocyte abnormality could be related to vascular diseases.

Von Willebrand Factor

Recently there have been increasing indications that after an endothelial injury, platelets and lipid entry in the arterial wall may be involved in the early stages of atherosclerosis. A recent important finding (by Ross and Vogel, 1978) is that a substance derived from platelets would be responsible for the smooth muscle cell proliferation of the atherosclerotic lesion. Fuster et al., (1978) using homozygotes von Willebrand pigs lacking this factor, have shown that such animals have a marked impairment in platelet attachment to the vascular wall. These pigs are resistant to the initiation and progression or atherosclerosis either spontaneous or induced by a mildly high-cholesterol diet. This contrasted with the heterozygous animals with milder impaired platelet function which were less resistant to atherosclerosis.

Leukocytes

In contrast to our increasing understanding of the mechanisms of platelet adherence, the specific factors that favor leukocytes adherence to the injured vascular wall are poorly understood although they may be quite important. We studied the effect of thrombocytopenia in rats, using an antiplatelet serum (Kovacs and Caen, 1979): examination of the micro-circulation exhibited a striking increase in the number of marginating, i.e. rolling, leukocytes. Such an increased adhesion of leukocytes to endothelial cells could have some relevance in the development of the ensuing microvascular lesions. Since this work was done, the discovery of leukotrienes (Samuelsson et al., 1979) and their potent biological activities (increased adhesion of leukocytes to endothelial cells, changes in vascular permeability) may bring a new insight in leukocyte - endothelial cells - interactions. In a recent work with Borgeat (Maclouf et al., 1982) we were able to show that platelets and leukocytes may cooperate for leukotrienes biosynthesis. We could show that platelet-derived lipoxygenase product, 12-HPETE, could initiate or amplify the leukotriene biosynthesis thus providing a new example of blood cells cooperativity.

CONCLUSIONS

In summary, it is quite clear that we have only surveyed part of the complex factors that play a role in arterial thrombosis. The brilliant, though so far incomplete PGI_2-TXA_2 balance hypothesis as governing platelet-vessel wall interactions has had the advantage of stimulating efforts in the cardiovascular research in biochemical, pathophysiological or pharmacological approaches. The cyclooxygenase metabolites are undoubtedly involved in the modulation of the normal homeostatic function of platelet-vessel wall interaction either by cAMP mediation or via the modulation of receptor sites of plasmatic macro-molecules such as fibrinogen or the Von Willebrand factor. Other cells such as red blood cells or leukocytes may also be of the upmost importance in the genesis of atherosclerotic disease. Blood cells cooperation such as platelet leukocyte interactions mediated by the non cyclooxygenase pathway, i.e. lipoxygenases, may also contribute to a more complex although more realistic picture of multifactorial causes of arterial thrombosis.

REFERENCES

Baumgartner, H. R., and Muggli, R., 1976, Adhesion and aggregation: morphological demonstration and quantitation in vivo and in vitro. Platelets in Biology and Pathology, J. L. Gordon, ed., pp23. Elsevier/North Holland Biomedical Press, Amsterdam.

Berlin, E., Matusik, E. J. Jr., and Young C. Jr., 1980, Effect of dietary fat on the fluidity of platelet membranes, Lipids 15:604.

Dyerberg, J., Bang, H. O., Stoffersen, E., Moncada, S., and Vane, J. R., 1978, Eicosapentaenoic acid and prevention of thrombosis and atherosclerosis, Lancet 2:117.

Fuster, V., Bowie, E. J. W., Lewis, J. C., 1978, Resistance to arteriosclerosis in pigs with von Willebrand's disease: Spontaneous and high cholesterol diet-induced arteriosclerosis, J.Clin.Invest., 61:722.

Gryglewski, R. J., Korbut, R., and Ocetkiewicz, A. C., 1978, Generation of prostacyclin by lungs in vivo and its release into arterial circulation, Nature 273:765.

Higgs, E. A., Moncada, S., Vane, J. R., Caen, J. P., Michel, H., and Tobelem, G., 1978, Effect of prostacyclin (PGI_2) on platelet adhesion to rabbit arterial subendothelium, Prostaglandins 16:17.

Hornstra, G., Christ-Hazelhof, E., Haddeman, E., Tenhoor, F., and Nugteren, D. H., 1981, Fish oil feeding lowers thromboxane and prostacyclin production by rat platelets and aorta and does not result in the formation of prostaglandin I_3, Prostaglandins 21:727.

Ingerman-Wojenski, C., Silver, M. J. Smith, J. B., and Macarak, E., 1981, Bovine endothelial cells in culture produce thromboxane as well as prostacylin, J.Clin.Invest., 67:1292.

Karniguian, A., Legrand, Y. J., and Caen, J. P., 1982, Prostaglandins: specific inhibition of platelet adhesion to collagen and relationship with cAMP level, Prostaglandins (in press).

Kovacs, I. B., and Caen, J. P., 1979, Increased interaction of vascular endothelium and leucocytes after administration of antiplatelet serum: role in the developing vascular defect, J.Clin.Pathol., 32:445.

Legrand, Y. J., Fauvel, F., Kartalis, G., Wautier, J. L., and Caen,
    J. P., 1979, Specific and quantitative method for estimation
    of platelet adhesion to fibrillar collagen, J.Lab.Clin.Med.,
    94:438.
Legrand, Y. J., Karniguian, A., Le Francier, P., Fauvel, F., and
    Caen, J. P., 1980, Evidence that a collagen-derived nona-
    peptide is a specific inhibitor of platelet-collagen inter-
    action, Biochem.Biophys.Res.Commun., 96:1579.
Levy-Toledano, S., Maclouf, J. Bryon, P., Savariau, E., Hardisty,
    R. M., and Caen, J. P., 1982, Human platelet activation in
    the absence of aggregation: a Ca^{2+} dependent phenomenon
    independent of thromboxane formation. Blood (in press).
Maclouf, J., Fruteau De Laclos, B., and Borgeat, P., 1982, Effects
    of 12-hydroxy-and 12-hydroperoxy-5,8,10,14-eicosatetraenoic
    acids on the synthesis of 5-hydroxy-6,8,11,14-eicosatetraenoic
    acid and leukotriene B_4 in human blood leukocytes. 3rd Inter-
    national conference on prostaglandins, Florence 18-21 May.
Moake, J. L., Tang, S. S., Olson, J. D., Troll, J. H. Cimo, P. L.,
    and Davies, P. J. A., 1981, Platelets, Von Willebrand factor,
    and prostaglandin I_2, Am.J.Physiol., 241:H54.
Moncada, S., Gryglewski, R., Bunting, S., and Vane, J. R., 1976,
    An enzyme isolated from arteries transforms prostaglandin
    endoperoxides to an unstable substance that inhibits platelet
    aggregation, Nature 263:663.
Moncada, S., Herman, A. G., Higgs, E. A., and Vane, J. R., 1977,
    Differential formation of prostacyclin (PGX or PGI_2), by
    layers of the arterial wall. An explanation for the anti-
    thrombotic properties of vascular endothelium, Thrombos.Res.,
    11:323.
Moncada, S., Korbut, R., Bunting, S., and Vane, J. R., 1978, Prosta-
    cyclin is a circulating hormone, Nature 273:767.
Ross, R., and Vogel, A., 1978, The platelet-derived growth factor.
    Cell 14:203.
Roth, G. J., and Majerus, P. W., 1975, The mechanism of the effect
    of aspirin on human platelets, J.Clin.Invest., 56:624.
Salzman, P. M., Salmon, J. A., and Moncada, S., 1980, Prostacyclin
    and thromboxane A_2 synthesis by rabbit pulmonary artery,
    J.Pharmacol.Exp.Ther., 215:240.
Samuelsson, B., Borgeat, P., Hammarström, S., and Murphy, R. C.,
    1979, Introduction of a nomenclature: Leukotrienes,
    Prostaglandins 17:785.
Siess, W., and Dray, F., 1982, Very low levels of 6-keto-prosta-
    glandin F_1 α in human plasma, J.Lab.Clin.Med., 99:388.
Sweetnam, P. M., and Elwood, P. C., 1982, "Aspirin and secondary
    mortality after myocardial infarction." The second MRC
    epidemiology unit trial in Cardiovascular Pharmacology of
    the Prostaglandins. Herman, A. G., Vanhoutte, P. M.,
    Denolin, H., and Goossens, A., Raven Press, New York, pp383.

Wautier, J. L., Paton, R. C., Wautier, M. P., Pintigny, D., Abadie, E., Passa, P., and Caen, J. P., 1981, Increased adhesion of erythrocytes to endothelial cells in diabetes mellitus and its relation to vascular complications, N.Engl.J.Med., 305:237.

Weksler, B. B., Marcus, A. J., and Jaffe, E. A., 1977, Synthesis of prostaglandin I_2 (prostacyclin) by cultured human and bovine endothelial cells, Proc.Natl.Acad.Sci.USA., 74:3922.

SYMPOSIA

INFLUENCE OF DIFFERENT FACTORS ON MILD HYPERTENSION

I. K. Shkhvatsabaya and A. L. Myasnikov

Institute of Cardiology
USSR Cardiology Research Sciences
Academy of Medical Sciences
Moscow, USSR

Mild hypertension (MH) should be considered according to two equally important aspects of arterial hypertension. One of them is directly associated with treatment of patients. Another aspect relates to the pathophysiological mechanisms of the disease and factors responsible for the process of subsequent evolution (progressing and regression of the disease). These two important aspects are determined by heterogeneity of cases which is reflected in clinical forms of the course of the disease with their own distinctive features, extent of involvement into the pathological process of vitally important organs, risk of complications, differences in prognosis.

The significance of the MH problem is especially well demonstrated in studies based on long-term observations (Veteran Administration Cooperative Study, 1972; US Public Health Service Hospitals, 1972; Kannel et al., 1980; Helgeland, 1981; Morgan, Meyers, 1981; etc.).

The main findings arising from these studies are the following.

It has been ascertained that moderately elevated level of blood pressure (BP) in adults is the most common medical problem in industrially developed countries (Epstein, 1979). Mild hypertension is heterogeneous by its course and prognosis. The latter depends not only on the degree of BP elevation, but rather on the range of BP fluctuations, age and previous injury of some vitally important organs (heart, brain, kidneys), on different risk factors (Veteran Administration Cooperative Study, 1972; Kannel et al., 1980). A very important conclusion has been drawn that some types of hypotensive therapy can differently influence the course and prognosis of the disease.

The results of these studies demonstrate the necessity of selection of MH patients for treatment and more careful choice of therapy. For example, myocardial infarction and sudden coronary death occurred more frequently in elderly patients (older than 65) with mild hypertension who were treated by diuretics (Morgan, Meyers, 1981). And it was indicated that during treatment by diuretics the development of hypertriglyceridemia and hyperuricemia was possible which could increase the risk of coronary complications. Taking into consideration that these patients were elderly it cannot be excluded that moderate BP elevation characteristic of patients with mild hypertension reflects a certain degree of adaptation of circulation system to the initial (or preexistent) organ disorders of atherosclerotic genesis. Due to this BP decrease could increase the vulnerability of patients to cardiovascular complications.

On the basis of the analysis of the data obtained in various studies on evaluation of the effectiveness of the long-term treatment of patients with mild hypertension, Alderman (1980) defines three groups of patients proceeding not from BP indices but rather from clinical characteristics, response to treatment and prognosis: group 1 - with no risk of sudden death and other complications, group 2 - with risk of complications and no results of treatment, group 3 - with risk of complications which can be modified and eliminated by active treatment. It is not excluded that these groups of patients have differences in the nature of the disease.

It is known that differentiation of patients on the basis of renin-sodium profile suggested by Laragh actually correlates with the extent of risk of complications (myocardial infarction, brain stroke) which has been shown in studies by Brunner et al. (1972).

From the presented data it is obvious that on the basis of the analysis of the results of long-term observations for MH patients it is possible to evaluate the natural course of the disease, to determine what external and internal factors can influence the disease including action of different drugs, to understand better the nature of the disease. In this connection it is reasonable to present the results of the studies performed at the A. L. Myasnikov Institute of Cardiology which demonstrate the effect of disorders of the heart, vascular wall, kidneys and excessive salt content in food on the course of mild hypertension.

We will consider consecutively the available data.

1. We carried out 3-5 year observations for 163 patients aged 25-54 with labile (LH) and stable (SH) hypertension without clinical signs of IHD and heart failure. In these patients we re-studied central hemodynamics and anatomo-functional state of the heart by echocardiography. It was found out that without regular treatment in 10% of patients with LH BP level came to normal, in 36% of patients progressing of the disease occurred, and in 54% the course of the

disease did not change. At the same time in 25% of patients with LH reverse development of left ventricular hypertrophy (LVH) occurred, i.e. left-ventricular myocardial mass (LVMM) decreased > 10 g. In 42% of patients we observed increase in LVH extent, mainly at the expense of increase of interventricular septum thickness (T_{ivs}), in 33% of patients LVMM did not change significantly.

In 60% of SH patients we observed LVH aggravation, in 33% - no changes and only in rare cases - LVH decrease. As for the course of the disease in these groups of patients, progressing signs were noted in 49%, the course did not change in 44% and improvement was observed in some patients.

The presented observations indicate that there was no direct parallel link between the dynamics of the disease course and changes in direction and manifestation of LVH. Thus, the known conclusion has been confirmed according to which LVH development in hypertension is not limited to the direct association with elevated BP, but has a more complicated mechanism (Tarazi and others). And changes in LVH extent occur more often and are found earlier than changes in the course of the disease. Nevertheless, the performed studies revealed the direct correlation between LVMM value and increase of systolic BP ($r = +0.58$, $p < 0.001$ - in LH; $r = +0.71$, $p < 0.001$ - SH). In cases of reverse LVH development in LH patients there were found its distinct correlations with decrease of the total peripheral vascular resistance ($r = +0.57$, $p < 0.05$). These findings are in agreement with literature data indicating relationship of LVH development with increase of systolic BP and LVH regression with initially lower diastolic BP (Inrahim et al., 1981). Besides the mentioned above data, the results on changes of some indices of intracardiac hemodynamics are also very important. Increase of end diastolic volume (EDV) and end diastolic size (EDS) of the left ventricle were observed initially, i.e. at the first examination, in cases of reverse development and also in progressing of LVH in patients with hyperdynamic type of circulation. LVH regression was characterized by subsequent increase of volume indices of the left ventricle in diastole. As known, EDV increase testifies to increased venous flow which in hypertension, especially at early stage in elevated cardiac output, was reported by many authors and associated with increase of central cardiopulmonary blood volume as a result of re-distribution of blood from periphery to the center due to venoconstriction. There are reasons to believe that at early stages of the disease the indicated hemodynamic shifts have a functional basis which determines predisposition of these patients to either progressing or reverse development of hypertension. It should be emphasized that subsequent development of the disease is not always combined with increase of LVH extent (as also, by the way, normalization of BP with LVH regression), but further LVH increase (according to LVMM, T_{ivs}) usually indicates to the progressing of the disease and this index should be taken into consideration in evaluation of the dynamics of the disease course.

It is a matter of principle to have objective criteria which could be used for prognosis of possible LVH evolution in arterial hypertension, especially in application of different hypotensive drugs which, as known from literature, are effective differently in respect of reverse LVH development (Tarazi et al., 1979). In this connection there should be mentioned the data obtained by our researchers. These findings testify to the direct and close correlation between LVMM changes and the values of intramyocardial stress of left ventricular wall (6). This has been well demonstrated in cases of reverse LVH development in patients treated by diuretics, beta-adrenal blocking agents (E. G. Diyakova, A. P. Yurenev), when decrease of 6_{max} value by more than 60% of the initial index preceded LVMM decrease. These observations are in an agreement with the data obtained by Ibrahim et al. (1981) on a higher dependence of LVMM on changes in the value of LV intramyocardial stress compared to other factors.

Taking into account the results of the effectiveness of long-term treatment with some hypotensive drugs (diuretics, in particular), a special attention should be paid to functional consequences of LVMM decrease and other shifts in the organic and systemic levels in decrease and normalization of previously elevated blood pressure. From this point of view the presented above data on the significance of studies of the value and dynamics of 6_{max} changes of left ventricle in treatment with hypotensive drugs are very important.

Other practically important data have been obtained by our researchers (A. A. Klembovsky, A. P. Yurenev). It was found that BP decrease by more than 25% of the initial level in patients with marked arterial hypertension and LVH under the effect of i/v injection of sodium diazoxide leads to decrease of myocardial contractile function.

2. Morphofunctional changes of vascular wall should be considered among other factors which are associated with manifestation and duration of arterial hypertension, on the one hand, and degree and rate of LVH development and other vascular and organic lesions, on the other hand.

Vascular system and heart in anatomo-functional relation represent a common system together with the mechanisms of their regulation, therefore it can be assumed that structural, in particular hypertrophic changes developing in hypertension are not limited to the heart but also spread to vascular wall. In fact, in studies of SH patients our researchers (V. V. Paniflov, N. N. Usubaliev) found close correlation between LVH (according to LVMM determined by echocardiography) and value of minimal resistance (R_{min}) reflecting ability of vessels to dilation in reactive hyperemia in response to limb ischemia performed by the method of venous occlusive plethysmography with tensio-transmitter. Thus, for the first time it was shown that LVH development and structural changes of vascular wall could occur simultaneously.

This means that LVMM determination to a certain extent can be used as an index of manifestation of hypertrophic changes of vascular wall in SH patients. At the same time indices characterizing anatomo-functional state of peripheral vessels restudied in dynamics can be also used in evaluation of the degree of progressing or possibility of reverse development of hypertension.

As for patients with mild hypertension, the obtained data indicate that in normokinetic type of hemodynamics there is statistically significant increase of vessel resistance in maximal vasodilation, i.e., signs of structurally adaptive changes of resistive vessels. In contrast, such changes were not observed in hyperkinetic type. It is not excluded that the revealed regularities can be in a certain extent connected with the nature of subsequent course of the disease. It is likely that patients with marked hypertrophic changes of the heart and vessels are prone to progressing of hypertrophy. However, long-term observations for the circulation dynamics are necessary to confirm this assumption.

We have gained some experience of dynamic studies in treatment with diuretics (Usubaliev N. N.) We have studied patients with mild (BP_d < 105 mm Hg) and stage II B (BP_d > 105 mm HG) hypertension aged 28-50. In these patients we determined peripheral blood flow and regional resistance of crus vessels by venous occlusive plethysmography.

According to the results of the study improvement of peripheral hemodynamics was observed only in SH (BP_d > 105 mm Hg) and in good hypotensive effect of short-term therapy (2 weeks) by furosemide and hypothiazide. This was expressed in decrease of vascular tension, significant R_{min} decrease indirectly indicating increase of vessel lumen resistance. Nevertheless, in spite of R_{min} decrease, i.e. increased ability to vasodilation, its values were higher than in the control.

It is true that decrease of vessel resistance at rest and maximal dilation under the effect of diuretics reflects increase of arteriole lumen due to normalization of water-electrolytic content of vascular wall and decrease of its swelling (Tobian, 1952). However, maintenance of higher R_{min} as compared to the control in patients treated with diuretics indicates the presence of structural changes of vascular wall of other nature not connected with water-saline disturbances.

3. Renal mechanisms play a key role in the development of a number of forms of arterial hypertension and in pathogenesis of hypertension, in particular. According to numerous literature data the kidneys and pathophysiological mechanisms connected with them widely participate in the onset, development and progressing hypertension.

We will discuss here only a number of questions directly related to pathogenesis and clinical aspects of mild hypertension.

we present data obtained in clinico-morphological study of kidneys
in hypertensive patients. 42 patients (26 women and 16 men, aged from
17 to 44) with mild hypertension (stage II A according to A. L. Myasnikov classification) were studied. All these patients underwent
percutenaous renal biopsy. The bioscopic material was studied by
light-optical and electron microscopic analysis. The patients were
followed-up for 3-5 years. Patients whose history data included
diseases which could cause renal changes were excluded from the study.
In all patients hypertension was diagnosed. The duration of the
disease varied from 2 to 6 years and was not accompanied by urinary
syndrome and any disturbances in renal function.

In all 42 patients bioscopic material was heterogeneous. In
9 cases it revealed a healthy kidney; in 19 patients we found insignificant changes such as roughness of mesangium in some glomeruli,
swelling of epithelium of proximal tubules in unchanged JGA, arteriole
hyalinosis with stenosis of their lumen at some points. In 1/3 of
cases (14 patients) we detected marked changes: some glomeruli had
initial elements of sclerosing, other glomeruli had partial hyalinosis
with replacement of one or several loops by hyaline, dystrophic changes
of tubule apparatus, and in some cases small foci of interstitial
sclerosis. In patients of this group we revealed sclerosing of renal
vessels with thickening of intima of arteries of medium and small sizes,
hyperelastosis, some lumen stenosis and initial arteriole hyalinosis.
6 out of 14 patients had morphological signs of JGA hyperfunction which
was judged by hypertrophy and hyperplasia of JGA, hypergranulation of
epithelioid cells.

Out of 42 cases 27 patients were followed-up for 5 years in an
out-patient clinic and were not treated regularly.

It can be seen that out of 5 patients with initially normal
kidneys in 4 cases AH course did not change, and 1 patient had further
development of hypertension.

Out of 11 patients with initially insignificant renal changes in
5 cases the course of the disease did not change, and 6 patients had
stabilization and progressing of AH. During all the period of observation the patients did not have changes in urine, renal function
was within normal levels, there were no complications in the brain
and heart. Progressing of the disease was determined only according to
BP indices and nature of AH course.

Fundamental differences in the course of the disease were found
in patients of group 3 with initially more marked morphological changes:
distant results were obtained in 11 patients (7 patients did not have
regular treatment, and 4 patients had regular treatment). It is
essential that out of all 11 patients in 10 cases we observed AH
stabilization at a higher level (BP_d > 110 mm Hg) and signs of progressing (increase of resistance to hypotensive therapy in the absence
of urinary syndrome). Especially distinct picture of progressing was
observed in cases of interstitial sclerosis.

Thus, it can be concluded that in patients with mild hypertension real danger of further development, and in some cases progressing of the disease, can occur in the presence of structural changes in glomeruli, tubules, renal vessels of medium and small sizes. And these patients do not have changes in urine, and irregular treatment by hypotensive drugs is of low effectiveness. The obtained data testify to the possibility of inclusion of renal factor in the process of formation of patients not only as functional shifts of renal blood flow, but also as structural changes of renal vessels. It cannot be excluded that in 1/3 of patients with morphologically marked JGA activation renin-angiotensin mechanism plays a certain role in progressing of the disease.

Not repeating well-known reports (Tobian, Laragh and others) on the important etiological and pathogenetic role of excessive salt content in food in arterial hypertension, we present summarized clinical data obtained in joint studies by researchers of A. L. Myasnikov Institute of Cardiology (A. A. Nekrasova, Yu. I. Suvorov, I. F. Patrusheva, S. E. Ustinova, N. A. Chernova) and Uzhgorod University (M. I. Fatula). We studied population of one of the rural regions of the Transcarpathians where NaCl content in water is from 2 to 5 times higher than in normal drinking water. Due to reduction of sensitivity of gustatory receptors to salt, people of this region usually add higher amounts of salt in food, consuming 400 mEq Na daily.

Among these people we observed elevation of BP > 160/95 mm Hg in 13.8%, in the boundary zone it was found in 13.2%, while these values were 3.4 and 7.4%, respectively, in the control group (normal salt consumption).

The population of this region was followed-up for 20 years. Studied subjects had excessive salt consumption and the first examination showed labile arterial hypertension > 160/95 mm Hg. These studies demonstrated that normalization of BP occurred in 7%, improvement - in 5.4%, progressing of the disease with stabilization and further elevation of arterial hypertension - in 10%. In 77% cases the course of the disease remained the same. Patients of the control group with labile elevation of BP > 160/95 mm Hg, but with normal salt consumption (< 180 mEq per day) had different dynamics of the disease: BP normalization - in 19.7%, improvement - 13.4%. progressing of the disease - in 2.6%, and the course did not change in 64%.

Thus, it was demonstrated that excessive salt consumption had unfavourable effect on hypertension course.

In the process of this study we revealed some peculiarities of systemic dynamics in excessive salt consumption, i.e. higher indices of total peripheral resistance as compared to the controls, decrease of cardiac output and increase of the volume of circulating blood.

Besides hemodynamic changes, prolonged excessive salt consumption causes changes in the functional state of renin-angiotensin-aldosterone system (RAAS). Such changes can even occur in healthy subjects subjected to chronic salt overloading and are aggravated in hypertensive patients with excessive salt consumption. This is expressed in the absence of decrease of plasma renin activity (PRA) and aldosterone concentration in blood plasma (ACBP) in high salt overloading or tendency to their increase in patients with labile (mild) hypertension, significant increase of PRA (instead of its decrease) by more than twice of the initial value in stable and high hypertension (BP$_d$ > 110 mm Hg). Complete dissociation in PRA and ACBP reactions is observed at different loadings in stable hypertension.

The indicated above changes of hemodynamics and RAAS in hypertensive patients in prolonged excessive salt consumption can, evidently, determine some clinical peculiarities of hypertension course in these cases, in particular predisposition to sodium retention, high total peripheral resistance and possibility for further progressing of the disease.

Studies based on the evaluation of water and sodium transport by the kidneys in hypertensive patients are very important taking into account the effect of salt consumption on the course of mild hypertension. According to the studies performed by our researchers, patients with labile hypertension have three types of reactions on salt loading. Two types of them (II and III) reflect disorders in regulation of sodium and water transport processes and are characterized in one subgroup of patients (II) by excessive natriuresis and diuresis (phenomenon of exaggerated natriuresis) with reduction of renal ability to concentrate urine on the 1st and 2nd days after salt loading, and in contrast, in another subgroup (III) they are characterized by significant decrease of sodium excretion in small urine volume of high concentration (osmomolarity).

It is assumed that in the first case the observed effect is associated not with structural changes of tubules, but with inadequate reaction of hypothalamo-hypophysial system on salt loading as insufficient ADH release in blood. In the second case such effect is, probably, connected with primary disorders of renal function regulation leading to increase of sodium reabsorption in proximal tubules or ascending part of Henle's loop. It is likely that these patients are especially sensitive to salt overloading which promotes not only further development but also progressing of the disease. Similar to reactions observed in experiments in rats with spontaneous hypertension (Yu. V. Postnov et al.), patients with this type of reaction on salt loading can be considered as subjects with hereditary predisposition to increased sensitivity to sodium. Thus, we assume that on the basis of response to salt loading in mild hypertensive patients it is possible to define two subgroups (2/3 of all patients with labile hypertension) of patients with functional disorders of sodium and water transport by the kidneys.

The presented data let us make some conclusions which may serve as a basis in discussion of questions related to nature, course, therapy and prognosis of mild hypertension.

1. Mild hypertension is not homogeneous by biochemical (hormonal) and functional (hemodynamic) indices, by extent of involvement of organs (heart, kidneys) into the process, response to treatment and by rates and direction of disease evolution.

2. Early involvement of the heart and kidneys in pathological process is prognostically significant for further development and possible progressing of the disease. This includes LVH and IVS combined with changes of cardiac volume indices per diastole, and different degrees of structural changes of glomerular and tubular apparatus of the kidneys, primary hyalinosis of renal arterioles, hyperplasia and hypertrophy of JGA, elements of interstitial sclerosis (by renal biopsy data).

3. Significance of chronic and prolonged salt overloadings is associated with existence of sensitive and insensitive groups of patients to sodium chloride which can be identified by nature and degree of diuresis and natriuresis in response to salt loadings.

4. In order to find methods for higher effectiveness of treat-ment and prevention of possible complications it is necessary to conduct long-term observations for patients with mild hypertension and define different clinical groups according to the course of the disease.

EPIDEMIOLOGY AND NATURAL PROCESS

OF MILD HYPERTENSION

P. Lund-Johansen

Cardiology Section, Medical Department A
University of Bergen
Bergen, Norway

INTRODUCTION

Most studies on the pathophysiology of essential hypertension have suffered from being done in selected subjects referred to hospitals or hypertension clinics. In 1963/64 a screening of the blood pressure (BP) in the Bergen population gave us the opportunity to start a long-term study of the natural process of mild hypertension in a small group of patients recruited from an epidemiological survey.

The BP was screened in 77% of the total adult population (92.000) and in 98.1% of a 10% random sample[1,2]. All subjects with diastolic BP above 120 mmHg and a randomly selected group with moderate and mild hypertension (diastolic 90-120 mmHg) were called for a diagnostic follow-up. Male subjects who at this follow-up and at one additional examination had mild or moderate previously untreated essential hypertension and no other diseases (obese subjects were excluded) were candidates for a study of the circulatory disturbances.

CENTRAL HEMODYNAMICS - CROSS SECTIONAL STUDIES

Central hemodynamics were studied at rest and during exercise in 77 hypertensives 17-66 years old and in 48 age matched normotensive controls[3]. In the youngest age group, 17-29 years, with a mean value of BP at rest sitting of 150/92 mmHg, the cardiac index (CI) was 13% higher (p<0.05) than in the age matched controls. The heart rate (HR) was 16% higher (p<0.01), and the stroke index (SI) was not significantly different. The total peripheral resistance index (TPRI) was not significantly different. In the hypertensives 30-39 years with BP 160/99 mmHg, the SI was subnormal, but since HR was increased, the CI was normal. The TPRI was significantly increased. In hypertensives in their 40-ties and 50-ties the cardiac index and stroke index were subnormal and the TPRI increased. Similar results have been found in studies from different parts of the world (reviews in 4, 5).

The high CI and HR in subjects supposed to be in the early phase of essential hypertension formed the concept of a hyperkinetic circulation with a "luxury" perfusion of the tissues at this stage of the disease. To protect the tissues from overirrigation the arteriolar resistance was then expected to increase and thus reduce the blood flow. The hypertension would then be maintained by the increase in TPRI (the "whole body autoregulation" theory). However, an argument against this theory is that our study as well as three others demonstrated an increased oxygen consumption (VO$_2$) (about 12%) in the young mildly hypertensive subjects, and the CI was not increased when related to the metabolic demands[5]. In other words, no overirrigation in the tissues seemed to take place and the whole body autoregulation theory can not explain the increased TPRI in established essential hypertension.

The cause of the high CI, HR and VO$_2$ in early essential hypertension is not known, but an overactivity in the sympathetic nervous system is usually postulated but difficult to demonstrate[6].

Studies in the spontaneously hypertensive rats (SHR), the animal model with many similarities to human essential hypertension, have shown that even in young, mildly hypertensive animals structural changes appear very soon in the heart and in the resistance vessels[7]. Based on our studies of hemodynamics during rest only, it might seem that the heart pump function and the arterioles are not affected in early human hypertension. However, studies performed during physical exercise change this picture. Even during mild exercise (50 Watt) the young hypertensives are definitely no longer hyperkinetic. The CI related to VO$_2$ is then subnormal. The HR is still increased but the SI is then subnormal. Furthermore TPRI does not fall to the same low levels as in normotensive controls. The exercise studies seem to indicate that structural changes are present in mild hypertension already in the third decade and recently a reduced compliance in the left ventricle has been demonstrated at an early stage of essential hypertension[8].

CENTRAL HEMODYNAMICS - PROSPECTIVE STUDIES

The results from cross-sectional studies should indicate that the circulatory system in essential hypertension would change from a "high-flow low-resistance" system in the early phase to a "low-flow high-resistance" system in the later. Our group of patients from 1964/65 who had been studied hemodynamically have now been followed for 17 years. After 10 years clinical data were available in 75 of the 77 subjects and 33 subjects who had been untreated, were restudied hemodynamically by the same methods as 10 years before. After 17 years clinical data were available in 75 and a third hemodynamic study in those still untreated have started. All living subjects have remained hypertensive over these 17 years.

10-year follow-up. In the two youngest age groups treatment had been started in four subjects while 28 were untreated, apparently healthy, and they were restudied hemodynamically. (One subject died from heart and lung insufficiency). In age group III (40-49 years) only 5 patients were untreated. All patients in the oldest group (50-66 years) started treatment and 12 of 16 had died after 10 years.

In age group I (17-29 years) the VO_2 during rest had decreased 8% (p<0.05) but was almost unchanged in group II. The BP at rest showed remarkably few changes. Only during 150 W exercise was there a significant increase in MAP from 133.1 to 141.0 mmHg (6%) in age group I, and from 140.7 to 147.3 mmHg (5%) in age group II. In spite of the small changes in BP the CI at rest had fallen in both age groups, 15% and 23%, respectively. During 150 W load the mean values had decreased about 15% in each age group. In both age groups the reduction in CI was associated with a significant decrease in SI of about 8-12% at rest and during exercise. The HR during rest and exercise showed only small changes. TPRI had increased significantly during rest sitting, the increase was about 25-30% in both age groups. Figure 1 shows the changes in age group 17-29 years. The small group of patients 40-49 years demonstrated the same changes as the two younger age groups, but the increase in TPRI and BP was much greater.

Thus the long-term study demonstrated that the expected increase in TPRI had indeed occurred, although the increase in BP was relatively modest.

17-year follow-up. For ethical reasons treatment has been started when diastolic BP has increased to > 100 mmHg. After the 10-year restudy and over the next 7 years the blood pressure has increased to such levels in most subjects and after 17 years only 6 out of 36 subjects in age group I and II are still untreated. Preliminary results from the third hemodynamic restudy in untreated subjects seem to indicate further decline in cardiac index and increase in total peripheral resistance.

CONCLUSION

The present and a few other long-term studies in untreated subjects with essential hypertension have demonstrated that mild hypertension is usually a progressive disorder with slowly developing pathological changes in the heart pump and in the resistance vessels,

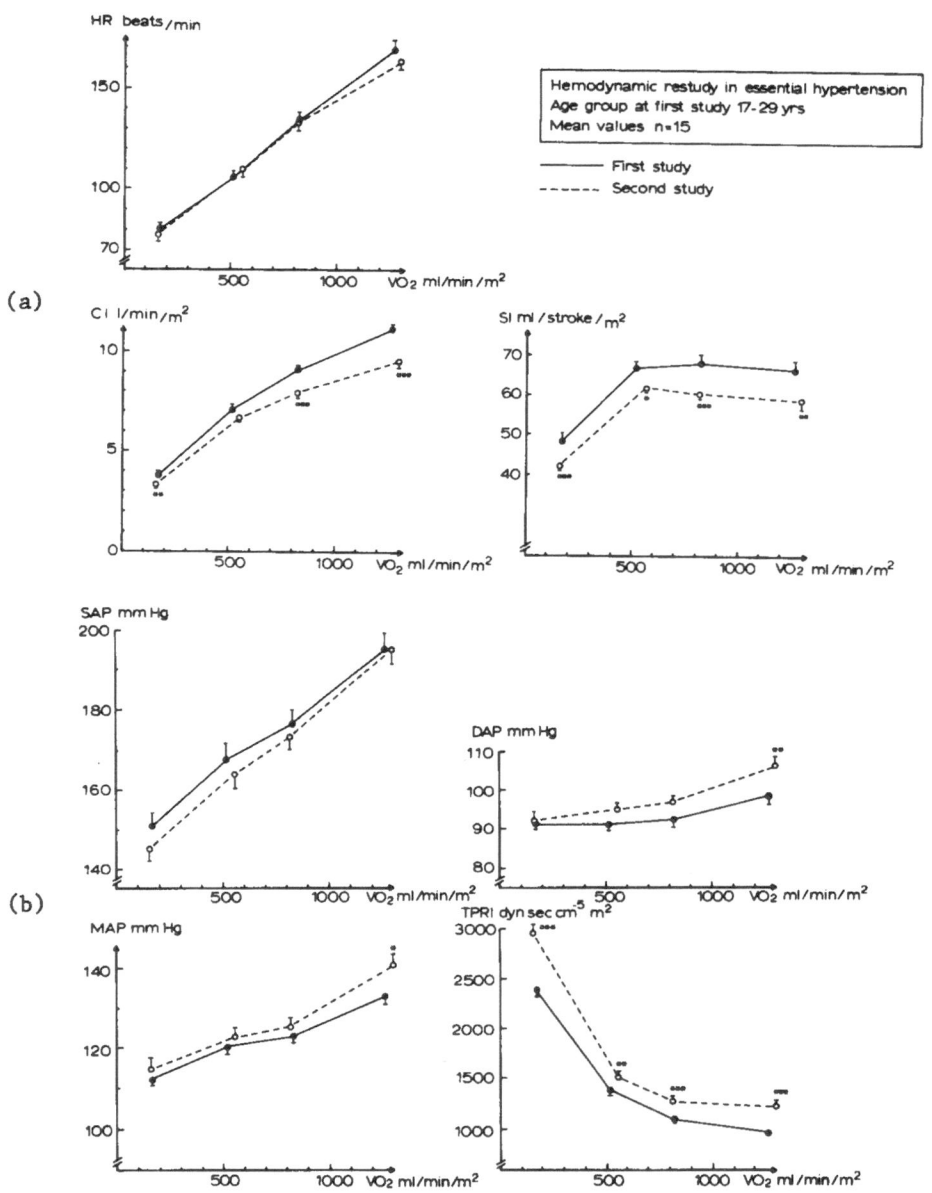

Fig. 1(a). Heart rate (HR), cardiac index (CI) and stroke index (SI)
in age group 17–29 years. Mean values and SEM. *p<0.05,
**p<0.01, ***p<0.001.

Fig. 1(b). Systolic (SAP), diastolic (DAP) and mean arterial pressure
(MAP) and total peripheral resistance index (TPRI) in age
group 17–29 years. Mean values and SEM. *p<0.05, **p<0.01,
***p<0.001.

although the increase in BP is usually not impressive in subjects in their 20-ties and 30-ties during the first 10 years. From then on increase in BP seems to be more common. Thus mild hypertension (defined as BP during rest 140/90 - 170/105 mmHg on several occasions, weeks apart) is perhaps a more important threat to the cardiovascular system than what is commonly believed. Our presently available antihypertensive agents reduce blood pressure through quite different mechanisms resulting in widely different hemodynamic patterns[9]. From a hemodynamic point of view, an antihypertensive agent, devoid of side-effects, correcting the hemodynamic disturbance would seem to be the logic approach to treatment of mild hypertension.

REFERENCES

1. E. Eilertsen and S. Humerfelt, The blood pressure in a representative population sample, Acta Med.Scand. 183:293 (1968).
2. I. Holme and H. Th. Waaler, Five-year mortality in the city of Bergen, Norway, according to age, sex and blood pressure, Acta Med. Scand. 200:229 (1976).
3. P. Lund-Johansen, Hemodynamics in early essential hypertension, Acta Med.Scand. Suppl.482:1 (1967).
4. W. H. Birkenhäger and M. A. D. H. Schalekamp, in: "Control Mechanisms in Essential Hypertension," Elsevier, Amsterdam-Oxford-New York (1976).
5. P. Lund-Johansen, State of the Art Review: Haemodynamics in essential hypertension, Clin.Sci. 59:343s (1980).
6. S. Julius, Abnormalities of autonomic nervous control in borderline hypertension, Schweizische Med.Wschr. 106:1698 (1976).
7. S. A. Lundin and M. Hallbäck-Nordlander, Background of hyperkinetic circulatory state in young spontaneously hypertensive rats, Cardiovasc.Res. 14:561 (1980).
8. F. M. Fouad, R. C. Tarazi, J. H. Gallagher, W. J. MacIntyre, and S. A. Cook, Abnormal left ventricular relaxation in hypertensive patients, Clin.Sci. 59:411s (1980).
9. P. Lund-Johansen, Haemodynamic effects of antihypertensive agents, in: "The Treatment of Hypertension," E. D. Freis, ed., MTP Press, Lancaster (1978).

MILD HYPERTENSION : TREATMENT AND PROGNOSIS

A.E. Doyle

University of Melbourne, Department of Medicine
Austin Hospital, Heidelberg
Victoria, 3084. Australia

Two major studies on the effects of antihypertensive drug
treatment in mild hypertension have recently been published. Both
have demonstrated that patients with mild hypertension treated with
antihypertensive drugs have a lower death rate and fewer vascular
complications than patients either untreated or less vigorously
treated.

The High Blood Pressure Detection and Follow-up Program[1] conducted a large study in several centers in the United States of
America. Patients with diastolic blood pressures above 90 mmHg
were admitted to the study. No patients were excluded because of
pre-existing vascular or associated disease. Patients were randomly
allocated to one of two groups. One of these, the "stepped care"
group were seen regularly in special treatment clinics and given
free aggressive anti hypertensive therapy. The other group, the
"referred care" group were referred back to their own doctors, who
may or may not have treated their hypertension. The mortability in
the stepped care group both from cardiovascular and non-cardiovascular
causes was lower than in the referred care. The reduction in all
cause mortality was larger in blacks than whites. The reduction
in mortality in the mild group, with diastolic pressures 90-105 mmHg
was 13 per 1,000 persons over five years. In the HDFP reduction
in stroke incidence was more obvious than reduction in ischaemic
heart disease.

The Australian Therapeutic Trial in Mild Hypertension[2] differed
in several important respects from the HDFP. Entry diastolic pressures were 95-109, using the average of six readings. The control
group received matching placebos and both groups attended the same
special clinics. Persons with evidence of previous stroke, myocardial

235

infarction, renal failure, diabetes or angina were excluded from the
study. In spite of the differences in design the Australian Study
and the HDFP came to broadly similar conclusions. Mortality from
cardiovascular disease was reduced in the Australian Study by 2 per
1,000 persons per annum, and morbidity, mainly from stroke, by 5 per
1,000 persons per annum. The major end points in both groups were
due to ischaemic heart disease, and in this category there were 33
myocardial infarctions in each group. The incidence of other manifestations of ischaemic heart disease was similar in both groups.

The total incidence of trial end points in the placebo treated
group was low. This seems to have been due to three factors.
Firstly, patients with pre-existing evidence of vascular complications
were excluded. Secondly in the placebo group 198 patients (12%)
whose diatolic pressures consistently rose above 110 mmHg were given
active treatment, but remained in their original randomization to
the placebo group. Finally, in all the patients receiving placebos,
diastolic pressures fell to levels below 95 mmHg.

Analysis of the relationship between the average levels of
blood pressure achieved during the period of observation showed
that in both the actively treated and placebo groups increasing
levels of diastolic blood pressure was associated with a higher rate
of trial end points. At the very lowest diastolic pressures the
rates in the active and placebo groups was almost identical. However, 87% of the actively treated group had average diastolic pressures below 94 mmHg, whereas 55% of the placebo group were in this
category. At higher average levels of diastolic pressure, the rate
of trial end point occurrence was higher in the actively treated
than in the placebo treated group, suggesting that if blood pressure
is not well controlled, the administration of antihypertensive drugs
may be associated with an additional risk, presumably related to
the drugs themselves. An alternative explanation is that the small
group of mild hypertensives apparently resistant to the antihypertensive effects of drugs may constitute a small sub group with a
worse prognosis than the average patient.

In the placebo group as a whole there was a fall of diastolic
pressure over a period of three years. Over half the placebo group
had diastolic pressures below 99 mmHg at three years, and 12% of the
group developed pressures persistently above 110 mmHg. On the
average those whose pressures fell below 95 mmHg had lower than
average pressures originally, while those whose pressures rose above
mild limits had higher than average initial pressures. No characteristics emerged, however, which allowed a prediction to be made in an
individual person as to whether the blood pressure would rise or fall.

SUMMARY AND CONCLUSIONS

1. Mild hypertension can be defined as the presence of diastolic
    blood pressures consistently between 95-109 mmHg.
2. In persons with mild hypertension prognosis is considerably
    better in those with no evidence of cardiovascular disease; in
    this group mortality is approximately 2 per 1,000 per annum.
    In persons with mild hypertension and pre-existing cardiovascular
    complications, mortality is much higher.
3. Ischaemic heart disease, which is the commonest complication of
    mild hypertension, is not significantly influenced by anti-
    hypertensive drug treatment.
4. The incidence of stroke is significantly reduced in treated
    mild hypertension.
5. A prolonged observation period is helpful in deciding which
    patients to treat. In over half the patients initially found
    to be mildly hypertensive, blood pressure falls to levels at
    which treatment provides no benefit.

REFERENCES

1. Hypertension detection and follow-up program co-operative group.
    Five year findings of the hypertension detection and follow-
    up program. I. Reduction in mortality of persons with high
    blood pressure including mild hypertension, JAMA 242:2562-
    2571 (1979).
2. Management Committee, The Australian Therapeutic Trial in Mild
    Hypertension, Lancet. 1:1261-12287 (1980).

ANTIHYPERTENSIVE THERAPY IN PATIENTS ABOVE AGE 60: A report of the

European Working Party on High Blood Pressure in the Elderly (EWPHE)

A. Amery[1], W. Birkenhäger[2], M. Bogaert[3], P. Brixko[4],
C. Bulpitt[5], D. Clement[3], P.de Leeuw[2], J.F.De Plaen[6],
M. Deruyttere[7], A.De Schaepdryver[3], R. Fagard[1],
F. Forette[8], J. Forte[9], R. Hamdy[10], J. Hellemans[1],
J.F. Henry[8], A. Koistinen[11], G. Leonetti[12], P. Lewis[5],
P. Lund-Johansen[13], J.P.R. MacFarlane[14], K. Meurer[15],
P. Miguel[9], J. Morris[16], A. Mutsers[4], A. Nissinen[11],
E. O'Brien[17], K. O'Malley[17], P. Omvik[13], J.C. Petrie[18],
L. Terzoli[12], J. Tuomilehto[11], B. Williams[14], P. Willemse[2]

The following centers are collaborating in the EWPHE:

1. University Hospital St. Raphael, Leuven, Belgium.
2. Zuiderziekenhuis, Rotterdam, The Netherlands.
3. University Hospital, Gent, Belgium.
4. Geriatric Hospital Le Valdor, Liège, Belgium.
5. Hammersmith Hospital, London, United Kingdom.
6. University Hospital St. Luc, Brussels, Belgium.
7. Medisch Centrum voor Huisartsen, Leuven, Belgium.
8. Hôpital Charles Foix, Ivry, France.
9. University Hospital Santa Maria, Lisboa, Portugal.
10. St. John's Hospital, London, United Kingdom.
11. North Karelia Project, Kuopio, Finland.
12. Istituto di Ricerche Cardiovascolari, Milano, Italy.
13. University Hospital Haukeland, Bergen, Norway.
14. Victoria Geriatric Unit, Glasgow, Scotland.
15. University Hospital Köln, West Germany.
16. St. Charles Hospital, London, United Kingdom.
17. Royal College of Surgeons, Dublin, Ireland.
18. Aberdeen Royal Infirmary, Aberdeen, Scotland.

Seven hundred and ninety two hypertensive patients above the
age of 60 have entered the double blind multicenter trial of the
European Working Party on High blood pressure in the Elderly (EWPHE).
Half were treated with one capsule daily containing 25 mg

hydrochlorothiazide and 50 mg triamterene and half were given placebo.
If blood pressure control was not adequate in those receiving active
treatment, a second capsule was given and if necessary up to 2 g of
methyldopa/day.

No significant differences between the groups were present prior
to randomization. A significant blood pressure difference of 25/10
mmHg was obtained between the groups and maintained during five years
of follow-up. No major disturbances in serum potassium or serum
sodium were noted.

On the other hand, during the initial phase an increase in
serum creatinine and serum uric acid was noted in the actively
treated group, which was maintained during the later years. This
increase in serum creatinine was related to the decrease in sitting
systolic blood pressure. Also, changes in serum uric acid correlated
with changes in serum creatinine both in the placebo and in the actively treated group, but were independent of the change in creatinine;
the serum uric acid was on average 1 mg higher in the actively treated
than in the placebo group.

Fasting blood glucose did not change significantly in the
placebo treated group, but it did so in the active treatment group.

A favorable influence on prognosis by active treatment can be
expected on the basis of the blood pressure reduction and in the
absence of major electrolytes disturbances. However, the balance
between this decreased risk and the increase produced by the rise in
blood glucose and the other treatment effects remains to be determined.
The trial continues and more patients are being admitted.

THE CLINICAL RELEVANCE OF PARTIAL AGONIST ACTIVITY OF BETA-ADRENOCEPTOR BLOCKING DRUGS

W. H. Aellig

Experimental Therapeutics Department
Clinical Research Division, Sandoz Ltd.
4002 Basel, Switzerland

Introduction

Beta-adrenoceptor blocking drugs are often considered first choice therapy in patients with mild hypertension who require medical therapy. This is due not only to their effectiveness but also to the low incidence of side-effects during long-term administration.

There is a general consensus that it is β-adrenoceptor blockade which is responsible for their therapeutic effectiveness in the treatment of hypertension as well as angina pectoris (Simpson and Waal-Manning, 1970; Prichard, 1974). Of the different ancillary properties, membrane stabilizing action seems to be of no practical relevance, whereas clinical advantages have been attributed to partial agonism - also called intrinsic sympathomimetic activity or ISA - and to β_1-adrenoceptor selectivity.

Partial Agonist Activity

The potential advantages of partial agonist activity long remained a matter of debate and only in recent years have the advantages theoretically to be expected been confirmed in the clinical situation.

A β-blocker with partial agonist activity occupies β-adrenoceptors in the same way as a drug without this property and effectively prevents the access of stimulatory agonists in a competitive manner. In addition it provides some stimulation to the receptors. The clinical pharmacological peculiarities of a β-adrenoceptor blocking drug with partial agonist activity have recently been reviewed (Aellig, 1982a).

Beta-adrenoceptor blocking drugs with partial agonist activity	Acebutolol
	Penbutolol
	Alprenolol
	Oxprenolol
	Practolol
	Bopindolol
	Pindolol

Fig. 1.

The stimulant action of the β-adrenoceptor blocking drugs listed in Figure 1 is either smaller than that provided by <u>normal</u> resting sympathetic activity (this applies to acebutolol, penbutolol, alprenolol, oxprenolol and practolol) or just about as high as resting sympathetic activity (bopindolol and pindolol). The stimulant action therefore totally or partly compensates for the loss of <u>resting</u> sympathetic drive resulting from β-adrenoceptor blockade. The effects of <u>increased</u> sympathetic stimulation during physical or mental stress, however, are reduced to the same extent as by drugs devoid of stimulant activity. One of the most obvious differences is therefore that drugs without ISA nearly always reduce resting heart rate - even if initial values are very low - whereas the effect of drugs with ISA depends on pre-existing sympathetic activity.

<u>Heart Rate at Rest</u>

An example for the correlation between the effect of a β-adrenoceptor blocking drug with partial agonist activity and resting

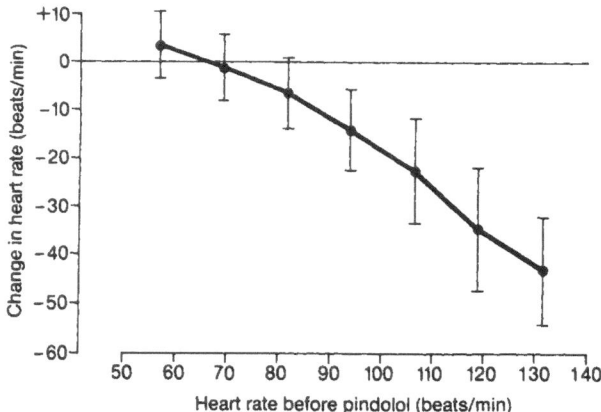

Fig. 2.   Changes in resting heart rate, related to pre-treatment values in patients with essential hypertension during oral therapy (mean ± s.e.). Reproduced from Rosenthal et al., 1979, with kind permission of British Journal of Clinical Practitioner.

heart rate is shown in Figure 2.   In a multicenter study Rosenthal
et al. (1979) studied over 7,000 hypertensive patients treated with
pindolol.   In patients with pre-treatment resting heart rates of
about 70 beats/min pindolol produced no net changes.   The ISA of the
drug therefore just about replaced the effect of resting sympathetic
activity.   The higher the pre-treatment heart rate, however, the
greater was its reduction.   When initial heart rate was low, the ISA
of pindolol led to a slight increase.

The maximum stimulant activity of the partial agonists currently
used is already reached with low therapeutic doses and is independent
of the dose over a range wider than that generally used in clinical
practice.   Carruthers and Twum-Barima (1981) studied oral doses of
pindolol from 2.5 to 57.5 mg, and found no difference in the effects
on resting heart rate.

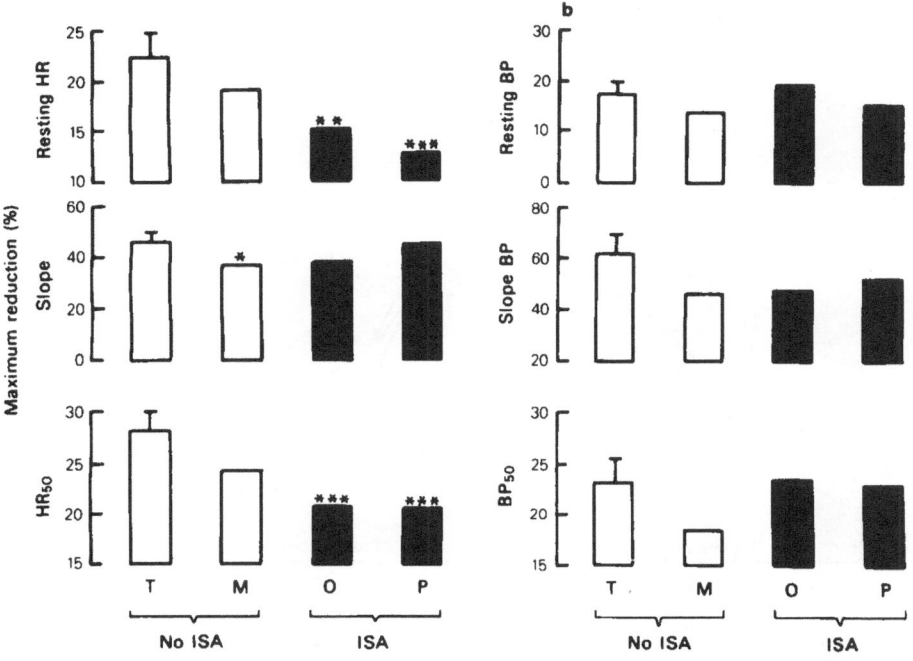

Fig. 3.   Maximum reduction in resting heart rate and blood pressure,
          in the slope of the heart rate and blood pressure rise
          during exercise and in the heart rate and blood pressure
          observed during 50% of working capacity after oral admin-
          istration of timolol (T), metoprolol (M), oxprenolol (O) and
          pindolol (P).   Error bars represent the standard error of
          the difference between any two columns (analysis of vari-
          ance).   **P < 0.01, ***P < 0.001 for difference from
          timolol.   Reproduced from Jennings et al., 1981, with kind
          permission of the British Journal of Clinical Pharmacology.

Exercise-induced Tachycardia

β-adrenoceptor blocking drugs with partial agonist activity
inhibit the effect of beta-adrenoceptor stimulation on the heart to
the same extent as drugs devoid of this property. Tachycardia due to
exercise or to infused isoprenaline is therefore reduced in a dose-
dependent manner (Aellig, 1982b). Four drugs with and without ISA
were compared by Jennings et al. (1981). Several doses were administered and the results in Figure 3 show the maximum effects reached
with each drug. As expected resting heart rate was more reduced by
timolol and metoprolol - drugs without ISA - than by oxprenolol and
pindolol - drugs with ISA, whereas resting blood pressure fell to the
same extent after all drugs. The reduction of the blood pressure and
heart rate rise during exercise was identical after all compounds,
whether they possessed ISA or not.

Erikssen et al. (1982) exercised 10 healthy subjects with increasing work loads before - and 24h after one week of oral treatment

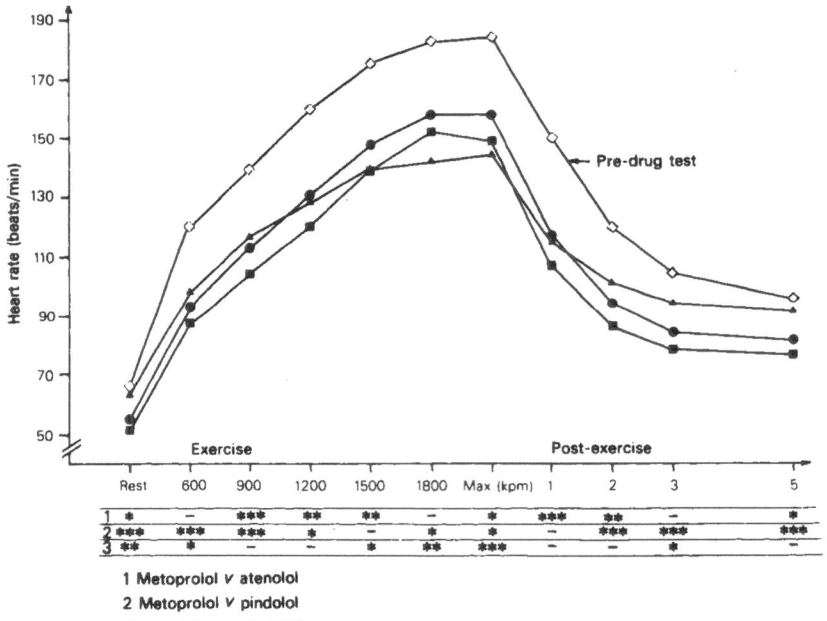

Fig. 4. Effects of metoprolol 300 mg/d (■), atenolol 100 mg/d (●)
and pindolol 15 mg/d (▲) on heart rate before, during, and
after exercise measured 24h after 6 days of therapy.
*P < 0.05, **P < 0.01, ***P < 0.001. Reproduced from
Erikssen et al., 1982, with kind permission of the British
Journal of Clinical Pharmacology.

(Figure 4). Metoprolol (300 mg/d) and atenolol (100 mg/d) reduced resting heart rate from about 65 to about 55 beats/min whereas pindolol (15 mg/d) was practically without effect. During exercise, however, the increase in heart rate was reduced after all three β-adrenoceptor blocking drugs and, in the doses used in this experiment which represent frequently used therapeutic doses, heart rate during maximum exercise was even lower after pindolol than after metoprolol and atenolol.

Thus, β-adrenoceptor blocking drugs with ISA reduce the effects of increased sympathetic activity as effectively as drugs lacking this property, but they do not interfere with cardiac function at rest.

Peripheral Resistance in Acute Studies

If resting heart rate is unchanged or only slightly reduced then cardiac output will be unchanged or only slightly lowered. As a result one would expect drugs with a clinically relevant ISA to produce little change in peripheral resistance.

In an experiment in 6 healthy volunteers blood flow in the lower extremities was measured using venous occlusion plethysmograph (Aellig, 1979). The results are summarized in Figure 5. After placebo blood flow was somewhat reduced during the 4 hours of observation. Blood flow values after 10 mg pindolol were practically identical to those after placebo. After 160 mg propranolol,

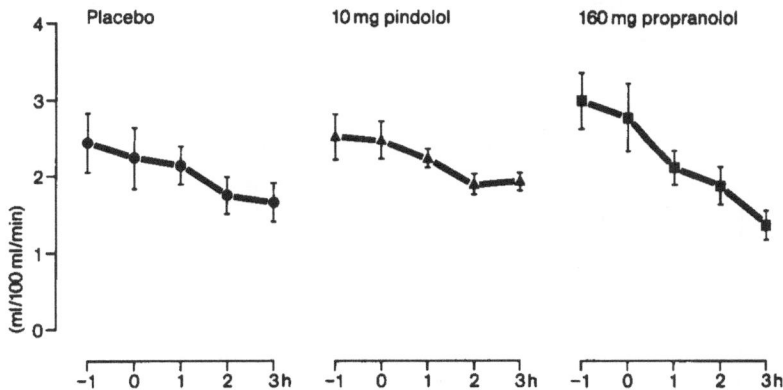

Fig. 5. Blood flow in the calf before and after oral administration of placebo, 10 mg pindolol or 160 mg propranolol to 6 healthy volunteers (mean ± s.e.). Data from Aellig, W. H., 3. Basel Hypertoni Symposiet, Stockholm, 1979, ed. L. Hansson and O. Thulesius.

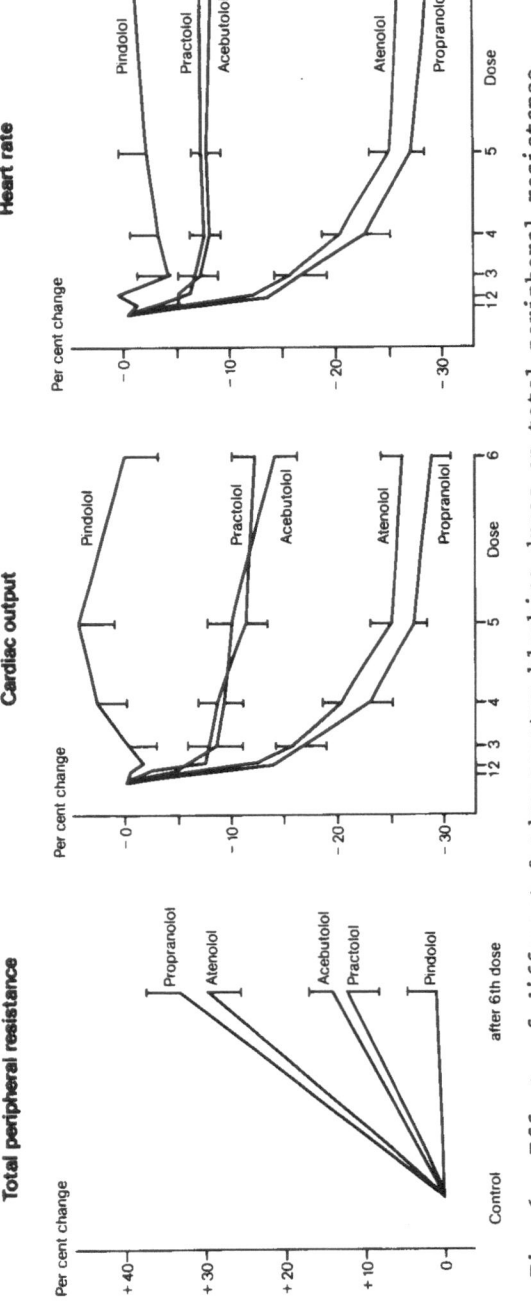

Fig. 6. Effects of different β-adrenoceptor blocking drugs on total peripheral resistance,
cardiac output, and heart rate after intravenous administration to patients with angina
pectoris.
After Svendsen et al., 1981, with kind permission of Clinical Pharmacology and
Therapeutics.

however, the reduction in peripheral blood flow was significantly greater than after either placebo or pindolol.

Svendsen et al. compared the acute haemodynamic effects of β-adrenoceptor blocking drugs with and without ISA or with β_1-selectivity in healthy volunteers (Svendsen et al., 1979) as well as in patients with angina pectoris (Svendsen et al., 1981). The results of the latter study are summarized in Figure 6. As expected, resting heart rate is only slightly influenced after pindolol but markedly reduced with propranolol and atenolol, drugs without ISA; practolol and acebutolol lie in between. Cardiac output is not reduced with pindolol and falls most markedly with propranolol and atenolol. Peripheral resistance, however, increased most markedly after propranolol and atenolol. The results with atenolol show that β_1-adrenoceptor selectivity does not protect against the increase in total peripheral resistance which is secondary to the reduction in cardiac output. Peripheral resistance was less influenced by practolol and acebutolol - which possess ISA - and remained un-altered after pindolol. Haemodynamic effects similar to those obtained in this study in man were reported by Clark et al. (1982) in dogs.

Peripheral Resistance During Treatment of Essential Hypertension

In the treatment of hypertension it is of course important to study the haemodynamic effects of a drug also during chronic oral therapy. Man in't Veld and Schalekamp (1982) analysed the literature on the acute and long-term haemodynamic effects of β-adrenoceptor blocking drugs in patients with essential hypertension. After acute administration blood pressure remained practically unaltered and drugs without ISA (timolol, atenolol, propranolol and metoprolol) markedly reduced cardiac output and increased peripheral resistance. Pindolol, with a marked ISA, had practically no influence on both parameters. Penbutolol, acebutolol, oxprenolol, practolol and alprenolol, with less ISA, showed an intermediate effect (Figure 7).

During chronic therapy, when blood pressure is reduced, at first sight the figure looks very similar (Figure 8). All peripheral resistance values, however, are now lower than in the acute situation. Timolol, propranolol, metoprolol and atenolol, which reduce cardiac output, still elevated peripheral resistance but less so than after acute administration. Pindolol and practolol, which did not reduce cardiac output, now exhibited a clear reduction in peripheral resistance below pre-treatment values. The drugs with a smaller degree of ISA showed intermediate effects.

During chronic therapy therefore β-adrenoceptor blocking drugs with ISA lower resistance to pre-treatment values or in the case of practolol and pindolol even to values clearly below pre-treatment

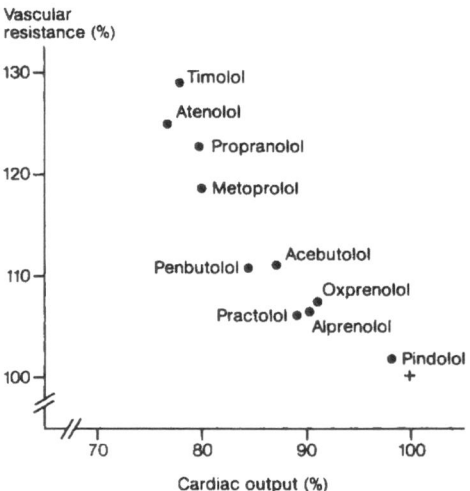

Fig. 7.   Acute haemodynamic effects of β-adrenoceptor blocking
          drugs in relation to pre-treatment values (indicated by
          the black cross). Reproduced from Man in't Veld and
          Schalekamp, 1982, with kind permission of the British
          Journal of Clinical Pharmacology.

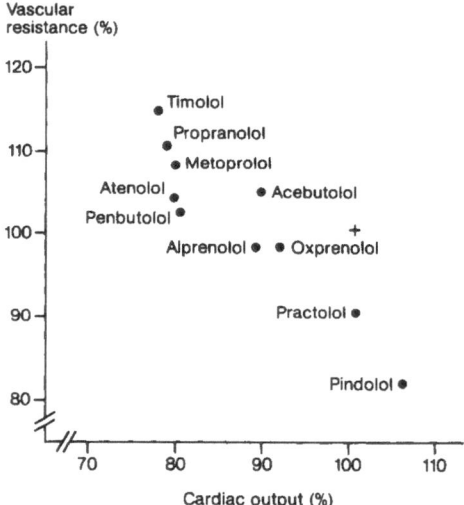

Fig. 8.   Long-term haemodynamic effects of β-adrenoceptor blocking
          drugs in relation to pre-treatment values (indicated by
          the black cross). Reproduced from Man in't Veld and
          Schalekamp, 1982, with kind permission of the British
          Journal of Clinical Pharmacology.

values. These differences are of potential clinical importance and drugs with a clinically relevant ISA appear to offer haemodynamic advantages in the treatment of hypertension.

Other Aspects

Other advantages have been attributed to ISA, for example that drugs with ISA do not unfavourably alter the ratio between HDL and LDL cholesterol (Pasotti et al., 1982; Leren et al., 1982; Lehtonen et al., 1982), that they are less likely to cause bronchoconstriction in susceptible patients (Louis and McNeil, 1982) and that they are less likely to give rise to a rebound phenomenon on sudden withdrawal (Walden et al., 1982; Rangno et al., 1982, Szecsi et al., 1982, Prichard, 1982).

An impairement of glucose metabolism in some insulin-dependent diabetics was reported during treatment with a β-adrenoceptor blocking drug (Waal-Manning, 1979). This effect was smaller with β_1-selective drugs. In order to establish whether the presence or

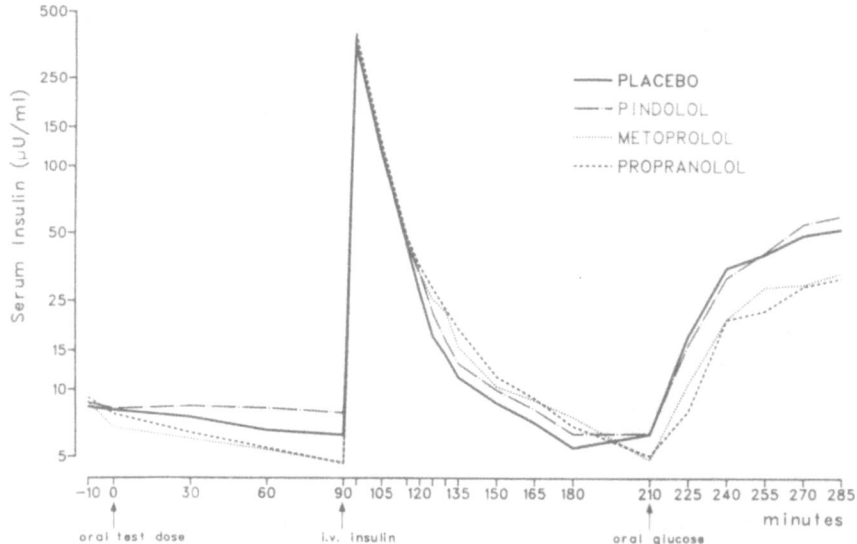

Fig. 9. Effects of an oral dose of placebo, pindolol (15 mg), metoprolol (200 mg) or propranolol (160 mg), during hypoglycaemia induced by insulin (0.1 U/kg body weight) and after an oral glucose load (100g) on serum insulin concentrations in volunteers (n = 8). Mean ± s.e. mean results. Reproduced from Schlüter et al., 1982, with kind permission of the British Journal of Clinical Pharmacology.

absence of ISA is relevant in this respect, Schlüter et al. (1982) administered oral doses of placebo, 15 mg pindolol, 200 mg metoprolol and 160 mg propranolol to 8 healthy volunteers. 90 min later insulin (0.1 U/kg body weight) was given intravenously. After identical serum insulin peaks, insulin levels underwent a slower decline after β-adrenoceptor blocking drugs (Figure 9). The effect was greatest after propranolol, smaller but significant after metoprolol (the relatively β₁-selective drug) and only slight and not significant after pindolol (the drug with ISA). When an oral glucose load was given two hours after insulin the rise of serum insulin was signifi- cantly delayed and reduced after propranolol and metoprolol, but not after pindolol.

The adrenaline peak during hypoglycaemia (Figure 10) was more than doubled after propranolol, less increased after metoprolol but not influenced after pindolol. These experimental studies in healthy subjects require confirmation in diabetic patients.

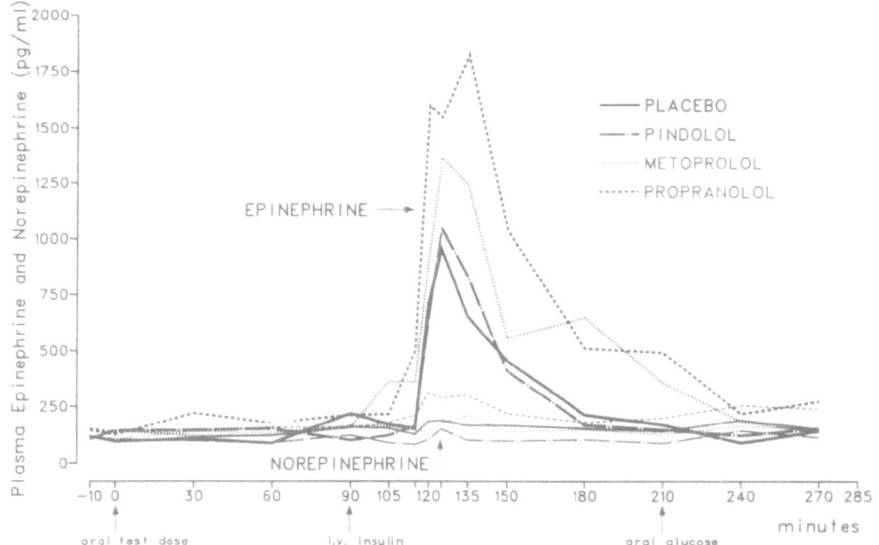

Fig. 10.   Effects of an oral dose of placebo, pindolol (15 mg), metoprolol (200 mg), or propranolol (160 mg) during hypoglycaemia induced by insulin (0.1 U/kg body weight) and after an oral glucose load (100g) on plasma adrena- line (epinephrine) and noradrenaline (norepinephrine) concentrations in volunteers (n = 8). Mean ± s.e. mean results. Reproduced from Schlüter et al., 1982, with kind permission of the British Journal of Clinical Pharmacology.

Conclusions

The results of the different clinical and clinical pharmacological studies reported here indicate that a β-adrenoceptor blocking drug with a clinically relevant ISA may have a series of therapeutically important advantages in the treatment of hypertension.

REFERENCES

Aellig, W. H., 1979, Nagra kliniskt farmakologiska experiment med β-adrenoceptorblockerande farmaka, in: 3. Basel Hypertoni Symposiet, pp.29-33, L. Hansson and O. Thulesius, eds.

Aellig, W. H., 1982a, Pindolol - A β-adrenoceptor blocking drug with partial agonist activity: clinical pharmacological consideration, Br.J.Clin.Pharmac.,13:187S-192S.

Aellig, W. H., 1982b, Clinical pharmacology of pindolol, Am.Heart J., 104:346.

Carruthers, S. G. and Twum-Barima, Y., 1981, Measurement of partial agonist activity of pindolol in man, Clin.Pharmac.Ther. 30: 581-586.

Clark, B. J., Menninger, K., and Bertholet, A., 1982, Pindolol - the pharmacology of a partial agonist, Br.J.Clin.Pharmac., 13:149S-158S.

Erikssen, J., Thaulow, E., Mundal, R., Opstad, P., and Nitter-Hauge, S., 1982, Comparison of β-adrenoceptor blockers under maximal exercise (pindolol v metoprolol v atenolol), Br.J. Clin.Pharmac., 13:201S-209S.

Jennings, G., Bobik, A., and Korner, P., 1981, Influence of intrinsic sympathomimetic activity of β-adrenoceptor blockers on the heart rate and blood pressure responses to graded exercise, Br.J.Clin.Pharmac., 12:355-362.

Lehtonen, A., Hietanen, E., Marniemi, J., Peltonen, P., and Niskanen, J., 1982, Effect of pindolol on serum lipids and lipid metabolizing enzymes, Br.J.Clin.Pharmac., 13:445S-448S.

Leren, P., Eide, I., Foss, O. P., Helgeland, A., Hjermann, I., Holme, I., Kjeldsen, S. E., and Lund-Larsen, P.G., 1982, Antihypertensive drugs and blood lipids: the Oslo study, Br.J.Clin.Pharmac., 13:441S-444S.

Louis, W. J., and McNeil, J. J., 1982, β-adrenoceptor blocking drugs: the relevance of intrinsic sympathomimetic activity, Br.J.Clin.Pharmac., 13:317S-320S.

Man in't Veld, A. J., and Schalekamp, M. A. D. H., 1982, How intrinsic sympathomimetic activity modulates the haemodynamic responses to β-adrenoceptor antagonists. A clue to the nature of their antihypertensive mechanism, Br.J.Clin.Pharmac., 13: 245S-257S.

Pasotti, C., Capra, A., Fiorella, G., Vibelli, C. and Chierichetti, S. M., 1982, Effects of pindolol and metoprolol on plasma lipids and lipoproteins, Br.J.Clin.Pharmac., 13:435S-439S.

Prichard, B. N. C., 1974, β-adrenoceptor blocking drugs in angina
     pectoris, Drugs, 7:55-84.
Prichard, B. N. C., Bhattacharjee, P., Tomlinson, B., and
     Walden, R. J., 1982, The withdrawal of β-adrenergic blocking
     drugs, (same volume).
Rangno, R. E., and Langlois, S., 1982, Comparison of withdrawal
     phenomena after propranolol, metoprolol and pindolol, Br.J.
     Clin.Pharmac., 13:345S-351S.
Rosenthal, J., Kaiser, H., Raschig, A., and Welzel, D., 1979,
     Treatment of hypertension with a β-adrenoceptor blocker. A
     multicenter trial with pindolol, Br.J.Clin.Pract., 33:165-
     174, 181.
Schlüter, K. J., Aellig, W. H., Petersen, K.-G., Rieband, H.-Ch.,
     Wehrli, A., and Kerp, L., 1982, The influence of β-adreno-
     ceptor blocking drugs with and without intrinsic sympatho-
     mimetic activity on the hormonal responses to hypo- and
     hyperglycaemia, Br.J.Clin.Pharmac., 13:407-417S.
Simpson, F. O., and Waal-Manning, H. J., 1970, Hypertension and
     β-adrenergic blockade, New Horizons Med., 1:59-72.
Svendsen, T. L., Hartling, O., and Trap-Jensen, J., 1979, Immediate
     haemodynamic effects of propranolol, practolol, pindolol,
     atenolol and ICI 89.406 in healthy volunteers, Eur.J.Clin.
     Pharmacol., 15:223-228.
Svendsen, T. L., Hartling, O. J., Trap-Jensen, J., McNair, A., and
     Bliddal, J., 1981, Adrenergic β-receptor blockade: Hemody-
     namic importance of intrinsic sympathomimetic activity at
     rest, Clin.Pharmacol.Ther., 29, 6, 711-718.
Szécsi, E., Kohlschütter, S., Schiess, W., and Lang, E., 1982,
     Abrupt withdrawal of pindolol or metoprolol after chronic
     therapy, Br.J.Clin.Pharmac., 13:353S-357S.
Waal-Manning, H. J., 1979, Can β-blockers be used in diabetic
     patients? Drugs, 17:157-160.
Walden, R. J., Bhattacharjee, P., Tomlinson, B., Cashin, J.,
     Graham, B. R., and Prichard, B. N. C., 1982, The effect of
     intrinsic sympathomimetic activity on β-receptor responsive-
     ness after β-adrenoceptor blockade withdrawal, Br.J.Clin.
     Pharmac., 13:359S-364S.

THE WITHDRAWAL OF BETA ADRENERGIC BLOCKING DRUGS

B. N. C. Prichard, P. Bhattacharjee,
B. Tomlinson and R. J. Walden

Department of Clinical Pharmacology
School of Medicine, University College London
The Rayne Institute, 5 University Street
London WC1E 6JJ

INTRODUCTION

It was found fairly soon after the introduction of beta adrenergic blocking drugs for the treatment of angina pectoris that when they were stopped abruptly an exacerbation of ischaemic symptoms sometimes occurred to above pre-beta blockade levels. The first report was in a trial of oxprenolol in angina where seven cases of status anginosus occurred out of nineteen patient in the trial when placebo was substituted for active treatment (Wilson et. al. 1969). Two cases of severe ischaemia were reported in a trial of propranol when placebo was substituted in twenty patients with angina. One patient required hospital admission for acute coronary insufficiency and one patient died from coronary occlusion the day after the propranolol (40 mg qds) was stopped (Zoster and Beanlands, 1969). In a multidose study of propranolol in angina pectoris the patients experienced a higher incidence of chest pains during the first week of placebo compared with the second week (Prichard and Gillam, 1971). Slome (1973) reported two cases of myocardial infarction that occurred when propranolol was stopped in patients with angina pectoris. Alderman et. al. (1974) described six cases of severe ischaemia in angina patients when propranolol (80 or 160 mg/day) was stopped. All of them experienced unstable angina, three had infarcts one of whom died; there was one case of sudden death, and one other developed multiple ventricular ectopics.

CLINICAL STUDIES WITH PROPRANOLOL

Miller et al., (1975a) reported a series of twenty patients with
stable angina where there were two ischaemic deaths, one sudden death,
one acute anterior infarct with shock, and four other serious reactions,
three cases of intermediate coronary syndrome and one ventricular tachycardia when propranolol was stopped. These patients had received
propranolol for a total period of twelve weeks; 160 mg daily for six
weeks and 320 mg a day for the final period. There were four additional patients who experienced increased angina attacks on placebo
compared to prior to propranolol administration. These ten patients
had significantly more severe angina (as suggested by more angina
attacks per week and trinitrin consumption) than the remaining ten
who had no excessive exacerbation of the manifestation of ischaemia
after propranolol was stopped. On the other hand they had not observed
any episodes in a "large number" of "symptomatic coronary patients"
who had propranolol stopped abruptly prior to cardiac catheterization.
This might be taken to suggest that it was the limitation of physical
activity that provided protection against serious exacerbations of
the disease on drug withdrawal. In a retrospective study in a series
of patients with angina, propranolol, average 149.2 mg (range 40-
320 mg) was abruptly stopped for coronary arteriography on fifty three
occasions in fifty one patients (Myers and Wisenberg, 1977). These
patients included fourteen with single vessel disease but with greater
than 70% stenosis, the rest had significant narrowing, ie. over 50%
of two or three vessels and all but four at least 70% stenosis. There
were two patients who had experienced unstable angina on propranolol,
one had a recurrence off propranolol which responded to restarting
propranolol, the other patient, however, experienced a fatal myocardial
infarction ten days after stopping propranolol. Again, as was the
case in the report of Miller et al., (1975a), these patients with
more severe disease appeared to be at greater risk. Mizgala and
Counsell (1976) reported fifteen acute coronary events in fourteen
patients with severe angina when propranolol was stopped, six transmural infections, three intramural infarctions with one ventricular
fibrillation and six episodes of acute coronary insufficiency.

Myers et al., (1979) reported a series of one hundred patients
with angina admitted to hospital for coronary arteriography. Propranolol was abruptly stopped after an average duration of treatment of
8.2 months and at an average dose of 216 mg. Three patients had
minor increases in chest pain and two patients had non-transmural
infarctions prior to the time propranolol was stopped; and the same
number of minor and major episodes occurred after the cessation of
the drug. The occurrence of ischaemic episodes was not related
to stopping propranolol but to the severity of the disease; all
four patients who developed non-transmural infarction had Class IV
New York Heart Association symptoms. In another survey, fifty five
patients who had propranolol, average dose 127 mg (range 20-320 mg)
stopped prior to cardiac catheterization revealed only one patient who

experienced any increase in pain. Another forty seven patients
continued on propranolol, average 143 mg (range 80-320 mg). The
overall incidence of chest pain in the two groups while they were in
hospital was 27% in those who stopped propranolol, and 28% in those
continuing propranolol. However, there was one patient in the group
which stopped propranolol who had a ventricular dysrhythmia and myocardial infarction, but this was following selective coronary artery
dye injection. The authors concluded that propranolol withdrawal
syndrome is infrequent in hospital patients (Shiroff et al., 1978).
In a study of blood pressure and incidence of atrial arrhythmias in
patients undergoing coronary bypass surgery (Kadish et al., 1979),
it was found that stopping propranolol 48 hours or 10 hours preoperatively was associated with a greater rise in blood pressure
during intubation and a higher incidence of post-operative atrial
arrhythmias than in patients who had half of their usual dose of
propranolol on the morning of operation and 1 mg iv qds in the intensive care unit.

WITHDRAWAL OF OTHER BETA BLOCKING DRUGS

The withdrawal of propranolol and metoprolol in twenty patients
with angina pectoris resulted in one patient experiencing a fatal
infarct when placebo was substituted for metoprolol and in the same
circumstances another patient experienced severe angina (Frich and
Luurila, 1976). Meinertz et al., (1979) also reported a case of
myocardial infarction in an anginal patient when metoprolol was
stopped; however, this coincided with the commencement of nifedipine
treatment which may have contributed as its administration can be
associated with a tachycardia (Beeley and Talbot, 1979).

THE EFFECT OF GRADUAL WITHDRAWAL OF BETA ADRENERGIC BLOCKING DRUGS

The withdrawal of propranolol which had been given for over three
months, over six days in one patient and nine days in two patients
was still associated with increase in sensitivity to isoprenaline
(Nattel and Rangno, 1978). However when fifteen hypertensive patients
given propranolol 80 mg qds for over a month were studied, the six
who had the dose reduced gradually to 10 mg qds for fourteen days
had no evidence of increase in sensitivity to isoprenaline or increase
in blood pressure or plasma catecholamines compared to the ultimate
stable levels in contrast to the nine patients in whom propranolol
was abruptly stopped (Rangno and Nattel, 1980). Similarly when metoprolol 300 mg/day was first reduced to 25 mg bd for ten days before
the drug was stopped only minimal sensitivity to isoprenaline was
seen (Rangno et al., 1982).

TIMING OF THE WITHDRAWAL PHENOMENON

There is some difficulty in being certain of the incidence of
delayed reactions after beta blockade withdrawal as ischaemic events
may occur due to reasons other than the recent administration of beta
blocking drugs. The timing however, seems to vary considerably from
one to fourteen (Miller et al., 1975; Mizgala and Counsell, 1976)
or possibly twenty one days (Alderman et al., 1974), after the cessation of beta blocking treatment.

WITHDRAWAL OF BETA BLOCKING DRUGS IN NON-ISCHAEMIC PATIENTS

Goldberg et al., (1977) performed continuous intra-arterial
monitoring studies that suggested that withdrawal of beta blocking
drugs (oxprenolol in seven patients, propranolol in one) in hypertensive patients was not associated with an overshoot of blood pressure
in contrast to clonidine. Other investigators have also found no
overshoot of blood pressure when propranolol was stopped (Vlachakis
and Aledort, 1980). However, hypertensive patients may complain of
palpitations, tremor, sweating and similar symptoms after the stopping
of beta blocking drugs metoprolol and propranolol (Pedersen et al.,
1979). Williams et al., (1979) have also described a hypertensive
patient who experienced palpitations associated with a tachycardia
and marked ST segment depression when metoprolol was stopped.

MECHANISM OF BETA ADRENERGIC WITHDRAWAL PHENOMENON

There have been several suggested mechanisms to explain the
withdrawal phenomenon.

EFFECT OF BETA ADRENERGIC RESPONSES

Boudoulas et al., (1977) observed an increase in sensitivity of
heart rate responses to isoprenaline infusions 24-48 hours following
the end of two days of administration of propranolol at a dosage of
40 mg qds to six normal volunteers aged 20-24. It was suggested that
the propranolol withdrawal phenomenon was the consequence of the
formation of additional beta receptors during propranolol therapy
which persisted on propranolol withdrawal for a short period leading
to augmented sympathetic responsiveness. Similarly the administration
of propranolol average 240 mg/day (range 160-320 mg) was stopped in
nine hypertensive patients who had been on treatment for at least
three months, an increased responsiveness to isoprenaline began
2-6 days later lasting for 3-13 days after propranolol was withdrawn
(Nattel et al., 1979). The average bolus dose of isoprenaline required
to produce an increase in heart rate of 25 beats/minute six days after
was 1.2 µg while it was an average of 2.3 µg after responses were

stabilized by day 14. In another investigation with the cardioselective agent metoprolol (300 mg/day) in eight hypertensives for over
six weeks a 52% average increase in cardiac sensitivity to isoprenaline
was seen 2-8 days after withdrawal (Rangno et al., 1982). In seven
other patients when metoprolol dosage was first reduced to 25 mg bd
only minimal hypersensitivity was seen.

In our studies in a between subject study in normal volunteers,
we titrated doses of propranolol (final average dose 614 mg/day)
atenolol (634 mg/day) and pindolol (18 mg/day), with drug administration for a total of about three weeks so that maximum inhibition
of exercise tachycardia was obtained. Isoprenaline hypersensitivity
was seen after atenolol (n=6) at some time in the withdrawal phase,
with measurements at 1 day and then alternate days until Day 13 post
drug. Hypersensitivity was observed with two of the six subjects
after propranolol but not after pindolol in any of the volunteers
(Walden et. al., 1982). In another study Rangno and Langlois (1982)
found a steady restoration of isoprenaline sensitivity in ten hypertensive subjects with no overshoot after pindolol was stopped.
Likewise after oxprenolol (160-320 mg given for 8-18 months) was
withdrawn in six hypertensive patients the sensitivity to isoprenaline
gradually increased with observations at 1, 2, 3, 6 and 13 days post
drug, there was no overshoot with hypersensitivity of heart rate
responses (Bolli et al., 1981).

Goldstein et al., (1981) studied normal volunteers (n=14) that
were given propranolol for 24 days in a dose (80-240 mg) sufficient
to reduce the exercising heart rate at 160 watts by 20 beats/minute.
Studies were performed 1, 2 and between 6-9 days after stopping
propranolol, no increase in isoprenaline sensitivity was seen.
These investigators gave infusions of isoprenaline, 4 minutes at
each dose level, sufficient to increase heart rate by 20 beats/minute
over preinfusion levels or to give a rate of 120 beats/minute.
Lindenfeld et al., (1980) administered infusions of adrenaline to
ten normal subjects and ten patients with angina; in neither group
was there an increase in the heart rate and systolic blood pressure
responses 4 days after two weeks of administration of propranolol
160 mg a day compared to control, or at least 6 days in the angina
group that was studied for a longer period.

Nattel et al., (1979) did not find any overshoot of heart rate
measured at rest. Likewise Lindenfeld et al., (1980) and Goldstein
et al., (1981) found no overshoot of supine heart rate after propranolol
was stopped. Ross et al., (1981) also observed no overshoot of heart
rate at rest supine or standing when propranolol 160 mg one day (80 mg
bd) was given for one week (n=6) or six weeks (n=12) to normal volunteers. On the other hand, Pedersen et al., (1979) found a significant
overshoot of standing heart rate with levels of 95 at 48 hours after
the last dose falling to 89 on the seventh day after metoprolol
(150-300 mg a day, n=5) or propranolol (160 mg daily, n=1).

Goldstein et al., (1981) observed an overshoot at higher levels of sympathetic activity. After tilt following stopping propranolol, an increase of heart rate of 6 beats over levels prior to propranolol was observed (p<0.05), following tilt plus the administration of atropine (0.8 mg iv), an increase of 8 beats/minute compared to before propranolol (p<0.02). There is some difficulty with these results as the subjects were in-patients (see below). When increased sympathetic activity was induced by vasodilation from 1 mg sublingual glyceryl trinitrate an enhanced tachycardia was seen in the immediate withdrawal phase before heart rates stabilized. There also appeared to be an enhancement of the tachycardia of Valsalva's manoeuvre in the withdrawal phase after six weeks propranolol (Ross et al., 1981). Other experiments suggested four days propranolol administration was not long enough for the withdrawal overshoot of post vasodilation tachycardia (n=6). However, although there was no peak followed by a decline after propranolol was stopped, in contrast to the other groups, the post vasodilation heart rate remained high (120/min) compared to the post six week propranolol group (100/min); control heart rates before beta blocking drug administration were not reported. Similar overshoot of the post vasodilation heart rate was seen in normal volunteers after atenolol 200 mg/day for six weeks (n=6), oxprenolol 160 mg/day for one week (n=6) and acebutalol 400 mg/day for one week (n=6). Overshoot of the post vasodilation heart rate was also seen in hyperthyroid patients with propranolol 160 mg/day for six weeks (n=6), and oxprenolol 160 mg/day for six weeks (n=6) (Ross et al., 1981).

Jackson et al., (1979) found a significant overshoot of exercise systolic blood pressure after propranolol (80 mg qds for one week) at 42 and 54 hours post drug, and after atenolol (100 mg daily for 1 week) at 66 hours, but no overshoot of heart rate was found. Goldstein et al., (1981) observed that the heart rate at 160 watts of exercise averaged 165 beats/minute, a rise of 12 over control (p<0.02) 48 hours after withdrawal of propranolol 80-240 mg daily. These results are difficult to interpret as the subjects were not trained, one baseline exercise being performed, one at 4 days or more on drug, one 2-7 days before propranolol was stopped, besides 1, 2 and 7 days after drug. Propranolol was given for 24-79 days, average 36 days. Throughout the subjects were in-patient, and although it is stated they maintained physical activity, being an in-patient represents the possibility of change of activity level, thus a 'negative' training effect seems possible. A higher exercising heart rate than control might be expected therefore once beta receptor occupation from propranolol had completely declined, ie. at Day 2, when overshoot was reported. Rangno and Langlois (1982) observed a tachycardia of exercise of 158 the second day after stopping pindolol (10 mg bd for one month in ten hypertensives), whereas the rate at Day 20 was 144. However, the probability of a training effect makes these results difficult to interpret as no readings were obtained until the day pindolol was stopped. However others have not

found an overshoot of the exercise tachycardia. It was not seen
after propranolol (160 mg/day) in ten normals with observations
made at 2 and 4 days post drug, or in ten patients with angina at
2, 4 and 6 days post drug (Lindenfeld et al., 1980). Walden et al.,
(1982) studied trained normals and overshoot was not seen with daily
observations for 13 days in the withdrawal phase after propranolol
(average 614 mg/day) atenolol (average 634 mg/day) or pindolol
(average 18 mg/day).

Experiments in animals have also revealed evidence of increased
beta responses after beta blockade withdrawal. Hypersensitivity was
seen after withdrawal of propranolol (120 mg qds) in dogs, to the
cardiac responses to isoprenaline (Webb et al., 1981). However no
evidence of post drug increased beta receptor sensitivity was seen
in dogs treated with four weeks oral propranolol at a dosage of
40 mg, 8 hourly (Myers and Horwitz, 1978). Experiments in rats also
showed a hypersensitivity to isoprenaline after propranolol withdrawal
(Botting and Gibson, 1979). Also in rats hypersensitivity to isoprenaline was seen after the administration of oxprenolol or meto-
prenolol. This response appeared to be oscillatory; on some days
hypersensitivity was seen but not on others (Manning et al., 1981).
While Le Roy et al., (1978) did not demonstrate any increase in the
amount of left ventricular cyclic AMP levels following the administration of isoprenaline in the mouse from 8-40 hours post propranolol
compared to saline, Manning et al., (1980) found an increase in
cyclic AMP and dP/dt max in rat hearts after the withdrawal of three
weeks oxprenolol or metoprolol. Hypersensitivity in rats to heart
rate responses to isoprenaline was confirmed with propranolol but
was not found after the administration of atenolol or LL 21,945,
a long acting non-selective beta blocking drug (Botting and Crook,
1981). Three to six days following the termination of three weeks
oral propranolol to guinea pigs, Dennis et al., (1980) found an
increase in incidence of arrhythmias during pre-ischaemic aerobic
perfusion; during re-perfusion the incidence of arrhythmias was increased and there was a large rise in the occurrence of ventricular
fibrillation.

BETA RECEPTOR POPULATION

A reduction in the number of frog erythrocyte beta receptors
has been found after the chronic administration of isoprenaline,
but propranolol administration failed to alter their number. However,
experiments in rats revealed an increase in beta adrenergic receptor
binding sites in ventricular membranes after two weeks administration
of propranolol, the receptor assay being made 8 hours after the last
dose of propranolol (Glaubier and Lefkowitz, 1977a). The reduction
of beta receptor stimulation from the administration of guanethidine
or 6-hydroxydopamine was also associated with an increase in beta
receptor population (Glaubiger and Lefkowitz, 1977b). Studies with

homogenized whole rat hearts however failed to reveal any increase in
receptor population after propranolol administration (Baker and Potter,
1980). Aarons et al., (1980) demonstrated with radioligand studies
in man a 43% average increase in beta receptor density in human lymphocytes that reached a maximum after 5 days of propranolol 160 mg
daily administration. This increase in receptor population declined
to pre-propranolol levels between 4 and 7 days after propranolol was
withdrawn. However, while others found an increase in beta receptor
population in human leucocytes during the administration of propranolol 240 mg/day for 4 weeks (Fraser and Wood, 1979), because levels
fell below control within 2 days of stopping propranolol it was felt
by these investigators that it was improbable that a continuing raised
beta receptor population was the explanation of the withdrawal phenomenon. Finally, Goldstein et al., (1981) in nine normal subjects
found no increase in white cell beta receptor sites or in cyclic
adenosine monophosphate produced in response to isoprenaline after
propranolol withdrawal. These subjects were in-patients during
propranolol administration and possibly relatively inactive; this
may therefore have influenced these results (see above).

CATECHOLAMINE LEVELS

     Catecholamines do not increase after beta blocker withdrawal.
Plasma levels of adrenaline and noradrenaline were not found to
increase after withdrawal of metoprolol (five patients), propranolol
(one patient) in a group of hypertensives (Pedersen et al., 1979).
Maling and Dollery (1979) in fact observed a fall in plasma noradrenaline in five hypertensive patients after propranolol average
dose 344 mg (range 240-640 mg) was stopped. Likewise Lindenfield
et al., (1980) found a fall in serum adrenaline levels back to control
after propranolol 160 mg daily for 14 days was stopped in ten normal
volunteers and ten patients with angina pectoris. Propranolol
blocked the adrenaline induced increase in free fatty acid levels,
which then returned to baseline with no overshoot when propranolol
was stopped. Similarly, measurements of both adrenaline and noradrenaline at 48 hours post propranolol (up to 240 mg daily for 6-
8 weeks) fell back to control (Vlachakis and Aledort, 1980). No
evidence ot overshoot of plasma noradrenaline when propranolol was
stopped was seen in seven normals studied by Goldstein et al. (1981),
in eight hypertensives after metoprolol (Rangno et al., 1982) or
in six hypertensives after oxprenolol Slow Release 160 of 320 mg.
(Bolli et al., 1981). Our investigations in normals with propranolol
(average 614 mg/day) atenolol (average 634 mg/day) or pindolol (18
mg/day) revealed a fall in serum noradrenaline with drug administration, and no overshoot at 5 or 7 days post drug (Walden et al.,
1982). Likewise work in animals has indicated that an overshoot
of noradrenaline does not occur when propranolol is stopped (Webb
et al., 1981). Vanillylmandelic acid (VMA) excretion was not found
to be increased after the administration of propranolol in normal
subjects (Pantano and Lee, 1976).

On the other hand, Nadeau et al., (1980) found a 55% (p<0.02) increase in urinary adrenaline levels 24 hours after the withdrawal of 4 weeks of propranolol 240 mg/day which returned to normal after 48 hours. The urinary noradrenaline levels showed no overshoot but were increased by 26% during propranolol treatment. Rangno and Nattel (1980) found an overshoot of plasma catecholamines when propranolol (80 mg qds for over one month) was withdrawn.

RENIN LEVELS

Plasma renin levels are reduced by beta adrenergic blocking drugs. No overshoot of renin levels was seen when oxprenolol was withdrawn in six hypertensives by Bolli et al., (1981), or in normal volunteers after atenolol, pindolol or propranolol (Walden et al., 1982).

THYROID HORMONES

Three cases, two hypertensives and one ischaemic patient were reported who developed symptoms after propranolol withdrawal confirmed by laboratory findings of thyrotoxicosis that apparently developed during propranolol treatment (Shenkman et al., 1977). There have been suggestions that increased levels of thyroid hormones may be at least partly responsible for increased beta receptor responsiveness. Free tri-iodothyronine levels were found to be raised in four out of five hypertensive patients who developed tachycardia, sweating, and tremor 2 to 6 days after propranolol (160-480 mg daily for 2 to 18 months) withdrawal, no change in thyroxine or total thyroid hormone levels were found (Kristensen et al., 1978). The increase in free tri-iodothyronine correlated with the serum propranolol concentration on its last day of administration. However, in this study no pre-propranolol or follow up levels of thyroid hormones were reported.

Ross et al (1980) did not observe any change in thyroid hormones in euthyroid subjects after propranolol (160 mg/day for 4 to 8 weeks) was stopped, but an increase in tri-iodothyronine and free tri-iodothyronine though not throxine or free thyroxine levels in hyperthyroid subjects so treated; again hormone levels before propranolol were not quoted. Lindenfeld et al., (1980) did not find any increase in tri-iodothyronine levels after 2 weeks of propranolol 160 mg daily was stopped, free tri-iodothyronine levels were not reported. We observed a fall in serum free T_3 in normals with the administration of atenolol, pindolol and propranolol, with a return to baseline after the drugs were stopped with measurements made 1,3,5,7,9 and 11 days post drug (Walden et al., 1982). Rangno et al., (1982) found no evidence of increased levels of serum T_3 and T_4 after withdrawal of metoprolol (300 mg/day) in eight hypertensive patients; likewise there

was no effect on these hormones after oxprenolol (160-320 mg daily)
was withdrawn in six hypertensives (Bolli et al., 1981).

EFFECT OF BETA ADRENERGIC BLOCKING DRUGS ON PLATELET AGGREGATION

    Observations in patients with angina pectoris indicate that they
have an abnormally low threshold to aggregation to adrenaline or
adenosine diphosphate (ADP) compared to age and sex matched normal
controls. Frishman et al., (1978) for instance found the average
concentration for the biphasic response and maximal platelet aggregation in ten normals at rest was 3.72 μM for ADP and 6.46 for
adrenaline. The corresponding figures for twenty patients with angina
at rest was 1.55 μM for the ADP and 1.26 μM for adrenaline. When
propranolol 160 mg daily for 16 weeks was given to ten of the ischaemic
patients, 3.43 μM ADP was then required for aggregation, ie. similar
to normal controls, compared to a control level of 1.32 μM (p<0.01)
in those patients; the results after 50 weeks were similar to those
at 16 weeks. After propranolol was stopped only 1.0 μM was required
for aggregation 48 hours later, but this was not significantly lower
than prior to propranolol. The responses to adrenaline showed a
similar pattern, after propranolol 12.9 μM of adrenaline was now
required for aggregation in contrast to 1.02 μM before propranolol
(p<0.01), then two days after propranolol was stopped an average of
0.57 μM adrenaline was required. These results were not significantly
different overall from pre-propranolol, but six patients were hyper-
aggregable compared to pre-propranolol. The ten ischaemic patients
who received placebo showed no change in their abnormally high degree
of sensitivity of platelet aggregation to ADP and adrenaline during
the period of observation. Studies in hypertensive patients revealed
an increase in the threshold to maximum platelet aggregation at rest
by adenosine diphosphate from propranolol (6-8 weeks) which declined t
control values two days after propranolol was stopped. Values
returned to control levels although some patients showed an increased
sensitivity compared to control (Vlachakis and Aledort, 1980).
Exercise resulted in a decrease in the amount of adenosine diphosphate
required for platelet aggregation both before (0.55 μM) and after
propranolol (0.25 μM), the differences were not significant. The
administration of propranolol 80-240 mg/day for 24 to 79 days in
normal subjects has indicated that platelet survival is reduced (7.8
days) during the withdrawal phase compared to control (10 days,
p<0.05) (Goldstein et al., 1981). Aggregation of platelets liberate
the prostaglandin thromboxane A_2 which is a coronary vasoconstrictor
(Ellis et al., 1976) this may be a possible basis for a platelet
dependent withdrawal phenomenon.

PROGRESSION OF THE DISEASE PROCESS

In some cases the withdrawal of beta blocking drugs after prolonged treatment could lead to the unmasking of underlying progression
of the disease process, at least as a contributing factor. In
the absence of β-blockade, oxygen supply might not be sufficient to
meet the requirements of the heart even at rest (Diaz et al., 1974).

EFFECT OF INTRINSIC SYMPATHOMIMETIC ACTIVITY

The beta adrenergic blocking drugs vary in their pharmacodynamic
properties, presence or absence of a number of associated properties,
intrinsic sympathomimetic effect, membrane stabilising activity and
cardio-selectivity, and this has been used as a basis of classification
(Prichard, 1978). It seems possible that post beta blockade sensitivity may be due to the generation of additional beta receptors,
thus a beta blocking drug with some partial agonist effect might
provide sufficient beta stimulation to prevent the generation of
additional beta receptors. There is evidence, as discussed above,
with the partial agonist beta blocking drugs pindolol and also oxprenolol, of the absence of post beta blockade hypersensitivity to
isoprenaline. However, in the case of oxprenolol, which possesses
less partial agonist effect, there have been reports of the withdrawal syndrome in ischaemic patients (Wilson et al., 1969).

CONCLUSION

There is little doubt that the beta blocker withdrawal syndrome
is a real phenomenon although the incidence may be low. In some
experimental studies this may be explained by the relatively short
period of observation. In addition to stopping the beta blocker,
exertion may usually be a prerequisite for the development of significant clinical consequences where serious reactions appear to
have occurred in patients with more severe ischaemic disease. When
it is necessary to stop a beta blocking drug, patients should have
the dose reduced gradually and be advised to minimise exertion as the
dose is reduced and for two to three weeks after the drug is stopped.
It is advisable to maintain the final low dose for at least two weeks.

The mechanism of the withdrawal phenomenon may be the generation
of additional beta receptors during the period of beta blockade, thus
when the beta blocker is withdrawn the increased beta receptor population readily results in excessive beta stimulation. This will
be important when the delivery and use of oxygen is finely balanced,
as frequently occurs in ischaemic disease. There is some evidence
that the possession of intrinsic sympathetic stimulating properties
by a beta blocking drug may no longer mean that additional receptors are formed during the administration of the beta blocking drug.

Acknowledgement

    We wish to thank Laetitia Fox for her assistance with this
paper.

REFERENCES

Aarons, R. D., Nies, A. S., Gal, J., Hegstrand, L. R. and Molinoff,
    P. B.,1980, Elevation of B-adrenergic receptor density in
    human lymphocytes after propranolol administration. J. of
    Clin. Investig.,65:949-957.
Alderman, E. L., Coltart, D. J., Wettach, G. E. and Harrison, D. C.,
    1974, Coronary artery syndromes after sudden propranolol
    withdrawal. Annals of Internal Medicine, 81:625-627.
Baker, S. P. and Potter, L. T., 1980, Effect of propranolol on B-
    adrenoceptors in rat hearts. Br. J. of Pharmacol., 68:8-10.
Beeley, L. and Talbot, J., 1979, Beta-blocker withdrawal syndrome?
    The Lancet, February 17, p.387.
Bolli, P., Buhler, F. R., Raeder, E. A., Amann, F. W., Meier, M.,
    Rogg, H., and Burckhardt, D., 1981, Lack of Beta-adrenoceptor
    hypersensitivity after abrupt withdrawal of long-term therapy
    with oxprenolol. Circulation, 64:6, 1130-1134.
Botting, J. H. and Gibson, A., 1979, Beta blocker withdrawal syndrome.
    The Lancet, 1:875-876.
Botting, J. H., and Crook, P., 1981, Effect of abrupt withdrawal of
    chronically administered β-blocking drugs on cardiac sensi-
    tivity in the rat. Experientia, 37:1320-1322.
Boudoulas, H., Lewis, R. P., Kates, R. E. and Dalamangas, G., 1977,
    Hypersensitivity to adrenergic stimulation after propranolol
    withdrawal in normal subjects. Annals of Internal Medicine,
    87:433-436.
Dennis, S. C., Manning, A. S., Hearse, D. J. and Coltart, D. J., 1980.
    Myocardial electrical instability after abrupt withdrawal of
    long term administration of propranolol to guinea pigs.
    Clinical Science, 59:No. 3, 207-209.
Diaz, R. G., Somberg, J., Freeman, E. and Levitt, B., 1974, Myocardial
    infarction after propranolol withdrawal. Am. Heart J., 88:
    257-258.
Ellis, E. F., Oelz, O., Jackson Roberts, L., Payne, N. A., Sweetman,
    B. J., Nies, A. S. and Oates, J. A., 1976, Coronary arterial
    smooth muscle contraction by a substance released from plate-
    lets: Evidence that it is thromboxane A_2. Science vol. 193:
    1135-1137.
Fraser, J. P. and Nood, A. J. J., 1979, Alterations in B-receptor
    density following prolonged propranolol treatment. Circulatio
    (Abstracts 59-60) 60 Supp. II, 274.
Frick, M. H. and Luurila, O., 1976, Double-blind titrated-dose com-
    parison of metoprolol and propranolol in the treatment of
    angina pectoris. Annals of Clin. Res., 8:385-392.

Frishman, W. H., Christodoulou, J., Weksler, B., Smithen, C., Killip, T., and Scheidt, S., 1978, Abrupt propranolol withdrawal in angina pectoris. Effects on platelet aggregation and exercise tolerance. Am. Heart J., 95:169-179.

Glaubiger, G. and Lefkowitz, R. J., 1977a, Elevated beta-adrenergic receptor number after chronic propranolol treatment. Biochemical and Biophysical Research Comm., 78:720-725.

Glaubiger, G. A., Lefkowitz, R. J. and Durham, N. C., 1977b, Increased B-adrenergic receptor number in rat hearts after chemical sympathectomy or propranolol treatment. Circulation, 56 No.4, Supp.3, 158.

Goldberg, A. D., Raftery, E. B. and Wilkinson, P., 1977, Blood pressure and heart rate and withdrawal of antihypertensive drugs. Br. Med. J., 1:1243-1246.

Goldstein, R. E., Corash, L. C., Tallman, J. F., Lake, C. R., Hyde, J., Smith, C. C., Capurro, N. L. and Anderson, J. C., 1981, Shortened platelet survival time and enhanced heart rate responses after abrupt withdrawal of propranolol from normal subjects. Am. J. of Cardiol., 47:1115-1122.

Jackson, G., Schwartz, J., Kates, R. E. and Harrison, D. C., 1979, Physiologic basis for B-blockade 'rebound'. Atenolol versus propranolol. Clin. Res., 27:44A.

Kadish, A., Oka, Y., Becker, R., Frater, R., Lin, Y. T. and Frishman, W., 1979, Propranolol withdrawal: Cause of post-coronary bypass arrhythmias and hypertension. Circulation, 60 No.4. Pt.2, 104.

Kristensen, B. Ø., Steiness, E. and Weeke, J., 1978, Propranolol withdrawal and thyroid hormones in patients with essential hypertension. Clin. Pharmacol. and Therap., 23:624-629.

Leroy, J., Myers, H., Browning, R. and Bundman, M., 1978, Left ventricular cyclic AMP levels following withdrawal from chronic propranolol. Circulation, 58, No.4. Pt.2, 185.

Lindenfeld, J., Crawford, M. H., O'Rourke, R. A., Levine, S. P., Montiel, M. M. and Horwitz, L. D., 1980, Adrenergic responsiveness after abrupt propranolol withdrawal in normal subjects and in patients with angina pectoris. Circulation, 62, No.4, 704-711.

Maling, T. J. B. and Dollery, C. T., 1979, Changes in blood pressure, heart rate and plasma noradrenaline concentration after sudden withdrawal of propranolol. Br. Med. J., 2:366-367.

Manning, A. S., Yellon, D. M., Coltart, D. J., and Hearse, D. J., 1981, Abrupt withdrawal of chronic beta-blockade: Adaptive changes in cyclic amp and contractility. J. of Mol. and Cell. Cardiol., 13:999-1009.

Manning, A. S., Yellon, D. M., Hearse, D. J. and Coltart, D. J., 1980, Chronic beta-blockade: Supersensitivity to catecholamine challenge following cessation of treatment. J. of Mol. and Cell. Cardiol., 12: Suppl. 1, 100.

Meinertz, T., Hajorg, J., Kasfer, W., Kersting, F., and Heinz-Brluing, K., 1979, Beta-blocker withdrawal syndrome? The Lancet, 1:270.

Miller, R. R., Olson, H. G., Amsterdam, E. A. and Mason, D. T., 1975a,
    Propranolol-withdrawal rebound phenomenon. Exacerbation of
    coronary events after abrupt cessation of antianginal therapy.
    New Eng. J. of Med., 293:416-418.
Mizgala, H. F. and Counsell, J., 1976, Acute coronary syndromes
    following abrupt cessation of oral propranolol therapy.
    Can. Med. Assoc. J., 114, No.12, 1123-1126.
Myers, J. H. and Horwitz, L.D., 1978, Hemodynamic and metabolic
    response after abrupt withdrawal of long term propranolol.
    Circulation, 58:196-201.
Myers, M. G. and Wisenberg, G., 1977, Sudden withdrawal of propranolol
    in patients with angina pectoris. Chest, 71:24-26.
Myers, M. G., Freeman, M. R., Juma, Z. A. and Wisenberg, G., 1979,
    Propranolol withdrawal in angina pectoris. A prospective
    study. Am. Heart. J., 97:298-302.
Nadeau, J. H., Fraser, J., Robertson, D. and Wood, A. J. J., 1980,
    Effect of chronic propranolol treatment and withdrawal on
    urinary epinephrine and norepinephrine levels. Clin. Res.
    28, No.2, 240A.
Nattel, S. and Rangno, R. E., 1978, Failure of gradual withdrawal
    of propranolol to prevent beta adrenergic supersensitivity.
    Circulation, 58, No.4, Pt.2, 103 (Abstracts).
Nattel, S., Rangno, R. E. and Van Loon, G., 1979, Mechanism of
    propranolol withdrawal phenomena. Circulation, 59:1158-1164.
Pantano, J. A. and Lee, Y-C, 1976, Abrupt propranolol withdrawal
    and myocardial contractility. Arch. of Intern. Med., 136:
    867-871.
Pedersen, O. L., Mikkelsen, E., Nielsen, J. L. and Christensen, N. J.,
    1979, Abrupt withdrawal of beta-blocking agents in patients
    with arterial hypertension. Effect on blood pressure, heart
    rate and plasma catecholamines and prolactin. Eur. J. of
    Clin. Pharmacol., 15:215-217.
Prichard, B. N. C., 1978, B-adrenergic receptor blockade in hyper-
    tension, past, present and future. Br. J. of Clin. Pharmacol.
    5:379-399.
Prichard, B. N. C. and Gillam, P. M. S., 1971, Assessment of propranolc
    in angina pectoris. Clinical dose response curve and effect
    on electrocardiogram at rest and on exercise. Br. Heart J.,
    33:473-480.
Rangno, R. E., Langlois, S., and Lutterodt, A., 1982, Metoprolol
    withdrawal phenomena: Mechanism and prevention. Clin.
    Pharmacol. and Therap., 31: 8-15
Rangno, R. E. and Langlois, S., 1982, Comparison of withdrawal after
    propranolol, metoprolol and pindolol. Br. J. of Clin.
    Pharmacol., 13:345s-351s.
Rangno, R. and Nattel, S., 1980, Prevention of propranolol withdrawal
    phenomena by gradual dose reduction. Clin. Res.,28, No.2,
    214A.
Ross, P. J., Jones, M. K. and John, R., 1980, Thyroid hormone levels
    after propranolol withdrawal. Clin. Science, 58:22P

Ross, P. J., Lewis, M. J., Sheridan, D. J. and Henderson, A. H.,
    1981, Adrenergic hypersensitivity after beta-blocker with-
    drawal. Br. Heart J., 45:637-642.
Shenkman, L., Podrid, P. and Lowenstein, J., 1977, Hyperthyroidism after
    propranolol withdrawal. J. of Am. Med. Assoc., 238, No.3,
    237-239.
Shiroff, R. A., Mathis, J., Zelis, R., Schenk, D. W., Babb, J. D.,
    Leaman, D. M. and Hayes, A. H.,1978, Propranolol rebound -
    A retrospective study. Am. J. of Cardiol., 41:778-780.
Slome, R., 1973, Withdrawal of propranolol and myocardial infarction.
    The Lancet, 1:156.
Vlachakis, N. D. and Aledort, L., 1980, Hypertension and propranolol
    therapy: Effect on blood pressure, plasma catecholamines and
    platelet aggregation. Am. J. of Cardiol., 45 (2) 321-325.
Walden, R. J., Bhattacharjee, P., Tomlinson, B., Graham, B. R.,
    Cashin, Jeanette and Prichard, B. N. C., 1982, The effect
    of intrinsic sympathomimetic activity on beta receptor
    responsiveness after beta blockade withdrawal. Br. J. of
    Clin. Pharmacol., 13:359s-364s.
Webb, J. G., Newman, W. H., Walle, T. and Daniell, H. B., 1981,
    Myocardial sensitivity to isoproterenol following abrupt
    propranolol withdrawal in conscious dogs. J. of Cardiovas.
    Pharmacol., 3:622-635.
Williams, L. C., Turney, J. H. and Parsons, V., 1979, Beta-blocker
    withdrawal syndrome. The Lancet, 1:494-495.
Wilson, D. F., Watson, O. F., Peel, J. S. and Turner, A. S., 1969,
    Trasicor in angina pectoris: a double-blind trial. Br. Med.
    J., 2:155-157.
Zsoter, T. T. and Beanlands, D. S., 1969, Propranolol in angina
    pectoris. Arch. of Intern. Med., 124:584-587.

.

THE MANAGEMENT OF HYPERTENSION

C.T. Dollery

Professor of Clinical Pharmacology
Royal Postgraduate Medical School
London

In his stirring remarks at the opening of the IXth World Congress
of Cardiology in Moscow Dr Mahler, Director General of the World
Health Organization, made some critical comments about high technology
medicine. He also made some favorable references to the results of
treating hypertension. Many will agree with Dr Mahler, but I see a
danger in his criticisms of modern technology, for it confuses ends
and means. The end is better prevention and/or treatment of disease
by simple, effective and, preferably, cheap methods. Evolution of
those methods may require application of the most sophisticated
technology. The treatment of hypertension is a case in point. The
medicinal chemistry, pharmacology, and clinical research that have
led to therapeutic use of antihypertensive drugs involved a great
deal of very sophisticated science. The output of that science may
have been in medicine that a nurse or medical assistant can use, but
if the resources of medical care had all been devoted to training
medical auxiliaries there would have been no medicines for them to
use.

In the case of hypertension the discovery of effective antihypertensive drugs has redefined the nature of the problem.

Over the past 30 years hypertension has evolved from a medical
emergency, patients presenting with left ventricular failure, renal
failure or hypertensive encephalopathy, to an exercise in preventive
medicine that tests the effectiveness of the medical care delivery
system as much as the clinical skill of the doctor. I can illustrate
this change by referring to the results of treatment in 660 severely
hypertensive patients who began treatment at the Hammersmith Hospital
Hypertension Clinic in the 5 year period between 1962 and 1966
(Bulpitt and Dollery unpublished). This was a time when treatment

269

methods had stabilised after the era of ganglionic blockade. The
patients had relatively severe hypertension with a mean pre-treatment
diastolic pressure in excess of 120 mmHg. They have now been followed
in the Hypertension Clinic for a minimum of 15 years. Those who
died have been ascertained by the Office of Population Censuses and
Surveys, the organization which maintains the mortality records in
the United Kingdom.

The survival of these patients has been remarkably good. In the
case of patients who were between 30 and 49 years old at diagnosis,
over 75% were still alive after 15 years. Thus these patients fell
into the pressure range of the first Veterans' Administration trial.
The data show that the favorable effects of treatment can be maintained over very long periods of time. Those who died had on average
a higher blood pressure, smoked more cigarettes, had a higher blood
urea, were older and included more males than those who lived. There
were two noteworthy exceptions to the profile of risk factors. The
mean serum cholesterol and body weight were slightly higher in those
who lived than in those who died. The survival of black patients
was also slightly better than of whites because fewer of them died
of myocardial infarction. In the white patients myocardial infarction
was the most important cause of cardiovascular death.

This and other studies have enabled us to redefine the problem
of hypertension. The acute bursting vascular pathology that leads
to cerebral haemorrhage or renal failure is readily controlled or
prevented by drug treatment. The strengthening of the heart and
blood vessels by hypertrophy of muscle is halted, and to some extent
reversed, by treatment. The same cannot be said for fibrous replacement of muscle in blood vessels and the heart. My own studies in
the retina and those of Dr Tarazi in the heart suggest that infiltration by collagen is not remodelled during treatment. This had
led to the rather fanciful terminology referring to the collagen
infiltrated heart of the treated hypertensive as a "beating scar".

The principal problem remaining is that of occlusive, especially
atheromatous, vascular disease. Much less progress has been made
with this condition and there is a distinct shortage of ideas about
how to tackle it. We may hope that earlier treatment of hypertension
and more effective antismoking measures may in time make an impact
on this problem. We shall need to pay attention to possible adverse
effects of drugs upon atheroma as a disease (e.g. the hypoglycaemia
and hyperuricaemia caused by thiazide diuretics, and the hyper-
lipidaemia caused by beta adrenergic blockade).

Finally, a word about the structure of this symposium. We have
deliberately not scheduled a standard talk about management of the
uncomplicated patient. Step care regimes which include a beta
blocker, a diuretic and a vasodilator, have been generally adopted.
Whether the beta blocker should be beta-1 selective or non selective,

the diuretic should be potassium conserving or not, and the precise type of vasodilator are a matter of personal preference. No clinical trials have been published which tell us which of these is best in terms of outcome. My own choice currently falls on atenolol as the beta blocker, moduretic as the diuretic, and hydrallazine or minoxidil as the vasodilator. I anticipate that the choice of vasodilator will move towards the calcium antagonists in the future. The role of angiotensin converting inhibitors remains to be defined. They appear to have fewer pharmacodynamic side effects than beta blocking drugs. However, the favorable pharmacodynamic effects of beta adrenergic blockade in patients who have suffered a myocardial infarction may not be shared by the angiotensin converting inhibitors.

For the future some of the most important arguments about the management of hypertension relate to the role of sodium, the use of angiotensin converting enzyme inhibitors, and beta adrenergic blocking drugs. The one aspect of atheromatous disease in which there have been favorable developments is the use of balloon dilatation of renal artery stenosis, and we are pleased to have Dr Heiss to address us on that topic.

SODIUM AND BLOOD PRESSURE IN HUMAN HYPERTENSION

D.L. Davies*, C. Beretta-Piccoli, K. Boddy**,
J.J. Brown, R. Fraser, A.F. Lever and J.I.S. Robertson

MRC Blood Pressure Unit, *Gardiner Institute Department
of Medicine, Western Infirmary, Glasgow and **The Scottish
Universities Research and Reactor Centre, East Kilbridge
Scotland

The role of sodium in the pathogenesis of hypertension is not
agreed. It is likely that excess dietary sodium or excessive retention of sodium is capable of raising blood pressure in some circumstances in man. In Conn's syndrome, for example, the body content
of sodium is abnormally increased, the increase is positively related
to arterial pressure[1], and both abnormalities are corrected by surgical removal of the causative tumour[1]. It is also well recognized
that increased dietary sodium can raise blood pressure in patients
with chronic renal failure[2]. However, in essential hypertension the
role of sodium is much less certain. Although blood pressure and
dietary sodium are higher and essential hypertension is commoner in
'civilized' than in primitive societies, within a civilized society
the essential hypertensives do not, as a rule, eat or excrete more
sodium than normal individuals[3]. Nor do patients with essential
hypertension have an excess of body sodium and yet amongst such
patients arterial pressure and body sodium are positively related,
while normal subjects show no correlation of arterial pressure and
body sodium[4,5] (Figure 1). Some workers consider it unlikely that
dietary sodium is important in the pathogenesis of essential hypertension[3,6], others have suggested that patients with essential hypertension differ from normal subjects in showing a greater change of
arterial pressure for a given change of dietary sodium (Figure 2).
It is the response to change of diet, not the magnitude of the change
of diet which is abnormal.

DIETARY SODIUM

An increase of dietary sodium raises blood pressure in some
patients with essential hypertension[8]; on decreasing dietary sodium

273

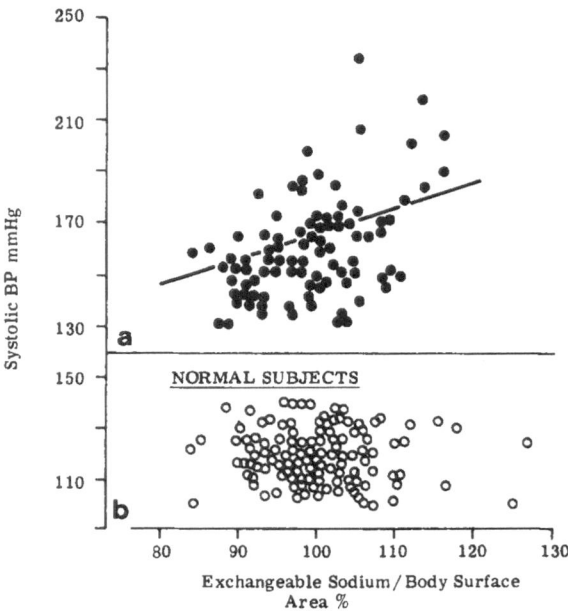

Fig. 1.   (a) Essential Hypertension.   (b) Normal Subjects.
Relation of systolic blood pressure with exchangeable
sodium in patients with untreated essential hypertension
and in normal subjects. Details of the patients and controls are given in refs. 4 and 5. The significance of
these and other correlations with arterial pressure are
given in the table.

blood pressure falls[7],[9] [10]. Changes of arterial pressure are less
marked in normal subjects during the same increase of dietary sodium[8].
This is compatible with the idea of an altered response but it does
not establish the point as the dietary studies referred to are of a
few days duration, while the hypertensive state presumably develops
over years. Also, the response of blood pressure to a particular
treatment is of limited value in identifying the cause of high blood
pressure. Arterial pressure is regulated by more than one mechanism
and essential hypertension can be corrected by drugs acting on different mechanisms. A patient with essential hypertension may respond
with a reduction of blood pressure when given a low sodium diet or
diuretic and when given inhibitors of the renin-angiotensin system
or agents which interfere with transmission in the peripheral and
central nervous systems. As the primary fault in essential hypertension is unlikely to lie in all these sites a good response to low
sodium diet does not necessarily prove that a high sodium diet is
the primary fault.

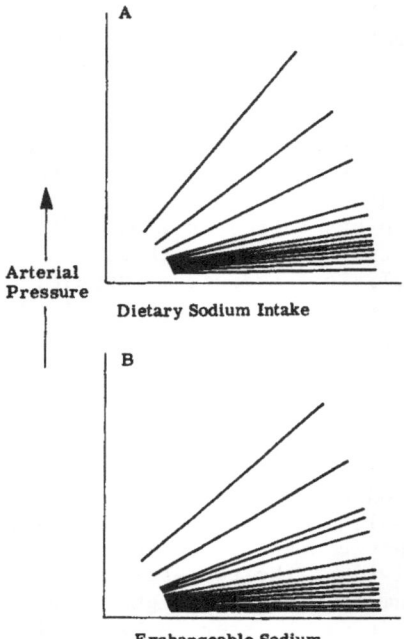

Fig. 2.   A. Hypothetical relation of arterial pressure and dietary
          sodium intake in different people, each represented by a
          single regression line. Most people show little or no in-
          crease in pressure on increasing sodium intake, while a
          few show a distinct increase.
          B. Hypothetical relation of arterial pressure with ex-
          changeable or total body sodium. Again, most people show
          little change on changing body sodium while a few show a
          distinct change.
          Reproduced from the Brit. Med.J. (ref.4) with permission.

        A practical issue arises from the success of low sodium diets
in essential hypertension. Most workers demonstrating a good response
to such diet recommend their adoption in the treatment of hypertension
as a more 'natural' alternative to treatment with hypotensive drugs.
Superficially this is an attractive idea but with every hypotensive
regime there are two points to be established: that the regime
lowers blood pressure and that the lowering of blood pressure reduces
the excess mortality associated with high blood pressure. The
second is more difficult to prove, but ultimately more important.
Before using earlier hypotensive regimes clinicians have insisted on
proof of benefit. Furthermore, demonstration of benefit from one
hypotensive agent has not been considered sufficient evidence to
recommend all agents. Separate tests of benefit were considered

necessary for treatment in severe and moderate hypertension[11], for
treatment in mild hypertension[12,13] for treatment in the elderly
and for treatment with beta-adrenergic blocking agents and thiazide
diuretics[12].

The attitude to testing benefit with low sodium diets in hypertension is different. As noted earlier, several studies have shown
that blood pressure can be reduced by a low sodium diet, but we
know of no study which has tested or aims to test the beneficial
qualities of such diets. Meanwhile, there are numerous recommendations, some from political agencies, suggesting that dietary sodium
should be reduced either in the whole population or in hypertensive
individuals[7,9,14,15]. A trial testing the assumption of these recommendations is needed urgently, in our view.

BODY SODIUM AND ARTERIAL PRESSURE

The content of sodium in the body can be measured by isotope
dilution as exchangeable sodium[16] and by activation analysis[17] which
measures the total body content of sodium. Where both methods are
used in the same individual the two estimates correlate well (Figure
3). Total body sodium is generally higher since some body sodium is
not exchangeable[16]. It can be seen in Figure 1 and in the Table 1
that total body sodium and NaE correlate significantly and positively
with arterial pressure in patients with essential hypertension, no
significant correlation of NaE and blood pressure emerging in normal
subjects. This is compatible with the idea that essential hypertensive individuals are those in whom a given change of body sodium
leads to a greater than normal change of arterial pressure. If true,
the hypothesis would explain both the rise of arterial pressure with
increasing dietary sodium and the response of hypertensive patients
to diuretic agents and low sodium diets. Data in Figure 4 are compatible with this since they show that changing body sodium leads to
a greater change of blood pressure in hypertensive than in normal
subjects, but it can be seen also that data derive from different
studies. Comparison of normal and hypertensive subjects in one laboratory would be a better test.

There are other important reservations. When our data are analysed in subgroups no correlation of blood pressure and body sodium
is found in women or in young hypertensives[4,5]. Thus, if essential
hypertension is a progressive illness and if the younger patients in
our study represent an earlier stage of the disease found in older
patients, the absence of the correlation between body sodium and
blood pressure in the young suggests that its presence is not the
primary fault leading to essential hypertension. Instead, the disease
may pass through several stages becoming progressively more dependent
on sodium[5].

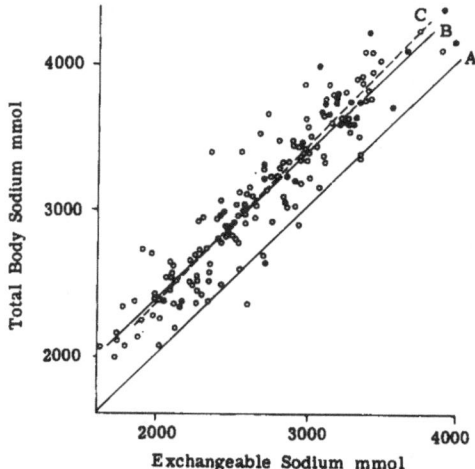

Fig. 3. Relation of exchangeable sodium and total body sodium
measured by activation analysis. Solid points are from 38
essential hypertensive patients having both measurements
(details of these patients are given in refs. 4 and 5).
Open circles are for all other measurements made in our
patients, most of whom have renal artery stenosis or Conn's
syndrome before and after treatment. 'A' is the line of
identity; 'B' the regression for the 38 essential hypertensives; 'C' the regression for other conditions.

Another point of interest is that in young patients with essential hypertension there is an abnormal relation of arterial pressure
with plasma potassium concentration (Table 1). There are links between the potassium concentration of extracellular fluid and the
activity of the autonomic nervous system and overactivity of the
autonomic nervous system is suspected by some workers as a pathogenic
factor in the early stages of essential hypertension[18,19].

IN SUMMARY

Excess dietary sodium and excess body sodium can lead to hypertension but patients with essential hypertension show no evidence of
either excess. This does not rule out a role for sodium since hypertensive individuals may be those in whom arterial pressure rises
when dietary sodium and body sodium are increased. This abnormality
is more likely to be present in old than in young patients. An abnormal mechanism involving potassium and autonomic nervous overactivity may be more important in the earlier stages.

Table 1. Body Sodium and Potassium and their relation with Blood Pressure

A. Mean ± SD

	Whole group		Age <35 yr		Age >50 yr	
	Normal	Essential Ht.	Normal	Essential Ht.	Normal	Essential Ht.
n	121	91	63	30	37	29
Blood pressure mmHg	120/76±11/9	160/102±20/15	118/73±11/10	154/98±14/3	126/80±11/8	165/104±21/13
Plasma Na mmol.l^{-1}	140.1±2.0	139.3±2.3*	140.7±1.5	138.3±2.4**	141.8±1.0	140.1±2.2*
Exchangeable Na						
% surface area	100.0±7.3	99.1±7.1	100.2±7.1	96.6±5.2*	99.1±8.0	102.6±7.7
% leanness index	100.0±7.3	97.8±6.6**	99.8±7.7	95.3±5.1**	99.4±7.9	101.3±7.0

B. Correlation with BP

	Whole group				Age <35 yr				Age >50 yr			
	Normal		Essential Ht.		Normal		Essential Ht.		Normal		Essential Ht.	
	Syst.	Diast.	Syst.	Diast.	Syst.	Diast.	Syst.	Diast.	Syst.	Diast.	Syst.	Diast.
Exchangeable Na												
% surface area	0.04	-0.03	0.44**	0.31*	-0.07	-0.09	0.12	0.05	-0.15	0.12	0.64**	0.48**
% leanness index	0.02	0.01	0.41**	0.33**	-0.03	-0.07	0.22	0.15	-0.08	0.16	0.69**	0.59
Total body Na			0.55***	0.44**								
Plasma potassium	0.17	0.09	-0.32**	-0.41***	-0.08	-0.13	-0.41*	-0.51**	0.11	0.13	-0.36	-0.16
KE	–	–	-0.28*	-0.28*	–	–	-0.39	-0.52*	–	–	-0.38	-0.27
Total body K	–	–	-0.38**	-0.39**	–	–	-0.32	-0.52**	–	–	-0.03	-0.14

Mean values ± SD are shown in the upper part of the table, *p <0.05; **p <0.01; ***p <0.001.
Total body sodium was measured in 38 patients.

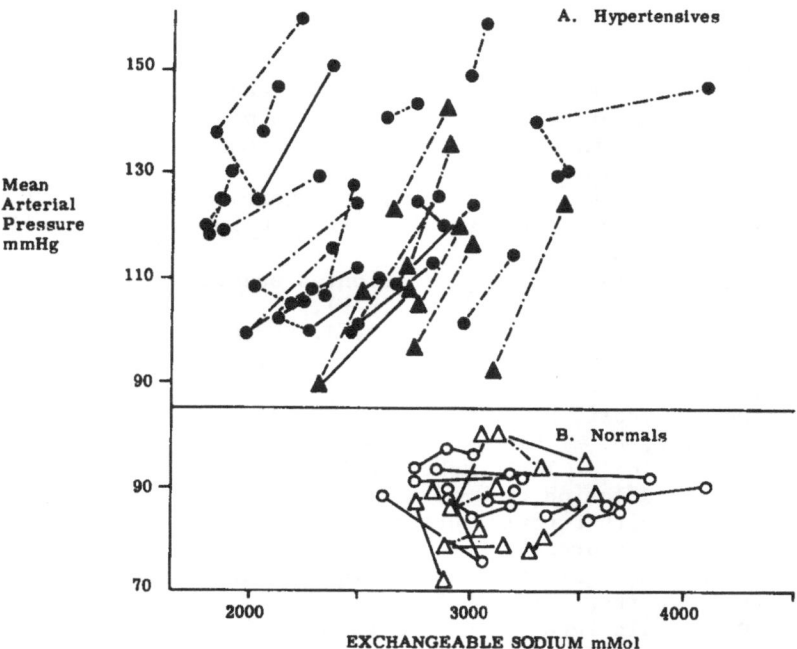

Fig. 4.   Relation between exchangeable sodium and mean arterial
          pressure before and during changes of dietary sodium intake.
          Open symbols, normal subjects; solid symbols, patients with
          essential hypertension.   Lines join measurements in the
          same individual.   A dashed line indicates measurements made
          during sodium restriction, a solid line, measurements made
          during sodium loading and a dotted line, measurements made
          under identical dietary circumstance.   Solid circles are
          from hypertensive patients studied by Dahl and his colleagues
          (refs. 19 and 20).   Solid triangles are for essential hyper-
          tensives studied in the Glasgow Unit; open circles are from
          normal subjects studied by Kirkendall and his colleagues
          (ref. 21); open triangles are from normal subjects studied
          in the Glasgow Unit.

ACKNOWLEDGEMENTS

We thank Miss Ann Matheson for secretarial help.

REFERENCES

1. C. Beretta-Piccoli, D. L. Davies, J. J. Brown, J. B. Ferriss,
    R. Fraser, A. F. Lever, J. J. Morton, and J. I. S. Robertson,
    The relation of arterial pressure with plasma and body elec-
    trolytes is similar in Conn's syndrome and essential hyper-
    tension, Clin.Sci. (in press).

2. F. C. Husted, K. D. Nolph, and J. F. Maher, $NaHCO_3$ and NaCl
    tolerance in chronic renal failure, J.Clin.Invest. 56:414
    (1975).

3. F. O. Simpson, Salt and hypertension: a sceptical review of the
    evidence, Clin.Sci. 57:463s (1979).

4. A. F. Lever, C. Beretta-Piccoli, J. J. Brown, D. L. Davies,
    R. Fraser, and J. I. S. Robertson, Sodium and potassium in
    essential hypertension, Brit.Med.J. 283:463 (1981).

5. C. Beretta-Piccoli, D. L. Davies, K. Boddy, J. J. Brown, A. M.
    M. Cumming, B. W. East, R. Fraser, A. F. Lever, P. L. Padfield,
    P. F. Semple, J. I. S. Robertson, P. Weidmann, and E. D.
    Williams, Relation of body sodium, body potassium, plasma
    potassium with arterial pressure in essential hypertension,
    Clin.Sci. (in press).

6. G. W. Pickering, Salt intake and blood pressure, Cardiovasc.
    Revs.& Reports. 1:13 (1980).

7. L. K. Dahl, Salt intake and hypertension, in: "Hypertension,
    Pathophysiology and Treatment," J. Genest, E. Koiw, and O.
    Kuchel, eds., McGraw-Hill Book Company, New York, 548 (1977).

8. J. M. Sullivan, T. E. Ratts, J. C. Taylor, D. H. Kraus, B. R.
    Barton, D. R. Patrick, and S. W. Reed, Hemodynamic effects
    of dietary sodium in man, Hypertension 2:506 (1980).

9. T. Morton, W. Adam, A. Gillies, M. Wilson, G. Morgan, and S.
    Carney, Hypertension treated by salt restriction, Lancet
    1:227 (1978).

10. G. A. MacGregor, F. E. Best, J. M. Cam, N. D. Markandu, D. M.
    Elder, G. A. Sagnella, M. Squires, Double blind randomised
    crossover trial of moderate sodium restriction in essential
    hypertension, Lancet 1:251 (1982).

11. Veterans Administration Cooperative Study Group on antihyper-
    tensive agents, Effects of treatment on morbidity in hyper-
    tension: results in patients with diastolic blood pressures
    averaging 115 through 129 mmHg, JAMA 202:1228 (1967).

12. MRC Working Party on mild to moderate hypertension. Randomized
    control trial of treatment for mild hypertension: design
    and pilot trial, Brit.Med.J. 1:1437 (1977).

13. R. Reader, The Australian therapeutic trial in mild hypertension,
    Report by the Management Committee, Lancet 1:1261 (1980).

14. Select Committee on Nutrition and Human Needs, "Dietary goals
    for the United States," United States Senate, Chairman, G.
    McGovern, U.S. Government Printing Office, 49 (1977).

15. Report of a Select Committee of Food and Drug Administration,
    "Evaluation of the health aspects of sodium chloride and
    potassium chloride as food ingredients," Washington DC (1979).

16. D. L. Davies, and J. W. K. Robertson, Simultaneous measurement of total exchangeable potassium and sodium using ^{43}K and ^{24}Na, Metabolism 22:133 (1973).

17. K. Boddy, J. J. Brown, D. L. Davies, A. Elliot, I. Harvey, J. K. Haywood, I. Holloway, A. F. Lever, J. I. S. Robertson, and E. D. Williams, Concurrent estimation of total body and exchangeable body sodium in hypertension, Clin.Sci.& Mol.Med. 54:187 (1978).

18. Z. Zadik, B. P. Hamilton, and A. A. Kowarski, Integrated concentration of epinephrine and norepinephrine in normal subjects and in patients with mild essential hypertension, J.Clin.Endocrinol.& Metab. 50:842 (1980).

19. I. J. Kopin, D. S. Goldstein, G. Z. Feuerstein, The sympathetic nervous system and hypertension, in: "Frontiers in Hypertension Research," J. H. Laragh, F. R. Buhler, D. W. Seldin, eds., Springer-Verlag, New York 283 (1981).

20. L. K. Dahl, B. G. Stall, and G. C. Cotzias, Metabolic effects of marked sodium restriction in hypertensive patients: changes in total exchangeable sodium and potassium, J.Clin. Invest. 33:1397 (1954).

21. V. P. Dole, L. K. Dahl, G. C. Cotzias, D. D. Dziewiatkowski, and C. Harris, Dietary treatment of hypertension. II. Sodium depletion as related to the therapeutic effect, J.Clin.Invest. 30:584 (1951).

22. W. M. Kirkendall, W. E. Connor, F. D. Abboud, S. P. Rastogi, T. A. Anderson, and M. Fry, The effect of dietary sodium chloride on blood pressure, body fluids, electrolytes, renal function and serum lipids of normotensive man, J.Lab.Clin. Med. 87:418 (1976).

INHIBITION OF THE RENIN ANGIOTENSIN SYSTEM

IN THE TREATMENT OF HYPERTENSION

R. Fagard, P. Lijnen, J. Staessen, and A. Amery

Hypertension and Cardiovascular Rehabilitation Unit
Dept. of Pathophysiology, Faculty of Medicine
University of Leuven, 3000 Leuven, Belgium

Renin is a proteolytic enzyme that is synthetized, stored and secreted mainly by the juxtaglomerular apparatus of the kidney. The release of renin is regulated a.o. by renal baroreceptors, by sodium-sensitive mechanisms at the level of the macula densa, by the sympathetic nervous system, prostaglandins and angiotensin II. Renin acts on its substrate, angiotensinogen, an alpha-2-globulin produced in the liver and present in the plasma to form the decapeptide angiotensin I, which is practically devoid of pressor activity. The converting-enzyme, a peptidyl-dipeptidase, converts angiotensin I to angiotensin II by splitting off the dipeptide histidyl-leucine at the C-terminal of the decapeptide. The pulmonary circulation is the main site of conversion, but converting-enzyme is also present in the plasma, in the splanchnic system, in the kidney and in several other tissues. Angiotensin II is the effector hormone of the system in man. Its most important actions are direct pressor effects on the arteriolar smooth muscle, stimulation of the aldosterone secretion by the adrenal gland, and effects on the central and peripheral nervous system; these actions result in an increase of blood pressure and in salt and water retention.

The renin-angiotensin system may be blocked more or less selectively at several levels. Pharmacological agents which depress sympathetic activity decrease renin release, as is the case with beta-adrenoceptor blocking agents. The action of renin on renin substrate has been antagonized by nonspecific proteases such as pepstatin, and antibodies to renin and to angiotensinogen as well as structural analogues of the latter have been developed. Peptide and nonpeptide converting-enzyme inhibitors interfere with the conversion of angiotensin I into angiotensin II, but also with the degradation of bradykinin. Angiotensin II analogues, acting as

283

antagonists by competing with angiotensin II at its receptor sites, have been synthetized, but are not completely devoid of agonist actions.

This paper will deal only with the angiotensin II analogues and with the converting-enzyme inhibitors.

ANGIOTENSIN II ANALOGUES

In the first approach to the development of angiotensin II antagonists a thorough study of structure activity relationships of angiotensin II was performed[1]. As a result of these studies, it was shown that the side group in position 8 on angiotensin II was responsible for the transmission of the information which caused smooth muscle contraction. The information led to the development of the 8-substituted analogues that are competitive inhibitors of angiotensin II. Moreover it was found that substitution of sarcosine in position 1 potentiates the biological activities already existing in the molecule.

The derivate of angiotensin II which has been used most in clinical and/or experimental studies is 1-sarcosine-8-alanine-angiotensin II (saralasin)[2]. This substance has antagonist properties, but also agonist angiotensin II-like activities which is not surprising for an agent that arose from modification of angiotensin II.

In a few studies[3-6] saralasin has been infused into supine sodium replete hypertensive patients, whose sodium intake was between 95 and 150 mmol/24 hours. A vasodepressor response, usually defined as a decrease of diastolic or mean arterial pressure of 7-8 mmHg, occurred in 0-40% of the patients. Differences between studies may be explained by the etiology of hypertension, prevailing plasma renin levels and possibly by differences in plasma volume which may have been decreased with a consequent rise in plasma renin in severe hypertensives[7]. Furthermore, stimulation of the renin-angiotensin system in the seated position[8] may increase the number of responders. In several studies saralasin was administered in both sodium replete and sodium depleted conditions[3-6]. Whereas in these studies 0-40% of the patients responded to saralasin with a significant vasodepressor response in sodium replete conditions, the percentage was 30-90% after sodium depletion. Differences between studies are mainly due to patient's selection, but also to the degree of sodium depletion. Indeed, the number of responders and the magnitude of the pressure fall rose with increasing degree of sodium depletion[6] and even low renin patients do respond to saralasin after severe sodium depletion[9]. When blood pressure decreases in response to saralasin this is usually related to a reduction of systemic vascular resistance[10].

The use of angiotensin II antagonists for the treatment of hypertension is up to now limited by the fact that they have to be administered parenterally. Therefore they can only be used for short periods of time. Brunner et al.,[11] reported that when given to seven patients with malignant or advanced hypertension, saralasin lowered blood pressure to close to normal levels in three patients, whose peripheral plasma renin activity was elevated, and reduced the blood pressure slightly or not at all in the remaining four with normal or low renin levels. A similar experience was reported by Streeten et al.,[12] but they found intravenous infusions of nitroprusside more reliable in those circumstances.

CONVERTING ENZYME INHIBITORS

The nonapeptide teprotide, which is found in snake venom, blocks the conversion of angiotensin I into angiotensin II but has to be administered intravenously. Recently orally active converting enzyme inhibitors have been synthetized, of which the most thoroughly investigated is captopril (2-D-methyl-mercaptopropanoyl-L-proline; SQ 14225).[13] It effectively inhibits the pressor effect of exogenous angiotensin I in man[14] and suppresses the levels of endogenous angiotensin II.[15] However the converting enzyme is also responsible for the degradation of bradykinin, and accumulation of kinins may contribute to the hypotensive response to captopril.[16] There are at present no convincing data that non specific mechanisms, independent of inhibition of converting enzyme are operational.[17]

Captopril lowers blood pressure to a variable extent in patients with hypertension.[18] When a group of subjects with a wide range of plasma renin or angiotensin II levels is studied, the hypotensive effect is correlated with these levels, but the relationship is better for the acute hypotensive effect than for prolonged treatment.[18,19] In sodium replete patients with uncomplicated essential hypertension blood pressure decrease averages 10 to 25%, and is comparable to the effects of thiazides or beta-blockers.[18] The response appears to be greater in patients with severe renovascular hypertension, in some with 'resistant' of 'malignant' hypertension, or after renin-stimulating procedures such as sodium depletion. In high-renin patients with contracted plasma volume dramatic blood pressure falls may however occur with the first dose of captopril.[20] The dose response curve of captopril in hypertensive man suggests that 3 x 50 mg per day guarantees effective biochemical expression of converting enzyme inhibition.[21] Smaller doses, even a few mg, are effective, but then the effect is only of short duration. Hemodynamically the fall in pressure is based on a reduction of systemic vascular resistance both at rest[19] and during exercise,[22] with little or no increase of heart rate and cardiac output; also pulmonary capillary wedge pressure falls with captopril.

Treatment with captopril has been associated with side effects such as rash and taste disturbance, hematological effects as neutropenia and agranulocytosis, and proteinuria.[18]

COMPARISON OF SARALASIN AND CAPTOPRIL

When saralasin and captopril are administered to slightly sodium-depleted hypertensive patients, the changes of pressure of both drugs are related to the prevailing plasma renin level. However, the hypotensive effect of captopril is about 10 mmHg greater than that of saralasin.[15] The difference may be due to the intrinsic pressor effect of saralasin, or to kinin accumulation during captopril.

These data indicate that there is still room for the development of more specific inhibitors of the renin angiotensin system.

REFERENCES

1. M. C. Khosla, R. R. Smeby, and F. M. Bumpus, Structure activity relationships in angiotensin II analogs, in: "Angiotensin," Springer, Berlin, p.162 (1964).
2. D. T. Pals, F. D. Masucci, G. S. Denning, F. Dipos, and D. C. Fessler, Role of the pressor action of angiotensin II in experimental hypertension, Circ.Res. 29:673 (1971).
3. L. Baer, J. Z. Parra-Carillo, and I. Radichevich, Angiotensin II blockade: Evidence for baroreceptor mediated renin release and the role of sodium balance, Kid.Int. 15:S60 (1979).
4. L. S. Marks, M. H. Maxwell, and J. J. Kaufman, Renin, sodium, and vasodepressor response to saralasin in renovascular and essential hypertension, Ann.Int.Med. 87:176 (1977).
5. R. Fagard, A. Amery, P. Lijnen, and T. Reybrouck, Effects of angiotensin II antagonist 1-sar-8-ala-angiotensin II in hypertension in man, Eur.J.Clin.Invest. 7:473 (1977).
6. C. Thananopavarn, M. S. Golub, P. Eggena, J. D. Barrett, and M. P. Sambhi, Angiotensin II, plasma renin and sodium depletion as determinants of blood pressure response to saralasin in essential hypertension, Circulation 61:920 (1980)
7. J. C. Romero, D. R. Holmes, and C. G. Strong, The effect of high sodium intake and angiotensin antagonist in rabbits with severe and moderate hypertension induced by constriction of one renal artery, Circ.Res. 40(Suppl.1):17 (1977).
8. D. B. Case, J. M. Wallace, H. J. Keim, J. E. Sealy, and J. H. Laragh, Usefulness and limitations of saralasin, a partial competitive agonist of angiotensin II, for evaluating the renin and sodium factors in hypertensive patients, Am.J.Med. 60:825 (1976).

9. H. Gavras, A. B. Ribeiro, I. Gavras, and H. R. Brunner, Reciprocal relation between renin dependency and sodium dependency in essential hypertension, New Engl.J.Med. 295: 1278 (1976).

10. R. Fagard, A. Amery, P. Lijnen, T. Reybrouck, J. V. Joossens, L. Billiet, E. Moerman, and A. De Schaepdryver, Effects of 1-sar-8-ala-angiotensin II on systemic and pulmonary haemodynamics in hypertensive patients, Clin.Exp.Physiol. Pharmacol. 5:457 (1978).

11. H. R. Brunner, H. Gavras, J. H. Laragh, and R. Keenan, Hypertension in man, exposure of the renin and sodium components using angiotensin II blockade, Circ.Res. 34(Suppl.1):35 (1974).

12. D. H. P. Streeten, G. H. Anderson, and T. G. Dalakos, Angiotensin blockade: its clinical significance, Am.J.Med. 60: 817 (1976).

13. M. A. Ondetti, B. Rubin, and D. W. Cushman, Design of specific inhibitors of angiotensin converting enzyme: new class of orally active antihypertensive agents, Science 196:441 (1977).

14. R. K. Ferguson, G. A. Turini, H. R. Brunner, and H. Gavras, A specific orally active inhibitor of angiotensin-converting enzyme in man, Lancet 1:775 (1977).

15. R. Fagard, A. K. Amery, P. J. Lijnen, and T. M. Reybrouck, Comparative study of an angiotensin II analog and a converting enzyme inhibitor, Kid.Int. 17:647 (1980).

16. O. A. Carretero, A. G. Scicli, and R. Maitra, Role of kinins in the pharmacological effects of converting enzyme inhibitors, in: "Angiotensin Converting Enzyme Inhibitors," Urban & Schwarzenberg, Baltimore-Munich, p.105 (1981).

17. B. Rubin, M. J. Antonaccio, and Z. P. Horovitz, The antihypertensive effects of captopril in hypertensive animal models, in: "Angiotensin Converting Enzyme Inhibitors," Urban & Schwarzenberg, Baltimore-Munich, p.27 (1981).

18. R. C. Heel, R. N. Brogden, T. M. Speight, and G. S. Avery, Captopril: a preliminary review of its pharmacological properties and therapeutic efficacy, Drugs 20:409 (1980).

19. R. Fagard, A. Amery, T. Reybrouck, P. Lijnen, and L. Billiet, Acute and chronic systemic and pulmonary hemodynamic effects of angiotensin converting enzyme inhibition with captopril in hypertensive patients, Am.J.Cardiol. 46:295 (1980).

20. R. Fagard, A. Amery, P. Lijnen, and J. Staessen, First dose effects of the oral angiotensin converting enzyme inhibitor captopril, Arch.Int.Pharmacodyn.Ther. (Suppl.):179 (1980).

21. P. Lijnen, R. Fagard, J. Staessen, L. J. Verschueren, and A. Amery, Dose response in captopril therapy of hypertension, Clin.Pharmacol.Ther. 28:310 (1980).

22. R. Fagard, C. Bulpitt, P. Lijnen, and A. Amery, Response of the systemic and pulmonary circulation to converting enzyme inhibition at rest and during exercise in hypertensive patients, Circulation 65:33 (1982).

CATHETER TREATMENT OF RENOVASCULAR HYPERTENSION

K. Mathias and H. W. Heiss

Department of Diagnostic Radiology
University of Freiburg

Renovascular hypertension can be treated effectively in nearly all patients with modern antihypertensive drugs. But medical therapy is accompanied by disadvantages such as lacking patient compliance, and side effects of the medication. Long-term medication - as necessary in younger patients - is expensive, and the reduced blood flow to the affected kidney is not improved. In the past vascular surgery was the treatment of choice in patients with renal artery stenosis with hyperreninemia and a short history of hypertension. Operative pain and risk, costs and an uncertain treatment result restricted vascular surgery to critically selected patients.

Four years ago percutaneous transluminal catheter dilatation (PTRD) was added to the therapeutic spectrum of renovascular hypertension.[2,3,5,7] In the meanwhile we treated 76 patients with this method and gained plenty of data to evaluate the benefits and limitations of the procedure.

INDICATIONS

PTRD is indicated in patients with a combination of hypertension, hyperreninemia, and renal artery stenosis regardless of its nature (Table 1). Age is no limiting factor for PTRD, but it may be difficult to dilate renal arteries in infants younger than 2 years because of the small vascular dimensions. In older children PTRD may be performed successfully.[8,9] In patients older than 60 years the blood pressure cannot be expected to return to normal values, but most of these patients are treated for renal insufficiency due to bilateral kidney disease.[4] Kidney grafts with anastomotic or post-anastomotic renal artery stenosis caused by intimal proliferation

289

Table 1.   Indications for PTRD in Renovascular Hypertension

Renal Artery Stenosis: 70% or more
      Atherosclerosis
      Fibromuscular Dysplasia
      Neurofibromatosis
      Intimal Proliferation in Kidney Graft
      Postoperative Anastomotic Stenosis
Renal Artery Occlusion
      Rarely in Atherosclerosis in
      Connection with Renal Insufficiency
Renal Insufficiency
      Caused by Stenosis or Occlusion

---

are suited for PTRD, but the success rate is not as high as in our
other patients depending on the implantation technique and anatomical
details.[6] Patients with post-traumatic or atherosclerotic renal
artery occlusions are furtheron candidates for surgery.[1]

PERFORMANCE

     PTRD is carried out in local anesthesia under light sedation.
Long acting antihypertensive drugs are discarded before the intervention to avoid threatening pressure drops. The blood pressure
should not exceed 200 mmHg during PTRD to prevent hemorrhage at the
puncture site. In critical patients this is achieved by sodium
nitroprusside infusion under continuous pressure surveillance.

     The normal approach for PTRD is the femoral artery at the
groin. A transaxillary route is chosen when the renal artery
originates with an acute angle from the aorta or when the iliac
arteries are obstructed.[10]

     Two catheter systems are available for PTRD.

1.   Single catheter technique: after probing of the renal artery
     with a diagnostic catheter a guide wire is placed with its tip
     beyond the stenosis, the diagnostic catheter is exchanged
     against a dilatation catheter (F-7 or F-5), and the stenosis
     is dilated.
2.   Coaxial catheter technique: a guiding catheter (F-9 or F-8) is
     placed before the ostium of the renal artery. A small di-
     latation catheter (F-4.5) is passed through it and enters the
     narrowed renal artery. Thereafter, dilatation is performed.

     The coaxial catheter set is advantageous when a high degree
stenosis cannot be overcome by the thicker single catheter, but will
produce a bigger puncture hole.

During PTRD the pressure is measured in the renal artery determining the pressure gradient before and after dilatation. At the end of the dilatation treatment a control angiogram is performed. On the first day the patients receive 20,000 U of heparine, and medication with platelet aggregation inhibitors is started, and should be continued for a least 6 months.

RESULTS

PTRD was attempted in 76 patients with 87 stenoses. The patients had a mean age of 45 years with a range from 5 to 75 years. The nature of the stenoses is shown in Table 2. PTRD was finished in 5 patients without success, in whom the obstruction could not be passed by the dilatation catheter (2 stenoses in fibromuscular dysplasia and 2 in kidney grafts, 1 renal artery occlusion). PTRD was technically successful in 82 of 87 stenoses (94%). In 19 patients hypertension persisted or recurred. In 14 of them a control angiogram was performed and revealed a normal renal artery in 9 and a recurrent stenosis in 5 patients. In 2 cases the recurrent stenosis was redilated improving the hypertension considerably. In all 3 patients with renal insufficiency the kidney function was improved by PTRD, but the blood pressure was not reduced significantly (Table 3).

Case 1:   22-year old woman with a blood pressure of 240/110 mmHg. Angiography revealed bilateral fibrodysplastic renal artery stenosis. The stenotic segment of the renal artery was dilated on both sides, and the blood pressure declined within 6 hours to 120/80 mmHg (Figure 1). The patient is normotensive for 8 months without medication.

Case 2:   58-year old man with a history of hypertension for 2 years and a renal artery stenosis on the left side. After PTRD a residual stenosis of 20% remained, but the blood pressure returned to normal values without any medication.

The patients came for follow-up studies every 3 months in the first year and every 6 months thereafter. The mean follow-up amounts to 23 months with a range from 1 to 58 months. The results were evaluated using the life table method. 24 of 76 patients were cured with blood pressure values below 150/95 mmHg without antihypertensive drugs. In 33 patients the blood pressure declined after PTRD, but the patients still need saluretics or β-blocking agents to keep the blood pressure in the normal range. Most of these patients belong to the group with an atherosclerotic stenosis and are older than 45 years. In 19 patients the blood pressure remained unchanged after PTRD. 7 of these patients had nearly normal renin values before

Table 2. Nature of Renal Artery Stenosis

Atherosclerosis	68	78%
Fibromuscular Dysplasia	13	15%
Kidney Graft	6	7%

Table 3. Results of PTRD

Patients	76	100%
Normotensive (<150/95 mmHg)	24	32%
Improved	33	43%
Hypertensive	19	25%
Dead	2	2.5%

PTRD and 3 patients suffered from terminal renal insufficiency. In 2 females with fibromuscular dysplasia hyperreninemia vanished, but hypertension persisted. In one patient with malignant hypertension cerebral hemorrhage occurred 2 months after PTRD, and had a fatal outcome.

Renin concentration was determined in renal vein blood samples before and after PTRD in 68 patients. Renin values were elevated in 51 of them (74%), 6ng/ml/h being the upper normal limit. The predictive implications were impressive: 90% of the patients with hyperreninemia had a blood pressure decrease after PTRD. But renin concentration and renin ratio are of little use for the indication of PTRD, because in 59% of the cases with normal to borderline renin values hypertension was improved after PTRD, too.

COMPLICATIONS

Complications were encountered in 3 patients (4%) and required surgical intervention in one case of renal artery dissection treated by an aortorenal bypass graft. Two patients developed a hematoma at the groin which was conservatively managed.

CONCLUSIONS

PTRD was performed in 76 patients with renovascular hypertension with a primary success rate of 94%, and a blood pressure decrease in 75% of the patients. 5 patients (6%) developed a recurrent stenosis during a mean follow-up of 23 months which was redilated in 2 of

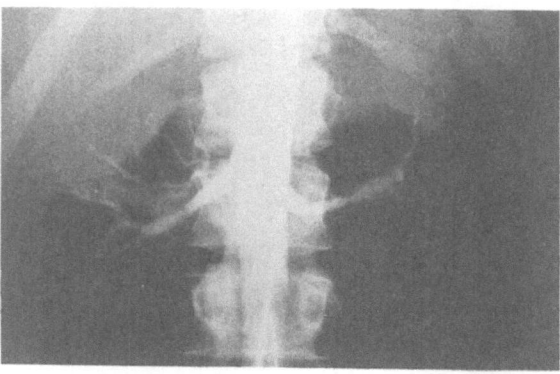

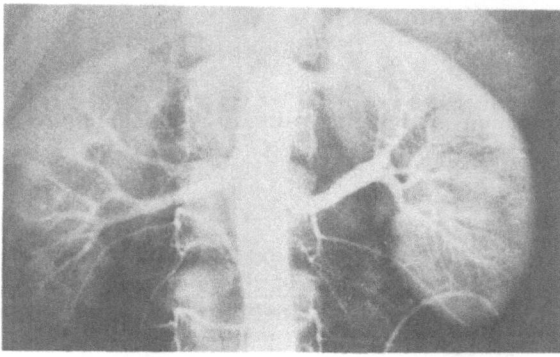

Fig. 1. 22-year-old female with bilateral fibrodysplastic renal artery stenosis which could be completely removed on both sides.

them (2.5%) with good result. These data, confirmed by other groups working with PTRD, underline the efficacy of the procedure in renovascular hypertension.[2,3,5,7]. Therefore, in our opinion there is enough evidence that PTRD should be attempted in all hypertensive patients with renal artery stenosis with a narrowing of more than 70%, regardless of renin values. Vascular surgery should be restricted to patients with additional vascular problems as aneurysm of the renal artery, aortic aneurysm or iliac artery occlusion, and to those with technical treatment failures of PTRD. Patients older than 60 years should be managed conservatively, and are only referred to PTRD when the blood pressure cannot be controlled sufficiently by antihypertensive medication or when renal insufficiency develops.

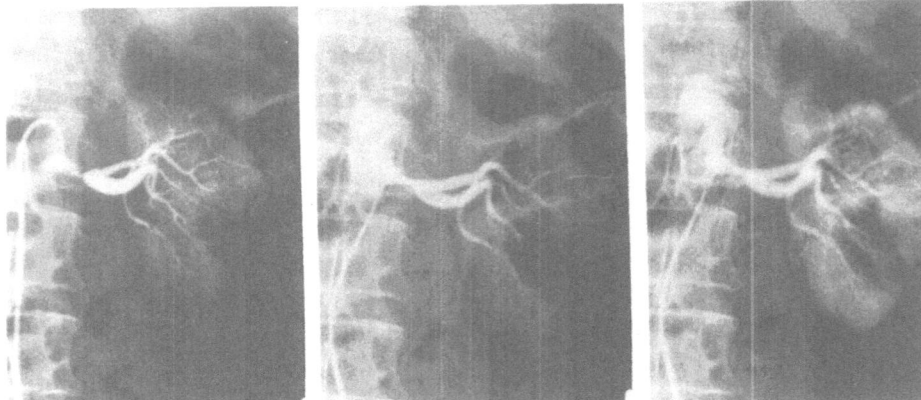

Fig. 2.   58-year-old man with left sided atherosclerotic renal
          artery stenosis, considerably improved by PTRD. Better
          filling of the intrarenal arterial braches after dilation.

REFERENCES

1. J. M. Barry and C. V. Hodges, Revascularization of totally
    occluded renal arteries, J.Urol. 119:412 (1978).
2. B. Katzen, J. Chang, G. H. Lukowsky, and E. G. Abramson, Percu-
    taneous transluminal angioplasty of renovascular hypertension.
    Radiology 131:53 (1979).
3. U. Kuhlmann, W. Vetter, J. Furrer, U. Lütlof, W. Siegenthaler,
    and A. Grüntzig, Renovascular hypertension: treatment by
    percutaneous transluminal dilatation, Ann.Intern.Med. 92:1
    (1980).
4. A. G. Logan, and M. I. Steinhardt, Restoration of renal function
    by unilateral percutaneous transluminal dilatation of stenosed
    renal artery, Canad.Med.Assoc.J. 122:910 (1980).
5. F. Mahler, A. Krneta, and M. Haertel, Treatment of renovascular
    hypertension by transluminal renal artery dilatation, Ann.
    Intern.Med. 90:56 (1979).
6. K. Mathias, W. Rau, and G. Kauffmann, Katheterdilatation einer
    Arterienstenose nach Nierentransplantation, Dtsch.Med.Wschr.
    104:437 (1979).
7. K. Mathias, P. Billmann, R. Liebig, T. Kröpelin, and K.
    Thierfelder, Behandlung der renovaskulären Hypertonie mit
    der Katheterdilatation, Radiologe 20:494 (1980).
8. K. Mathias, E. Struck, F. Schindera, and B. Urbanyi, Percutaneous
    treatment of renovascular hypertension, Pediatr.Radiol. 11:154
    (1981).
9. T. A. McCook, S. R. Mills, D. R. Kirks, D. K. Heaston, H. F.
    Seigler, and R. B. Malone, Percutaneous transluminal renal

artery angioplasty in a 3½-year-old hypertensive girl, J. Pediatr. 97:958 (1980).

10. Ch. J. Tegtmeyer, C. A. Ayers, and H. A. Wellons, Axillary approach to percutaneous renal artery dilatation, Radiology 135:775 (1980).

PATHOGENETIC MECHANISMS IN ESSENTIAL HYPERTENSION

Franz H. Messerli and Edward D. Frohlich

Department of Internal Medicine
Section on Hypertensive Diseases
Ochsner Medical Institutions
New Orleans, Louisiana

INTRODUCTION

Major parts of the etiology and pathogenesis of hypertension remain fragmentary and hypothetical. Over the past few years,[1-5] investigative attention has focused more and more on the hypothesis of Dahl[6] that a circulating natriuretic substance might be the culprit of the increase in arterial pressure. This concept proposes that a genetic defect of sodium metabolism causing a discrete positive sodium balance might stimulate secretion of a naturiuretic hormone. Thus, normal sodium balance in the prehypertensive patient could be achieved by continuous high levels of naturiuretic hormone. However, sodium transport inhibition would occur not only along the nephron but in other tissues as well.[4,7,8] In vascular smooth muscle it would increase the reactivity and tone of arteriolar and venous smooth muscle, thereby elevating arterial pressure and diminishing the venous compliance. Constriction of capacitance vessels would, in turn, shift the total blood volume from the periphery toward the cardiopulmonary area. This expansion of cardio-pulmonary volume would further perpetuate the secretion of the sodium transport inhibitor from the hypothalamus (even in the presence of a normal or contracted total blood volume) and a vicious circle would ensue.

This hypothesis is supported by hemodynamic, fluid volume, and endocrine changes that have been documented over the natural history of arterial hypertension as it evolves from its prehypertensive state to borderline and established hypertension, and reaches its

final stage in congestive heart failure. The following is a review
of this pathogenetic sequence that takes place as hypertensive cardiovascular disease progresses.

PREHYPERTENSION

Dysregulatory mechanisms leading to established essential hypertension may have their onset in early childhood. Normotensive
children or adolescents of hypertensive parents are at an increased
risk of developing high blood pressure at a later stage and thus
provide a study population that is to some extent prehypertensive.
In borderline or established hypertension, alterations in the
activity of the sympathetic nervous system, in hemodynamics, in
endocrine factors, or in vascular reactivity could represent the
consequence rather than the cause of the disease. In contrast, in
these prehypertensive adolescents secondary effects of an elevated
arterial pressure are absent. Several subtle alterations have indeed been documented over the past few years: offspring of parents
with essential hypertension have been found to have abnormalities
of sodium transport in white and red blood cells which possibly
reflect a generalized defect in cellular sodium transport. [8] Also,
Falkner et al [9] demonstrated that normotensive adolescents who had
a significant family history of hypertension showed a sustained
diastolic pressure response to mental stress which was similar to
patients with borderline hypertension and different from normotensive subjects without a positive family history. Moreover,
these prehypertensive subjects had significantly elevated plasma
catecholamines levels after mental stress.[9]

Similarily, McCrory et al[10] found abnormalities in blood
pressure and plasma catecholamines response to orthostatic stress
in normotensive siblings of hypertensive children. Thus, some
normotensive adolescents who have a genetic risk of essential
hypertension exhibit a hemodynamic and endocrine response to stress
that is similar to the one observed in borderline hypertension.
This clearly indicates that similar adrenergic dysfunction can be
even encountered already in the normotensive prehypertensive stage
and does not arise as a consequence of the blood pressure elevation.

BORDERLINE HYPERTENSION AND OBESITY HYPERTENSION

Non-obese young patients with borderline hypertension are
characterized by an elevated cardiac output and cardiac index, an
increase in heart rate, and an augmented renal blood flow.[11-20]
Symptoms and signs of an increased sympathetic outflow such as
palpitations, chest pain, and mitral prolapse are common.[21,22]
Total blood volume is slightly contracted and redistributed to the
cardiopulmonary circulation.[12,17,21,23] At the same time, higher

circulating norephinephrine levels can be observed.[21,24] Although
total peripheral resistance has been found to be numerically normal
in these patients, it is still inappropriately elevated with regard
to their level of cardiac output.[12,25] These hemodynamic changes
with cardiopulmonary translocation of the intravascular volume
suggest vasoconstriction in the arteriolar as well as the venous
vascular bed. An increase in tone in vascular smooth muscle together
with elevated heart rate and cardiac contractility reflects enhanced
participation of the sympathetic nervous system or decreased parasympathetic tone.[27-29] Thus, an adrenergic dysfunction seems to
be the predominant underlying mechanism for the discrete elevation
of arterial pressure in these young borderline hypertensive
patients.

Obese normotensive persons are also at a higher risk of developing established hypertension than comparable lean subjects.[30,31]
Obesity, therefore, represents another prehypertensive state. However, in contrast to the hyperadrenergic borderline hypertensive
state, described above, the elevated cardiac output in obese patients
is associated with an expanded intravascular volume but a normal
distribution within the central and peripheral circulation.[21]
Cardiac output in obesity parallels the expansion of total blood
volume and both seem at a first glance to merely reflect the increase
in metabolic requirements that occur because of the additional
(adipose) body mass. However, we have recently shown that the augmented cardiac output observed in obese patients cannot be explained
by the increased requirements due to adipose perfusion alone.[21]
Thus, the elevation in cardiac output seems inappropriate with regard
to the amount of fat tissue. These hemodynamic changes of obesity
with an elevated cardiac output, expanded total blood volume, and
a decreased peripheral resistance are remarkably similar to the
experimental situation that occurs initially with salt-loading in
a partially nephrectomized dog (Fig 1). Many experiments have
shown (in this model) that an expanded blood volume associated with
renal arterial constriction will result in arterial hypertension.[32-34]

Transition to Established Hypertension (Fig 2)

When hyperadrenergic borderline hypertensive patients grow
older and their disease progresses to established hypertension,
cardiac output falls toward normal values and total peripheral resistance continues to rise.[19,35-37] As a consequence, intravascular
volume becomes progressively more contracted.[38] This shift in the
hemodynamic profile from a high cardiac output hypertension to high
vascular resistance hypertension could be mediated through changes
in receptor responsiveness or receptor density and/or by progressively
increasing circulating norephrinephrine levels.[19,24,39] Thus, the
hemodynamic pattern in established essential hypertensive patients
is characterized by normal cardiac output, contracted intravascular
volume, and elevated total peripheral resistance.[40-42] Renal

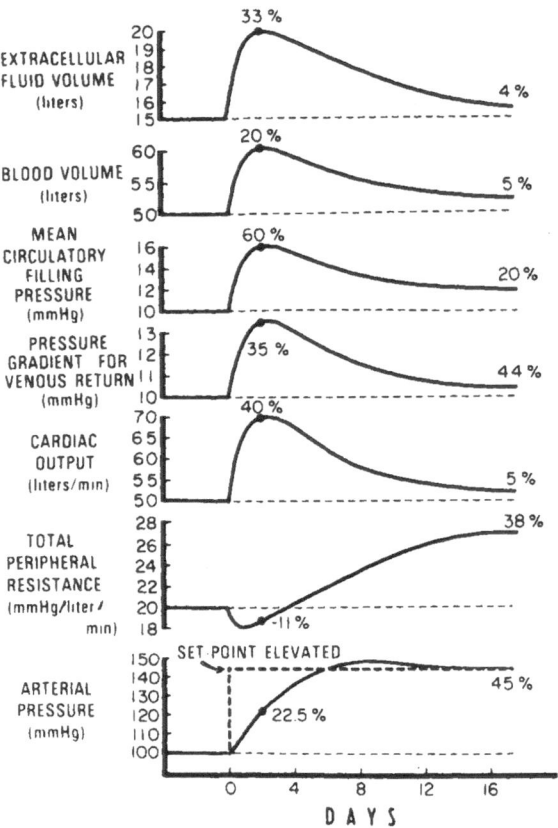

Fig. 1.   Pathogenesis of hypertension with salt-loading in partially
          nephrectomized dogs (from Guyton AC, Circulation 64:1079,
          1981, with permission)

blood flow seems to fall relatively early in the disease process,
whereas glomerular filtration rate remains normal.[43,44] As a
consequence, filtration fraction becomes elevated. Circulating
norepinephrine levels, although progressively increasing with age,
[19,24,39] are most often within normal range.

     Obese patients progress from the normotensive to the hyper-
tensive stage by a progressive vasoconstriction without change in
cardiac output.[45] Vasoconstriction seems to be a response to the
chronically inappropriately elevated systemic blood flow (i.e.,
cardiac output) in obesity. Consequently, the low total peripheral
resistance progressively increases and the initially expanded intravascular volume becomes smaller.[45] Since the effects of obesity

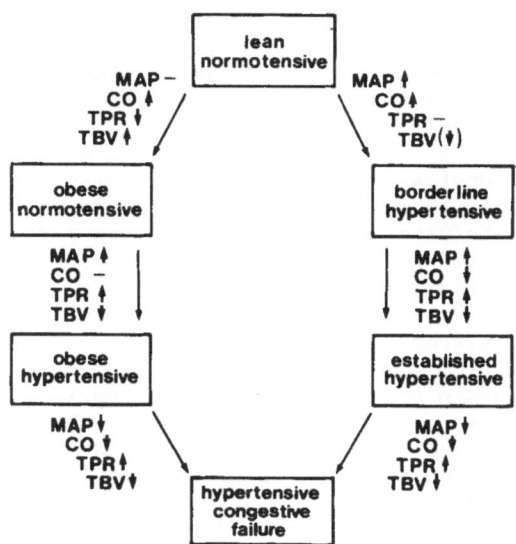

Fig. 2. Pathogenesis and evolution of arterial hypertension in
obese and nonobese patients
MAP: Mean arterial pressure
CO: Cardiac output
TPR: Total peripheral resistance
TBV: Total blood volume

and arterial hypertension on intravascular volume and total peripheral resistance offset each other, an obese hypertensive patient may be characterized by a high cardiac output, normal total peripheral resistance and a normal total blood volume.[46] However, as hypertensive cardiovascular disease becomes more severe, intravascular volume becomes contracted and total peripheral resistance elevated. Cardiac output has a tendency to fall in patients with morbid obesity because of early left ventricular dysfunction.[47] Thus, the transition of hemodynamic profile from the obese normotensive to the obese hypertensive patient seems to be mediated predominantly by volume and autoregulatory mechanisms without much involvement of the autonomic nervous system. Perhaps then, the pathogenesis of obesity hypertension in man may represent the clinical counterpart of the famous Guytonian model[35] of experimental hypertension in the salt-loaded, partially nephrectomized dog.

HYPERTENSION IN THE ELDERLY AND CONGESTIVE HEART FAILURE

As the patient grows older, blood pressure increases progressively and target organ involvement progresses. The hemodynamic picture of the nonobese patient is characterized by a high vascular resistance and a normal to low cardiac output.[40] As a consequence of long-standing elevated vascular resistance, target organ damage such as nephrosclerosis, systemic vascular disease, and retinopathy may develop. In constrast, since obesity is associated with a lower vascular resistance, it can be expected, at least to some extent, to mitigate systemic vascular disease.[48] These pathophysiologic observations lend credence to the findings of Pererra et al of a higher prevalence of accelerated hypertension (as characterized by retinopathy and arteriolar necrosis on renal biopsies) in lean than in moderately obese women.[48]

However, although obesity may exert a beneficial effect on systemic vascular disease, it greatly enhances the risk of congestive heart failure. The increased stroke volume and the increase in end-diastolic pressure result in a high preload to the left ventricle that is already burdened by a high afterload of arterial hypertension.[46] The heart adapts to this double burden with eccentric hypertrophy. The two evils, hypertension and obesity, take a heavy toll of the heart and distinctly increase the longterm risk of congestive failure. Not surprisingly, obese hypertensive patients have been documented to be at a high risk of premature congestive failure regardless of their level of arterial pressure.[49,50]

Irrespective of body weight, a progressive increase in arterial pressure will ultimately lead to congestive failure. At that stage, cardiac output declines and total peripheral resistance becomes greatly elevated. For this prefinal stage the term "decapitated" hypertension has been used: the left ventricle is no longer able to maintain the arterial pressure at its high level and a fall in pressure ensues. Although intravascular volume still may be contracted, activation of the renin-angiotensin-aldosterone system occurs and thereby promotes progressive sodium and fluid retention. Consequently the classical clinical picture of congestive failure with low cardiac output, impaired organ perfusion and generalized edema ensues.

THE HYPERADRENERGIC VS THE AUTOREGULATORY PATHWAY

From a study of the two extremes, hypertension in the lean and hypertension in the obese, a dissection can be made of a predominantly hyperadrenergic mechanism from one that seems to involve more volume and autoregulation (Fig. 3.). Thus, in lean patients in a very early phase of the disease, evidence of increased adrenergic activity can be documented. Conceivably, the blood pressure may be maintained at a high level by an enhanced adrenergic outflow with relatively little or no involvement of volume factors. On the other

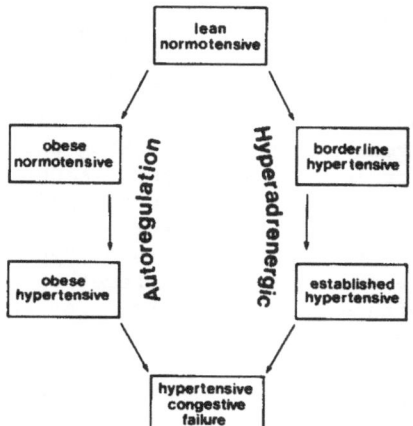

Fig. 3. The hyperadrenergic versus the volume/autoregulatory
pathway in the pathogenesis of essential hypertension.

hand, in the distinctly obese patient, an evolution as originally
proposed by Guyton may take place.[34] Volume expansion and an
elevated cardiac output lead by an autoregulatory process to a
progressively increasing peripheral resistance which thereby
elevates arterial pressure. Both pathogenetic pathways are comparable with Dahl's hypothesis:[6] the rise in vascular resistance could
be triggered and/or accelerated by increased circulating levels of
sodium transport inhibitor.

However, pathogenesis of arterial hypertension in the very
lean and in the very obese patient merely represent two extremes
of a continuing spectrum. Since most patients with essential
hypertension are somewhat overweight, it is fair to assume that
generally a combination of both pathophysiologic mechanisms may
be operating. Established essential hypertension most probably
represents the end result of a pathogenesis that involves the
hyperadrenergic as well as the autoregulatory pathway.

SUMMARY

Disparate pathogenetic mechanisms are involved in essential
hypertension in lean and in obese patients. In lean subjects,
evidence of early adrenergic dysfunction with elevated cardiac output, venous constriction and expanded cardiopulmonary volume as well

as increased circulating norepinephrine levels can be demonstrated.
In contrast, obese subjects are characterized by volume expansion,
lower vascular resistance although their cardiac output may be
elevated to a similar level as in lean borderline hypertensive
patients. It is proposed that blood pressure elevation is maintained by enhanced adrenergic outflow causing postcapillary venoconstriction without or less apparent involvement of volume factors
in lean subjects. However, volume and autoregulatory mechanisms
are more apparent in the mediation of the pathogenesis of hypertension in obese patients. Pathogenesis of hypertension in the
very lean and the very obese are two extremes of a continuum.
Since most patients with essential hypertension are somewhat overweight, generally a combination of both pathophysiologic mechanisms
may be operating.

REFERENCES

1.   F. J. Haddy and H. W. Overbeck, The role of humoral agents in
     volume expanded hypertension. Life Sci. 19:935-948 (1976).
2.   M. P. Blaustein. Sodium ions, calcium ions, blood pressure
     regulation, and hypertension: A reassessment and a hypo-
     thesis. Am J. Physiol. 232: C165-C173 (1977).
3.   H. E. deWardener, G. A. MacGregor, Dahl's hypothesis that
     a saluretic substance may be responsible for a sustained
     rise in arterial pressure: Its possible role in essential
     hypertension. Kidney Int. 18: 1-9 (1980).
4.   L. Poston, R. B. Sewell, S. P. Wilkinson et al, Evidence for a
     circulating sodium transport inhibitor in essential hyper-
     tension. Br. Med J. 282: 847-849, (1981)
5.   G. A. MacGregor, S. Fenton, J. Alaghband-Zadeh et al, Evidence
     for a raised concentration of a circulating sodium transport
     inhibitor in essential hypertension. Br. Med. J.283
     1355-1357 (1981).
6.   L. K. Dahl, K. D. Knudsen, J. Iwai, Humoral transmission of
     hypertension. Circulation Res 1 (Suppl. 24/25): 21-31,
     (1969).
7.   E. Ambrosioni, F. C. Costa, L. Montebugnoli, F. Tartagni, B.
     Magnani, Increased intralymphocytic sodium content in
     essential hypertension: An index of impaired Na^+ cellular
     metabolism. Clin Sci 61:181-186, (1981).
8.   P. Meyer, R. P. Garay, Genetic markers in essential hypertension.
     Clin Exp Hyper 3:4, (1981).
9.   B. Falkner, H. Kushner, B. Onesti, E. T. Anselakos, Cardio-
     vascular characteristics in adolescents who develop essential
     hypertension. Hypertension 3(5): 521-527, (1981).
10. W. McCrory, A. A. Klein, R. A. Rosenthal, Blood pressure,
     heart rate, and plasma catecholamines in normal and hyper-
     tensive children and their siblings at rest and after
     standing. Hypertension 4(4):507-513 (1982)

11. J. Widimsky, M. D. Fejfarova, Z. Fejfar, Changes in cardiac output in hypertensive disease. Cardiologia 31:381,(1957).

12. E. D. Frohlich, V. J. Kozul, R. C. Tarazi, H. P. Dustan, Physiological comparison of labile and essential hypertension. Circ Res 27:55, (1970).

13. R. Sannerstedt, Hemodynamic response to exercise in patients with essential hypertension. Acta Med Scand 180 (suppl 458):1, (1966).

14. O. Lund-Johansen, Hemodynamics in early essential hypertension. Acta Med Scand 181 (suppl 482): 1, (1967).

15. M. E. Safar, J. P. Fendler, B. Weil, J. M. Idatte, P. Veauve-Mayr, P. Milliez, Etude hemodynamique de l'hypertensioin arterielle labile. Presse Med 78:111 (1970).

16. S. Julius, A. V. Pascual, R. Sannerstedt, C. Mitchell, Relationship between cardiac output and peripheral resistance in borderline hypertension. Circulation 43:382 (1971)

17. M. E. Ulrych, E. D. Frohlich, R. C. Tarazi, H. P. Dustan, I. H. Page, Cardiac output and distribution of blood volume in central and peripheral circulations in hypertensive and normotensive man. Br Heart J 31:370 (1969).

18. J. M. Kioschos, W. M. Kirkendall, M. R. Valenca, A. E. Fitz, Unilateral renal hemodynamics and characteristics of dye-dilution curves in patients with essential hypertension and renal disease. Circulation 35:229 (1967).

19. F. H. Messerli, E. D. Frohlich, D. H. Suarez, et al, Borderline hypertension: Relationship between age, hemodynamics and circulating catecholamines. Circulation 64:760-764 (1981)

20. N. K. Hollenberg, J. P. Merrill, Intrarenal perfusion in the young "essential" hypertensive: A subpopulation resistant to sodium restriction. Trans Assoc Am Physicians 83:93 (1970).

21. F. H. Messerli, H. O. Ventura, E. Reisin et al, Borderline hypertension and obesity: Two prehypertensive states with elevated cardiac output. Circulation 66: 55-60, (1982).

22. J. G. R. deCarvalho, F. H. Messerli, E. D. Frohlich, Mitral valve prolapse and borderline hypertension. Hypertension 1:518-522, (1979).

23. C. N. Ellis, S. Julius, Role of central blood volume in hyperkinetic borderline hypertension. Br Heart J 35:450-455 (1973).

24. O. Bertel, F. R. Buhler, W. Kiowski, B. E. Lutold, Decreased beta-adrenergic responsiveness as related to age, blood pressure, and plasma catecholamines in patients with essential hypertension. Hypertension 2:180, (1980).

25. Y. Miura, K. Kobayashi, H. Sakuma, H. Tomioka, M. Adachi, K. Yoshinaga, Plasma noradrenaline concentrations and haemodynamics in the early stage of essential hypertension. Clin Sci and Mol Med, 55 (Suppl. 4): 69s-71s, (1978).

26. E. D. Frohlich, Hemodynamics of hypertension. In: Jacques
    Genest, Erick Koiw and Otto Kuchel (eds.) "Hypertension",
    New York, McGraw-Hill, (1977).

27. S. Julius, J. Conway, Hemodynamic studies in patients with
    borderline blood pressure elevation. Circulation 38:
    282-288, (1968).

28. S. Julius, M. Elser, Autonomic nervous cardiovascular
    regulation in borderline hypertension. Am J. Cardiol 36:
    685-695, (1975).

29. S. Julius, Abnormalities of autonomic nervous control in
    borderline hypertension. Schweiziersche Medizinische
    Wochenschrift, 106: 1698-1705, (1976).

30. S. Heyden, H. A. Tyroler, C. G. Hames, et al, Diet
    treatment of obese hypertensives. Clin Sci Mol Med
    45:209s, (1973).

31. W. B. Kannel, N. Brand, J. J. Skinner Jr., T. R. Dawber,
    P. M. McNamara, The relation of adiposity to blood pressure
    and development of hypertension. The Framingham study.
    Ann Intern Med 67:48, (1967).

32. J. B. Langston, A. C. Guyton, B. H. Douglas, P. E. Dorsett,
    Effect of changes in salt intake on arterial pressure and
    renal function in partially nephrectomized dogs. Circ
    Res 12: 508-513, (1963).

33. A. W. Cowley Jr., A. C. Guyton, Baroreceptor reflex effects
    on transient and steady-state hemodynamics of salt-loading
    hypertension in dogs. Circ Res 36:536-546, (1975).

34. A. C. Guyton, The relationship of cardiac output and arterial
    pressure control. Circulation 64:1079-1088, (1981).

35. Y. A. Weiss, M. E. Safar, G. M. London, A. C. Simon, J. A.
    Levenson, P. M. Milliez, Repeat hemodynamic determinations
    in borderline hypertension. Am J Med 64:382, (1978).

36. A. R. Cournand, L. Riley, E. S. Breed, W. F. Baldwin, D. W.
    Richards Jr, Measurements of cardiac output in man using
    the technique of catherization of the right auricle or
    ventricle. J. Clin Invest 24-106 (1945).

37. M. Brandfonbrener, M. Landowne, N. W. Shock, Changes in cardiac
    output with age. Circulation 12:557, (1955).

38. R. C. Tarazi, E. D. Frohlich, H. P. Dustan. Plasma volume in
    man with essential hypertension. N Engl J Med 278:762-765,
    (1968).

39. C. R. Lake, M. G. Ziegler, M. D. Coleman, I. J. Kopin, Age-
    adjusted plasma norepinephrine levels are similar in normo-
    tensive and hypertensive subjects. N Engl J Med 296:298,
    (1977).

40. E. D. Frohlich, R. C. Tarazi, H. P. Dustan. Reexamination of
    the hemodynamics of hypertension. Am J Med Sc 257:9-23,
    (1969).

41. R. Sannerstedt, Differences in haemodynamic pattern in various
    types of hypertension. Triangle 9:293-299, (1970).

42. P. Lund-Johansen, Haemodynamics in essential hypertension. Clin Sci 59:343s-354s, (1980).

43. F. C. Reubi, P. Weidmann, J. Hodler, P. T. Cottier, Changes in renal function in essential hypertension. Am J Med 64(4): 556-563, (1978).

44. M. Friedman, A. Selzer, H. Rosenblum, The renal blood flow in hypertension as determined in patients with variable, with early and long-standing hypertension. JAMA 17: 92-95, (1941).

45. F. H. Messerli, K. Sundgaard-Rise, E. Reisin, et al, Disparate cardiovascular obesity and arterial hypertension. Am J Med 1882 (in press).

46. F. H. Messerli, Cardiovascular effects of obesity and hypertension. Lancet 1167-1168, (1982).

47. O. Divitis, S. Fazio, M. Petitto, G.Maddalena, F. Contaldo, M. Mancini, Obesity and cardiac function. Circulation 64:447-482, (1981).

48. G. A. Perera, A. Damon, Height, weight, and their ratio in the accelerated form of primary hypertension. Arch Int Med 100:263-265, (1957).

49. J. K. Alexander, J. R. Pettigrove, Obesity and congestive heart failure. Geriatrics 22:101-106, (1967).

50. T. Gordon, W. B. Kannel. Obesity and cardiovascular disease: the Framingham Study. Clin Endocrinol Metabol 5:367-374, (1976).

NEURAL FACTORS IN ESSENTIAL HYPERTENSION

Giuseppe Mancia

Istituto di Clinica Medica IV
Università di Milano
Centro di Fisiologia Clinica e Ipertensione
Ospedale Maggiore
Milano and C.N.R., Italy

Since the discovery that the autonomic nervous system represents a mechanism of primary importance in the regulation of circulation the idea that essential hypertension might depend on a derangement in neural cardiovascular control has been a leading one in the investigation related to this pathological condition.

This presentation will not touch all complex and controversial aspects of this topic but rather concentrate on a few points derived from studies on both experimental and human hypertension. It is hoped that these points will show some of the basic information that has been gained during these years, but also underline the limitation in our knowledge of this field.

Mention of results obtained in studies on experimental hypertension is important because this approach has answered two key questions that are still unsolved in human hypertension. The first question is whether neural factors may produce a condition of high blood pressure, i.e. whether they may have an initiating role in this disease. By showing that in several animal species a variety of neuropsychological manipulations can produce a permanent blood pressure elevation this question has received a positive answer. The following are a few examples:

(a) a prolonged blood pressure rise has been shown to occur in monkeys subjected to adverse conditioning, i.e. to a stressful procedure that requires the animals to act in a way that can avoid them the delivery of unpleasant stimuli[1,2];

(b) a hypertension has been shown to occur in male mice which behave
     as dominant within their colony, in contrast to the lower blood
     pressure values (and the lower incidence of cardiovascular com-
     plications) of other mice of the colony whose social behaviour
     appears to be subordinate to the dominant ones;[3]

(c) neural factors have also appeared to be responsible for the
     initiation of the hypertensive state in the Okamoto strain of
     rats. It has been shown[4] that these rats display exaggerated
     pressor responses to stressful stimuli even at an age that pre-
     cedes the development of hypertension. Furthermore such devel-
     opment has been shown to be prevented or slowed either by early
     treatment with "antisympathetic" drugs or by a drastic reduction
     in the amount of natural stimuli that occur in rats' lives.
     Thus, this hypertension model has reproduced the condition that
     is believed to characterize essential hypertension, i.e. an
     interaction between environmental and inherited factors.[5] It
     has also shown that the latter may consist in a hyperactivity of
     the neural structures involved in the integration of the defence
     mechanisms, the permanent blood pressure elevation being prob-
     ably the consequence of behaviourally-induced excessive phasic
     blood pressure rises.

The second question is whether neural influences, beside being
capable of playing an initial role, are important as secondary factors, i.e. whether they represent a mechanism that maintains blood
pressure high in non-neurally initiated hypertensions. Animal
studies have provided a positive answer also to this question. For
example, destruction of sympathetic nerve structures either at a
peripheral or a central site has been shown to be followed by a large
blood pressure reduction not only in neurally induced hypertensions
but also in hypertension models of a non-neural origin (DOCA hypertension, renovascular hypertension, etc.).[6] Furthermore, the development of renovascular hypertension in rats has been slowed or prevented not only by diffuse sympathetic destruction, but also by
restricted lesions placed centrally in the hypothalamus.[7] Finally,
data of our group have shown that in secondary hypertension normalization of blood pressure values can be achieved also by spontaneous
reduction of the existing sympathetic vasoconstrictor tone.[8] These
findings are exemplified in Figure 1 which represents average blood
pressure values recorded intra-arterially during a large number of
wakefulness-sleep cycles in a normotensive and a renovascular hypertensive cat. Both animals had been subjected to sino-aortic denervation to allow an unbuffered depression of sympathetic vasoconstrictor tone to occur during sleep, particularly during its REM
phase.[8] In the normotensive cat the REM sleep-induced sympathetic
depression reduced blood pressure to low values. The same low
values, however, were attained during REM sleep by the renovascular
hypertensive cat, whose blood pressure elevation thus depended on
activation of sympathetic tone. The mechanisms through which stenosis of renal arteries or DOCA injections lead a sympathetic acti-

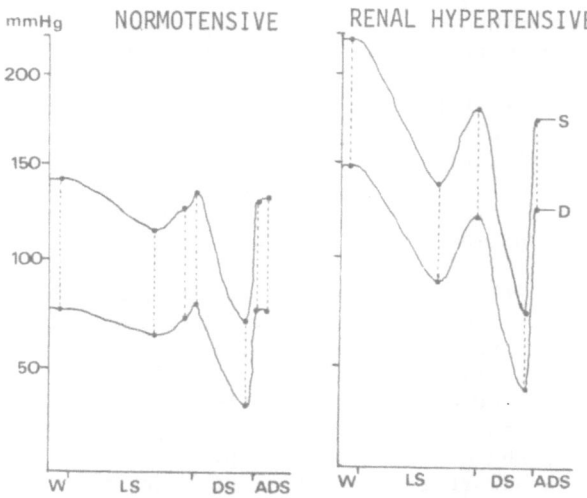

Fig. 1.   Systolic (S) and diastolic (D) blood pressure during the
          wakefulness-sleep cycle in a normotensive and a renovas-
          cular hypertensive cat, both with sino-aortic denervation.
          W: wakefulness; LS: light or synchronized sleep; DS:
          deep or REM sleep; ADS: after deep sleep. Each point
          represents the average of 10 different episodes. (From
          Mancia and Zanchetti, "Physiology during Sleep", p.1, 1980,
          Academic Press, by permission).

vation that takes over the responsibility of the hypertensive state
represent a third basic question. This question is still unanswered. Current hypotheses focused on the relationship between
sodium and norepinephrine stores and release in the nerve terminals[6]
and on the stimulating properties of angiotensin II at various central and peripheral sympathetic sites.[9,10]

     Coming to neural factors in human hypertension it is important
to emphasize that this field is encompassed with two methodological
difficulties. The first difficulty is represented by the fact that
in humans hypertension is commonly seen at a variably advance stage
from its inception which prevents the separation between primary and
secondary factors that has been so profitably applied in experimental animal models. The second and more important difficulty is that
the approaches that have so far been employed to quantitate neural
cardiovascular influences have major limitations. This applies to
old approaches (personality patterns, assessment of haemodynamic
responses to stress, assessment of depressor responses to "anti-
sympathetic" drugs, basal haemodynamics, etc.) but also involves the
new ones. For example measurement of plasma norepinephrine levels,
though capable of signaling large and diffuse stimulation or

depression of sympathetic activity, may represent a relatively insensitive index of more moderate alterations in sympathetic tone,
particularly when comparisons have to be made among subjects.[11,12]
Direct assessment of this tone in skeletal muscle circulation, besides representing only a fraction of the overall sympathetic activity, may also be difficult to quantitate and compare among subjects.
Due to these limitations it is not surprising that studies on the
importance of neural factors in essential hypertension have produced
many conflicting and inconclusive results.

There is a further approach to this problem, however, that
avoids the elusive quantitation of sympathetic activity and addresses
to clarification of the mechanisms that are involved in neural
cardiovascular regulation of human beings and to their evaluation in
normotensive and hypertensive individuals. A mechanism that has been
extensively investigated is the reflex control of the cardiovascular
system exerted by the arterial baroreceptors. Several studies that
have examined the baroreceptor control of heart rate have shown that
in hypertension its range is reset towards the elevated blood pressure values and its sensitivity is reduced.[14] These studies have
raised the possibility that essential hypertension is due to a reduction in the reflex inhibition that physiologically modulates
sympathetic noradrenergic activity.

However, data obtained recently by us and by others[15,16] do not
support this possibility. If a reduction in baroreflex sensitivity
were important in producing hypertension, baroreceptor denervation
should be followed by a permanent blood pressure elevation. Table 1
shows that this may not be the case. In unanaesthetized unrestrained
cats blood pressure was continuously recorded for several hours
before and a week after section of the sino-aortic nerves. Computer
analysis of the tracings showed that blood pressure was much more
variable after than before the sino-aortic nerve section, a
finding to be expected in consideration of the buffering role of the

Table 1. Effects of Sino-aortic Denervation Alone or Combined
          with Vagotomy on Blood Pressure Mean Values and Blood
          Pressure Variability*

	n = 8			n = 6		
	Intact	SAD	P<	SAD	SAD+vagot	P<
Mean arterial pressure (mmHg)	99±7	93±7	NS	103±8	101±6	NS
Variation coefficient (%)	6±1	12±2	.01	13±2	12±6	NS

*Data represent means (±SE) from recording performed in unanaes-
 thetized, unrestrained cats.

arterial baroreceptor afferents on the blood pressure oscillations. However, mean blood pressure values did not differ significantly in the two conditions. This was the case even when, in another series of cats, blood pressure recordings were performed first after sino-aortic denervation and then 1-7 days after bilateral vagotomy, a procedure which removed the residual inhibitory influence reflexly exerted on sympathetic tone, namely that arising from cardiopulmonary receptors.[17] Thus even complete baroreceptor denervation (a condition that might be equated to "0 sensitivity" of the baroreflex) does not appear capable of producing hypertension.

Further evidence against involvement of the arterial baroreflex in essential hypertension was obtained in human studies through the use of the neck chamber technique, which allows carotid transmural pressure to be increased or reduced in a measurable and gradual amount, and to relate these alterations to the resulting mean arterial pressure responses, thereby obtaining the sensitivity of the most important baroreflex function, i.e. blood pressure control[18]. A study performed in normotensive subjects and in subjects with moderate and severe essential hypertension[19] showed that (a) in normotensive subjects the blood pressure changes caused by reducing carotid transmural pressure, i.e. by deactivating baroreceptors, were greater than the blood pressure changes caused by increasing carotid transmural pressure, i.e. by stimulating baroreceptors, (b) the blood pressure effects of baroreceptor deactivation progressively fell, and those of baroreceptor stimulation progressively increased in size on going from normotensive to moderate and severe hypertensive subjects, (c) the sums of the blood pressure effects of baroreceptor deactivation and stimulation, and the maximal slopes of these responses, were similar in the three groups (Figure 2). These findings indicate that, at variance with heart rate control, baroreceptor control of blood pressure is largely preserved in essential hypertension. They confirm that a resetting of the baroreflex occurs in this condition and suggest that this phenomenon may be so marked as to displace the set-point of the reflex in a direction opposite to that predictable, on the basis of the blood pressure elevation, i.e. towards threshold rather than towards saturation.[20] In a further study we were able to show that an unchanged sensitivity and a marked resetting of the baroreceptor-blood pressure control also characterize subjects with renovascular hypertension.[21] Taken together these findings do not support the possibility that the arterial baroreflex represent a causal factor in essential hypertension. They do show, however, that an important modification of the baroreflex, namely a marked resetting, can occur as a result of blood pressure elevations. Such resetting may represent a factor that defends the raised blood pressure and secondary contributes to this condition. It may also be viewed, however, as an adjustment that preserves the baroreflex ability to protect hypertensive subjects against further acute pressure rises and that by favouring maintainance of sympathetic vasoconstrictor tone allows the antihypertensive action of sympathetic agents to take place.

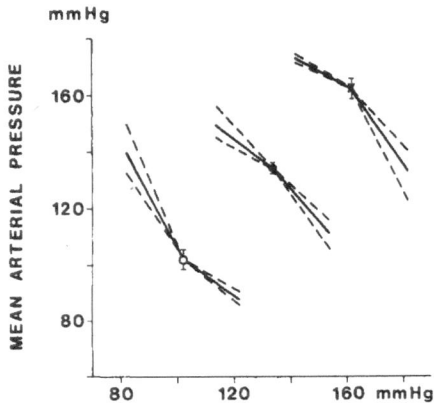

Fig. 2. Reductions and increases in mean arterial pressure (verti-
         cal line) induced by increases and reductions in carotid
         transmural pressure (horizontal line). Data represent
         average values from a group of normotensive subjects
         (n = 11), a group of subjects with moderate essential
         hypertension (n = 18) and a group of subjects with severe
         essential hypertension (n = 17). The open circle, closed
         circle and the cross represent average (±SE) baseline mean
         arterial pressure of the 3 groups respectively. The con-
         tinuous lines departing from these symbols represent the
         slopes of the mean arterial pressure in relation to the baro-
         receptor stimuli, the dashed lines representing the standard
         errors. Note the reverse asymmetry of the pressor and de-
         pressor responses in the severe hypertensive as compared
         to the normotensive subjects (adapted from Mancia et al.,
         Circ. Res. 43:170, 1977, by permission).

     Another approach we have followed is analysis of spontaneous
blood pressure variability due to the demonstration that this phenomenon may be largely neural in nature. Figure 3 shows the results
obtained in an ambulant subject in which blood pressure was invas-
ively monitored for 24 hours by the Oxford technique.[22] The blood
pressure signal was analyzed by a computer which provided mean and
standard deviation values of each of the 48 half hours of the 24 hour
period. Average of the 48 standard deviations was then calculated
and used as an index of the blood pressure variability within half
hours, i.e. a rather short-term variability. The standard deviation
observed by averaging the 48 mean values was also calculated and used
as an index of the blood pressure variations among half hours, i.e. a
longer-term variability. The same analysis was performed for heart
rate. In 38 subjects blood pressure variabilities showed a weak and
often non-significant correlation with the arterial baroreflex sensitivity, suggesting that the differences in the buffering action of
this mechanism that may exist within the population may not be

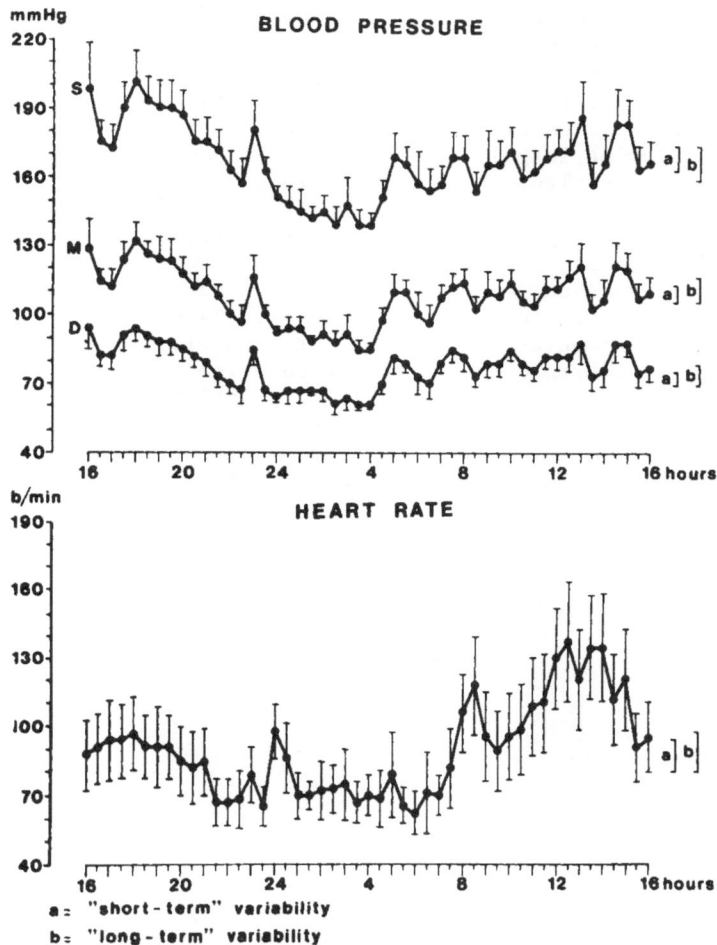

Fig. 3. Computer analysis of systolic blood pressure, diastolic
blood pressure, mean arterial pressure and heart rate obtained during a 24 hour intraarterial blood pressure monitoring in an ambulant subject. The blood pressure signal
was sampled by a computer every 60 msec. Data are expressed as mean values and standard deviations for each
of the 48 half hours of the recording. a: standard deviation within half hour, i.e. short-term variability;
b: standard deviation among half hour, i.e. long-term
variability. For further explanations see text.

crucial in determining the extent of this phenomenon.[23] On the other
hand the short-term blood pressure variability showed a striking
reduction during sleep and its changes throughout the 24 hours were

closely paralleled by alterations in short-term heart rate variability. Blood pressure and heart rate mean values also showed a
concomitant close parallelism. These findings can be explained by
postulating the existence of central influences affecting consen-
sually cardiac and vascular targets whose importance in daily cardiovascular modulation largely predominates over negative feed-back
systems that would alter these targets in opposite directions.

If blood pressure and heart rate variabilities mainly reflect
centrally originated influences, their comparisons at normal and high
blood pressure may bear a special interest. Such comparison was made
in subjects classified on the basis of their 24 hour mean arterial
pressure values as being normotensive or as having an essential
hypertension of moderate or severe degree.[23,24] Figure 4 shows that
short-term absolute mean arterial pressure variability (i.e. standard
deviation within half hours) showed a tendency to increase progress-

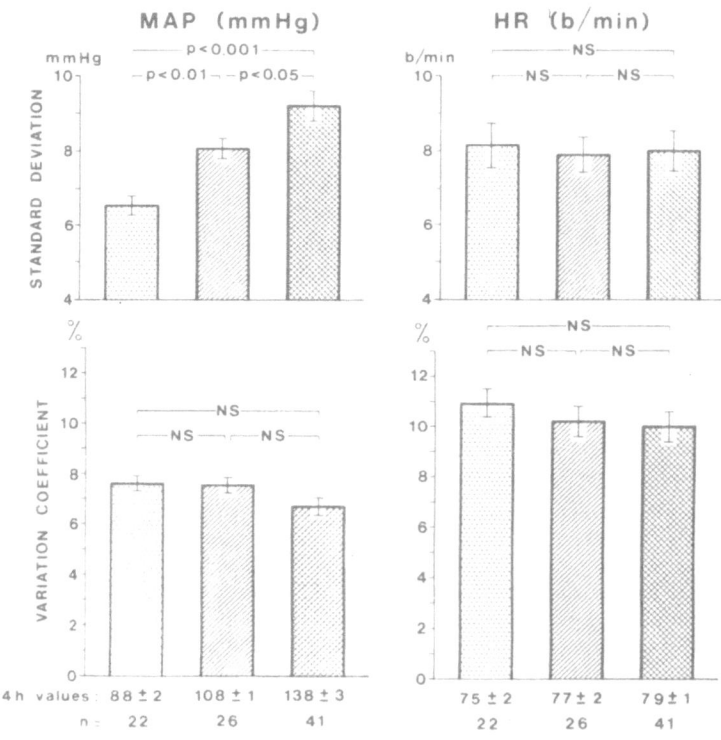

Fig. 4.   Short-term mean arterial pressure and heart rate in 3
          groups of subjects with normal blood pressure, moderate
          and severe essential hypertension. Figures at the bottom
          represent 24 hour average mean arterial pressure and heart
          rate values. Age was similar in the 3 groups.

ively to normotensive to severe hypertensive subjects. However, when relative variability was used instead, namely when variation coefficient was adopted to correct for differences in baseline blood pressure values, such tendency was lost and variability appeared to be similar in the various groups. This was the case for systolic and diastolic blood pressure, and also occurred when the analysis was performed on long-term blood pressure variability. Heart rate variabilities, either absolute or relative, also were similar regardless of the 24 hour mean blood pressure values. From the postulate outline above one might conclude that there is no alteration in central modulation of circulation in essential hypertension. This feature, and the reset but unimpaired baroreceptor-blood pressure control, might also allow to conclude for an overall normality of neual cardiovascular control in this condition. Whether this normality is the result of a secondary adjustment or truly reflects lack of participation of neural factors in the genesis of this disease remains to be clarified.

REFERENCES

1. J. A. Herd, W. H. Morse, R. T. Kelleher and L. G. Jones, Arterial hypertension in the squirrel monkey during behavioral experiments, Am.J.Physiol. 217:24 (1969).
2. R. P. Forsyth and R. E. Harris, Circulatory changes during stressful stimuli in Rhesus monkeys, Circ.Res. 26, Suppl.1: 13 (1970).
3. J. P. Henry, P. M. Stephens and G. A. Santisteban, A model of psychosocial hypertension showing reversibility and progressions of cardiovascular complications, Circ.Res. 36:156 (1975).
4. B. Folkow, Central neurohormonal mechanisms in spontaneously hypertensive rats compared with human essential hypertension, Clin.Sci.Mol.Med. 84, Suppl. 2:205 (1975).
5. G. W. Pickering, "The nature of essential hypertension," Churchill Ltd., London (1961).
6. J. De Champlain, Experimental aspects of the relationships between the autonomic nervous system and catecholamines in hypertension, in:"Hypertension," J. Genest, E. Koiw and O. Kuchel, eds., McGraw-Hill, New York, p.76 (1977).
7. M. L. Brody, G. D. Fink, J. Buggy, J. R. Haywood, F. J. Gordon and A. K. Johnson, The role of the anteroventral third ventricle (AV3V) region in experimental hypertension, Circ.Res. 43, Suppl. 1:2 (1978).
8. G. Mancia and A. Zanchetti, Cardiovascular regulation during sleep, in:"Physiology during Sleep," J. Orem and C. D. Barnes, Academic Press, New York, p.1 (1980).
9. C. M. Ferrario, K. L. Barnes, S. E. Szilagyi and K. B. Brosnihan, Physiological and pharmacological characterization of the area postrema pressor pathways in the normal dog, Hypertension 1:235 (1979).

10. B. G. Zimmerman, T. F. Rolewicz, E. W. Dunham and J. L. Gisslen, Transmitter release and vascular responses in skin and muscle of hypertensive dogs, J.Pharmacol.Exp.Therap. 163:320 (1968).

11. A. Zanchetti, G. Mancia and G. Leonetti, Humoral markers in hypertension, in "Radioimmunoassay of Drugs and Hormones in Cardiovascular Medicine," A. Albertini, M. Da Prada and B. A. Peskar, eds., North Holland Elsevier, Amsterdam, p.3 (1979).

12. G. Mancia, G. Leonetti, G. B. Picotti, A. Ferrari, M. D. Galva, L. Gregorini, G. Parati, G. Pomidossi, C. Ravazzani and A. Zanchetti, Plasma catecholamines and blood pressure responses to the carotid baroreflex in essential hypertension, Clin. Sci. 57:165s (1979).

13. W. Delius, K. E. Hagbarth, A. Hongell and G. B. Wallin, General characteristics of sympathetic activity in human muscle nerves, Acta.Physiol.Scand. 84:65 (1972).

14. P. Sleight, Reflex control of the heart rate, Am.J.Cardiol. 44: 889 (1979).

15. A. Ramirez, G. Bertinieri, L. Belli, A. Cavallazzi and G. Mancia, Effect of arterial and cardiopulmonary receptor denervation on blood pressure and heart rate control in conscious cats, manuscript in preparation.

16. A. W. Cowley, J. F. Liard and A. C. Guyton, Role of baroreceptors in daily control of arterial blood pressure and other variables in dogs, Circ.Res. 32:564 (1973.

17. G. Mancia, R. R. Lorenz and J. T. Shepherd, Reflex control of circulation from heart and lungs. " Int. Review Physiol., Cardiovasc. Physiol. II," Vol. 9, A. C. Guyton and A. W. Cowley eds., University Park Press, Baltimore, p.11 (1976).

18. J. Ludbrook, G. Mancia, A. Ferrari and A. Zanchetti, The variable-pressure neck-chamber method for studying the carotid baroreflex in man, Clin.Sci.Mol.Med. 53:165 (1977).

19. G. Mancia, J. Ludbrook, A. Ferrari, L. Gregorini and A. Zanchetti, Baroreceptor reflexes in human hypertension, Circ.Res. 43:170 (1978).

20. G. Mancia, A. Ferrari, L. Gregorini, G. Parati, M. C. Ferrari, G. Pomidossi and A. Zanchetti, Control of blood pressure by carotid sinus baroreceptors in human beings, Am.J.Cardiol. 44:895 (1979).

21. G. Mancia, A. Ferrari, G. Leonetti, G. Pomidossi and A. Zanchetti, Carotid sinus baroreceptor control of arterial pressure in renovascular hypertensive subjects, Hypertension 4:47 (1982).

22. F. D. Stott, V. G. Terry and A. J. Honour, Factors determining the design and construction of a portable transducer system, Postgrad,Med.J. 52, Suppl. 7:97 (1976).

23. G. Mancia, A. Ferrari, L. Gregorini, G. Parati, G. Pomidossi, G. Bertinieri, G. Grassi and A. Zanchetti, Blood pressure, variability in man: its relation to high blood pressure, age and baroreflex sensitivity, Clin.Sci. 59:401s (1980).

24. G. Mancia, Blood pressure variability at normal and high blood pressure, Chest, in press.

RENOVASCULAR HYPERTENSION:

NEW ASPECTS OF PATHOGENESIS AND TREATMENT

J. J. Brown, W. B. Brown, G. P. Hodsman,
A. G. Lever, Dorothea McAreavey, J. J. Morton,
Elizabeth C. M. Wallace, and J. I. S. Robertson

Medical Research Council Blood Pressure Unit
Western Infirmary, Glasgow, United Kingdom

Although it is now nearly half a century since Goldblatt and his colleagues demonstrated that hypertension could be produced experimentally by the application of a constriction to a renal artery,[1] the pathogenesis of this condition remains imperfectly understood. The issue is clinically relevant, because in man hypertension is often associated with renal artery stenosis, and in a proportion of such patients, although by no means all, blood pressure can be lowered either by renal arterial reconstruction or by excision of the kidney distal to the stenosis. The importance of the renin-angiotensin system in initiating and maintaining renovascular hypertension remains particularly controversial.

In 1974 we proposed[2] a schema relating the evolution of renovascular hypertension to changes in the renin system. In the first phase, which appears within minutes of the application of a renal artery stenosis, plasma renin and angiotensin II, and arterial pressure, rise together, and fall, also in parallel, if the stenosis is relieved. Within days this is succeeded by a second phase in which, while blood pressure remains high, plasma renin and angiotensin II are proportionately less markedly elevated. This dissociation has cast doubt on the importance of the renin system in phase II, although blood pressure may still be lowered either by correction of the renal artery stenosis or removal of the affected kidney. Clinical renovascular hypertension is not often observed earlier than phase II. Much later a third phase supervenes in which blood pressure remains high while the renin system continues relatively suppressed; in phase III surgical measures are ineffective in lowering arterial pressure. Almost certainly the renin-angiotensin system is not pathogenically relevant in phase III. Clini-

319

cally, the distinction between phases II and III is of major importance in deciding on surgical measures.

Recent studies in this department[3] have attempted to define
more precisely the evolution of renovascular hypertension in relation
to the renin-angiotensin system. Rats with both kidneys remaining
were studied, a unilateral renal artery clip being applied to one
group, while control animals had a sham operation. In an attempt to
minimise artifacts, blood samples for the assay of plasma renin and
angiotensin II, and arterial pressure measurements, were obtained
in conscious animals.

On the day after operation, when the first measurements were
made, blood pressure, plasma renin and plasma angiotensin II concentrations were significantly elevated in the rats with unilateral
renal artery stenosis. Two weeks after operation, however, plasma
renin and angiotensin II had subsided in the clipped rats to values
no different from those seen in the controls, although blood pressure
remained significantly elevated. From the fourth week after operation
onwards, plasma renin and angiotensin II again rose in the rats with
unilateral renal artery stenosis, and to a very variable extent in
different animals, while the hypertension became more severe. Blood
pressure, renin and angiotensin II remained significantly elevated
in the clipped rats up to 20 weeks from operation, when the study
was terminated. A significant positive correlation was demonstrable
($r = 0.48$, $n = 21$, $p<0.05$) between plasma angiotensin II and arterial
pressure in measurements made on the first and second days after
applying the unilateral renal artery clip.

We have previously shown[4] similar related changes in blood
pressure and plasma angiotensin II immediately after renal artery
constriction in conscious dogs; in these dog studies an almost identical relationship between blood pressure and angiotensin II was obtained during acute intravenous infusions of exogenous angiotensin
II. Thus it appears that in the first phase of renovascular hypertension, the blood pressure increase can be explained by the immediate rise in plasma renin, and hence the direct pressor effect
of the resultant increase in plasma angiotensin II.

Between 8 and 20 weeks after clipping, in the rats,[3] endogenous
plasma angiotensin II was also significantly correlated with arterial
pressure ($r = 0.51$, $n = 47$, $p<0.001$), and the regression was no different in slope from that describing the similar relationship at 1
and 2 days after clipping. However, at 8-20 weeks, blood pressure
was markedly higher for concurrent plasma angiotensin II than was
the case 1 and 2 days after clipping.

These findings in the rat corroborate and extend our earlier
observations in man.[2,5] In a series of untreated patients with
hypertension associated with a renal or renal arterial lesion, a

significant positive correlation was found between endogenous plasma angiotensin II and arterial pressure; however, for any given value of plasma angiotensin II, blood pressure was distinctly higher than could be achieved by brief elevation of plasma angiotensin II during intravenous infusions of the peptide.

What are the possible factors involved in the upward shift of angiotensin II: blood pressure relationship during the evolution of renovascular hypertension? This changed relationship could well be independent of any alterations in the renin-angiotensin system. However, two observations raise the possibility that chronic but perhaps quite modest elevation of plasma angiotensin II might be responsible for resetting its own pressor dose-response curve.

First, in a patient with a renin-secreting tumour,[6] in whom there was chronic elevation of plasma angiotensin II, and in whom this increase was almost certainly the sole ultimate cause of the hypertension, a similarly enhanced angiotensin II : blood pressure relationship was seen. Removal of the tumour restored both plasma angiotensin II and blood pressure to normal. Second, infusion of angiotensin II into conscious dogs for 2 weeks, at a dose which elevated mean plasma angiotensin II only from around 25 to 50 pg/ml - well within the physiological range - caused a progressive rise in arterial pressure and advancing elevation of the angiotensin II: blood pressure dose-response curve.[7]

These considerations therefore sustain the possibility that the renin-angiotensin system could still be centrally involved in the second phase of renovascular hypertension. Raised plasma angiotensin II might both begin and maintain hypertension due to renal artery stenosis. Nevertheless, this remains far from certain and the resetting of the angiotensin II : pressor dose-response curve could have other causes. Several possible mechanisms of this resetting, some of which might be angiotensin II-dependent, have been considered.

First, Folkow[8] has emphasised the structural changes in arterial and arteriolar walls in hypertension, and has pointed out that an increased wall : lumen ratio can per se have a progressive pressor effect. Such structural alterations could be initiated and perpetuated by increased levels of angiotensin II.

Second, Cowley and DeClue[9] found that part of the pressure increase seemed to result from a rise in cardiac output, possibly as a consequence of decreased vascular compliance.

Third, angiotensin II has a variety of central and peripheral sympathetic nervous actions that might well potentiate its initial pressor effect.[10,11] These include an excitatory action on the area postrema; stimulation of the adrenal medulla and sympathetic ganglia; potentiation of postganglionic neurotransmitter biosynthesis and release; and inhibition of neurotransmitter re-uptake.

Fourth, the prolonged infusion of angiotensin II at a low dose is accompanied by resetting of the baroreceptors.[9]

Fifth, chronic exposure of the adrenal cortex to increased levels of angiotensin II potentiates the aldosterone-stimulant effect of angiotensin II.[12] In renal hypertension in man there is evidence that the plasma aldosterone concentration is higher for a given plasma angiotensin II concentration than in normal subjects acutely infused with angiotensin II.[13] Such a phenomenon would require corresponding elevation of arterial pressure to balance the resultant tendency to retain sodium. Furthermore, the enhanced aldosterone level might lead to increased sodium accumulation in vascular walls that in turn could raise the wall : lumen ratio in resistance vessels, and also enhance the response to circulating vasoconstrictors. This effect on aldosterone might be relevant to renal hypertension in man, but it is unlikely to explain the progressive pressor effect of angiotensin II in the chronically infused dogs,[7] because in the latter plasma aldosterone was not significantly raised. However, in renal hypertension, an increase in plasma aldosterone concentration is not theoretically an obligatory requirement for a heightened tendency for sodium retention,[14] either in the entire body, or selectively in vascular walls, and hypertension can develop in adrenalectomised dogs maintained on constant replacement therapy.[15]

Sixth, Lucas and Floyer[16] have provided evidence of a hormone, of renal origin, that is responsible for altering tissue compliance, and whose release is inhibited in renal hypertension. It is possible that angiotensin II might modify the release of this hypothetical hormone.

In summary, it appears that circulating angiotensin II is entirely responsible, by acute vasoconstrictor effect, for the initial rise in pressure that follows renal artery constriction. Later, other mechanisms come into play. However, angiotensin II has undoubted pressor actions of slow onset, and these could, at least in part, be responsible for later phases of renal hypertension, both clinical and experimental; this remains unproved.

Sodium retention seems not to be a necessary accompaniment of evolving renovascular hypertension. In the one-clip two-kidney rat model, no differences in exchangeable sodium between hypertensive and sham-operated animals were seen up to 7 weeks after operation.[17] In man, renovascular hypertension shows indeed a tendency to sodium depletion, with a significant inverse relationship between arterial pressure and exchangeable sodium in a series studied by us.[18] With severe unilateral renal artery stenosis or occlusion, pronounced sodium depletion with secondary aldosterone excess may present as a striking hyponatraemic syndrome.[19]

If the renin-angiotensin system is involved in phase II of renovascular hypertension, antagonists and inhibitors of the system might be expected to correct the high blood pressure. The acute effects of agents such as saralasin – a competitive antagonist of angiotensin II – or captopril – an angiotensin I converting enzyme inhibitor – are consistent. With both types of drug an immediate fall in blood pressure is seen, in proportion to the pre-treatment plasma level of renin or angiotensin II.[20,21] In the case of captopril, the acute blood pressure fall is also in proportion to the acute fall in plasma angiotensin II.[21]

Although interesting, however, such immediate changes are not necessarily relevant to a slow pressor component of the action of angiotensin II, to unmask which more prolonged inhibition of the renin system might well be required.

Riegger et al.,[22] studying rats with one-clip two-kidney hypertension 28-60 days after operation, found that infusion of saralasin or of converting enzyme inhibitor for 11 hours slowly returned blood pressure to normal, while brief administration did not have this effect. This slow antihypertensive effect was not significantly related to pre-treatment plasma renin value.

The availability of orally-active converting enzyme inhibitors such as captopril and enalapril has permitted an evaluation of prolonged suppression of angiotensin II formation in renovascular hypertension in man.[23,24] Long-term administration of both of these agents has been shown to cause sustained reduction of plasma angiotensin II with converse increases in circulating renin and angiotensin I concentrations. The initial blood pressure reduction was proportional to the initial fall in angiotensin II but this early blood pressure change often related poorly with the long-term response.

Some severely hypertensive sodium-depleted patients had a very marked initial blood pressure fall,[19,23] while the long-term effect, after sodium balance was restored, was more modest. By contrast, other patients showed a gradual reduction in pressure over 1-3 weeks of continuous converting enzyme inhibition.[23] This latter type of response was observed in some patients whose pre-treatment plasma angiotensin II concentrations were within or just above the upper part of the normal range, and the effect might therefore have been due to reversal of the slow pressor component of angiotensin II. However, the converting enzyme inhibitors might lower blood pressure by mechanisms additional to suppression of angiotensin II formation, so that interpretation must, of necessity, be cautious.

Can long-term inhibition of the renin-angiotensin system aid in the selection of those patients with renal artery stenosis whose hypertension will respond to renal or renovascular surgery? In particular, can such a measure help distinguish between phases II and III of renovascular hypertension?

The issue is an important and difficult one. As we have commented elsewhere[25] "..... patients whose blood pressure will fall most after surgery are likely to have hypertension of recent onset, to be young, to have fibromuscular hyperplasia, to have increased renin, angiotensin II and aldosterone in peripheral blood with high renal vein renin ratio, reduced blood flow in the affected kidney, and well-maintained flow in the untouched kidney. At the opposite end of the spectrum, surgery is likely to fail in elderly patients with long-standing hypertension caused by atheromatous renal artery stenosis, with other vascular disease, impaired renal function, reduced blood flow in the untouched kidney, a normal renin in peripheral blood, and a normal renal vein renin ratio. The decision on surgery is not difficult in extreme examples of this sort. In practice most patients fall between, with a mixture of favourable and unfavourable features." Is it possible that the long-term use of captopril or enalapril might summate the varied effects of all these factors?[23]

In a small series, we found the initial response to captopril a poor guide to eventual surgical outcome.[23] However the long-term captopril response related well with the later response to renal arterial reconstruction or nephrectomy, predicting, in absolute terms of systolic and diastolic pressure, successes and failures alike. Interpretation must necessarily be cautious with the few patients studied; if however, the early promise were fulfilled in larger series, it could have not only prognostic value but also important pathophysiological implications concerning the role of renin in pathogenesis.

REFERENCES

1. H. Goldblatt, J. Lynch, R. Hanzal, and W. W. Summerville, Studies on experimental hypertension. I. The production of persistent elevation of systolic blood pressure by means of renal ischemia, J.Exp.Med. 59:347 (1934).
2. J. J. Brown, V. Cuesta, D. L. Davies, A. F. Lever, J. J. Morton, P. L. Padfield, J. I. S. Robertson, and P. Trust, Mechanism of renal hypertension, Lancet i:1219 (1974).
3. J. J. Morton and E. C. H. Wallace, Changes in blood pressure, renin and angiotensin II in the two-kidney one-clip Goldblatt rat: the importance of angiotensin II in the development and maintenance of hypertension. Submitted for publication. (1982).
4. A. M. Caravaggi, G. Bianchi, J. J. Brown, A. F. Lever, J. J. Morton, J. D. Powell-Jackson, J. I. S. Robertson, and P. F. Semple, Blood pressure and plasma angiotensin II concentration

after renal artery constriction and angiotensin II infusion in the conscious dog, Circ.Res. 38:315 (1976).

5. J. J. Brown, J. Casals-Stenzel, A. M. M. Cumming, D. L. Davies, R. Fraser, A. F. Lever, J. J. Morton, P. F. Semple, M. Tree, and J. I. S. Robertson, Angiotensin II, aldosterone and arterial pressure: a quantitative approach, Hypertension 1:159 (1979).

6. J. J. Brown, R. Fraser, A. F. Lever, J. J. Morton, J. I. S. Robertson, M. Tree, P. R. F. Bell, J. K. Davidson, and I. S. Ruthven, Hypertension and secondary hyperaldosteronism associated with a renin-secreting renal juxtaglomerular cell tumour, Lancet ii:1228 (1973).

7. B. L. Bean, J. J. Brown, J. Casals-Stenzel, R. Fraser, A. F. Lever, J. A. Millar, J. J. Morton, B. Petch, G. Riegger, J. I. S. Robertson, and M. Tree, Relation of arterial pressure and plasma angiotensin II concentration: a change produced by prolonged infusion of angiotensin II in the dog, Circ.Res. 44:452 (1979).

8. B. Folkow, Cardiovascular structural adaptation: its role in the initiation and maintenance of primary hypertension, Clin.Sci. 55 (Suppl.4):3 (1978).

9. A. W. Cowley and J. W. DeClue, Quantification of baroreceptor influence on arterial pressure changes seen in primary angiotensin-induced hypertension in dogs, Circ.Res. 39:779 (1976).

10. K. L. Barnes, K. B. Brosnihan, and C. M. Ferrario, Animal models, hypertension and central nervous system mechanisms, Mayo Clin.Proc. 52:387 (1977).

11. A. Zanchetti and C. Bartorelli, Central nervous mechanisms in arterial hypertension: experimental and clinical evidence, in: "Hypertension," J. Genest, E. Koiw, and O. Kuchel, eds., New York, McGraw-Hill, p.59. (1977).

12. W. Oelkers, M. Schöneshofer, G. Schultze, J. J. Brown, R. Fraser, J. J. Morton, A. F. Lever, and J. I. S. Robertson, Effect of prolonged low-dose angiotensin II on the sensitivity of the adrenal cortex in man, Circ.Res. 36,37 (Suppl.1):49 (1975).

13. D. G. Beevers, J. J. Brown, R. Fraser, A. F. Lever, J. J. Morton, J. I. S. Robertson, P. F. Semple, and M. Tree, The clinical value of renin and angiotensin estimations, Kidney Internatl. 8 (Suppl.5):181 (1975).

14. A. C. Guyton, T. G. Coleman, A. W. Cowley, K. W. Scheel, R. D. Manning, and R. A. Norman, Arterial pressure regulation: overriding dominance of the kidneys in long-term regulation and in hypertension, Am.J.Med. 52:584 (1972).

15. B. E. Watkins, J. O. Davis, R. H. Freeman, and G. A. Stephens, Production of renal hypertension in adrenalectomised dogs on constant hormone replacement therapy, Proc.Soc.Exp.Biol. Med. 157:116 (1978).

16. J. Lucas and M. A. Floyer, Changes in body fluid distribution and interstitial compliance during the development and

reversal of experimental renal hypertension in the rat,
Clin.Sci. 47:1 (1974).

17. D. McAreavey, W. Brown, and J. I. S. Robertson, Exchangeable
     sodium in rats with Goldblatt two-kidney one-clip hyper-
     tension, Clin.Sci. (in press). (1982).

18. D. L. Davies, K. McElroy, A. B. Atkinson, J. J. Brown, A. M. M.
     Cumming, R. Fraser, B. J. Leckie, A. Mackay, J. J. Morton,
     and J. I. S. Robertson, Relationship between exchangeable
     sodium and blood pressure in different forms of hypertension
     in man, Clin.Sci. 57 (Suppl.5):69 (1979).

19. A. B. Atkinson, J. J. Brown, D. L. Davies, A. F. Lever, J. J.
     Morton, R. Fraser, and J. I. S. Robertson, Hyponatraemic
     hypertensive syndrome with renal artery occlusion corrected
     by captopril, Lancet ii:606 (1979).

20. J. J. Brown, W. C. B. Brown, R. Fraser, A. F. Lever, J. J.
     Morton, J. I. S. Robertson, E. A. Rosei, and P. M. Trust,
     The effects of the angiotensin II antagonist saralasin on
     blood pressure and plasma aldosterone in man in relation to
     the prevailing plasma angiotensin II concentration, Prog.
     Biochem.Pharmacol. 12:230 (1976).

21. A. G. Atkinson, J. J. Morton, J. J. Brown, A. F. Lever, R.
     Fraser, and J. I. S. Robertson, Captopril in clinical hyper-
     tension: changes in components of the renin-angiotensin
     system and in body composition in relation to the fall in
     blood pressure, Brit.Ht.J. 44:290 (1980).

22. A. J. G. Riegger, A. F. Lever, J. A. Millar, J. J. Morton, and
     B. Slack, Correction of renal hypertension in the rat by
     prolonged infusion of angiotensin inhibitors, Lancet ii:1317
     (1977).

23. A. B. Atkinson, J. J. Brown, A. M. M. Cumming, R. Fraser, A. F.
     Lever, B. J. Leckie, J. J. Morton, and J. I. S. Robertson,
     Captopril in renovascular hypertension: long-term use in
     predicting surgical outcome, Brit.Med.J. 284:689 and 1557
     (1982).

24. P. Hodsman, J. J. Brown, D. L. Davies, R. Fraser, A. F. Lever,
     J. J. Morton, G. D. Murray, and J. I. S. Robertson, The
     converting enzyme inhibitor enalapril (MK421) in the treat-
     ment of hypertension with renal artery stenosis. Submitted
     for publication. (1982).

25. J. J. Brown, A. F. Lever, and J. I. S. Robertson, Renal hyper-
     tension: diagnosis and treatment. In: Renal Disease, 4th
     edition. Edited by Sir Douglas Black and N. F. Jones, p.731
     (1979).

ALTERATION OF CELL MEMBRANES IN PRIMARY HYPERTENSION

Yu. V. Postnov and S. N. Orlov

Central Research Laboratory
USSR Ministry of Public Health
Moscow, USSR

The past few years have witnessed a rapid accumulation of facts which give reason to believe that primary hypertension (essential hypertension in humans as well as spontaneous hypertension in Kyoto-Wistar rats) is causally associated to a wide-spread alteration of the cell membrane's regulation of intracellular free calcium and transport of univalent cations. In 1975-1978 we suggested that the hypertensive syndrome in primary hypertension is the manifestation of a certain type of membrane pathology[19-21]. Within a short period of time this hypothesis gradually began to gain ground. Below we present our data.

Erythrocytes

The first findings on the disturbance of the cell plasma membrane function of non-cardiovascular tissues in primary hypertension were obtained in studies of erythrocyte permeability. It was found that the rate constant of steady-state Na^+/Na^+ exchange through the erythrocyte membrane is increased both in spontaneous hypertension in rats (SHR, Kyoto-Wistar) and in essential hypertension[29,25,31]. These alterations are not connected with the Na-pump function[25,31], but are due to an increase of passive membrane permeability and/or to disturbances in the systems of counter-transport[3] and co-transport[7] of cations.

It is known that transmembrane transport of univalent cations is controlled by the concentration of free calcium in the cytoplasm[18,32]. This control is evidently achieved by changes in calcium content on the inner membrane surface[18]. Therefore, our further studies were directed to the study of intracellular calcium distribution. It was found that in both forms of primary hypertension the Ca-binding

327

ability of erythrocyte ghosts was reduced[26], which was due to a decrease in the number of calcium binding sites on the inner membrane
surface[24]. Similar data for rats with spontaneous hypertension were
also obtained by Devynck et al.[5] The technical difficulties in the
determination of free calcium-concentration in the cytoplasm are well
known. Quite recently Losse[10] laboratory developed microelectrodes
which allowed to solve this problem for erythrocytes. It was found
that free calcium concentration in the cytoplasm in erythrocytes
of spontaneously hypertensive rats was 50-60 times higher than in
normotensive control rats[10]. In erythrocytes this parameter is
determined by the rate of calcium influx into cells along the electro-
chemical gradient and by the rate of Ca^{2+} efflux at the expense of
Mg-Ca-ATPase activity[34]. The latter system is controlled by calmodulin[33].

In studies of the rate of [45]Ca influx into the erythrocytes of
SHR no differences were found[5]. There were also no differences in
the Mg-Ca-ATPase activity of erythrocyte membranes pre-treated with
EGTA[30]. However, both in spontaneous hypertension[16] and in patients
with essential hypertension (Table 1) the calmodulin effect on the
rate of [45]Ca accumulation by the inside-out vesicles was significantly
less than that of controls. In this connection it can be assumed that
the alteration of calmodulin interaction with Mg-Ca-ATPase is the
most probable cause of the Ca^{2+} concentration increase in the erythrocyte cytoplasm in primary hypertension.

Adipose Tissue

Compartmentation analysis of the kinetics of [45]Ca efflux was
used in studies of calcium distribution in adipose tissue. In these
experiments it was demonstrated that the content of intra-cellular
exchangeable calcium is increased at the expense of a higher calcium
content in mitochondria[23], both in spontaneous hypertension in rats[22]
and in essential hypertension[27]. Calcium overload of adipose tissue
in primary hypertension can probably be explained, as in the case of
erythrocytes, by a decrease of the calmodulin-dependent component of
Mg-Ca-ATPase activity of the adipocytes' plasma membrane. The presence
of the defect itself in the plasma membrane of adipocytes is confirmed
by the decrease of their Ca-binding ability[23] similar to that found
in erythrocytes,

Vascular Smooth Muscles

The existence of alterations in the excitation-contraction
coupling mechanism for vascular smooth muscle cells in hypertension
was revealed from numerous experiments on the variation in their
contractility, reactivity and sensitivity (see review[15]). Later on
it was shown that these changes in SHR are due to a disturbance of

Table 1. Affinity of Ca-pump to Ca^{2+} (K_m) and its Maximal Activity (V_{max}) in Erythrocyte Membranes in Essential Hypertension

Groups	n	Calmodulin 1.2×10^{-7}	K_m (μM)	V_{max} nmol Ca (mg protein IOV)$^{-1}$ min^{-1}
1. Control (normotensive patients)	11	–	1.72 ± 0.09	5.32 ± 0.61
2. Control (normotensive patients)	11	+	0.33 ± 0.04	25.11 ± 1.17
3. Essential hypertension	10	–	1.68 ± 0.10	4.98 ± 0.50
4. Essential hypertension	10	+	0.52 ± 0.04	10.32 ± 0.71
P$_{1,3}$			non-significant	
P$_{2,4}$			0.001	0.001

Erythrocyte membranes were treated with EGTA at the stage of isolation. IOV – inside-out vesicles. n – number of examined patients.

univalent cation transport[8] and also, as in the case of erythrocytes, are not related to a disturbance in the Na-K-ATPase activity, but to an increase in the rate of cation passive transport[1]. Calculations by Jones[9] showed that these disturbances lead to a partial depolarization of the sarcolemma and to enhanced excitability of SHR vascular smooth muscle cells.

In addition to disturbances of univalent cation transport in cells of SHR vascular smooth muscles, changes in their Ca-binding and Ca-accumulating systems were also found. Decrease by 40-60% of the ^{45}Ca accumulation rate was observed for crude cell microsome fractions of SHR aorta smooth muscles[2]. In subsequent studies similar alterations were also described for the sarcolemma fraction, where the decrease of Ca-binding ability of SHR membranes was detected together with a reduction of the ATP-dependent accumulation of ^{45}Ca[17,35].

Synaptosomes

Already the alteration of the plasma membrane function in erythrocytes, in adipose tissue cells and in vascular smooth muscles indicates the wide-spread character of the membrane defect in both forms of primary hypertension. Moreover, the decrease of plasma membrane's Ca-binding was observed in rats with spontaneous hypertension in cardiomyocytes, hepatocytes and synaptosomes of the brain[6]. The latter observation is especially important since it indicates the possibility of changes in the mechanism of neurotransmitter secretion by nerve terminals, which largely accounts for increases of vascular tone in primary hypertension. To elucidate the state of plasma membranes in the cells of the central nervous system in spontaneously hypertensive rats, we studied transport systems of Ca influx and efflux in isolated synaptosomes and microsomes from the brain tissue. It is known that the activity of these systems determines the cytoplasm calcium balance and finally, neurotransmitters output and reuptake by nerve endings. These studies were carried out jointly with G. M. Kravtsov and N. I. Pokudin.

It was found that basal calcium uptake (i.e. calcium uptake in physiological concentrations of sodium and calcium in incubation medium) in SHR synaptosomes was 1.5-2 times higher than in normotensive Kyoto-Wistar rats (Figure 1). The differences remained during membrane depolarization obtained by lowering the extracellular K^+ concentration and disappeared in saturated concentrations of this cation. It can be assumed that the initial difference in Ca uptake is due to the existence of a constant partial depolarisation of the plasma membrane of nerve cells in SHR. The following data have been obtained to prove this assumption.

1. Calcium uptake by synaptosome of SHR and control rats does not differ if a specific inhibitor of potential-dependent Ca-channels (verapamil) is present in the incubation medium.

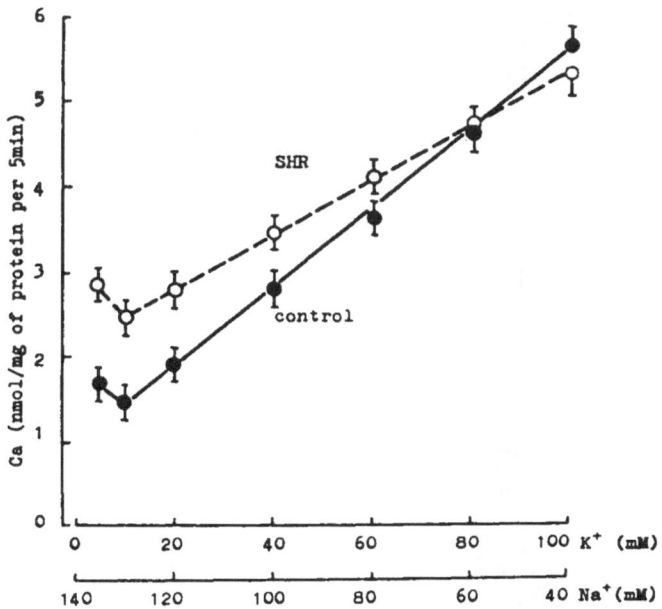

Fig. 1. Dependence of calcium uptake by synaptosomes in rats with
spontaneous hypertension (SHR) and normotensive controls
(NKWR) on the ratio of sodium and potassium concentration
in the incubation media.

2. Synaptosome permeability for Na^+ (the most important factor
for the formation of action potential in excitable tissues) is significantly increased in SHR as compared to normotensive controls
(Figure 2).

In subcellular brain tissue fractioning, besides the mitochondria,
one more membrane fraction with ATP-dependent calcium uptake ability
was found. According to the distribution of marker enzymes (presence
of Na-Ca exchange system, K^+-dependent Ca^{2+} uptake and calmodulin
effect on ATP-dependent calcium uptake), this fraction was characterized as a fraction of plasma membrane fragments of nerve cells and
their dendrites. In studies of the dependence of the ^{45}Ca uptake
rate of this fraction on Ca^{2+} concentration in the incubation medium
(Figure 3), it was found that the maximal rate of ^{45}Ca uptake in SHR
was 40% lower than in the controls. It should be emphasized that,
similarly to the Ca-transporting erythrocyte system, the calmodulin
effect on Ca^{2+} transport in the plasma membranes in SHR's brain was
significantly lower than that of normotensive animals (Figure 3).

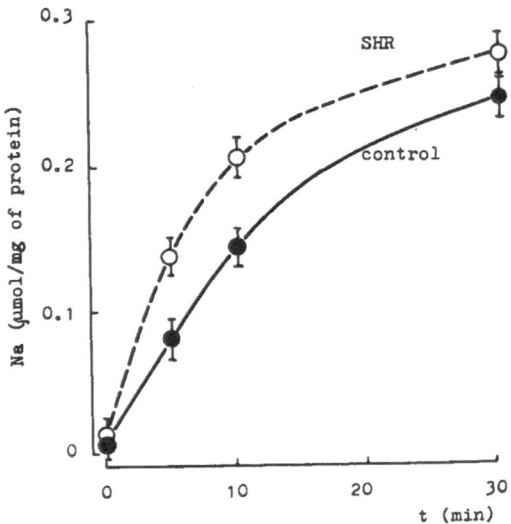

Fig. 2. The kinetics of sodium uptake by synaptosomes in rats with
         spontaneous hypertension (SHR) and normotensive control
         rats (NKWR).

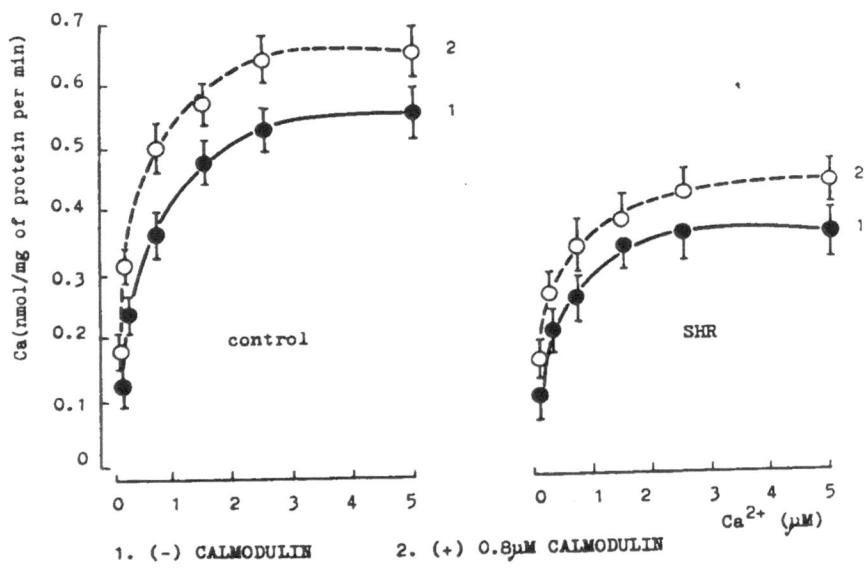

1. (-) CALMODULIN   2. (+) 0.8µM CALMODULIN

Fig. 3. Dependence of the rate of calcium accumulation by microsome
         from the brain of spontaneously hypertensive rats (SHR) and
         normotensive control rats (NKWR) on calcium concentration.
         1) without calmodulin; 2) +0.8 uM calmodulin.

The presented data give reasons to suggest that free calcium concentration in the cytoplasm of nerve terminals in SHR is increased. This may serve as one of the main causes of the increased activity of peripheral part of the sympathetic nervous system in SHR and, evidently, in essential hypertension in humans as well.

Molecular Mechanisms of Membrane Defect

The first attempts to study this problem were started simultaneously in our laboratory and in the laboratory of Prof. Meyer[11] by the technique of fluorescence probes. Using diphenyl-hexatrien, whose fluorescence polarization is determined by the rate of rotational diffusion of molecules in the hydrophobic regions of the membrane, an increase of microviscosity of these parts of erythrocyte membrane was observed in rats with spontaneous hypertension[11,12]. A reduction in the rate of lateral diffusion of molecules (especially significant in the region of protein-lipid contact) was found by means of another probe – pyrene both in spontaneous hypertension in rats[12] and in essential hypertension in humans[14]. Now some data are available indicating that the defect of structure of plasma membrane is not limited to erythrocytes, but also manifests itself in the plasma membranes of hypatocytes, synaptosomes and cardiomyocytes[4]. It can be assumed that the defect in the structure of the plasma membrane is the cause of disturbances of its cation-binding and cation-transporting function.

Conclusion

The present paper contains a short review of data on the studies of cell membranes in primary hypertension. These data confirm a wide-spread, if not universal, alteration of cell plasma membranes in primary hypertension, both in rats and in man. In excitable and non-excitable cells alterations in plasma membrane structure, alteration of the membrane's permeability to monovalent cations, decrease of its Ca-binding ability in combination with a disorder of the Ca-transporting systems were found. This is the basis of the membrane defect, which is manifested in the insufficiency of membrane control over free calcium concentration in the cytoplasm.

The membrane defect was observed at stages previous to the development of the hypertensive syndrome[25]; it was not detected in secondary hypertension both in experimental models[13,26] and in patients with chronic renal hypertension[14]; there was no dependence of the membrane defect on the activity of the sympathetic nervous system[28] and the secretory function of the adrenal cortex[22,25].

It should be noted that the wide-spread (not limited to one type of cell) membrane alteration in primary hypertension and its

obvious genetic origin are indicative of the fact that the initial
inherent defect of the genetic apparatus concerns the few basic genes
unaffected by repression during tissue differentiation.

As for the pathogenesis of hypertension, the following consequences of the alteration of cell membranes should be taken into
consideration:

1. the disturbance in the excitation – contracting coupling in
contractile cells of the cardiovascular system;

2. the alteration of Ca transport in the neurolemma (presynapti(
membrane), indicating the presence of an increased free calcium
concentration in nerve endings, intensifying neuromediator quantation
and changing synaptic transmission.

3. the change in cell calcium distribution in tissues which are
the target for the sympathetic nervous system, serving as the basis
for the alteration of its functional status (since both sensitivity a￼
reactivity of such targets are changed).

REFERENCES

1. J. Altman, R. Carry, A. Papadimitriou and M. Worcel, Alterations
   in ^{22}Na fluxes of arterial smooth muscle of spontaneously
   hypertensive rats, Brit. J. Pharmacol., 59:416 (1977).
2. K. Aoki, N. Ikedo, K. Yamashita, K. Tazumi, I. Sato and K. Hotta,
   Cardiovascular contraction in spontaneously hypertensive rats:
   Ca^{2+} interaction of myofibrils and subcellular membrane of
   heart and arterial smooth muscle, Jap. Circul. J. 38:1115 (197
3. M. Canessa, N. Adragna, H. S. Solomon, T. M. Connolly and D. C.
   Testeson, Increased sodium–lithium counter transport in red
   cells of patients with essential hypertension, New England I.
   Med. 302:772 (1980).
4. M. A. Dovynck, M. G. Pernollet, A. M. Numez, I. Aragon, T. Monten
   C. Helene and P. Meyer, Biophysical and biochemical demonstration of a diffuse alteration of plasma membrane in SHR's,
   in: "Abstr. of 8th Meet. of Intern. Soc. of Hypertension",
   Milan, Italy, R 107 (1981).
5. M. A. Devynck, M. G. Pernollet, A. M. Nunez and P. Meyer, Analysi
   of calcium handling in erythrocyte membranes of genetically
   hypertensive rats, Hypertension 3:397 (1981).
6. M. A. Devynck, M. G. Pernollet, A. M. Nunez and P. Meyer, Calciun
   binding alteration in plasma membrane from various tissues on
   spontaneously hypertensive rats, Clin. Exper. Hypertension
   3:787 (1981).
7. R. P. Garay, G. Dagher, M. G. Pernollet, M. A. Devynck and P.
   Meyer, Inherited defect in Na^+, K^+-co-transport system in
   erythrocyte from essential hypertensive patients, Nature
   (L) 284:281 (1980).

8. A. M. Jones, Altered ion transport in vascular smooth muscle from spontaneously hypertensive rats. Influence of aldosteron, norepinephrine and angiotensin, Circul Res. 33:563 (1973).

9. A. W. Jones, Reactivity of ions fluxes in rat aorta during hypertension and circulatory control, Federat. Proc. 33:133 (1974).

10. H. Losse, W. Zidek, H. Zumkley, F. Wessels and J. Vetter, Intracellular Na^+ as a genetic marker of essential hypertension, Clin. Exper. Hypertension 3:627 (1981).

11. T. Montenay-Garestier, I. Aragon, M. A. Devynck, P. Meyer and C. Helene, Evidence for structural changes in erythrocyte membranes of spontaneously hypertensive rats. A fluorescence polarization study, Biochem. Biophys. Res. Comm. 100:660 (1981).

12. S. N. Orlov, P. V. Gulak, Z. V. Karagodina and Yu. V. Postnov, The features of erythrocyte membrane structure in rats with spontaneous hypertension, Cardiology (in Russian) 21:108 (1981).

13. S. N. Orlov, Z. V. Karagodina, Ca-binding ability and erythrocyte membrane structure in rats with experimental hypertension, Cardiology (in Russian) 22 (3):106 (1982).

14. S. N. Orlov, Z. V. Karagodina, I. Yu. Postnov, N. I. Pokudin, and Yu. V. Postnov, Calcium binding and erythrocyte membrane structure in essential and secondary hypertensions, Cardiology (in Russian) 22 (5):124 (1982).

15. S. N. Orlov, N. I. Pokudin and Yu. V. Postnov, Permeability to monovalent ions, intracellular calcium distribution and contractility of vascular smooth muscle in arterial hypertension, Cardiology (in Russian) 18 (3):131 (1978).

16. S. N. Orlov, N. I. Pokudin and Yu. V. Postnov, Calcium transport in erythrocytes of rats with spontaneous hypertension: the features of interaction with calmodulin, Cardiology (in Russian) 22 (7):107 (1982).

17. S. N. Orlov and Yu. V. Postnov, Calcium accumulation and calcium binding by the cell membranes of cardiomyocytes and smooth muscle of aortas in spontaneously hypertensive rats, Clin. Sci. 59:207, suppl. (1980).

18. S. N. Orlov and A. S. Shevchenko, The effect of membrane-bound calcium on the activity of adenosine triphosphatase and erythrocyte permeability to monovalent cations, Biochemistry (in Russian) 44:208 (1978).

19. Yu. V. Postnov, Essential hypertension as a membrane pathology, Cardiology (in Russian) 15 (8):18 (1975).

20. Yu. V. Postnov, Pathology of cell membranes and the role of kidneys in essential hypertension, Ther. Arch. (in Russian) 49 (10):45 (1977).

21. Yu. V. Postnov and S. H. Orlov, Alteration of cell membranes in hypertension: role of altered membrane control over intracellular calcium, in: "Proc. of 1st Joint US-USSR Symp. of Hypertension", Sochi, USSR, NIH Publ. No 79-1272 (1979).

22. Yu. V. Postnov and S. N. Orlov, Features of intracellular calcium distribution in the adipose tissue of spontaneously hypertensive rats (SHR), Experientia 35:1480 (1979).

23. Yu. V. Postnov and S. N. Orlov, Evidence of altered calcium
    accumulation and calcium binding by the membranes of adipo-
    cytes in spontaneously hypertensive rats, Pflügers Archiv.
    385:85 (1980).

24. Yu. V. Postnov and S. N. Orlov, Alteration of membrane control
    over intracellular calcium in essential hypertension and in
    spontaneously hypertensive rats, in: "Intracellular Electro-
    lytes and Arterial Hypertension", H. Sumkley and H. Losse,
    (eds.), George Thiene Verlag, Stuttgart-New York (1980).

25. Yu. V. Postnov, S. N. Orlov, P. V. Gulak and A. S. Shevchenko,
    Altered permeability of the erythrocyte membrane for sodium
    and potassium in spontaneously hypertensive rats, Pflügers
    Archiv. 365:257 (1976).

26. Yu. V. Postnov, S. N. Orlov and N. I. Pokudin, Decrease of
    calcium binding by the red blood cell membrane in spontaneous
    hypertensive rats and in essential hypertension, Pflügers
    Archiv. 379:191 (1979).

27. Yu. V. Postnov, S. N. Orlov and N. I. Pokudin, Alteration of
    intracellular calcium distribution in the adipose tissue of
    patients with essential hypertension, Pflügers Archiv. 388:
    89 (1980).

28. Yu. V. Postnov, S. N. Orlov and N. I. Pokudin, Alteration of the
    intracellular calcium pool of adipose tissue in spontaneously
    hypertensive rats. No effect of peripheral immunosympathec-
    tomy, Pflügers Archiv. 390:256 (1981).

29. Yu. V. Postnov, S. N. Orlov and A. S. Shevchenko, Alteration of
    membrane permeability of erythrocytes in rats with spontaneou
    hypertension, Cardiology (in Russian) 15 (10):88 (1975).

30. Yu. V. Postnov, S. N. Orlov and A. S. Shevchenko, Ca^{2+}-binding
    alteration and Na-K-ATPase activity in the erythrocytes of
    patients with essential hypertension, Bull. Exp. Biol. Med.
    (in Russian) 84:41 (1977).

31. Yu. V. Postnov, S. N. Orlov, A. S. Shevchenko and A. M. Adler,
    Altered sodium permeability, calcium binding and Na-K-ATPase
    activity in the red blood cell membrane in essential hyper-
    tension, Pflügers Archiv. 371:263 (1977).

32. P. J. Romero, Role of membrane bound Ca in ghost permeability
    to Na and K, J. Membrane Biol. 29:329 (1976).

33. B. Sarkadi, T. Szacz and G. Gardas, Calcium and calmodulin in
    the regulation of blood cell function, Haematologia 14:121
    (1981).

34. H. J. Schatzmann, Active calcium transport across the plasma
    membrane of erythrocytes, in: "Calcium Transport in Contrac-
    tion and Secretion", E. Carafoli et al., (eds.) Amsterdam-
    Oxford (1975).

35. W. J. Wei, R. A. Janis and E. E. Daniel, Calcium accumulative
    activities of subcellular fractions from aortas and ventricl
    of spontaneously hypertensive rats, Circulat. Res. 39:133
    (1976).

HIGH DENSITY LIPOPROTEINS AND ATHEROSCLEROSIS

A. N. Klimov

Institute of Experimental Medicine

Leningrad, USSR

The change in the ratio between lipoprotein (LP) concentration with the density higher or lower than 1.063 g/ml was first observed in patients with ischemic heart disease as early as 1951[1]. Later Gofman et al.[2] also pointed to the increased blood concentration of low density lipoproteins (LDLP) and decreased content of high density LP (HDLP) in patients with clinical atherosclerosis. However, at that time attention was paid to the increasing level of LP in atherosclerosis leaving in shade the low levels of LP.

In 1970 T. N. Lovyagina and E. B. Ban'kovskaya[3] found that in man or animals (rabbit, guinea-pig, pig, monkey) with spontaneous or easily induced experimental atherosclerosis greater part of plasma cholesterol is contained by LDLP or very low density lipoproteins (VLDLP). In case of animals (suslik, rat, cat, dog) which never suffer from spontaneous atherosclerosis and are resistant or immune to experimentally induced atherosclerosis the major part of cholesterol is contained by HDLP. It is characteristic that such cholesterol distribution is preserved in the above mentioned animals (rat excluded) fed cholesterol-rich diets. It is interesting to note, that in case of cholesterol fed susliks the plasma cholesterol concentration level amounted to extremely high figures (more than 700 mg/dl), but the atherosclerosis did not develop in these animals since most of the cholesterol taken up by the organism was used to form HDLP. Soret et al.[4] reported on the lame attempt to induce atherosclerosis under experimental conditions in chinese hamsters, probably, also due to high HDLP blood level.

In 1975 G. Miller and N. Miller[5] reported that in patients with coronary atherosclerosis the level of HDLP cholesterol was evidently lower and that this might be important in pathogenesis.

Further clinical and population studies carried out in many countries of the world, due to the simplicity and availability of the CD-HDLP determination method, showed the lower cholesterol content of HDLP in ischemic heart disease (IHD) patients than in patients without any IHD signs (see review N 6). The often observed difference in the CS concentrations of HDLP of 3-6 mg/dl proved to be statistically significant. Thus, the population study of more than 7000 male sex residents of Moscow and Leningrad, aged 40 to 59, with signs of IHD (according to ECG at rest and Rose questionnaire) showed that the mean level of CS-HDLP amounted to 49.6 ± 17.2 mg/dl, while in persons without IHD it amounted to 53.5 ± 17.2 mg/dl (p < 0.001). So the difference is 3.9 mg/dl.

In line with the published data, HDLP cholesterol as an IHD predictor proved to be eightfold more sensitive than the total CS concentration and fourfold more sensitive than LDLP cholesterol[7]. We have suggested to calculate the so-called cholesterol coefficient of atherogeneity as the "predictor" which is represented by the following ratio[8,9]:

$$C = \frac{\text{LDLP cholesterol} + \text{VLDLP cholesterol}}{\text{HDLP cholesterol}}$$

In clinic it is more convenient to calculate this coefficient by determining the total and HDLP cholesterol:

$$C = \frac{\text{Total CS} - \text{HDLP CS}}{\text{HDLP CS}}$$

The higher the coefficient is (in healthy persons it does not exceed 3 units), the higher is the danger of IHD. In IHD patients the value of the coefficient often amounts to 5-6 and more units.

If at the beginning of the study of the physiologic role of HDLP they were termed "non-atherogenic" LP contrary to LDLP and VLDLP, there are all grounds now to consider them "anti-atherogenic". In this context, the mechanism of antiatherogenic HDLP action assumes special concern.

ON ANTIATHEROGENIC HDLP ACTION

At present, there is no unified theory to explain the anti-atherogenic action of HDLP or their subspecies.

One of the first viewpoints on this question[10,11] assumed the competition between HDLP and LDLP for the receptors on the cell surface and the higher the blood HDLP concentration is the fewer LDLP (and consequently less CS) penetrate into the cell. However, HDLP affinity for cell receptors appeared to be on the whole 200-fold lower as compared to that of LDLP[12]. Yet this affinity increases with the increase of apoprotein E concentration in HDLP and it is represented to a greater extent in $HDLP_c$ (c means cholesterol in-duced)[13].

The following facts may be opposed to the attempt aimed at explaining HDLP antiatherogenic action by their competition with LDLP for cell receptors. It is known that the receptor-bound cel-lular uptake to LDLP helps the blood LP homeostasis[12]. Receptor function disorders result in the increase of CS and LDLP blood levels. Thus, the competitive LDLP prevention from the receptor-bound cellular uptake must lead to the development of atherosclerosis rather than to its inhibition as it occurs in the hereditary receptor insufficiency[12].

Moreover, as the studies by Miller[14] have shown the increase instead of the inhibition of LDLP uptake by cells through the re-ceptor mechanism which followed the preincubation of human skin fibroblasts with HDLP. Cholesterol removal from the cells during their preincubation with HDLP stimulated the receptor synthesis and the uptake of additional amounts of LDLP.

Unfortunately, there are no data as to the HDLP influence on non-specific endocytosis LDLP uptake by the cells, particularly, by endothelial cells, in other words the effect on the process which is likely to promote the unregulated LDLP and CS accumulation in the endothelial and intimal cells.

In 1968, Glomset[15] presupposed that HDLP are involved in the removal of excess CS from the peripheral tissues and its transport to the liver for subsequent oxidation to bile acids. If we combine this hypothesis with receptor hypothesis of Goldstein and Brown[16], there appears the general pattern of CS transport into the cell by VLDLP-LDLP system and the reverse CS transport by HDLP (Figure 1). Evidently, at the insufficient blood level of HDLP they fail to remove CS from the cell.

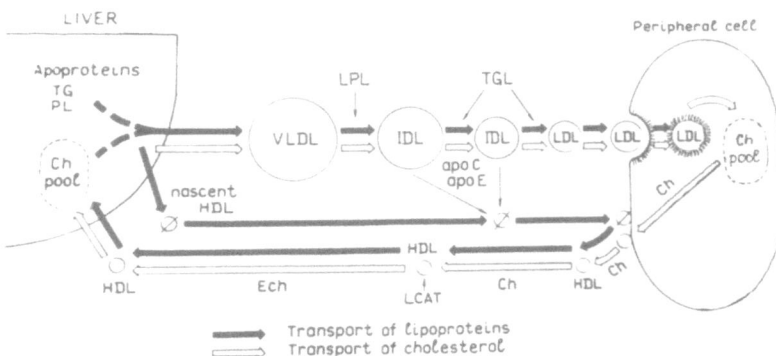

Fig. 1.   Transport of cholesterol from the liver into the peripheral
          cell and the reverse cholesterol transport.

     Analogously, the antiatherogenic HDLP action may be assumed
to result from partial cellular uptake of CS by these LP due to
their easy penetrability into the arterial wall, and CS removal
through the paravasal system of adventitia[8]. This conception is
supported by the studies showing that as a result of the interaction
in vitro between HDLP and CS the former are capable of dissolving
CS crystals[17], and due to the interaction with liposomes[18] and
erythrocytes[19] they are capable of removing from them a part of CS.
It is significant that HDLP fractions accepting a part of CS from
the erythrocyte membrane, augmented in size[19]. It is likely, that
in the studies mentioned above the main acceptors of CS were HDLP$_3$
and the formed large particles - HDLP$_2$. Further, the data obtained
in our laboratory[20] showed that during incubation of HDLP with
intima isolated from human aorta afflicted by atherosclerosis the
enrichment of HDLP$_3$ and to a much lesser extent of HDLP$_2$ by non-
esterified CS took place. So, one of the HDLP subspecies, namely
HDLP$_3$, is capable of binding additional amounts of CS. Alongside
this it is significant that being saturated with non-esterified
CS, HDLP$_3$ fractions became lighter and were translated to HDLP$_2$-
like particles. We cannot still define to what extent the capability
of HDLP$_3$ to bind non-esterified CS is manifested in vivo, though
it is worth mentioning the study of Sarma et al.[21] who showed that

in perfusion of pug coronary artery by homologous plasma with the addition of HDLP to it, inhibited the penetration of the labeled CS into the arterial wall.

Another possible mechanism of antiatherogenic HDLP action is connected with the fact established by Nikkila[22]: at high HDLP blood level the highest rate of the lipolysis of triglyceride (TG)-rich lipoprotein is observed. This is in accord with many studies showing the reciprocal correlation between the HDLP level (or CS HDLP) and TG VLDLP. A decrease in the content of the latter in blood caused by various means (the lowering of body mass, physical exercise, chlorphibrate intake) leads to the increase of HDLP level. All these data served as the ground for the assumption and then demonstration of direct VLDLP-HDLP interaction[23]:

$$VLDLP + HDLP_3 \xrightarrow{\text{lipoproteinlipase}} HDLP_2 + LDLP$$

As a result of this reaction catalyzed by lipoproteinlipase the decrease of the VLDLP level is observed. Is it of any importance to the organism? VLDLP according to Zilversmit[24], penetrates into the arterial wall primarily as highly atherogenic remnant particles.

In line with our data[25] among all the LP species VLDLP have most pronounced autoantigeneity leading to the formation of the autoimmune complex VLDLP-IgG circulating in blood. Like all other autoimmune complexes it may afflict the endothelium initiating the development of atherosclerotic process. In line with the above mentioned, it is possible to assume that the decrease of the VLDLP level favors the prevention of atherosclerosis. However, the reaction mentioned above results in the formation of LDLP which according to generally accepted viewpoints are the most atherogenic. So it is difficult to determine whether or not the reaction plays a protective role in atherogenesis. Nevertheless, it is likely to assume that the formed $HDLP_2$ are more antiatherogenic than $HDLP_3$. In connection with such an assumption there are some population and clinical data. It is known, for instance, that the difference in HDLP blood levels in men and women concern mainly $HDLP_2$. Long-distance runners have an increased level of $HDLP_2$ instead of $HDLP_3$. Just the same increase of the $HDLP_2$ level is observed with the administration of drugs decreasing the TG blood level. Namely this LP subspecy, contrary to $HDLP_3$ increased in hyper-α-lipoprotein-emia. On the other hand, the increase in the $HDLP_2$ level may be treated as a result of the antiatherogenic action either of nascent (disco-like) HDLP or other products on the way of formation of native HDLP or, finally, $HDLP_3$. Similar conception was put forward by Assman[26], for instance. It is also probable that $HDLP_2$ and $HDLP_3$ extracted by preparative ultracentrifuging, are not quite

equal to those HDLP circulating in blood. No doubt, additional
studies are necessary to determine the most antiatherogenic subspecy
of HDLP.

As was noted above, $HDLP_3$ are capable of non-esterified CS
binding. It can be CS from cell membranes, CS settled extra-cellularl
in the intima of arterial wall, or either CS released upon the hydrolysis of triglyceride-rich LP in plasma. Evidently, physico-chemical
composition and structure of $HDLP_3$ particles lead to such an uptake
of CS irrespective of its source. As $HDLP_3$ with taken CS transfer
to $HDLP_2$ or the similar particles the process of $HDLP_3$ regeneration
must occur in the organism. Nikkila et al.[27] assume, that the
inverse process of $HDLP_2$ metabolism to $HDLP_3$ takes place in the liver
involving the hepatic lipase in it.

The whole cycle of HDLP metabolism is in general represented
by the following scheme:

Inside the liver   Outside the liver

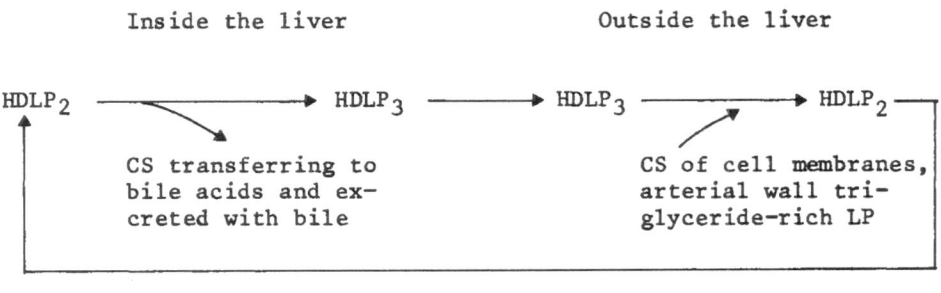

Scheme of possible $HDLP_2 \rightleftharpoons HDLP_3$ metabolism

In conclusion we would like to mention our lame attempt to
inhibit the development of experimentally-induced atherosclerosis
in rabbits by multiple intravenous administrations of heparologic
(horse) HDLP[28]. Despite the fact that on the whole within 10 weeks
each animal received 58 intravenous injections with 3143 mg of HDLP
(as protein), the experimentally-induced atherosclerosis was not inhibited, but on the contrary its development intensified. It is chara
teristic that in animals injected with HDLP the level of total CS and
especially of TG was low. By the end of the experiment the plasma of
the animals injected with HDLP was transparent (probably, due to the
lower content of VLDLP), whereas plasma of the control animals was
turbid. Probably in these experiments the effect of immunologic factors was clearly seen, conditioned by the manyfold administration of
heterologic HDLP which was followed by the intensification of atherosclerosis. HDLP extracted from plasma were likely to have weak antiatherogenic action either because of the lack of nascent HDLP among

them or the loss of antiatherogenic properties during isolation (LCAT etc.).

Finally, it is worth noting that rabbits possess extremely low activity of hepatic lipase (triglyceride lipase) in blood both basal and postheparin[29]. If this enzyme is involved in the $HDLP_2 \longrightarrow HDLP_3$ metabolism in the liver[27], one may assume that the low rate of metabolism in the rabbit liver does not lead to enough regeneration of $HDLP_3$ and their uptake by the blood. Probably, this leads to the easy development of experimentally induced atherosclerosis in rabbits.

We failed to delay the development of the experimentally induced atherosclerosis in rabbits by administrating homologous HDLP (unpublished data). In these experiments within 10 months each animal was subjected to 60 intravenous injections of HDLP, isolated from plasma of a great amount of healthy rabbits with the density ranging from 1.063 to 1.210. Each rabbit received totally 290 mg HDLP (as protein). As upon the administration of heterologous LP, the evident decrease of the total CS and TG content was observed in plasma of animals.

Though the experiments on the delay of the development of experimental atherosclerosis were not a success the obtained results showed that artificially induced increase in the blood level of HDLP in rabbits by multiple intravenous administration of heterologous homologous HDLP leads to the decrease of the total content of CS and TG which is in accord both with the above scheme put forward by Patsch et al.[23] and with general ideas about the scavenger activity of HDLP - i.e. the ability to utilize and accelerate CS catabolism and lipids upon the lipolysis of triglyceride-rich LP in blood[30].

The antiatherogeneity of HDLP is accepted to depend on the concentration ratio of $HDLP_3$ and $HDLP_2$ in it, free and esterified CS, phospholipids, apoproteins as well as the activity of LCAT and lipoprotein lipase in plasma and lipase in the liver.

The following hypothesis attempting to explain antiatherogenic HDLP action should be noted: inhibitory effect of HDLP on proliferation of aortic smooth muscle cells induced by LDLP[31]; inhibiting of the synthesis of glycosaminoglycans in aortic smooth muscle cells[32]; solubilization of glycosaminoglycan-LDLP complexes in arterial wall by HDLP[33]; the decrease in the thrombogenic LDLP action[34]; stimulation of the oxidation of CS to bile acids in the liver[35] etc.

CONCLUSION

There is yet no unified theory to explain the role of HDLP in the pathogenesis of atherosclerosis. The theories and hypotheses put forward consider the atherogenic action of HDLP at different physiologic levels - individual cell, arterial wall and plasma. Special attention is paid to the possible involvement of HDLP in CS removal from tissues, interference of HDLP into cellular uptake of CS and interrelation between HDLP and triglyceride-rich lipoproteins in plasma.

No matter what kind the atherogenic action of HDLP, of their subspecies or precursors was, we may consider as clearly established the low blood level of HDLP which reflects the state promoting the development of atherosclerosis and ischemic heart disease while the high blood level inhibits them. Probably, dislipoproteinemia characterized by both high blood level of LDLP or VLDLP and low blood level of HDLP, is the most dangerous for the organism.

REFERENCES

1. D. P. Barr, E. M. Russ and H. A. Eder. Protein-lipid relationshi in human plasma. 2.-In: Atherosclerosis and related conditions Am. J. Med., v. II, p. 480-493 (1951).
2. J. W. Gofman, W. Young and R. Tandy. Ischemic heart disease, atherosclerosis and longevity. Circulation, v. 34, p. 679-697 (1966).
3. T. N. Lovyagina and E. B. Ban'kovskaya. Plasma and aortic cholesterol and lipoproteins of various types of animals in the norm and hypercholesterolemia. Zhurnal evoluts. biokhim. fisiol., v. 3, p. 255-261.
4. M. G. Soret, M. C. Blanks, G. C. Gerritsen, C. E. Day and E. M. Block. Diet-induced hypercholesterolemia in the diabetic and non-diabetic chinese hamster. - In: Atherosclerosis Drug Discovery. C. E. Day (ed.), New York, Plenum Press, p. 329-343 (1976).
5. G. J. Miller and N. E. Miller. Plasma high density lipoprotein concentration and development of ischemic heart disease. Lancet, v. I, p. 16-19 (1975).
6. G. Heiss, N. J. Johnson, S. Reiland, C. E. Davis and H. A. Tyrole The epidemiology of plasma high-density lipoprotein cholester(levels. Circulation, v. 62 (suppl. 4), p. 116-136 (1980).
7. T. Gordon, W. P. Castelli, M. C. Hjortland, W. B. Kannel and T. Dawber. High density lipoproteins as a protective factor against coronary heart disease. Am. J. Med., v. 62, p. 707-714 (1977).
8. A. N. Klimov. Causes and conditions of atherosclerosis developm(In: Preventive cardiology, G. I. Kositsky (ed.), Medicina, Moscow, p. 260-321 (1977).
9. A. N. Klimov. The significance of lipid infiltration of artery intima at early stages of atherogenesis. Dt. Z. Verdau-u. Stoff-wechselkr., B. 38, s.231-233 (1978).
10. T. E. Carew, Y. Koschinsky, S. B. Hayes and D. Steinberg. A mechanism by which high density lipoprotein may slow the athe1 genic process. Lancet, i., p. 1315-1317 (1976).

11. O. Stein, Y. Stein and P. Goren. Metabolism and metabolic role of serum high density lipoproteins. In: High Density Lipoproteins and Atherosclerosis. A. M. Gotto, N. E. Miller and M. F. Oliver (eds.). Amsterdam. Elsevier, p. 37-49 (1978).

12. M. S. Brown and J. L. Goldstein. Analysis of mutant strain of human fibroblasts with a defect in the internalization of receptor-bound low density lipoproteins. Cell, v. 9, p. 663-674 (1976).

13. R. W. Mahley. Alterations in plasma lipoproteins induced by cholesterol feeding in animals including man. In: Disturbances in Lipid and Lipoprotein Metabolism. J. M. Dietschy, A. M. Gotto and J. A. Ontko (eds.). American Physiological Society, Bethesda, p. 181-197 (1978).

14. N. E. Miller. Induction of low density lipoproteins receptor synthesis by high density lipoproteins in cultures of human skin fibroblasts. Biochim. Biophys. Acta, v. 529, p. 131-137 (1978).

15. J. A. Glomset. The plasma lecithin: cholesterol acyltransferase reaction. J. Lipid Res. v. 9, p. 155-168 (1968).

16. J. L. Goldstein and M. S. Brown. The low-density lipoprotein pathway and its relation to atherosclerosis. Ann. Rev. Biochem. v. 46, p. 897-930 (1977).

17. C. W. M. Adams and Y. H. Abdulla. The action of human high density lipoproteins on cholesterol crystals. Atherosclerosis, v. 31, p. 465-471 (1978).

18. A. Jonas, L. K. Hesterberg and S. M. Drengler. Incorporation of excess cholesterol by high density serum lipoproteins. Biochim. Biophys. Acta, v. 528, p. 47-57 (1978).

19. A. N. Klimov, G. E. Shmelev, V. A. Noekin, I. F. Mamontova, L. G. Petrova-Maslakova and N. S. Parfenova. Measurement of human plasma lipoprotein distribution by dimensions. Biofisika, v. 27 (1982).

20. A. N. Klimov, L. G. Petrova-Maslakova, I. F. Mamontova, N. S. Parfenova, I. G. Kovaleva and V. F. Tryufanov. Interaction of high density lipoproteins and their subfractions with intima of atherosclerotic human aorta. Vopr. med. khimii, v. 28, N 2, s.122-125 (1982).

21. J. S. M. Sarma, G. V. Tschurtshenthaler and R. J. Bing. Effect of high density lipoproteins on the cholesterol uptake by isolated pig coronary arteries. Artery, v. 4, p. 214-223 (1978).

22. E. A. Nikkila. Metabolic and endocrine control of plasma high density lipoprotein. In: High Density Lipoproteins and Atherosclerosis. A. M. Gotto, N. E. Miller and M. F. Oliver (eds.), Amsterdam, Elsevier, p. 177-192 (1978).

23. J. R. Patsch, A. M. Gotto, T. Olivecrona and S. Eisenberg. Formation of high density lipoprotein$_2$-like particles during lipolysis of very low density lipoproteins in vitro. Proc. Natl. Acad. Sci. USA, v. 75, p. 4519-4523 (1978).

24. D. B. Zilversmit. A proposal linking atherogenesis to the inter-
    action of endothelial lipoprotein lipase with triglyceride-
    rich lipoproteins. Circulation Res. v. 33, p. 633-638 (1973).
25. A. N. Klimov, Yu. N. Zubzhitsky and V. A. Nagornev. Immuno-
    chemical aspects of atherosclerosis. Atherosclerosis Rev.
    v. 4, p. 119-156 (1979).
26. G. Assaman. The metabolic role of high density lipoproteins:
    Perspectives from Tangier disease. In: High Density Lipo-
    proteins and Atherosclerosis. A. M. Gotto, N. E. Miller
    and M. F. Oliver (eds.), Amsterdam, Elsevier, p. 77-89 (1978).
27. E. A. Nikkila, T. Kuusi and M. -R. Taskinen. Role of lipoprotein
    lipase and hepatic endothelial lipase in the metabolism of high
    density lipoproteins: a novel concept on cholesterol transport
    in HDL cycle. In: Metabolic Risk Factors in Ischemic Cardio-
    vascular Disease. L. A. Carlson and B. Pernow (eds.), New
    York Raven Press, p. 205; 215 (1982).
28. A. N. Klimov, L. G. Petrova-Maslakova, G. G. Chetchinashvili,
    L. M. Tchichatarashvili, V. A. Nagornev and V. F. Tryufanov.
    Effect of plasma lipoextraction and infusion of heterologous
    HDL on the development of experimental atherosclerosis in
    rabbits. In: Atheroslerosis, A. M. Gotto, L. C. Smith and
    B. Allen (eds.), New York, Springer-Verlag, p. 83-85 (1980).
29. I. B. Soliternova and N. G. Nikulitcheva. Lipoprotein lipase and
    hepatic triglycerin lipase in rabbit and rat plasma after
    heparin administration. Vopr. med. khimii, v. 28, N.I, p.
    87-92 (1982).
30. R. I. Levy and B. M. Rifkind. The structure, function and meta-
    bolism of high density lipoproteins: a status report.
    Circulation, v. 62, (suppl. 4), p. 4-8 (1980).
31. Y. Yoshida, K. FisheroDzoga and R. W. Wissler. Effects of
    normolipidemic HDL on proliferation of monkey aortic smooth
    muscle cells induced by hyperlipemic LDL. Circulation,
    Abstract, No. 383 (1977).
32. M. Tammi, T. Rönnemaa, T. Vihersaari, A. Lehtonen and J. Viikari.
    High density lipoproteinemia due to vigorous physical work
    inhibits the incorporation of [^{3}H] thymidine and the synthesis
    of glycosaminoglycans by human aortic smooth muscle cells in
    culture. Atherosclerosis, v. 32, p. 23-32 (1979).
33. M. Bihari-Varga. Influence of serum high density popoproteins
    on the low density lipoprotein-aortic glycosamino-glycan
    interactions. Artery, v. 4, p. 504-511 (1978).
34. A. Nordoy, B. Svensson, D. Wiebe and J. C. Hoak. Lipoproteins
    and the inhibitory effect of human endothelial cells on plate-
    let function. Circ. Res., v. 43, p. 527-534 (1978).
35. L. G. Halloran, C. C. Schwartz, Z. R. Vlahcevic, R. M. Hisman
    and L. Swell. Evidence for high density lipoprotein-free
    cholesterol as the primary precursor for bile acid synthesis
    in man. Surgery, v. 84, p. 1-7 (1978).

REGULATION OF PLASMA HIGH DENSITY LIPOPROTEIN CONCENTRATION BY LIPOPROTEIN LIPASE AND HEPATIC ENDOTHELIAL LIPASE

Esko A. Nikkilä

Third Department of Medicine
University of Helsinki
Helsinki 29, Finland

A number of epidemiologic and angiographic studies have established that the risk of developing ischemic heart disease (IHD) and the extent of coronary atherosclerosis bear a direct relationship to plasma LDL cholesterol concentration but are inversely correlated to HDL cholesterol.[1,2] The latter association seems to be mostly mediated by the HDL_2 subfraction.[3] The question on the possible additional role of elevated plasma triglyceride and VLDL levels in increasing the risk of IHD has remained controversial.[4] Many authors agree that hypertriglyceridemia is common among patients with IHD and also predicts the risk of developing new IHD[5,6] but multivariate analyses considering also plasma HDL have consistently eliminated triglycerides as an independent risk factor.[4] In other words, elevated VLDL indicates an increased risk of IHD only because of its close inverse association with HDL. Thus, high VLDL is not atherogenic if not accompanied by low HDL. It is also evident that the significance of HDL as a protective factor of IHD increases with increasing LDL cholesterol concentration. Accordingly, among populations with low LDL levels (usually due to diet) a simultaneous low HDL cholesterol is not atherogenic.

Many of the factors which are known to be positively or negatively associated with IHD are also related to plasma HDL cholesterol and influence it in such direction that HDL can be thought to be the biochemical link between the primary risk factor and the IHD. To mention a few examples, it is well documented that alcohol, estrogenic hormones and endurance exercise all increase the plasma HDL and decrease the risk of developing IHD whereas smoking, overweight, low physical activity and progestin-containing oral contraceptive pills tend to decrease HDL and increase the incidence of IHD.

The mechanism(s) by which the HDL or HDL_2 (or even a subfraction of the latter particle) inhibits the accumulation of lipids into arterial intima is not completely understood. Of plasma lipoproteins only HDL can promote efflux of cholesterol from cultured cells in vitro[7] and it is currently believed that the "reverse transport" of cholesterol from extrahepatic tissues to liver is the function of HDL which best accounts for its antiatherogenic effect.

Irrespective of the underlying mechanism the strong evidence relating low HDL cholesterol to atherosclerotic heart disease has raised major clinical interest for factors regulating plasma HDL (HDL_2) levels and for possibilities to increase low HDL by dietary or pharmacologic measures. It has been established that the metabolism of HDL particles is a complex process involving enzymes, transfer proteins and nonenzymatic exchange reactions most of the events occurring in circulating blood. This paper will review only the role of two endothelial lipolytic enzymes in the regulation of HDL levels. These are lipoprotein lipase and hepatic lipase (known also as hepatic endothelial lipase to avoid mixing with other lipases of the liver).

LIPOPROTEIN LIPASE AND PLASMA HDL (HDL_2)

Lipoprotein lipase (LPL) is a lipolytic enzyme bound to endothelial surface of capillaries in extrahepatic tissues, mainly adipose tissue, skeletal muscle and myocardium. It is released by heparin and can be assayed in postheparin plasma or in heparin eluates of tissues in vitro. The enzyme hydrolyzes triglycerides in chylomicrons and VLDL. During the course of this hydrolysis the surface phospholipids, cholesterol and apoproteins of these lipoproteins become fused with HDL increasing the total HDL mass and causing a shift from HDL_3 to less dense HDL_2 particles.[2] The rate of both hydrolysis of triglyceride-rich particles and of the formation of HDL or HDL_2 is dependent on the activity of LPL which enzyme thus is in key position in the metabolism of all these lipoproteins. In the presence of LPL deficiency (genetic or experimentally induced by specific antiserum) chylomicron and VLDL concentrations are much elevated while HDL is reduced to very low level and increases upon reactivation of LPL.[9] In normal human subjects the concentrations of total HDL cholesterol and of HDL_2 cholesterol and phospholipid are positively correlated with LPL activity measured either from tissue eluates or from postheparin plasma.[10,11] In contrast, no such relationship can be found between HDL_3 cholesterol and the LPL activity.[11] The metabolic linkage between VLDL and HDL at the LPL reaction explains well the known inverse correlation between the plasma concentrations of these two lipoproteins.

Many of the known influences on HDL cholesterol levels by physiological variables, pharmacologic agents or disease states can

be accounted for by corresponding changes in LPL activity. A number
of these factors are listed in Table 1.

Following the puberty women have higher levels of HDL than males
at all ages. The sex difference is present only in the HDL_2 subfraction. Women have also higher LPL activity than men in adipose
tissue and in postheparin plasma but not in skeletal muscle.[10]
Aerobic type exercise training increases both LPL activity of tissues
and plasma HDL[12,13] whereas anaerobic training does not influence
either LPL or HDL.[12] During immobilization both HDL_2 and HDL_3 are
decreased[14] and it is possible that lack of physical activity is a
major underlying cause of the low HDL levels reported in patients
with ischemic cerebral disease or claudication and other conditions
which restrict mobility. It is possible that also the IHD patients
of prevalence studies have shown reduced HDL levels because of poor
physical activity.

The low HDL cholesterol associated with obesity is hardly explained by a decreased LPL activity or low removal of VLDL. Even
though the LPL activity in adipose tissue of obese subjects is at
low side the total body LPL activity is normal or even increased.
The production rate of VLDL triglycerides is increased in obesity
but the turnover of non-triglyceride components of VLDL may be normal
or low thus leading to reduced transfer of material from VLDL to
HDL. For a similar reason the production of HDL through the lipolytic
pathway may be diminished during low fat – high carbohydrate diet
when little chylomicrons are being synthesized and therefore the
HDL level falls.

HEPATIC ENDOTHELIAL LIPASE AND PLASMA HDL (HDL_2)

Hepatic lipase (HL) is a phospholipase located at the endothelial
cells surrounding the liver sinusoids. It is probably bound to the
luminal surface in a similar fashion as the LPL since it is also
released by heparin and can be determined in postheparin plasma.
This enzyme was formerly thought to be active in the hepatic uptake
of chylomicron remnants but more recent findings of several laboratories have favored the view that the physiological function of HL
is hydrolysis and uptake of HDL_2. The evidence is based on following data. The HDL and HDL_2 cholesterol and phospholipid concentrations of experimental animals are increased after blocking the
HL activity in vivo by a specific antiserum.[15,16] Purified HL hydro-
lyses HDL_2 phospholipids in vitro at a much higher rate than phospholipids of other lipoproteins.[17] In normal human subjects an inverse correlation can be demonstrated between the HDL_2 and the
postheparin plasma HL activity.[18]

Some of the variations of HDL and HDL_2 cannot be related to
changes of LPL but seem to be associated with alterations of HL
activity. These are listed in Table 2.

E. A. NIKKILA

Table 1. Factors and conditions modulating plasma HDL or selectively HDL$_2$ levels presumably by changing lipoprotein lipase activity

Variable	Lipoprotein Lipase	HDL or HDL$_2$
Sex: Female/Male	High/Low	High/Low
Endurance training	Increase	Increase
Immobilization	Decrease?	Decrease
Regular use of alcohol	Increase	Increase
Caloric restriction	Decrease	Decrease
Clofibrate	Increase	Increase
Nicotinic acid	Increase	Increase
Probucol	Decrease	Decrease
Interferon	Decrease	Decrease
Insulin deficiency (diabetes)	Low	Low
Insulin resistance (diabetes, obesity)	Normal or low	Low
Insulin treated diabetes	Normal or high	Normal or high
LPL deficiency or apo C-II deficiency	Very low	Very low
Type 4 or 5 hypertriglyceridemia	Normal or low	Low
Uremia	Low	Low
Septic conditions, exdotoxins	Low	Low

The HL is evidently regulated by sex steroids. Women have significantly lower HL activity than men which difference may contribute to the higher HDL levels observed in women. Upon administration of estrogens the HL activity falls and the HDL is increased. Progestins with androgenic activity have an opposite effect increasing HL and decreasing the HDL and HDL$_2$ levels while medroxyprogesterone acetate which is weakly androgenic does not significantly influence HL activity and causes also little change in HDL concentration.[19] An anabolic steroid oxandrolone is a powerful inducer of HL[20] and its administration is followed by decrease of HDL.[21]

THE IMPORTANCE OF THE LPL AND HL IN TRANSPORT FUNCTION OF HDL

In spite of some similarities between LPL and HL the two enzymes appear to be regulated independently and to function separately without any mutual feedback system. In such situation where two enzymes responsible for production and removal of one metabolite vary independently, it may be difficult to demonstrate correlations between the concentration of the metabolite and the activity of either enzyme. This can be done either by selecting subjects who have almost similar activity of one of the enzymes but show a wide range of variation in the other. It can be shown that the correlation coefficient between HDL and LPL in different cohorts increases with decreasing variability of HL activity. For example, in obese subjects who show a very wide range of HL activities there is no significant correlation between LPL activity and HDL level whereas in hypothyroid patients who have a consistently low HL activity the correlation between LPL activity and HDL cholesterol concentration is of the order of + 0.85. Analogously, comparing individuals at similar LPL activity level a rather close correlation between the HDL$_2$ concentration and HL activity can be revealed.

It is important to realize that HDL and HDL$_2$ levels are determined by several factors other than the activity of the two enzymes. However, both LPL and HL appear to be important for the cholesterol transport function of HDL and for development of atherosclerosis. We have previously formulated a hypothesis on HDL cycle.[22] This concept involves, (1) secretion of new HDL particle by the liver, and rearrangement in circulation to HDL$_3$, (2) addition of phospholipid, protein and cholesterol to this (HDL$_3$) as products of breakdown of triglyceride-rich lipoproteins by LPL, (3) uptake of cholesterol from peripheral cells by the phospholipid-enriched HDL$_2$ (not excluding a similar function for HDL$_3$) and, ultimately, (4) degradation and uptake of HDL$_2$ by HL in the liver with possible (not established) re-entry of HDL particle (HDL$_3$?) into circulation and excretion of cholesterol into bile.

It seems that a high activity of LPL is advantageous in leading to accelerated production and increased concentration of HDL and

Table 2. Factors causing reciprocal changes in plasma
HDL or HDL_2 and hepatic lipase activity

Variable	Hepatic lipase	HDL or HDL_2
Sex: Female/Male	Low/High	High/Low
Exercise	Decrease	Increase
Obesity	High	Low
Estrogenic hormones	Decrease	Increase
Progestational hormones	Increase	Decrease
Anabolic steroids	Increase	Decrease
Androgens	Increase?	Decrease

HDL_2 but it is more difficult to conclude whether a high HL is also
antiatherogenic by increasing the hepatic uptake of HDL_2 cholesterol
but by simultaneously leading to decrease of HDL concentration. It
remains for future studies to explore whether there are two separate
entities of hypo-HDL-emia, one caused by low production rate and
another by a rapid removal of HDL, and whether these have different
impact on atherosclerosis.

Acknowledgements

The work presented in this paper has been supported by grants
from Finnish State Medical Research Council, Sigrid Juselius
Foundation and Yrjö Jansson Foundation, Helsinki, Finland.

REFERENCES

1. G. J. Miller, The epidemiology of plasma lipoproteins and
atherosclerotic disease, in: "Lipoproteins, Atherosclerosis
and Coronary Heart Disease," N. E. Miller and B. Lewis, eds.,
Elsevier/North Holland, Biomedical Press (1981).
2. N. E. Miller, Coronary atherosclerosis and plasma lipoproteins:
Epidemiology and pathophysiology considerations, J.Cardiovasc.
Pharmacol. 4:suppl.2:190 (1982).
3. N. E. Miller, F. Hammet, S. Rao, H. van Zeller, J. Coltart, and
B. Lewis, Relation of angiographically defined coronary
artery disease to plasma lipoprotein subfractions and
apolipoproteins, Br.Med.J. 282:1741 (1981).
4. K. Lippel, H. Tyroler, H. Eder, A. Gotto Jr., and G. Vahouny,
Relationship of hypertriglyceridemia to atherosclerosis,
Arteriosclerosis 1:406 (1981).
5. L. A. Carlson, L. E. Böttiger, and P. -E. Åhfeldt, Risk factors
for myocardial infarction in the Stockholm Prospective Study,
Acta Med.Scand. 206:351 (1979).

6. R. Pelkonen, E. A. Nikkilä, S. Koskinen, K. Penttinen, and S. Sarna, Association of serum lipids and obesity with cardio-vascular mortality, Br.Med.J. 2:1185 (1977).

7. C. J. Fielding and P. E. Fielding, Evidence for a lipoprotein carrier in human plasma catalyzing sterol efflux from cult-ured fibroblasts, and its relationship to lecithin : chol-esterol acyltransferase activity, Proc. Natl.Acad.Sci.USA 78:3911 (1981).

8. J. R. Patsch, A. M. Gotto Jr., T. Olivecrona, and S. Eisenberg, Formation of high density lipoprotein-like particles during lipolysis of very low density lipoproteins in vitro, Proc. Natl.Acad.Sci.USA 75:4519 (1978).

9. N. E. Miller, S. N. Rao, P. Alaupovic, N. Noble, L. Slack, J. Brunzell, and B. Lewis, Familial apolipoprotein C II deficiency: Plasma lipoproteins and apolipoproteins in heterozygous and homozygous subjects and the effects of plasma infusion, Eur.J.Clin.Invest. 11:69 (1981).

10. E. A. Nikkilä, M. -R. Taskinen, and M. Kekki, Relation of plasma high-density lipoprotein cholesterol to lipoprotein lipase activity in adipose tissue and skeletal muscle of man, Atherosclerosis 29:497 (1978).

11. M. -R. Taskinen and E. A. Nikkilä, High density lipoprotein subfractions in relation to lipoprotein lipase activity of tissues in man - evidence for reciprocal regulation of HDL_2 and HDL_3 levels by lipoprotein lipase, Clin.Chim.Acta 112: 325 (1981).

12. E. A. Nikkilä, M. -R. Taskinen, S. Rehunen, and M. Härkönen, Lipoprotein lipase activity in adipose tissue and skeletal muscle of runners: Relation to serum lipoproteins, Metabolism 27:1661 (1978).

13. P. D. Wood and W. L. Haskell, The effect of exercise on plasma high density lipoproteins, Lipids 14:417 (1979).

14. E. A. Nikkilä, T. Kuusi, and P. Myllynen, High density lipo-protein and apolipoprotein A-I during physical inactivity: Demonstration of low levels in patients with spine fracture, Atherosclerosis 37:457 (1980).

15. T. Kuusi, P. K. J. Kinnunen, and E. A. Nikkilä, Hepatic endo-thelial lipase antiserum influences rat plasma low and high density lipoproteins in vivo, FEBS Lett. 104:384 (1979).

16. A. van Tol, T. van Gent, and H. Jansen, Degradation of high density lipoprotein by heparin-releasable liver lipase, Biochem.Biophys.Res.Commun. 94:101 (1980).

17. K. Shirai, R. L. Barnhart, and R. L. Jackson, Hydrolysis of human plasma high density $lipoprotein_2$-phospholipids and triglycerides by hepatic lipase, Biochem.Biophys.Res.Commun. 100:591 (1981).

18. T. Kuusi, P. Saarinen, and E. A. Nikkilä, Evidence for the role of hepatic endothelial lipase in the metabolism of plasma high density $lipoprotein_2$ in man, Atherosclerosis 36:589 (1980).

19. M. J. Tikkanen, E. A. Nikkilä, T. Kuusi, and S. Sipinen,
     Different effects of two progestins on plasma high density
     lipoprotein (HDL$_2$) and postheparin plasma hepatic lipase
     activity, Atherosclerosis 40:365 (1981).
20. C. Ehnholm, J. K. Huttunen, P. K. Kinnunen, T. A. Miettinen,
     and E. A. Nikkilä, Effect of oxandrolone treatment on the
     activity of lipoprotein lipase, hepatic lipase and phos-
     pholipase A$_1$ of postheparin human plasma, N.Engl.J.Med.
     292:1314 (1975).
21. T. Tamai, T. Nakai, S. Yamada, T. Kobayashi, T. Hayashi, Y.
     Kutsumi, and R. Takeda, Effects of oxandrolone on plasma
     lipoproteins in patients with type IIa, IIb and IV hyper-
     lipoproteinemia: Occurrence of hypo-high density lipo-
     proteinemia, Artery 5:125 (1979).
22. E. A. Nikkilä, T. Kuusi, and M. -R. Taskinen, Role of lipo-
     protein lipase and hepatic endothelial lipase in the metab-
     olism of high density lipoproteins: A novel concept on
     cholesterol transport in HDL cycle, in: "Metabolic Risk
     Factor in Ischemic Cardiovascular Disease," L. A. Carlson,
     and B. Pernow, eds., Raven Press, New York (1982).

PECULIARITIES OF COMPOSITION AND PROPERTIES OF HIGH-DENSITY LIPOPROTEINS IN PATIENTS WITH CORONARY ATHEROSCLEROSIS

E. Gerasimova, Kh. Kurdanov, L. Matveyeca,
N. Perova and E. Ruuge

Cardiology Research Centre
Academy of Medical Sciences
Moscow, USSR

Epidemiological studies in various countries of the world have shown that lowering of HDL Ch level is a risk factor for coronary heart disease.[1,2,3,4] It has been found that the incubation of HDL with a smooth muscle cell culture results in the decrease of Ch level in the latter, while HDL Ch level increases.

At present an opinion has formed that antiatherogenic HDL properties are linked to the ability of these blood plasma proteins to remove Ch excess from membranes, including the membranes of smooth muscle and endothelial cells.[4,5] This unique property of high density lipoproteins is due to at least two characteristics of their composition.[6,7]

Firstly, HDL contain much more protein and phospholipids than other lipoproteins;

Secondly, apo-A-I apoprotein accounts for 70% of the protein while in other lipoproteins only traces of it can be found.

About 70% of all HDL phospholipids at normal HDL Ch are made up by lecithin and 12% - by sphingomyelin.

In model systems lecithin liposomes effectively bind cholesterol; that is also characteristic of apo-A-I, and the degree of binding increases if lecithin is added.[8]

It was also demonstrated that spirality of A-I apoprotein increases from 55 to 69%[9] if it is reconstructed with lecithin.

The results of these model experiments made it possible to assume that organization of HDL particles and performance of their antiatherogenic functions may also depend on phospholipid composition, amount of apo-A-I, and interaction of apo-A-I and phospholipids in the surface monolayer of the particles.

However, to perform continuously their cholesterol acceptor functions HDL need free Ch esterification. Free Ch comes to the surface monolayer from the membranes of smooth muscle and endothelial cells as well as from VLDL in the course of their catabolism in blood plasma. During esterification fatty acid is transferred only from lecithin to cholesterol by lecithin-cholesterolacyltransferase (LCAT).[10] The enzyme is activated by apo-A-I.

HDL consist of two main subclasses - HDL_2 and HDL_3. During the incubation of HDL_3 with lecithin and/or apo-A-I free Ch is esterified and particles of HDL_2 density are formed.[11]

It has been shown in a number of studies including our own that a reduction of HDL Ch in the blood plasma of patients with coronary heart disease is usually due to the decrease of HDL_2 Ch.[12,13] That is especially important since Ch esters contained by HDL_2 are transported into the liver for subsequent excretion from the organism. Though, molecular mechanisms responsible for the reduction of HDL antiatherogenic properties remained unclear.

Thus, we were interested whether in HDL_2 and/or HDL_3 of CDH patients with low HDL Ch there are:

1) any peculiarities is phospholipid composition

2) differences in apo-A-I amount;

3) changes in physico-chemical parameters and, specifically, in the surface monolayer fluidity of the particles, and whether

4) activity of LCAT-reaction, which transforms free Ch into esters and facilitates the transformation of HDL_3 into the particles of HDL_2 density, is changed in the plasma.

Finally, in connection with the data on the interplay between the platelet Ch content and their ability to aggregate, we tried to find out whether:

5) aggregational characteristics of platelets change after the incubation with HDL.

To clarify these questions all the patients observed (n=60) were divided into two groups: with normal and low HDL Ch. In both groups total plasma Ch and TG levels were within the limits of normal values. Reduction of HDL Ch was accompanied by the statistically significant increase of plasma TG, though their level remained within normal values.

In each of these groups we determined the amount of main phospholipids (lecithin and sphingomyelin), apo-A-I content in HDL_2 and HDL_3, and the activity of LCAT-reaction according to Stokke and Norum.

In patients with coronary atherosclerosis as compared with the control a decrease of HDL Ch was accompanied by the reduction of lecithin percentage, lecithin/sphingomyelin ratio, and the increase of sphingomyelin percentage in HDL_2. The same changes were registered in HDL_3 but they were less pronounced; lecithin/sphingomyelin ratio was significantly decreased only at low HDL Ch.

Then we selected the groups of patients with a strongly marked TG level increase (IV type of hyperlipoproteinemia-HLP) as well as patients with an increase of total plasma Ch only, i.e. with HLP of IIA type.

At low HDL Ch and HLP of IIA type small differences in HDL_3 and HDL_2 phospholipid composition were detected as compared with the control. Considerable changes were registered in the properties of main phospholipids of patients both with low HDL Ch and IV type HLP and those with the normal lipid plasma level: decreased lecithin %, increased sphingomyelin % and decreased lecithin/sphingomyelin ratio in HDL_2 and HDL_3. Since in type IV HLP lipoprotein lipolysis is considerably lower than in IIA type, one can assume that changes in the composition of the particles are not due to the association of secondary remnants formed in the course of lipoprotein lypolysis.

Comparison of the discovered differences in phospholipid composition with apo-A-I level shows that at low HDL Ch in HDL_2 and HDL_3 the decrease of lecithin/sphingomyelin ratio in subjects both with normal plasma Ch and TG levels, and with type IV HLP is accompanied by the decrease of apo-A-I, which is contained both by HDL_2 and HDL_3. Along with these changes, we found a decrease in the amount of free Ch, esterified Ch, and LCAT-reaction activity in the blood plasma of patients with low HDL Ch.

Thus, in CHD patients with low HDL Ch we have found the changes in phospholipid composition and apo-A-I amount, i.e. the parameters which determine molecular organization of HDL_2 and HDL_3 surface monolayer.

Next part of this study was aimed at investigation of HDL_2 and HDL_3 physico-chemical parameters in CHD patients with low HDL Ch. The parameters which reflect physico-chemical characteristics, specifically, HDL surface monolayer fluidity, were measured using ESR-spectroscopy of spin labels.

The paper gives the parameters of spin-mobility of hydrophobic spin labels incorporated into HDL_2 and HDL_3. The values of these parameters for HDL_2 and HDL_3, isolated from the blood plasma of CHD patients with low HDL Ch, reflect the decrease in spin-label surroundings in both particles as compared with the control. These differences are more pronounced in HDL_2 and HDL_3. The alterations were also found in the values of critical temperatures, which characterize phase transitions or phase separations of the label lipid surroundings in HDL_2 and HDL_3 surface monolayer. The alterations indicate the decrease of fluidity of HDL_2 and HDL_3 surface monolayer in CHD patients with low HDL Ch.

The differences in spectral parameters of spin-labels registered in HDL of patients with low HDL Ch are likely linked to the changes in lipid and protein content of HDL_2 and HDL_3, which were given in the first part of the paper. Evidently, they are accounted for by the alterations in the character of protein-lipid interactions in the surface monolayer of these particles.

ESR-spectroscopy analysis of HDL (isolated from the plasma of healthy subjects with normal HDL Ch) after incubation with spin-labeled Ch showed that there were two components in ESR-spectrum of HDL_2 and HDL_3, which indicates the incorporation of spin-labeled Ch into two loci of these particles with different organization of microsurroundings.

At low HDL Ch one component was missing in ESR-spectrum of HDL_2, which indicates a decrease of its cholesterol-acceptor functions, while HDL_3 completely failed to incorporate spin-labeled Ch.

Comparison of the results obtained by chemical methods with ESR-spectroscopy data made it possible to assume that changes in HDL_2 and HDL_3 composition and characteristics likely result in the decrease of cholesterol-acceptor properties of these particles. That is manifested by the lowering of HDL Ch in blood plasma of most IHD patients.

Subsequently, we made a simple test which allows to detect alterations in HDL cholesterol-acceptor characteristics. HDL_2 and HDL_3 were incubated with platelets whereupon aggregational ability of the latter was measured. The in vitro experiments (14), which showed that the accumulation of Ch in platelet membranes is accompanied by the alteration in adenilatcyclase activity and ATP-induced aggregation, were a prerequisite for this part of our study. HDL were isolated both from the plasma of control group subjects and IHD patients.

Necessary amounts of lipoproteins (LP) were added to the suspension of washed platelets from the plasma of normal subjects to obtain the final concentration similar to a normal LP concentration in blood plasma. After 10, 20, 30 and 60 min of incubation at 37° platelets were precipitated by centrifugation and resuspended in autologous plasma. In the obtained suspension ATP-induced platelet aggregation was measured.

HDL_2 and HDL_3 of patients with coronary atherosclerosis in concentrations similar to those of the HDL subfractions of healthy subjects did not inhibit aggregation.

On the contrary, the incubation of platelets with low and very low density lipoproteins (LDL and VLDL) isolated from plasma of IHD patients enhanced platelet aggregation.

Degree of the discovered effects both for HDL_2/HDL_3, and LDL/VLDL was proportional to the concentration of Ch in these lipoproteins.

A decrease in aggregational ability of platelets following the incubation with HDL of healthy subjects may be linked to their ability to accept Ch from the plasma membrane of platelets.

The absence of any effect of HDL_2 and HDL_3 isolated from blood plasma of IHD patients is of special interest. Likely, that may be accounted for by the decrease in HDL cholesterol-acceptor ability due to an alteration of chemical composition of HDL surface monolayer in IHD patients; lecithin/sphingomyelin is decreased due to reduced lecithin percentage and increased sphingomyelin percentage. The latter makes the structure of HDL surface monolayer more rigid.

Thus we have found that decreased HDL Ch level in blood plasma of patients with coronary atherosclerosis is accompanied by the alteration in a number of parameters of HDL_2 and HDL_3 surface mono-layer molecular organization, namely, in phospholipid composition and amount of apo-A-I. These alterations result in the decrease of HDL antiatherogenic function and manifest themselves in:

1) decreased ability of HDL to accept Ch from the membranes of smooth muscle and endothelial cells, from platelets and VLDL in the course of their metabolism in blood plasma;

2) reduced activity of LCAT-reaction, whereby free Ch is transformed into esters and HDL_3 - into the particles of HDL_2 density, which transport Ch into the liver for excretion from the organism.

REFERENCES

1. B. Lewis, A. Chait, C. M. O. Oakley, J. D. P. Wootton, A. Onitiri, G. Sigurdson and A. February. Serum lipoprotein abnormalities in patients with ischaemic heart disease: comparison with a control population. Brit.Med. J., V.3, p. 489-493. (1974).

2. O. Wiklund, A. Gustafson, and L. Wilhelmsen. Lipoprotein cholesterol in men after myocardial infarction compared with a population sample. Artery v.1, p. 339-405. (1975).

3. P. C. Castelli, J. T. Doyle, T. Gordon, C. G. Hames, M. C. Hjortland, S. B. Hulley, A. Kagan, and W. J. Zukel. HDL and other lipids in coronary heart disease. The cooperative lipoprotein pheno-typing study. Circulation v.55 p. 767-772 (1977).

4. G. J. Miller, N. E. Miller. Plasma high-density lipoproteins, atherosclerosis and coronary heart disease. In:"High-density lipoproteins". Day C.E. (ed), New York and Basel, Marcel Dekker, p. 435-462 (1981).

5. Y. Stein, M. C. Glangeaud, M. Fainara, and O. Stein. The removal of cholesterol from aortic smooth muscle cells in culture and Landschutz ascites cells by fractions of human high-density apolipoprotein. Biochem. Biophys. Acta, v.380, p.106-118 (1975).

6. V. P. Skipski, M. Barclay, R. K. Barclay, V. A. Fetzer, J. J. Good, and F. M. Archibald. Lipid composition of human serum lipoproteins. Biochem. J.,1 v. 104, p. 340-352

7. E. J. Schaefer, S. Eisenberg, R. J. Levy. Lipoprotein apoprotein metabolism. J. Lipid Res., v. 19, p. 667-687 (1978).

8. R. L. Jackson, A. M. Gotto, O. Stein and Y. Stein, A comparative study on the removal of cellular lipids from Landschutz ascites cells by human plasma apolipoproteins. J. Biol. Chem. v. 250, p. 7204-7209, (1975).

9. S. E. Lux, R. Hirz, R. J. Shrager, A. M. Gotto. The influence of lipid on the conformation of human plasma high density apolipoproteins. J. Biol. Chem.,v. 247, p. 2598-2606,(1972).

10. J. A. Glomset, E. T. Janssen, R. Kennedy and J. Dobbins. Role of plasma lecithin: cholesterol acyltransferase in the metabolism of high desntiy lipoproteins. J. Lipid Res., v.7, p. 639-648, (1966).

11. A. R. Tall, Conversion of HDL_3 into HDL_2 - like particle in vitro. Circulation, v.59-60, suppl.11, p.72, abstr. 275 (1979).

12. D. W. Anderson. HDL-cholesterol: the variable components. Lancet v.1, p. 819-820, (1978).

13. N. V. Perova, E. N. Gerasimova, V. A. Polessky, et al. Determination of cholesterol in subfractions of high density lipoproteins. Bulletin of the USSR Cardiology Research Center, USSR AMS, N.2 p. 55-60 (1979).

14. S. J. Shattil, R. A. Cooper, Membrane microviscosity and human platelet function. Biochemistry v. 15, p. 4832-4837, (1976).

BLOOD LIPIDS AND ANTIHYPERTENSIVE DRUGS: THE OSLO STUDY

Paul Leren, Ivar Eide, Olav P. Foss, Anders Helgeland,
I. Hjermann, I. Holme, Sverre E. Kjeldsen, and Per G.
Lund-Larsen

Ullevaal Hospital, Oslo, Norway

Epidemiologic studies have repeatedly shown a positive correlation between blood pressure and both coronary and cerebral
mortality. Moreover, there is also a positive correlation between
serum cholesterol and blood pressure. Nevertheless, randomised,
controlled drug treatment hypertension trials have failed to
achieve a favorable reduction of the incidence of coronary heart
disease (CHD), in contrast to cerebral artery disease which has
been significantly reduced by drug treatment.

The reason for this challenging observation is not known.
There might be many explanations. Recently attention has been
drawn to blood lipids and the effects of antihypertensive drugs
on the metabolism of lipoproteins.

In the Oslo Study we have undertaken some studies of the
effect on blood lipids in drug treatment of hypertension. Most
of these studies are of short duration and involve few patients,
which calls for some caution when drawing conclusions. On the
other hand, the studies were done in homogeneous groups of persons,
all men in a steady metabolic state. All were healthy and at work,
only suffering from mild, symptomfree hypertension. No other
drugs than the test drug were taken - given in a pre-fixed,
unchangeable dose - and a randomized drug approach was used, only
with one exception - the 3-year study in which the test groups
were matched. We have used both cross-over designs and parallel
groups.

In this way we have studied 4 beta-blockers, the alpha-blocker,
prazosin, and a thiazide, separately, and 5 combinations of two
drugs.

Of the beta blockers (Table 1) only pindolol was lipid neutral, probably due to its pronounced intrinsic symptomimetic activity, while propranolol, atenolol and oxprenolol lower HDL cholesterol and increased serum triglycerides. Hydrochlorothiazide (HCTZ) did not influence blood lipids. Prazosin lowered serum LDL + VLDL cholesterol and total triglycerides.

Table 1. Oslo Study. Metabolic effects (%change) of some antihypertensive drugs. Hypertension WHO 1. Men 47-55.

	Praz n=23 8 w	HCTZ n=10 10 w	Pind n=10 10 w	Aten n=9 16 w	Oxpren n=10 16 W	Prop n=23 8 w
Total chol	-8.9***	ns	ns	ns	ns	ns
LDL+VLDL chol	-10.1***	ns	ns	ns	ns	ns
HDL chol	ns	ns	ns	-16.7*	-11.5*	-13.0***
Chol ratio (1)	+7.0*	ns	ns	-19.2**	-13.7*	-15.2***
Total trigl	-16.2***	ns	ns	+17.9^{ns}	+19.4^{ns}	+24.0***
Uric acid	ns	ns	ns	ns	ns	+10.4**

*** $p < 0.001$
** $p < 0.01$
* $p < 0.05$
ns not significant
(1) $\dfrac{\text{HDL chol}}{\text{Total chol} - \text{HDL chol}}$

The combination of pindolol + prazosin lowered LDL + VLDL cholesterol by 12% (Table 2). Propranolol + HCTZ lowered HDL cholesterol and increased triglycerides. Propranolol + prazosin lowered HDL cholesterol. Methyldopa + HCTZ, and HCTZ + amiloride had no effect on blood lipids.

The clinical consequences of these metabolic changes are uncertain. The lipid effect might be of importance in long-term treatment of hypertension, especially for young people.

Table 2. Oslo Study. Metabolic effects (% change) of some anti-
          hypertensive drug combinations. Hypertension WHO 1.
          Men 40-55

	Praz Pind n=10 14 w	Praz Prop n=22 8 w	HCTH Amil n=10 14 w	M.dopa HCTH n=33 3 yrs	Prop HCTH n=33 3 yrs	Untr contr n=33 3 yrs
Total chol	ns	ns	ns	ns	ns	ns
LDL+VLDL chol	-12.0*	ns	ns		**	
HDL chol	ns	-7.5**	ns	ns ⊛	-18.1 ⊛	ns ⊛
Chol ratio	ns	ns	ns			
Total trigl	ns	ns	ns	ns	+44.3**	ns
Uric acid	+7.3*	+13.6**	+13.9*	ns	+21.8*	ns

** p < 0.01
* p < 0.05
ns not significant
⊛ Difference from mean of two treatment and a control group.

ENDOGENOUS REGULATION OF PROSTACYCLIN

SYNTHESIS IN ARTERIAL SMOOTH MUSCLE CELLS

J. Larrue, D. Daret, B. Dorian
J. Henri, and H. Bricaud

U. 8 de recherches de Cardiologie
I.N.S.E.R.M.
Avenue du Haut-Lévêque 33600 Pessac

The physiological and pathological roles of prostacyclin* (PGI_2) and thromboxane A_2 have attracted much attention in atherosclerosis.[1] Many investigations support the hypothesis that the loss of balance between these two prostaglandins is involved in vascular disease.[2] The capacity of the vascular wall to produce PGI_2 was reported originally for the intimal surface,[3] but medial smooth muscle cells also produce significant quantities both in vivo[4,5] and under culture conditions.[6] This capacity seems to be of importance especially after endothelial injury, such a situation probably involved in the atherosclerotic process.[7] Using arterial smooth muscle cells in culture, we have previously demonstrated that, in comparison with healthy cultured cells, cells originating from atherosclerotic aortas have a decreased capacity to produce PGI_2.[8] Such a reduced prostacyclin formation has been reported in aged aortic smooth muscle cells[9] associated with an increased PGE_2 synthesis. Despite this, the regulative mechanisms of PGI_2 generation in arterial cells remains unclear.

In the present report, evidences are presented which indicate that:

1. Several prostaglandins are produced by cultured smooth muscle cells.

---

*Abbreviations used:- PGI_2 : Prostaglandin I_2 (prostacyclin); $PGF_{2\alpha}$, PGE_2 : Prostaglandins $F_{2\alpha}$, E_2; 6 $KPGF_{1\alpha}$: 6-Keto Prostaglandin $F_{1\alpha}$; A.A. : Arachidonic Acid; HETE : Hydroxyeicosatetraenoic acid; TLC : Thin Layer Chromatography; HPLC : High Performance Liquid Chromatography; GC-MS : Gas Chromatography-Mass Spectrometry; SMC : Smooth Muscle Cells.

2. The release of A.A. from phospholipids is not a limiting factor
    for the prostaglandins secretion by smooth muscle cells.
3. Both cycloxygenase and PGI_2 synthetase activities are depressed
    in atherosclerotic cells.
4. Significant amounts of HETEs were formed in arterial smooth
    muscle cells.

On the basis of these findings, it is suggested that endogenous
lipoxygenase activities, either by some competitive mechanism with
cyclooxygenase or, by the way of endogenous hydroperoxydes intermediates, or both, may be implicated in the regulation of the vascular PGI_2 synthesis.

METHODOLOGICAL APPROACH

Rabbits were made atherosclerotic using an alternate, moderately
hypercholesterolemic diet (500 mg cholesterol/day) over a period of
1 year. At the end of the experimental period, the animals had
developed fibrous lipidic plaques.[10] Aortic SMC were obtained from
medial explants of both normal and atherosclerotic animals essentially
as described by Ross[11] and used in subcultures, at confluency, as
previously described.[8] These cells retained a number of metabolic
features concerning growth, collagen synthesis and arachidonic acid
metabolism which were in good agreement with those observed in
vivo.[12,13]

Arachidonic acid conversion was studied either using intact
$1.^{14}C$ A.A. prelabeled SMC or cell homogenates incubated with the
labeled precursor as described.[14] Incubation media were acidified
and extracted with ethyl acetate, then analysed either by TLC for
prostaglandins, or HPCL for lipoxygenase derivatives. In each
case, results were confirmed using GC-MS determination.

PROSTAGLANDIN PRODUCTION BY AORTIC SMOOTH MUSCLE CELLS

Rabbit vascular SMC in subculture synthesized radiolabeled
prostaglandins from both endogenous (Table 1) or exogenous (Table 2)
substrates. PGI_2 (measured as 6 Keto $PGF_{1\alpha}$, its stable degradation
product in vitro) appeared as the main derivative formed. The relative distribution of the 3 metabolites (PGI_2, $PGF_{2\alpha}$, and PGE_2) correlated well with that obtained from freshly isolated aortic tissue
(Table 3), despite the unexpected finding, that, in cell homogenates,
PGE_2 constituted a minor component as compared to intact cells.

INHIBITION OF PROSTAGLANDINS PRODUCTION IN ATHEROSCLEROTIC SMOOTH MUSCLE CELLS

Rings of aortic tissue originated from the media of atherosclerotic rabbits showed a reduce capacity to produce PGI_2 and $PGF_{2\alpha}$ (Table 3), accordingly, estimation of prostaglandin production in subcultures of SMC originated from atherosclerotic media showed that both PGI_2 and primary prostaglandin formations were significantly depressed (Table 4). When compared to healthy cells, the ratios of Prostaglandin formation by intact SMC incubated with labeled A.A. were found to be 0.37, 0.43, 0.54 for 6 Keto $PGF_{1\alpha}$, $PGF_{2\alpha}$ and PGE_2 respectively, in atherosclerotic cells. These results were confirmed in cell homogenates. So, despite an enhanced percentage of primary prostaglandins (50 vs 37%), and a relative increase of PGE_2 concentrations as compared to total prostaglandins formed in normal cells (40 vs 28%), a significantly lower prostaglandin biosynthetic capacity appeared in atherosclerotic smooth

Table 1. Prostaglandin production from endogenous arachidonic acid

	Percent of the Total Radioactivity Released			
	6 K $PGF_{1\alpha}$	$PGF_{2\alpha}$	PGE_2	Free A.A.
Healthy cells	15.3 ± 0.7	2.4 ± 0.5	6.0 ± 2.7	15.1 ± 3.1

1h. prelabeled cell layers were washed then activated by scraping in 5 ml of Tris NaCl buffer pH 7.5. The mixture was centrifuged and supernatant was extracted. Results expressed as percent of total radioactivity recovered for each compound are the mean of three experiments.

Table 2. Exogenous arachidonic acid conversion

Cell Type	Percent Transformation of A.A.*		
	6 K $PGF_{1\alpha}$	$PGF_{2\alpha}$	PGE_2
Intact S.M.C.**	8.87 ± 1.54	1.61 ± 0.56	4.20 ± 1.76
S.M.C. Homogenate***	2.58 ± 0.34	0.80 ± 0.27	0.36 ± 0.05

*   10nM 1.^{14}C A.A.;
**   2 ± 0.2 10^6 cells maintained in the cultured flask;
*** 1 mg protein.
     Results are expressed as mean ± SD from five different experiments.

Table 3. Exogenous arachidonic acid conversion by freshly isolated
          aortic tissue

	Percent Transformation of A.A.*		
	6 Keto PGF$_{1\alpha}$	PGF$_{2\alpha}$	PGE$_2$
Healthy aortic Media**	7.8 ± 1.1	1.03 ± 0.4	0.8 ± 0.3
Atherosclerotic aortic Media***	3.4 ± 1.1	0.4 ± 0.3	0.8 ± 0.5

*   10 nM of 1.^{14}C A.A.;
**   100 mg (w/w);
*** Atherosclerotic area defined by histologic examination after
     incubation.
     Results are expressed as mean ± SD from ten different experiments.

muscle cells, without any compensatory activation of PGE$_2$ formation,
clearly suggesting that PGI$_2$ synthetase and cyclooxygenase activities
were depressed.

These results indicate that, either the rate of formation of
endoperoxydes or the activity of the prostaglandin I$_2$ synthetase or
both are critical steps in atherosclerotic cells. Lipid peroxydes
resulting from the lipid accumulation in atherosclerotic arteries
have been previously shown as specific inhibitors of the prostacyclin
synthetase activity[15] and are candidates to explain the difference
observed. However, under the experimental conditions described,
neither the lipid concentrations in the culture or incubation media
nor the lipid composition of the two types of cells were different.
The previous identification of a lipoxygenase activity in vascular
tissue[16] led us to perform experiments to investigate the possibility
of such an activity in cultured SMC.

LIPOXYGENASE ACTIVITIES IN CULTURED SMOOTH MUSCLE CELLS

Homogenates from cultured SMC were incubated under the presence
of 1.^{14}C A.A. After ethyl acetate extraction, the extracts were
analysed by TLC. A significant lipoxygenase activity was observed.
The rate of formation of monohydroxylated derivatives (HETEs) expressed as percent of the total A.A. conversion raised from 0.8 in
healthy cells to 2.4 in atherosclerotic cells (Table 5). HPLC and
GC-MS determinations indicated that several mono-HETEs derivatives
are formed, namely 15 HETE and 12 HETE. Both of them have been
previously recognized as efficient inhibitors of PGI$_2$ synthesis.[17]

Table 4. Arachidonic acid conversion by cultured smooth muscle
cells originated from atherosclerotic aortas

Type of Experiment	Percent Transformation of A.A.		
	6 Keto $PGF_{1\alpha}$	$PGF_{2\alpha}$	PGE_2
Prelabeled cells	7.0 ± 1.0	3.5 ± 2.0	3.2 ± 3.3
Intact cells	3.31 ± 0.94	0.70 ± 0.35	2.70 ± 0.52
Cells homogenates	0.94 ± 0.21	0.47 ± 0.08	0.39 ± 0.07

Experimental conditions are identical as described in Table 1 and 2.
Results are expressed as mean ± SD from 3 (prelabeled cells) or 5
different experiments.

Table 5. Lipoxygenase activity in cultured arterial
smooth muscle cells

	Lipoxygenase	HETEs
	Activity*	6 K $PGF_{1\alpha}$
Healthy cells	0.85 ± 0.42	0.22 ± 0.03
Atherosclerotic cells	2.42 ± 0.61	1.20 ± 0.24

Homogenates of cultured smooth muscle cells (1 mg Protein)
were incubated with 10 nM 1.^{14}C A.A. as described.
* Lipoxygenase activity is expressed as percent A.A.
transformation.
Results are expressed as mean ± SD from three different
experiments using the same cellular types.

CONCLUDING REMARKS

The capacity of the vascular wall to produce prostacyclin seems
to be of importance as a protective mechanism against atherosclerosis.
The decreased generation of PGI_2 by arterial SMC may be significantly
involved in the progression of the atherosclerotic process. However,
the regulative mechanisms of PGI_2 production in arterial cells remains unclear as yet. Since the participation of extracellular
hydroperoxydes (HPETE) to the inhibition of the vascular PGI_2 formation appears unlikely,[18] an enhanced lipoxygenase activity in SMC
leading namely to the formation of monohydroxy derivatives (15 and
12 HETE) may contribute either by some competitive mechanism with
cyclooxygenase or by the way of endogenous hydroperoxy intermediates
(HPETE) or both, to the progression of the atherosclerotic process.

REFERENCES

1. R. J. Gryglewski, A. Dembinska-Kièc, A. Zmuda and T. Gryglewska, Prostacyclin and thromboxane A_2 biosynthesis capacities of heart arteries and platelets at various stages of experimental atherosclerosis in rabbits, Atherosclerosis 31:385 (1978).

2. S. Moncada, R. J. Gryglewski, S. Bunting, and R. J. Vane, An enzyme isolated from arteries transforms prostaglandin endoperoxydes to an unstable substance that inhibits platelet aggregation, Nature 263:663 (1976).

3. A. G. Herman, S. Moncada, and R. J. Vane, Formation of prostacyclin (PGI$_2$) by different layers of the arterial wall, Arch.Int.Pharmacodyn. 227:162 (1977).

4. S. Moncada, A.G. Herman, E. A. Higgs, and R. J. Vane, Differential formation of prostacyclin by layers of the arterial wall. An explanation for the anti thrombotic properties of vascular endothelium, Thromb.Res. 11:323 (1977).

5. G. Hornstra, E. Haddeman, and J. A. Don, Some investigations on the role of prostacyclin in thromboregulation, Thromb.Res. 12:367 (1978).

6. N. L. Baenziger, M. J. Dillender, and P. W. Majerus, Culture human skin fibroblasts and arterial cells produce a labile platelet inhibitory prostaglandin, Biochem.Biophys.Res.Comm. 78:294 (1977).

7. R. Ross and J. A. Glomset, The pathogenesis of atherosclerosis, N.Engl.J.Med. 295:369 (1976).

8. J. Larrue, M. Rigaud, D. Daret, J. Demond, J. Durand, and H. Bricaud, Prostacyclin production by cultured smooth muscle cells from atherosclerotic rabbit aorta, Nature 285:480 (1980).

9. W. C. Chang, S. I. Murota, J. Nakao, and H. Orimo, Age-related decrease in prostacyclin biosynthetic activity in rat aortic smooth muscle cells, Biochim.Biophys.Acta 620:159 (1980).

10. J. Larrue, G. Razaka, D. Daret, J. Demond, and H. Bricaud, Biosynthèse de la matrice extracellulaire dans les aires athéroscléreuses d'aortes de lapins in vitro, Arterial Wall 6:85 (1980).

11. R. Ross, The smooth muscle cell. II. Growth of smooth muscle in culture and the formation of elastic fibers, J.Cell Biol. 50:172 (1971).

12. M. Aumailley, T. Krieg, J. Larrue, and H. Bricaud, Synthesis of collagen in atherosclerosis. Studies in organ and cell culture, Arterial Wall 4:289 (1978).

13. J. Larrue, B. Dorian, J. Demond-Henri, and H. Bricaud, Endogenous arachidonic acid metabolism by cultured arterial smooth muscle cells, Biochem.Biophys.Res.Comm. 1011:861 (1981).

14. J. Larrue, C. Leroux, D. Daret, and H. Bricaud, Decreased prostaglandin production in cultured smooth muscle cells from atherosclerotic rabbit aorta, Biochim.Biophys.Acta 710:257 (1982).

15. S. Moncada, R. J. Gryglewski, S. Bunting, and R. J. Vane, A lipid peroxyde inhibits the enzyme in blood vessels microsomes that generates from prostaglandin endoperoxydes the substance which prevents platelet aggregation, Prostaglandins 12:715 (1976).
16. J. E. Greenwald, J. R. Bianchine, and L. K. Wong, The production of the arachidonate metabolite HETE in vascular tissue, Nature 281:588 (1979).
17. E. A. Ham, R. W. Egan, D. D. Soderman, P. H. Gale, and F. A. Kuchl Jr., Peroxidase-dependant deactivation of prostacyclin synthetase, J.Biol.Chem. 254:2191 (1979).
18. J. Turck, A. Wyche, and P. Needleman, Inactivation of vascular prostacyclin synthetase by platelet lipoxygenase products, Biochem.Biophys.Res.Comm. 95:1628 (1980).

PLATELETS, MEGAKARYOCYTES AND VASCULAR DISEASE

John F. Martin

University of Sheffield, Department of Medicine
Royal Hallamshire Hospital
Sheffield S 10 2JF
United Kingdom

There is now much evidence from man and animals that platelets
play an essential role in the production of atheroma. Pigs suffering
from von Willebrand's disease have a defect in platelet function. In
normal pigs atheromatous plaques can be produced in arteries by high
cholesterol diet, but if the same diet is fed to pigs with von
Willebrand's disease no atheroma is produced. Platelet dysfunction
protects the pigs against atheroma[1]. Likewise atheroma may be produced
in rabbits by high cholesterol diet but they may be protected against
it by thrombocytopenia produced in them by injection of antiplatelet
antibodies[2]. If baboons are injected intravenously with homocistine
they suffer endothelial damage firstly and later atheromatous lesions
in arteries. If the baboons are pre-treated with dipyridam, which
reduces platelet reactivity, then the baboons still suffer endothelial
damage from homocistine but atheromatous plaques do not develop.[3]
Although Eskimos are heavy smokers they have a very low incidence of
myocardial infarction and atheroma. They also have a long bleeding
time and decreased platelet aggregation. The explanation for this
probably lies in the large amount of eicosapentaenoic acid in their
diet[4]. There is therefore evidence from both animal experiments
and the Eskimo that platelets are necessary for the production of the
atheromatous lesion no matter what other conditions may also be
necessary.

Despite its importance, much concerning the physical nature of
the platelet is still under dispute. One view holds that the platelet
is produced from the bone marrow as a dense cell which becomes lighter
as it circulates[5]. Another that platelets are produced in a variety
of densities and volumes from the bone marrow and circulate without
undergoing significant change in normal function[6]. Clearly resolution

of this problem is important since if the differences between platelets in volume, density and reactivity are a consequence not of
ageing but of production then there is the possibility that if different types of platelets can be produced from the bone marrow then
disease states may be related to alterations in platelet production.
To observe changes in platelet density and volume platelets must
be separated by using density gradients for the former, or counter-
current centrifugation or cell sorting for the latter. Workers
holding different views about the relationship between platelet
density and ageing have all used density gradient centrifugation as
evidence for their conclusions. Table 1 shows that a variety of
different conditions have been used by various workers yet it has
recently been demonstrated that for a particular type of gradient only
one set of conditions can give actual separation by density[15]. It
is therefore possible that different conclusions about platelet
density in the literature may arise from methodological problems.

Table 1[*]

Author		Date	Medium	[+]D/C	g	t(mn)	gxt
Booyse	(7)	1968	Sucrose	D	14,650	45	1,600,000
					35,200	150	2,200,000
Karpatkin	(8)	1969	Oil	D	5,900	4	23,600
Minter	(9)	1971	Silicone	D	9,500	2	19,000
Ginsberg	(10)	1972	Oil	–	micro-haematocrit centrifuge	10	–
Bonneu	(11)	1973	Sucrose	D	55,000	60	3,300,000
Busch	(12)	1973	Ludox PVP	C	800	60	4,800
Charmatz	(13)	1974	Albumin	D	7,000	20	140,000
Penington	(6)	1976	Ludox PVP	C	10,180	5	50,900
Corash	(5)	1977	Stractan	D	52,951	30	1,600,000
Cieslar	(14)	1979	Stractan	D	2,000	45	90,000

[*] Conditions used by authors to separate platelets by density
[+] D = continuous gradient
   C = discontinuous
gxt = measure of the force used in the separation procedure

PLATELET DENSITY

If density is measured by continuous gradients of low viscosity
media under conditions of isopicnic centrifugation then a bell-shaped
distribution is observed that approaches the normal distribution
(Figure 1). The mean density is approximately 1.062 gml^{-1}. The
range of density is very small indicating that platelet density may
not be an important physiological variable. The shape of the curve
is argument that platelets are produced in all densities from megakaryocytes. If they were produced only as light cells that became
dense or dense cells that became light then they would have to alter
their rate of change of density in one direction and then the other
along lines demanded by the normal distribution. It is more reasonable
to assume that the shape of the curve is produced by random distribution of granules and mitochondria that are known to be denser than
the rest of the platelet constituents[16].

[75]SE Selenomethionine is an isotope-labelled aminoacid which
is rapidly cleared from the blood, does not label circulating
platelets and is taken up by megakaryocytes and incorporated into
cytoplasmic protein. Platelets released into the circulation thereafter are labelled with selenomethionine. This tool could therefore
be used to investigate whether platelets are produced from megakaryocytes in all densities. Figure 2 illustrates that if platelets
are produced in all densities from megakaryocytes then radioactive
platelets will be found in all densities as soon as radioactive
platelets are produced from the megakaryocytes; but if only light
cells or dense cells are produced then radioactivity will only
be found in the appropriate area of the gradient. When such an
experiment was carried out using rats, radioactive platelets were
indeed found among all densities from one to five days after selenomethionine was injected intravenously.

In a second experiment a representative platelet population was
taken from adolescent male monkeys and labelled with chromium
([51]CR) and then re-injected. The following day blood was taken from
the animals, fractionated into density subpopulations and radioactivity
and number measured. It was observed that the [51]CR labelled platelets
were distributed throughout all density subpopulations. Platelet
life span in the monkey is similar to that of man (8 days) and when
blood was again taken on the 5th day after labelling it was seen that
the [51]CR labelled platelets were again distributed throughout all
density subpopulations but there had been a significant yet small
increase in platelet density among the [51]CR labelled platelets.
The increase is approximately 5%, (Figure 3). The reason for this
increase is not clear but it may be that platelets take up a heavy
constituent as they circulate. These two experiments add evidence to
the argument that platelets are produced from the megakaryocyte in all
densities and circulate with only very slight increase in density as
they do so.

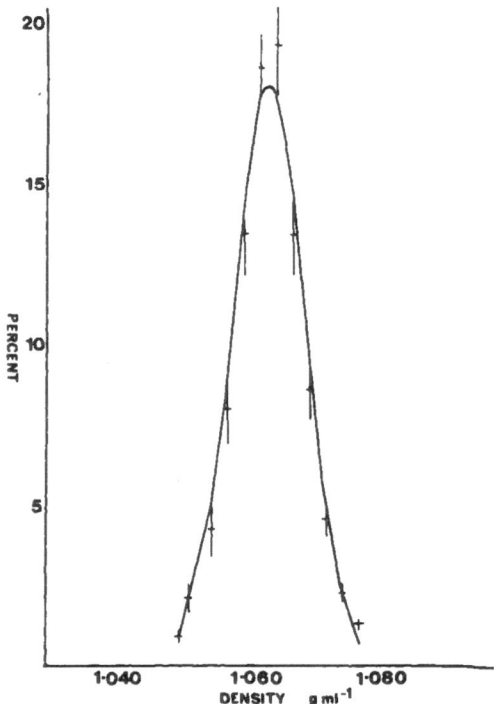

Fig. 1.   A single platelet volume distribution from a normal
          male. The crosses indicate the position of the curve
          had it been normal (or Gaussian). The approximation
          is very close. A single curve is shown as the mean of
          many curves would tend towards the normal as predicted
          by the central limit theorem.

PLATELET VOLUME

        Platelet volume distribution is unique among cellular volume
distributions in that it is log normal (Figure 4). The platelet
is unique in that it is not produced by mitosis. The two phenomena
are linked in the physical fragmentation theory of platelet production[18,17]. Unlike platelet density, platelet volume is a variable
of wide range and therefore may have physiological significance.
The origin of changes in the volume distribution is found in the
volume distribution of megakaryocyte cytoplasm[18]. If density
determined subfractions of platelets have their volume distribution
measured then it is seen that platelets of all volumes are found
within each density subpopulation. Applying this knowledge to the
experiments above it can be deduced that platelets of all volumes
are produced at thrombopoesis and that they do not substantially
change their volumes as they circulate under normal conditions.

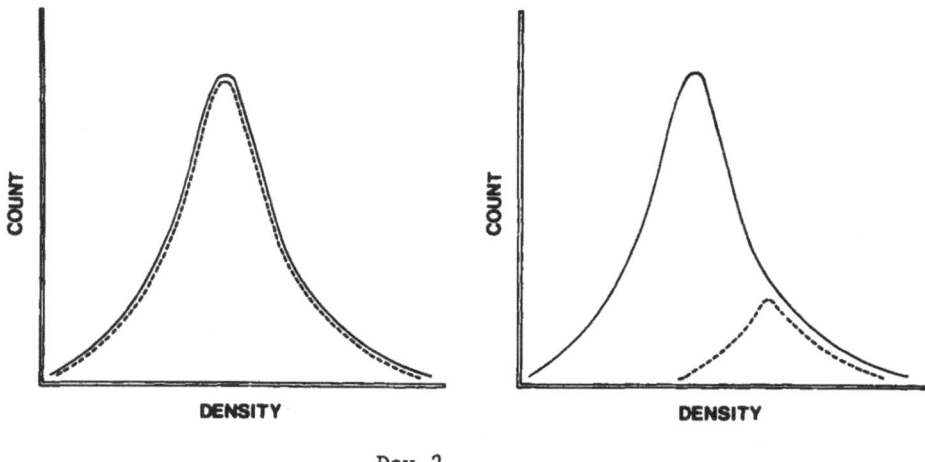

Day 2

Fig. 2. A sketch plan of possible results on the second day following the injection of [75]SE selenomethionine as described in the text. If platelets are produced from megakaryocytes only as dense cells, then radioactivity would only be found in the dense part of the platelet density distribution curve (on the right). If platelets are produced in all densities then, on day 2, radioactivity would be found in platelets of all densities (as on the left). If the radioactivity curve and the platelet number curve fit exactly then their index of concordance is 1. The actual indices of concordance for days 1-5 of the experiment were 0.992, 0.998, 0.995, 0.995 and 0.993.

If thrombocytopenia is induced very large platelets are produced immediately afterwards[18]. Large platelets are more reactive than small[19], and it could be that the major response to thrombocytopenia is the production of large platelets and secondarily of production of an increased number of platelets.

MEGAKARYOCYTE POLYPLOIDY

Apart from the normal ploidy number of a 2N complement of chromosomes megakaryocytes exhibit polyploidy: they can increase their nuclear DNA concentration up to 128N. This phenomena, rare in mammalian biology, allows rapid increase in cell size without the need to undergo mitosis which is time and energy consuming. Larger megakaryocyte cytoplasm then gives larger platelets[18]. The steady state mean ploidy number in the mammal is 16N; after thrombocytopenia this can increase to a mean of 32N with the appearance of ploidy numbers not usually seen. This mechanism is probably under hormonal control[20].

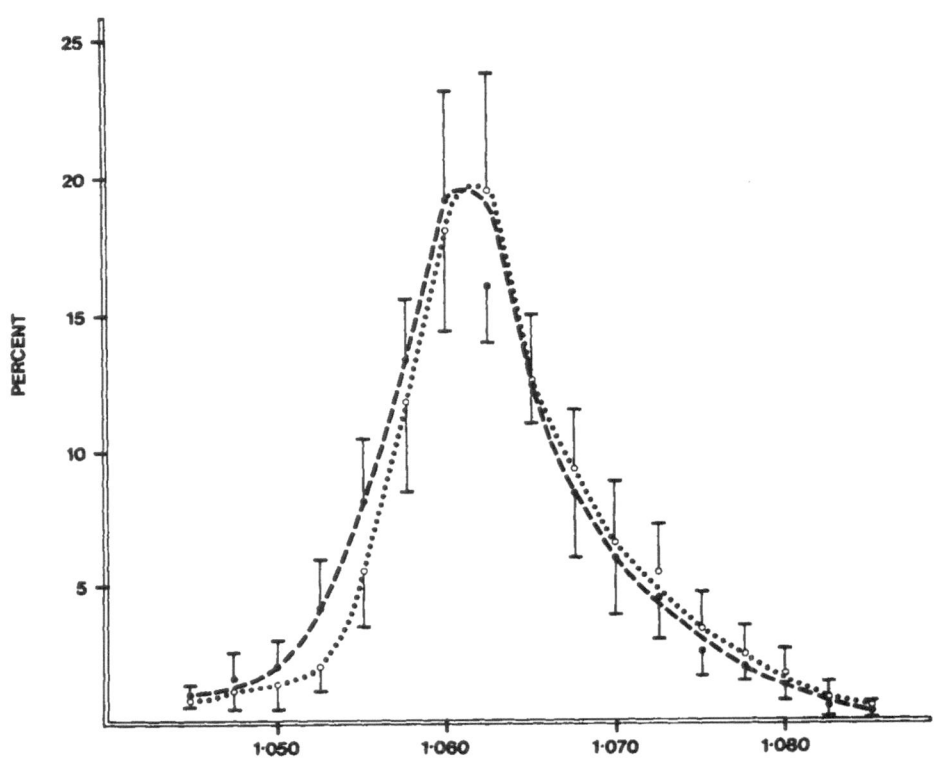

Fig. 3.   Platelet number (---) and ^{51}CR radioactivity (●●●) (mean
          ± SEM, n = 12) against platelet density in blood taken from
          monkeys 5 days after the injection of an autologous repre-
          sentative population of ^{51}CR labelled platelets. There
          has been a very small, yet significant, increase in plate-
          let density since the radioisotope labelled platelets were
          re-injected. (p<0.001 X^2 test).

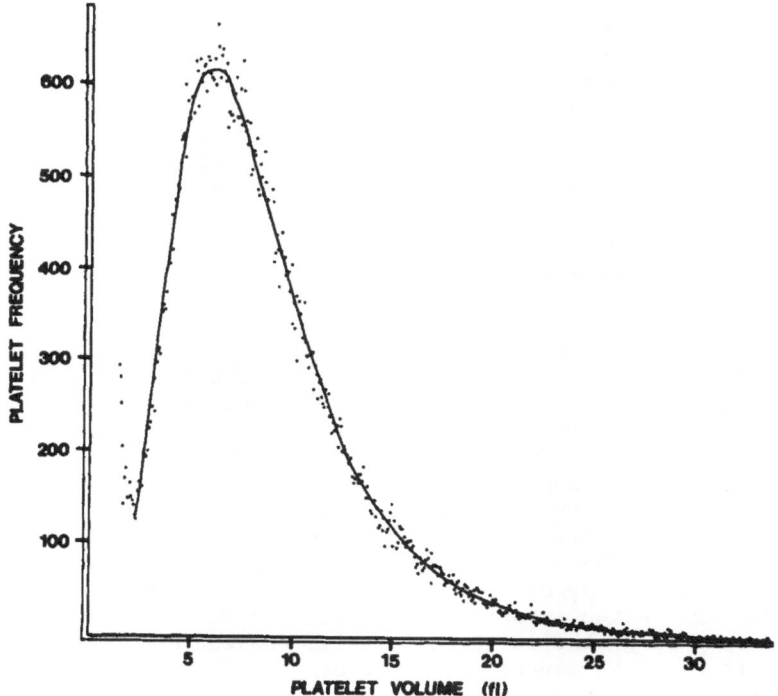

Fig. 4. The platelet volume distribution from a representative
         platelet population from a normal male. The curve is
         log normal i.e. when the log of platelet volume is plotted
         the curve becomes normal (Gaussian). Cells produced by
         mitosis have a normal volume distribution. The log normal
         platelet volume distribution is unique and reflects the
         platelet's unique mode of production.

MYOCARDIAL INFARCTION

A malfunction of the physiological system described here may
be involved in disease, either as cause or effect. Platelet volume
and density were therefore measured in men suffering myocardial
infarction. If platelets are heterogeneous cells then any study
must isolate a truly representative population. Since platelets
are separated from whole blood by physical means, their particular
biophysical variables may be preselected by the separation method.
In this study >93% of the platelet population in whole blood was
isolated by use of self generated sigmoidally shaped gradients of
polyvinyl pyrrolidone-coated silica (Percol) onto which whole blood
was layered and then subjected to velocity centrifugation. If the
rate of recovery of platelets from whole blood was any less than
90% then the volume differences reported below were not seen, as
the large platelets were lost in the velocity separation procedure.
Mean platelet volume and density in 15 men with evidence of myocardial
infarction from history (of less than 12 hours duration) and classical
electrocardiographic and cardiac enzyme changes were compared to
an age matched control group admitted to the same coronary care unit
with chest pain but without evidence of myocardial infarction.
Mean platelet volume was increased in the myocardial infarct group
($p < 0.0005$ Mann & Whitney u test) Figure 5. Platelet density was
slightly increased ($p < 0.005$), probably as a consequence of the increase in platelet volume Figure 6. Eleven of the test group and
22 of the control group were again tested 6 weeks later. The myocardial infarction group still had a significant increase in mean
platelet volume compared to controls (Figure 7). It may be argued
that mean platelet volume is increased in men with myocardial
infarction before the infarct occurs because, 1) since the platelet
survival in man is approximately 8 days most of the platelets circulating 12 hours after infarct would have been produced before the
infarct occurred 2) the increase is still present at 6 weeks when
the infarct might be expected to have healed, 3) because the log
normality of the platelet volume distribution was maintained in
the test group (Figure 8).

CONCLUSIONS

Platelet volume (and density) are determined at the time of
platelet production. There is evidence that platelets are involved
in atherogenesis and arterial thrombosis. Platelets are larger than
normal in myocardial infarction and this change may have a causal
role in the vascular pathology. Men suffering myocardial infarction
may have altered megakaryocytes that determine changes in their
circulating platelets.

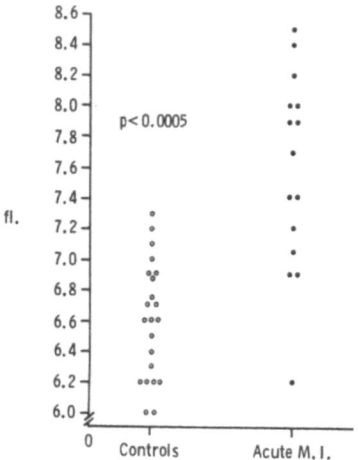

Fig. 5. Mean platelet volume in men suffering acute myocardial
infarction (MI) and in controls. Blood was taken within
12 hours of onset of symptoms.

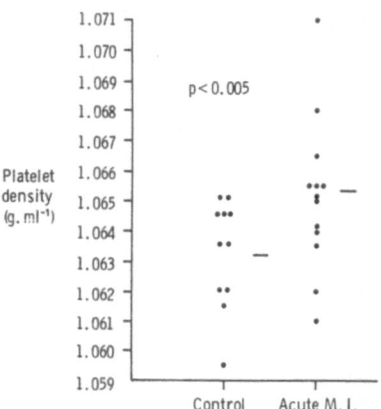

Fig. 6. Mean platelet density in the acute MI and control group.

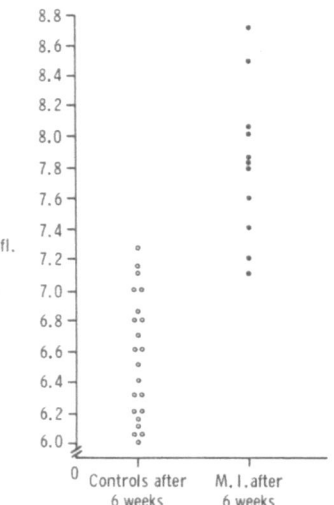

Fig. 7. Mean platelet volume in men 6 weeks following MI (●) and
         controls (○). Platelets are larger in MI group (p<0.001,
         Mann & Whitney u test).

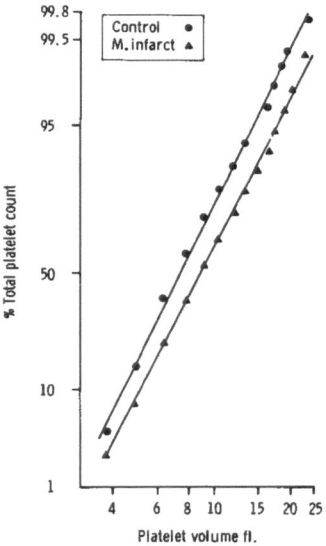

Fig. 8. Log probability plot of mean platelet volume in men suffering
         myocardial infarction (▲) and in the control group (●). The
         log normality of the platelet volume distribution is main-
         tained after myocardial infarction.

ACKNOWLEDGEMENTS

    Experimental work referred to here was done both with Professor
D. G. Penington and his colleagues, in the University of Melbourne
Department of Medicine, St. Vincent's Hospital, Fitzroy, Australia
and with my colleagues in the University of Sheffield Department
of Medicine.

REFERENCES

1. F. Foster, E. J. W. Bowie, J. C. Lewis, D. N. Fass, C. A. Owen
    and A. L. Brown, Resistance to arteriosclerosis in pigs
    with von Willebrand's disease. J. Clin. Invest.61:722 (1978).
2. R. J. Friedman, M. B. Stemerman, B. Wenz, S. Moore, J. Gauldie,
    M. Gent, M. L. Tiell and T. H. Spaet, The effect of thrombo-
    cytopenia on experimental arteriosclerosis lesion formation
    in rabbits. J. Clin. Invest.60:1191 (1977.
3. L. A. Harker, R. Ross, S. J. Slichter and C. R. Scott, Homo-
    cistine-induced arteriosclerosis. The role of endothelial
    cell injury and platelet response in its genesis. J. Clin.
    Invest. 58:731 (1976).
4. J. Dyerberg, H. O. Bang, E. Stoffersen, S. Monada and J. R. Vane,
    Eicospaentaenoic acid and prevention of thrombosis and athero-
    sclerosis. The Lancet. 11:117 (1978).
5. L. Corash, B. Shafter and M. Perlow, Heterogeneity of human whole
    blood platelet subpopulations. II. Use of a subhuman primate
    model to analyze the relationship between density and platelet
    age. Blood 52:726 (1978).
6. D. G. Penington, N. L. Y. Lee, A. E. Roxburgh and J. R. McGready,
    Platelet density and size: The interpretation of hetero-
    geneity. Br. J. Haematol. 34:365 (1976).
7. F. M. Booyse, D. Zschocke, T. P. Hoveke and M. E. Rafelson Jr.,
    Studies on human platelets. IV. Protein synthesis in maturing
    human platelets. Thromb. Diath. Haemorrh. 26:167 (1971).
8. S. Karpatkin, Heterogeneity of human platelets. I. Metabolic
    and kinetic evidence suggestive of young and old platelets.
    J. Clin. Invest. 48:1073 (1969).
9. F. Minter and M. Ingram, Platelet volume: density relationships
    in normal and acutely bled dogs. Br. J. Haematol. 20:55 (1971).
10. A. D. Ginsberg and R. H. Aster, Changes associated with platelet
    ageing. Thromb. Diath. Haemorrh. 27:407 (1972).
11. B. Boneu, A. Boneu, C. I. Raisson, R. Guiraud and R. Bierme,
    Kinetics of platelet "populations" in the stationary state.
    Thromb. Res. 3:605 (1973).
12. C. Bush and P. S. Olson, Density distribution of ^{51}Cr-labelled
    platelets within the circulating dog platelet population.
    Thromb. Res. 3:1 (1973).

13. A. Charmatz and S. Karpatkin, Heterogeneity of rabbit platelets.
     I. Employment of an albumin density gradient for separation
     of a young platelet population, identified with Se^{75}-seleno-
     methionine. Thromb. Diath. Haemorrh. 31:485 (1974).

14. P. Ceislar, J. P. Greenberg, M. L. Raud, M. A. Packham, R. L.
     Kinbough-Rathbone and J. F. Mustard, Separation of thrombin
     treated platelets from normal platelets by density-gradient
     centrifugation. Blood 53 :867 (1979).

15. J. F. Martin and E. A. Trowbridge, Theoretical requirements for
     the density separation of platelets, with comparison of
     continuous and discontinuous gradients. Thromb. Res. in press
     (1982).

16. A. J. Marcus, D. Zucker-Franklin, L. B. Safier and H. L. Ullman,
     Studies on human platelet granules and membranes. J. Clin.
     Invest. 45:14 (1966).

17. E. A. Trowbridge, J. F. Martin and D. N. Slater, Evidence for
     a theory of physical fragmentation of megakaryocytes,
     implying that all platelets are produced in the pulmonary
     circulation. Thromb. Res. in press (1982).

18. J. F. Martin, E. A. Trowbridge, G. L. Salmon and D. N. Slater,
     The relationship between platelet and megakaryocyte volumes.
     Thromb. Res. in press (1982).

19. C. B. Thompson, K. A. Eaton, S. M. Princiotta, C. A. Rushin and
     C. R. Valeri, Size dependent platelet subpopulations:
     relationship of platelet volume to ultrastructure, enzymatic
     activity and function. Brit. J. Haematol. 50:509 (1982).

20. W. Nagl, "Endopolyploidy and polyteny in differentiation and
     evolution" North Holland Publishing Co., Amsterdam (1978).

EFFECTS OF BETA RECEPTOR BLOCKING DRUGS ON PROSTACYCLIN (PGI$_2$) AND THROMBOXANE A$_2$ (TXA$_2$) BIOSYNTHESIS AS A NEW ASPECT OF THEIR MODE OF ACTION

W. Förster

Department of Pharmacology and Toxicology
Martin Luther University
4020 Halle/S, GDR

The discovery of TXA$_2$ and PGI$_2$ with their antagonistic actions on vessel wall and platelets were unquestionably milestones that fundamentally altered the prevailing ideas on pathophysiology and therapy of cardiovascular diseases.

In animals with acute coronary ligation and in patients with ischemic heart disease and angina pectoris the ratio PGI$_2$/TXA$_2$ is altered in favor of TXA$_2$.[1,2] If disorders in this ratio are considered as a general pathogenetic mechanism the clinically used antianginal drugs should normalize this disturbed ratio.

In earlier investigations[3,4] could be shown that some clinically used antianginal drugs increase the PGI$_2$ biosynthesis, thus restoring the normal PGI$_2$/TXA$_2$ ratio. A second possibility is the selective inhibition of the TXA$_2$ synthesis with a concomitant promotion of the PGI$_2$ synthesis. These effects show some other antianginal drugs.[5,6] Open was the question whether beta receptor blocking drugs act only as adrenolytic substances or influence also the synthesis of eicosanoids.[7]

In 1981 we[5] reported on an inhibition of the malondialdehyde generation by pindolol whereas this effect could not be evoked by propranolol even in a dose one power of ten higher. In a comparative study with propranolol and pindolol both substances enhanced the PGI$_2$ release from guinea pig Langendorff hearts when applied in concentrations evoking a negative inotropic effect (Figure 1).

Considering the arachidonic acid (AA)-induced aggregation in rabbit PRP 0.1 - 1.0 mmol/l propranolol diminished the aggregation in a dose dependent manner (Figure 2) whereas the biosynthesis

385

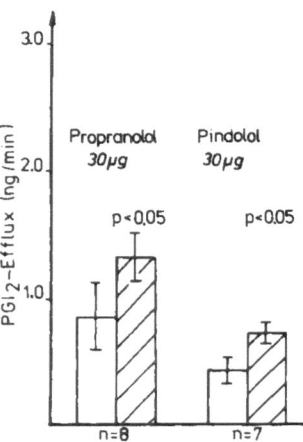

Fig. 1.   Influence of Propranolol and Pindolol on the PGI_2-Efflux
          from Langendorff Hearts of Guinea Pigs.

of TXA_2 was not influenced. Higher concentrations up to 5 mmol/l -
not shown in the figure - inhibited also the TXA_2 formation. Experiments with human PRP revealed a complete inhibition of the AA-induced
aggregation already with about 0.6 mmol/l. The lowest TXA_2 inhibiting
concentration was 1 mmol/l. Both experiments show that an inhibition
of the TXA_2 biosynthesis could be proved only with concentrations
distinctly higher than those which completely inhibited the AA-induced aggregation. Contrary to propranolol, pindolol inhibited the
AA-induced aggregation as well as the TXA_2 synthesis in a dose dependent manner (Figure 3). Effective concentrations were 0.1 mmol/l
or more. Both isomers of pindolol had approximately the same antiplatelet and TXA_2 synthesis inhibiting effects although in all concentrations used the (-) isomer was somewhat more effective than the
(+) isomer. There were no distinct differences between both isomers
of propranolol, too.

     The cause of the inhibition of TXA_2 by pindolol may be found in
its relatively potent inhibition of the cyclooxygenase: 10 uM inhibited it by about 60% and 200 uM by 76-83%. By comparison,
indomethacin was about one power of ten more potent. In contrast
to pindolol, propranolol even in the concentration of 200 uM did
not significantly inhibit the cyclooxygenase and showed with 1 mM
only a slight inhibition.

     Other differences of pindolol and propranolol were seen in
different incluences on platelet aggregation induced with the PG
endoperoxide analogue U-46619. Propranolol exerted an inhibition
one power of ten more potent than pindolol (Figure 4).

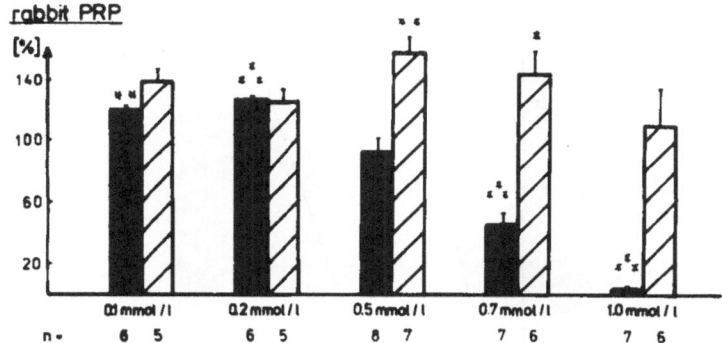

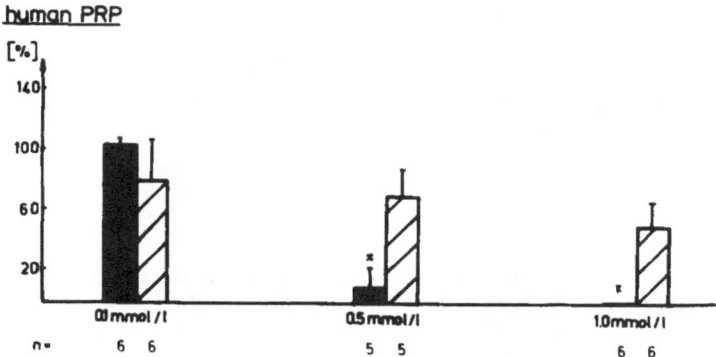

Fig. 2.   Effect of Propranolol on Arachidonic Acid-induced
         Aggregation and TXA_2 Formation (Rabbit and Human PRP,
         TXA_2-Bioassay) Aggregation ■ TXA_2 □.

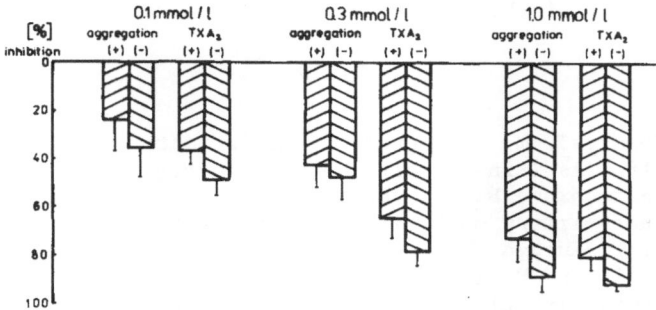

Fig. 3.   Effect of Pindolol-Isomers on Aggregation and TXA_2
         Formation (Rabbit-PRP, AA-induced Aggregation, TXA_2
         Bioassay).

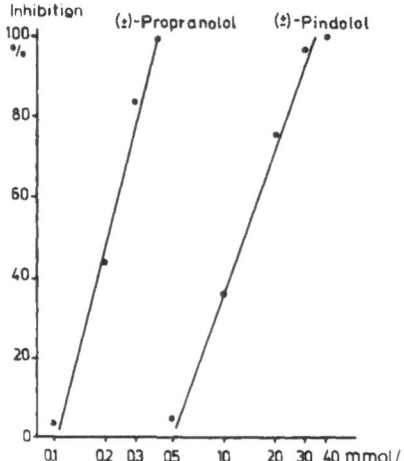

Fig. 4.   Effect of (±)-Propranolol and (±)-Pindolol on U-46619-
          induced Aggregation (Human-PRP).

SUMMARY

     Only one part of the mechanism of action of beta receptor
blocking drugs can be explained via their β-adrenolytic effect. The
antihypertensive and antiplatelet action is induced by influences
on the formation of eicosanoids. Pindolol seems to be a prototype
with a potent TXA_2 synthesis inhibiting effect probably via a relatively potent cyclooxygenase inhibition. Propranolol has a more
potent antagonistic effect on "TXA_2- receptors" than on TXA_2 synthesis. Both drugs stimulate the PGI_2 synthesis in coronary walls.
In this combination of the adrenolytic effect with the antiplatelet
and anti-TXA_2 actions we might have found the clue for the potent
clinical efficacy of the beta adrenergic blocking drugs.

REFERENCES

    1.   S. J. Coker, J. M. Ledingham, J. R. Parratt, and I. J.
         Zeitlin, Aspirin inhibits both the early myocardial release
         of thromboxane B_2 and ventricular ectopic activity following
         coronary artery occlusion in dogs, Scot.Med.J. 26:169 (1981).
    2.   M. Tada, T. Kuzuya, M. Inoue, K. Kodama, M. Mishima, M. Yamada,
         M. Inui, and H. Abe, Elevation of thromboxane B_2 levels in
         patients with classic and variant angina pectoris,
         Circulation 64:1107 (1981).
    3.   W. Förster, Effect of various agents on prostaglandin bio-
         synthesis and the antiaggregatory effect, Acta Med.Scand.
         (Suppl.)642:35 (1980).

4. P. Mentz, K. Pönicke, H. U. Block, Ch. Gießler, K. -E. Blass, B. -L. Bayer, and W. Förster, Stimulierung der prostazyklin-biosynthese als möglicher wirkungsmechanismus van dipyridamol, Arzneim.-Forsch. 31:2075 (1981).

5. W. Förster, Influence of cardiovascular drugs on platelet aggregation, Adv.in Myocardiol. (in press).

6. H. -U. Block, W. Förster, and I. Heinroth, SIN-1, the main metabolite of molsidomine inhibits prostaglandin endoperoxide analogue - and arachidonic acid-induced platelet aggregation as well as platelet thromboxane A_2 formation, Arzneim.-Forsch. 32:189 (1982).

7. W. Sziegoleit, J. Rausch, M. György, E. Dekov, and M. Békés, Influence of acetylsalicylic acid on acute circulatory effects of pindolol in hypertensive patients, in: "Prosta-glandins and Thromboxanes," W. Förster, ed., Pergamon Press, (1981).

PLATELET SPREADING AND THROMBI-FORMATION IN VITRO

V. Leytin, S. Domogatsky, V. Koteliansky, A. Mazurov
F. Misselwitz, O. Merzlikina, E. Podrez
K. Taube* and W. Forster*

USSR Cardiology Research Center, Academy of Medical
Sciences, Moscow, USSR
*Institute of Pharmacology and Toxicology of Martin
Luther University, Halle-Wittenberg, Halle, GDR

INTRODUCTION

The present paper deals with three main problems. In the first
section we consider platelet interaction with surfaces coated with
genetically distinct types of human collagen, which makes a part of
various vessel wall structures. The main stages of platelets-
collagenous substrates interaction are described: a) initial
attachment of platelets to the substrate, b) platelet spreading on
the substrate, and c) formation of thrombi-like aggregates adherent
to the substrate.

In the second section we dwell in more detail on the process of
platelet spreading and a possible role of spread platelets in mural
thrombi formation.

Finally, in the third section we consider: a) the induction of
spreading and adherent thrombi-like aggregates formation on collagen
by arachidonic acid and stable prostaglandin endoperoxides analogues,
and b) the inhibition of the processes by antithromboxane agent
Trapidil and stable prostacyclin analogues.

PLATELET INTERACTION WITH COLLAGEN SUBSTRATES FORMED BY GENETICALLY DISTINCT TYPES OF HUMAN COLLAGEN

Four types of collagen have been found in human and animal
vessels: I, II, IV, and V. These collagens differ in chain compo-

sition, the ability to form fibrils, and localization in the vessel
wall. Many researches have investigated the ability of different
collagen types to induce platelet aggregation in suspension. It was
concluded that the above mentioned types of collagen in fibrillar
form induce platelet aggregation while those in amorphous or
monomeric form are not capable of being aggregation inducers.

Platelet interaction with collagen-coated surfaces differs from
platelet-collagen interaction in suspension by a number of parameters. Thus, we studied how platelets would interact with various
types of human collagen if the collagens are immobilized on the
surface.

Monomeric collagen of different types was isolated from human
placenta and immobilized on the surface in two different ways (Figure
1). Procedure I: collagen was added into the wells of multiwell
tissue culture plates; fibril formation was performed in suspension
at 37°C and neutral pH with subsequent immobilization of fibrils on
well bottoms. Procedure II: collagen in monomeric form was directly
adsorbed on the well bottoms at 4°C. Thus, two types of surfaces
were formed; one coated with fibrillar collagen, another with
monomeric collagen. Human platelets separated from plasma by gel-
filtration were added into thus prepared wells and incubated with
rotation for 40 min. at 37°C. After removing nonadherent platelets
and washing the wells, adhesion was analyzed by scanning electron
microscopy (SEM) (Figure 1).

Figure 2 shows the interaction of platelets with a surface
coated with type III collagen. The coating was produced in two ways:
1) collagen fibrils with an average diameter of 100 nm, which covered
well bottoms by a dense multilayer network, were formed (Figure 2,a);
2) fibrillogenesis was not carried out and well bottoms were covered
with amorphous collagen (Figure 2,b). Though, regardless of absence
or presence of collagen fibrils adherent platelets form on the substrate large multilayer aggregates, which resemble thrombi (Figure
2,a,b).

Platelet interaction with the surface covered with type III
collagen also results in intensive platelet spreading (Figure 3).
Platelets spread on collagen are a highly attractive substrate for
the platelets from suspension; they readily bind to the upper surface
of spread platelets (Figure 3). Sheets of confluent spread platelets
form the basis of thrombi-like structures (Figure 4).

Type I collagen used as a substrate behaves in a similar way.
Both in amorphous and fibrillar form this type of collagen stimulates
thrombi-like aggregate formation and platelet spreading.

Completely different picture of adhesion is observed when type V
collagen is used as a substrate (Figure 5,a). In this case platelet

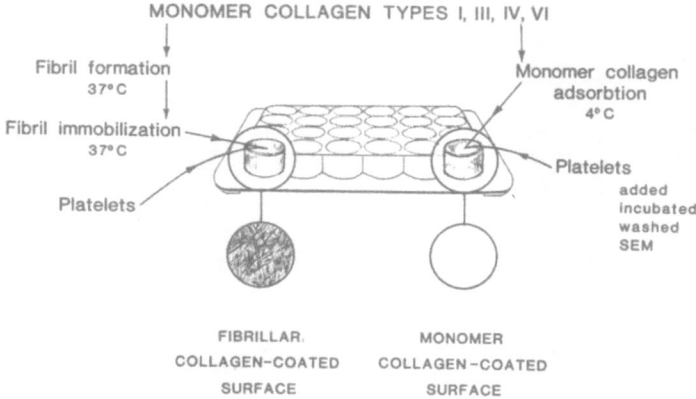

MONOMER COLLAGEN TYPES I, III, IV, VI

Fibril formation
37°C

Monomer collagen
adsorbtion
4°C

Fibril immobilization
37°C

Platelets

Platelets
added
incubated
washed
SEM

FIBRILLAR
COLLAGEN-COATED
SURFACE

MONOMER
COLLAGEN-COATED
SURFACE

Fig. 1.   General scheme of experimental studies of platelet interaction with surfaces covered with genetically distinct
types of human collagen. Well bottoms of Multiwell culture plates were covered with fibrillar or monomeric collagens (0.6 - 0.8 mg per well) of type I, II, IV, and V,
isolated from human placenta. Gel-filtered human platelets were added into the wells (I-I,5 x 10^8/ml, 0.2 ml
per well) and incubated for 40 min. at 37°C with rotation
in a horizontal incubator-shaker at 36 rev./min. Then,
nonadherent platelets were removed, the wells washed, and
the adhesion was studied by scanning electron microscopy
(SEM).

adhesion level is 20-100-fold lower for type I and III collagens.
Adherent platelets are usually at the stage of initial attachment and
have discoid or spheroid shape. There is no platelet spreading and
adherent aggregates formation on this substrate (Figure 5,a). If
type I and type V collagens are mixed in the ratio 4:I the resulting
substrate looks like the one made of pure type I collagen (Figure
5,b), while platelet adhesion is practically the same as that to the
purified type V collagen (Figure 5,b). Likely, type V collagen when
bound to type I collagen blocks its sites responsible for the formation of thrombi-like aggregates and platelet spreading.

While interacting with the surface covered with type IV collagen
in amorphous form, platelets spread (Figure 6,a) and make up small
aggregates, which are localized on the upper surface of spread
platelets (Figure 6,b). Similar picture of adhesion is observed when
type IV collagen is immobilized in fibrillar form.

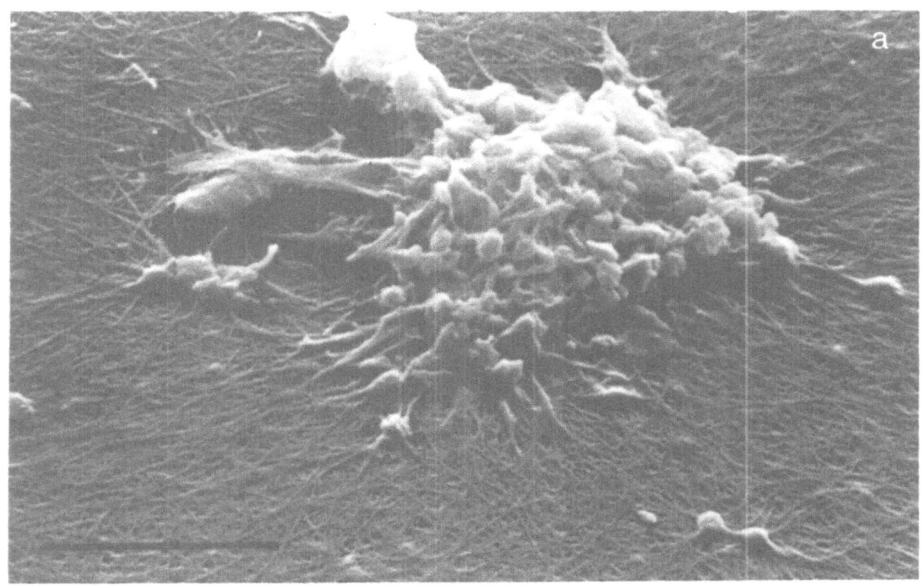

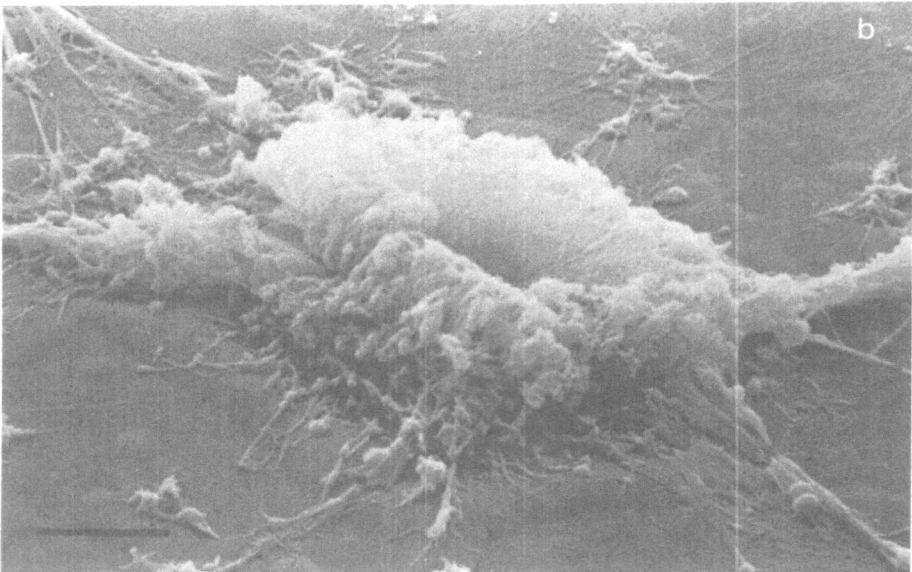

Fig. 2. Formation of thrombi-like aggregates on surfaces covered
with type III human collagen in fibrillar (a) or monomeric form. Irrespective of the presence (a) or absence
(b) of fibrils, large multilayer thrombi-like platelet
aggregates are deposed on the surface. Scale bar - 10μm.

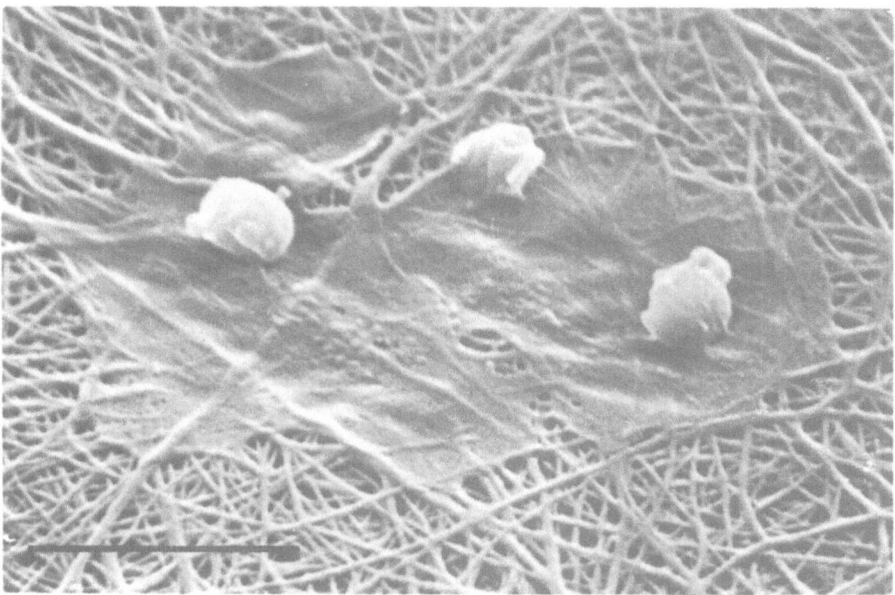

Fig. 3. Platelet spreading on the surface covered with type III
         fibrillar collagen and adhesion of platelets from suspen-
         sion to the upper surface of spread platelets. The
         micrograph shows three completely spread platelets; two
         of them have adherent spheroid platelets from suspension
         on the upper surface. Scale bar - 5 μm.

     Thus, various types of collagen substrates have different
thrombogeneity with respect to platelets (Table 1). Type V collagen
is an athrombogenic substrate characterized by low level of adhesion,
and adherent platelets are nonactivated or low activated. Type IV
collagen is a substrate of moderate adhesiveness; platelets spread on
it and form small aggregates. Type III and I collagens are
thrombogenic substrates whereon all stages of platelet activation,
even thrombi-like structures formation, are observed (Table 1).

     It should be underlined that during the interaction of platelets
with immobilized collagen surface the degree of substrate thrombogeneity is mainly determined by the genetic type of collagen and does
not depend on whether collagen is in fibrillar of amorphous form
(Figure 2,6). On the contrary, it is only fibrillar forms of
collagen that induce platelet aggregation in suspension. The reason
for these differences is likely accounted for by the fact that the
substrate formed both by fibrillar and monomeric collagen offers a

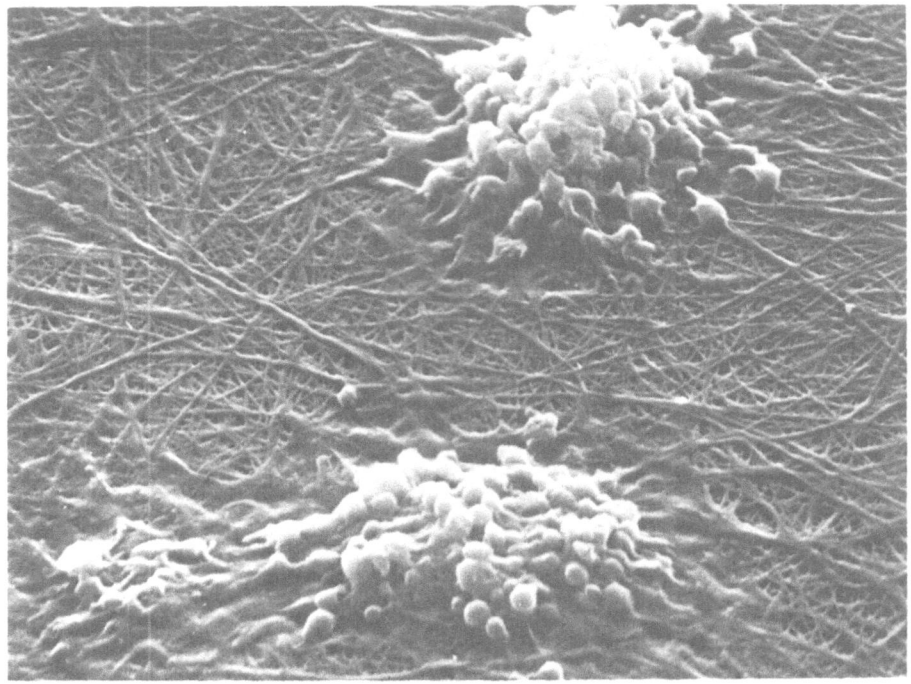

Fig. 4.   Sheets of confluent spread platelets at the basis of
          thrombi-like aggregates adherent to type III fibrillar
          collagen.   Scale bar — 10 μm.

great number of platelet-binding sites concentrated on the surface
available for the simultaneous interaction with platelets.   In suspension a similar "concentration" of platelet-binding sites can be
obtained only if monomeric collagen is organized into fibrils.

    The obtained data elucidate the differences in thrombogenic
characteristics of various anatomic structures of the in vivo vessel
wall.   Taking into account the localization of the above mentioned
collagen types with respect to the luminal surface one can better
understand: athrombogenity of the endothelial lining of undamaged
vessel, moderate thrombogeneity of basal membrane in shallow vessel
wall injuries, and high thrombogeneity of subendothelial intimal
layer, media and adventitia, which are exposed in deep injuries and
frank trauma of the vessel (Table 1).   The interaction of thrombogenic and athrombogenic collagen types may also play an important
role in mural thrombi formation (Figure 5).

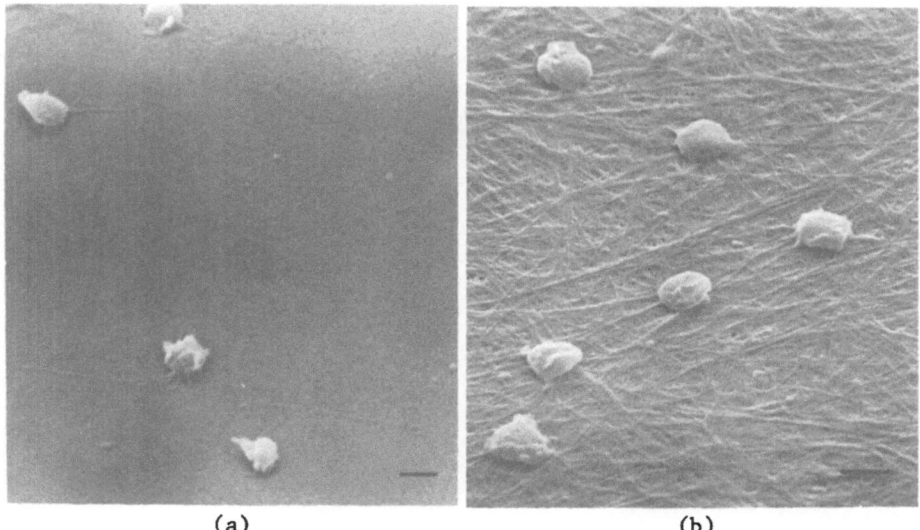

(a)   (b)

Fig. 5. Platelet adhesion to the surfaces covered with type V
         collagen (a), and a mixture of type I and type V col-
         lagens in the ratio 4:1 (b). The first substrate is
         amorphous (a), the latter is fibrillar (b). In both
         cases adherent platelets are at the stage of initial at-
         tachment; there is no spreading and thrombi-like aggre-
         gate formation. Scale bar - 2 µm.

SPREAD PLATELETS AND THEIR POSSIBLE ROLE IN MURAL THROMBI FORMATION

     In the series of experiments described we used commercial acid
soluble calf skin collagen (CSC) to cover the well bottoms of multiwell tissue culture plates (Figure 1). Reactivity of the collagen
with respect to platelets strongly resembles human type IV collagen.
Similar to type IV collagen platelet interaction with the surface
covered with CSC involves three main processes: 1) platelets from
suspension attach to the collagen substrate, 2) then they spread, and
3) platelets from the suspension attach to the upper surface of
spread platelets. That results in the formation of small aggregates
on spread platelets; large multilayer thrombi-like aggregates are not
formed. Thus, calf skin collagen is a fitting substrate to study in
vitro the initial stages of thrombogenesis, i.e. platelet spreading
and attachment of platelets from suspension to the upper surface of
spread platelets.

     Figure 7 shows one of the mechanisms of platelet spreading on
the substrate. It is clearly seen as membranous web spreads between
two pseudopods of a spheroid platelet (Figure 7,a). At later stages

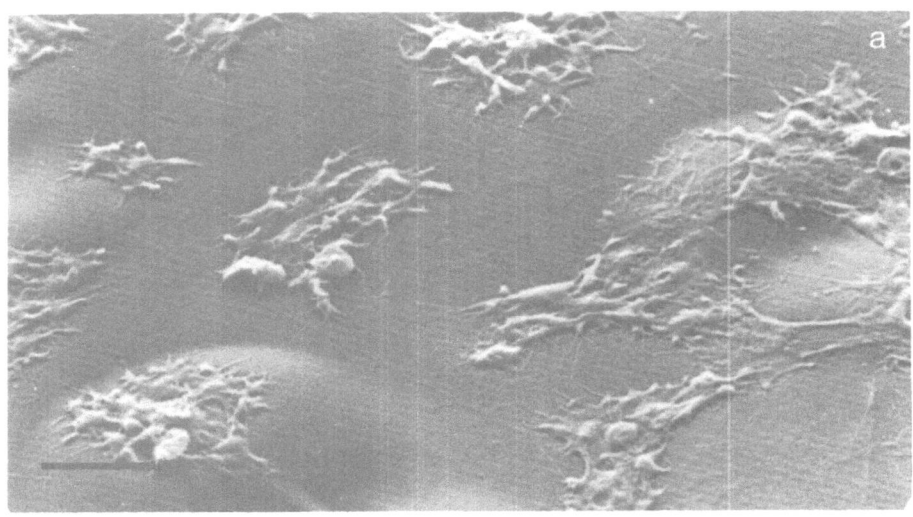

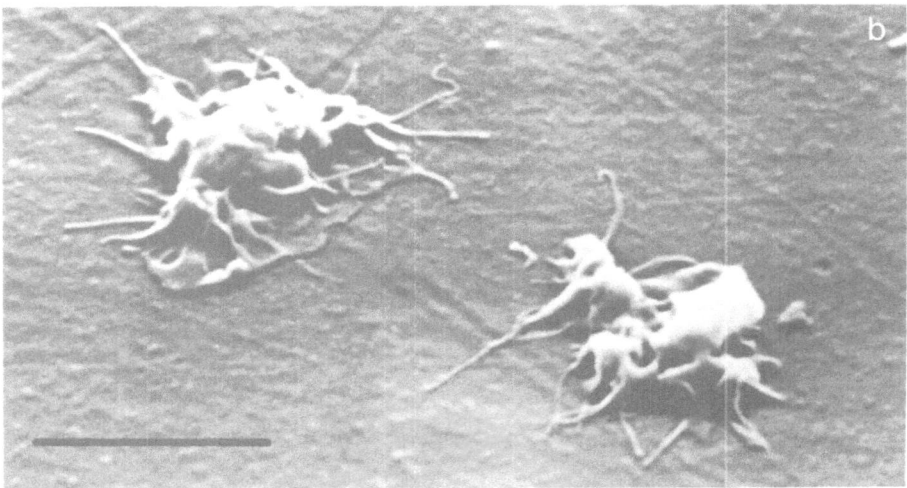

Fig. 6. Platelet adhesion on the surface covered with amorphous
         type IV collagen. Platelets actively spread on the col-
         lagen substrate; single platelets (a) and microaggregates
         (b) bind to the upper surface of spread platelets. Scale
         bar - 5 μm.

Table 1. Summation of Experimental Data on Platelet Interaction with
          the Substrates Formed of Genetically Distinct Types of
          Human Collagen (Fig. 2-6)

Collagenous substrate	Platelet-collagen interaction		Main localization of collagen in the vessel wall (I - 3)
	Adhesion level	Shape change, Aggregation	
V	low	Initial attachment, formation of pseudopods	Liminal surface of endothelial cells
IV	moderate	Spreading, moderate aggregation	Basal membrane
III	high	Spreading, aggregation, formation of thrombi-like structures	Subendothelium
I	high		Media, adventitia

of spreading the platelet comes into close contact with the substrate, radial spreading of webs between other pairs of pseudopods
takes place (Figure 7,b) and thus a well-spread platelet is formed
(Figure 7,c). The analysis of spreading kinetics shows that in our
model system this process takes about 10 min.

Another stage of platelet interaction with a collagen-covered
surface is the adhesion of platelets from suspension to the upper
surface of spread platelets (Figure 8,a). Adherent platelets may be
organized into aggregates (Figure 8,b). Sometimes several spread
platelets fuse forming local cell sheets whereto the platelets from
suspension are attached (Figure 8,c,d). The density of adhesion of
platelets from suspension per an area unit of the spread platelet
exceeds that of fibrillar collagen regions by 10-30, and in certain
experiments, by 50-100-fold. These data demonstrate that spread
platelets can be a substrate for mural thrombi formation.

To what extent does the nature of a substrate determine the
processes of platelet spreading and subsequent adhesion of platelets
to their surface? To answer the question important for the understanding of thrombogenetic mechanisms we have studied how these
processes develop on two substrates: calf skin collagen and collagen
treated with plasma fibronectin - a glycoprotein, which actively
stimulates the attachment of various nucleated cells to a collagen
substrate.

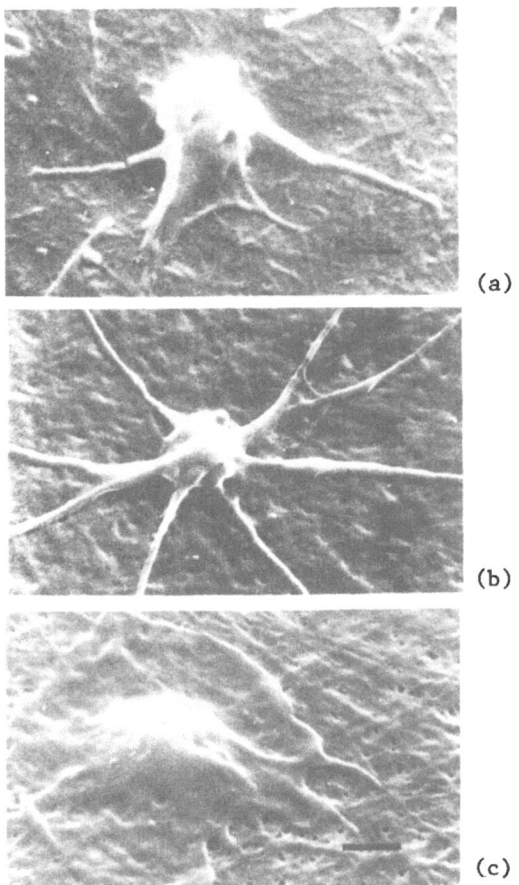

(a)

(b)

(c)

Fig. 7. The mechanism of platelet radial spreading on collagen
         substrate. For the experiments shown in Figure 7-16
         wells covered with CSC (Sigma, C-35II) were used. (a) -
         a spheroid platelet at early stage of spreading. A mem-
         brane "web" is being formed between the two pseudopods.
         The edges of pseudopods and the web are in contact with
         the substrate; (b) subsequent stage of spreading. Radial
         spreading of webs between three pairs of pseudopods
         (arrows). Close contact of platelets with the substrate
         along the whole lower surface of pseudopods and webs; (c)
         - platelet spreading is coming to an end. There is a
         flat circle of lamellar cytoplasm (hyalomer) on the per-
         iphery of the platelet and granulomer hillock in the
         center which indicates the transfer of platelet granules
         from the periphery to the center. Granulomer hillock
         disappears with complete platelet spreading and exocy-
         tosis of granules (Figure 3,8,a). Scale bar - I μm.

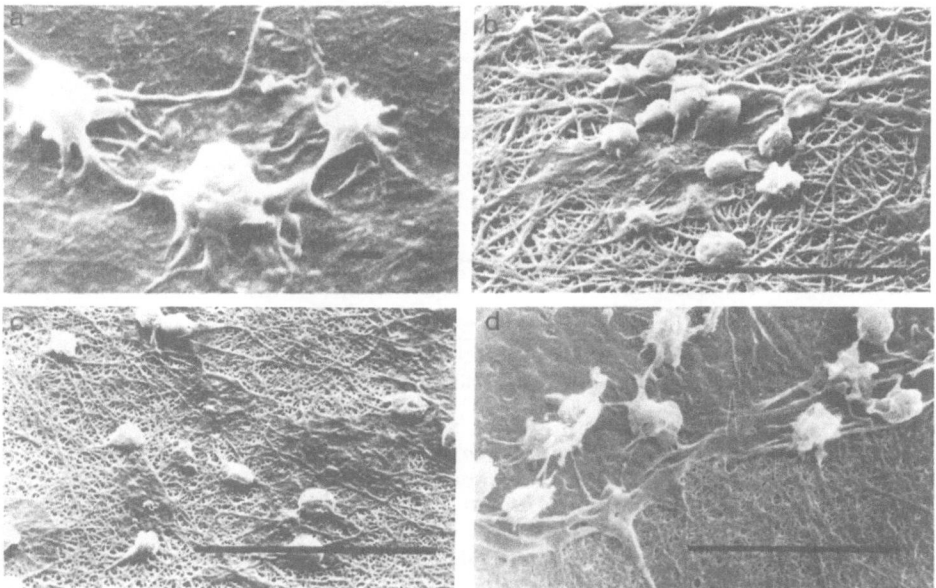

Fig. 8. Adhesion of platelets from suspension on the upper
         surface of spread platelets. (a) - three single spheroid
         platelets adherent to the upper surface of a completely
         spread platelet with irregular jagged shape (scale bar -
         I μm); (b) - formation of microaggregates of spheroid and
         discoid platelets on the spread platelet surface; (c,d) -
         local cellular layers of confluent spread platelets with
         single adherent platelets and micro-aggregates. Collagen
         covered regions neighboring spread platelets have con-
         siderably fewer adherent spheroid and discoid platelets
         (a-d). Scale bar - 10 μm.

     It was found that pretreatment of collagen substrate with
fibronectin increases platelet spreading by 8-9-fold (Figure 9).
Such stages of platelet activation as disc-to-sphere transformation
and formation of pseudopods, which precede platelet spreading, are
stimulated by fibronectin to a considerably lesser extent (Figure 9).

     It is very important that fibronectin treatment sharply reduces
the adhesion of platelets from suspension to the upper surface of
spread platelets (Figure 10). We estimated this effect by measuring
the percentage of the so-called adhesive spread platelets, i.e. the
platelets, which have adherent platelets on their upper surface. It
has been established that after fibronectin treatment the relative
number of adhesive spread platelets decreases from 45% to 10-12%
(Figure 10).

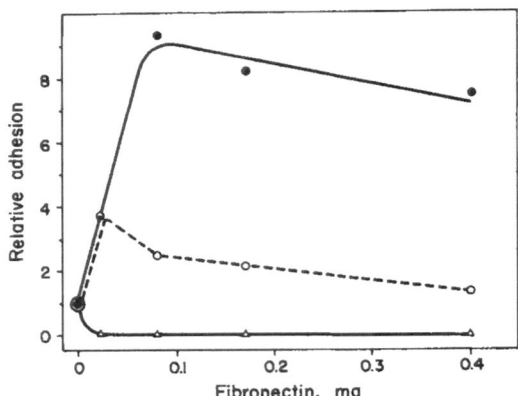

Fig. 9. Fibronectin effect on the spreading of platelets on col-
         lagen substrate. CSC covered wells were pretreated with
         different doses of fibronectin and washed, and adhesion
         was measured by SEM. ●———● - spread platelets; ○———○ -
         activated unspread platelets (discs with pseudopods, spheres
         and spheres with pseudopods); △———△ - inactivated platelets-
         discs.

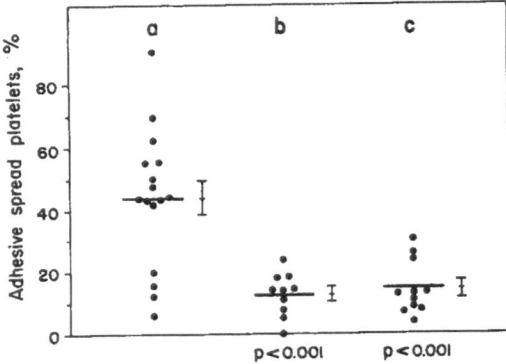

Fig. 10. Fibronectin effect on the binding of platelets from sus-
          pension with the upper surface of platelets spread on
          collagen. Adhesion was carried out in CSC-covered wells
          non-treated (a) or pretreated (b,c) with fibronectin.
          Prior to the addition of platelets unbound fibronectin
          was either removed from the incubation mixture (b) or
          not (c). The ability of spread platelets to bind the
          platelets from suspension was determined by measuring
          the percentage of adhesive spread platelets, i.e. the
          platelets with adherent platelets on the upper surface.
          The total number of spread platelets was taken for 100%.
          Mean values ± standard errors are given. Statistic sig-
          nificance of differences between the means (p) in ex-
          periments (b) and (c) as compared with the experiment
          (a) was calculated using Student's t-test.

The obtained data indicate that while increasing with fibronectin the ability of a collagen substrate to spread platelets one
can simultaneously decrease the adhesiveness of the upper surface of
spread platelets for the platelets from suspension. It is possible
that one of the physiological functions of fibronectin is to stimulate the formation of "pseudoendothelial" carpet of unadhesive spread
platelets in deendothelialized zones of the vessel wall by binding to
these zones.

Is it a specific effect of fibronectin or a general phenomenon
accounted for by the fact that platelets better spread on attractive
substrates and become less adhesive for the platelets from suspension? To investigate the problem we have compared platelet spreading
and adhesion on spread platelets in two substrates: 1) collagen and
2) activated polystyrole, a material used for multi-well culture
plates, which has high adhesiveness for a wide variety of cells. It
turned out that platelets spread on polystyrole more actively than on
collagen. This is manifested by a 2-fold increase of the spread
platelets fraction and mean area of one spread platelet (Table 2).
Besides, there is a considerable difference in the shape of spread
platelets. The calculation of the so-called two-dimensional form
parameter, i.e. the ratio of figure area to its squared perimeter,
showed that on polystyrole the shape of spread platelets approximates
a circle, while on collagen they have irregular jagged shape (Table
2). The result demonstrates that polarization of spreading, i.e.

Table 2. Binding of Platelets to CSC and Activated Polystyrole.
Platelet Spreading and Adhesion of Platelets from
Suspension to the Upper Surface of Spread Platelets.

| Substrate | Spread platelets | | | Adhesion on spread platelets |
	per cent*	mean area, $\mu km^2{}^+$	form para-meter[+], F	x $10^{-3}/nm^2$
Collagen	30.6 ± 6.0	13.4 ± 0.7	0.42 ± 0.01	22.4 ± 5.2
Plastic	62.1 ± 12.8	25.6 ± 1.0	0.85 ± 0.01	3.5 ± 1.2
	p < 0,05		p < 0,01	p < 0.001

Platelets were added into uncovered wells of Multiwell (Falcon) and
CSC-covered wells. *Spread platelets - % of the total number of
adherent platelets. [+] Mean area and two-dimensional form parameter
(F) of spread platelets were measured in MOP-3 (Reichert-Jung,
Austria), $F = \dfrac{4TS}{U^2}$, where S - figure area, U - figure perimeter.
For a circle F = I; for markedly irregular figures (elongated or
jagged) F approximates to 0. Mean ± standard error is given for 7
experiments. Statistic significance of differences between the means
(p) was calculated using Student's t-test.

selection of major directions for spreading is quite different on collagen and plastic.

A 6.5-fold fewer number of platelets from suspension attach to the platelets spread on polystyrole as compared with the platelets spread on collagen (Table 2). That seems to be the most important result of these experiments. Thus, just as in case of fibronectin the platelets spread on attractive substrate are characterized by a decreased adhesiveness for platelets from suspension. This phenomenon may be possibly accounted for by the existence of certain common proteins within receptor complexes responsible for the inter-action of spread platelets both with the substrate and platelets from suspension. An increase in collagen substrate adhesiveness con-ditioned by fibronectin or the use of a more attractive substrate (polystyrole) results in the migration of these proteins from the upper surface of spread platelets onto the surface facing the sub-strate. Such a redistribution leads to the decrease of spread platelets adhesiveness for the platelets from suspension, which in its turn reduces a possibility of mural thrombi formation on spread platelets.

These data make it possible to broaden the approach to selection of artificial biomaterials for vascular grafts and prosthetic heart valves. Probably, along with the search for new low adhesive materials researchers should turn to those that facilitate intensive platelet spreading. In this way surfaces covered with a carpet of nonadhesive spread platelets may be obtained.

MODULATION OF PLATELET SPREADING AND OF FORMATION OF THROMBI-LIKE AGGREGATES ADHERENT TO COLLAGEN SUBSTRATE

Platelet spreading and adherent thrombi-like aggregate formation were stimulated by exogenous platelet activators - arachidonic acid and stable methano-epoxy-analogue of prostaglandin endoperoxides (U46619). Inhibition of these processes was studied using Trapidil, U46619 antithromboxane agent, and stable prostacyclin analogues - carbacyclin and $6\beta - PGI_I$.

Calf skin collagen was used as a substrate. In the absence of platelet activators an ordinary picture of adhesion to this type collagen is observed: adhesion of single platelets, moderate spread-ing and adhesion to spread platelets (Figure 11,a). Adhesion in the presence of arachidonic acid or U46619 results in surface accumu-lation of thrombi-like aggregates alternating with thrombi-free areas (Figure 11,b). Such distribution pattern makes it possible to quantitate thrombi formation by counting the number of adherent thrombi-like structures.

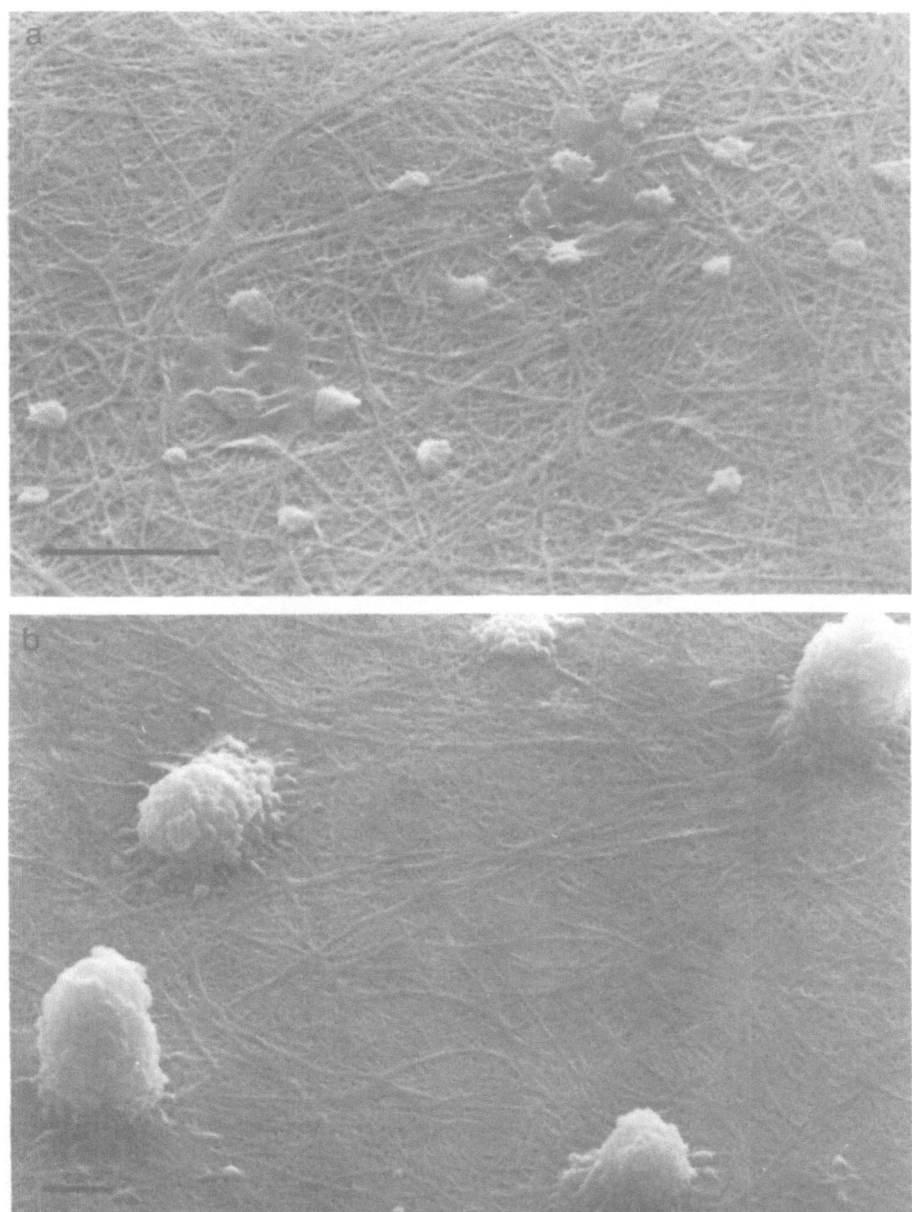

Fig. 11. U46619-induced formation of thrombi-like aggregates adherent to collagen. The binding of platelets with CSC-
covered surface was performed in the absence of the inducer (a) or with I μm of U46619 (b). U46619 was added

(continued)

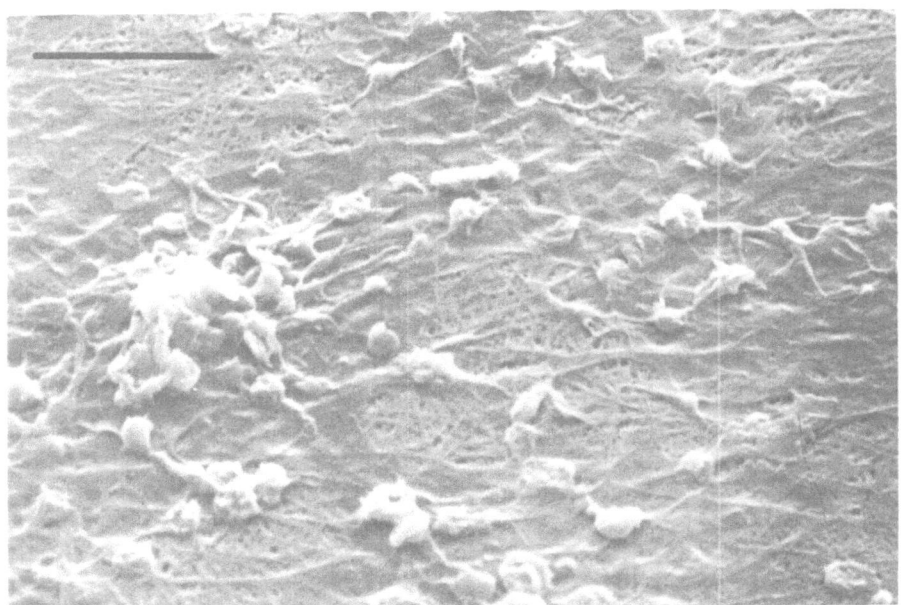

Fig. 12.   Induction of platelet spreading on collagen substrate by
            arachidonic acid. Arachidonic acid (200 μM) was added
            into CSC-covered wells 3-5 min. prior to platelets.
            Intensive platelet spreading results in the formation of
            vast cell sheets on the substrate whereto single plate-
            lets from suspension, microaggregates and thrombi-like
            structures are binding. Scale bar - 10 μm.

Fig. 11 (continued)

            into the wells 3-5 min. before the platelets and direct-
            ly prior to stirring. In the absence of the inducer
            platelet interaction with CSC-substrate is characterized
            by initial attachment to the substrate, moderate spread-
            ing, and the adhesion of platelets from suspension to
            spread platelets (a). The inducer action leads to for-
            mation of thrombi-like structures discretely distributed
            on the substrate (b) and fields of confluent spread
            platelets (Figure 12). Scale bar - 10 μm.

The above mentioned activators also induce intensive platelet spreading (Figure 12). Spread platelets fuse and form the sheets covering up to 50% of collagen substrate. Single platelets, aggregates and thrombi-like structures bind to the upper surface of spread platelets (Figure 12).

Antithromboxane agent Trapidil (Rocornal) completely inhibits platelet spreading and thrombi-like aggregate formation on CSC (Figure 13). Trapidil also has antithrombotic effect when thrombogenic human Type I collagen is used. At the same time Trapidil inhibits arachidonic acid-induced thromboxane A_2 synthesis in platelets only by half (Figure 14). These data indicate that antithrombotic Trapidil action cannot be fully accounted for by the inhibition of thromboxane A_2 snythesis in platelets.

We have studied antithrombotic action of carbacyclin and 6β - PGI_I, chemically stable prostacyclin analogues. According to the data of other authors, carbacyclin and 6β - PGI_I prevent platelet aggregation induced by U46619 and arachidonic acid in human platelet-rich plasma. 10 ng/ml dose of carbacyclin and 50 ng/ml dose of 6β-PGI_I produce a half inhibiting effect. Complete inhibition is caused by 30 and 100 ng/ml, respectively (Figure 15). The effect of prostacyclin analogues on adherent thrombi-like structures formation

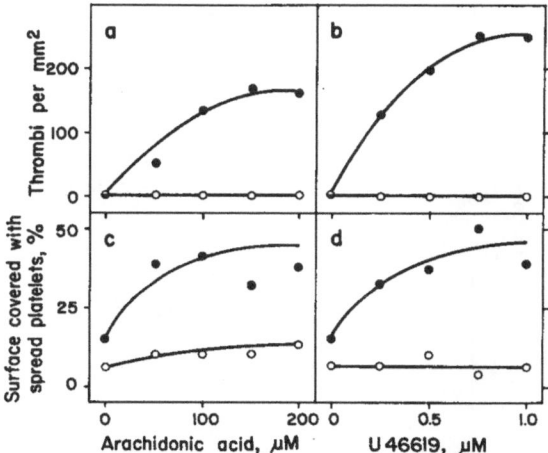

Fig. 13. Formation of thrombi-like aggregates adherent to collagen (a,b) and platelet spreading (c,d) induced by arachidonic acid and U46619. Inhibitory Trapidil effect. Trapidil, 1 μM (o——o) or the buffer (•——•) were added into CSC-covered wells. Then, after 3-5 min. intervals platelets and different doses of arachidonic acid (a,c) or U46619 (b,d) were added following each other. The formation of thrombi-like aggregates and spreading were measured by SEM.

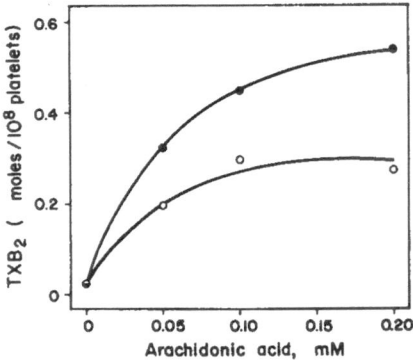

Fig. 14. Trapidil effect on arachidonic acid-induced thromboxane
          B$_2$ synthesis in platelets. The conditions under which
          the adhesion was carried out are given in the legend to
          Figure 13. Thromboxane B$_2$ was determined by radioimmu-
          noassay in the unadherent platelets fraction in the
          absence (●——●) and in the presence (○——○) of 1 mM
          Trapidil.

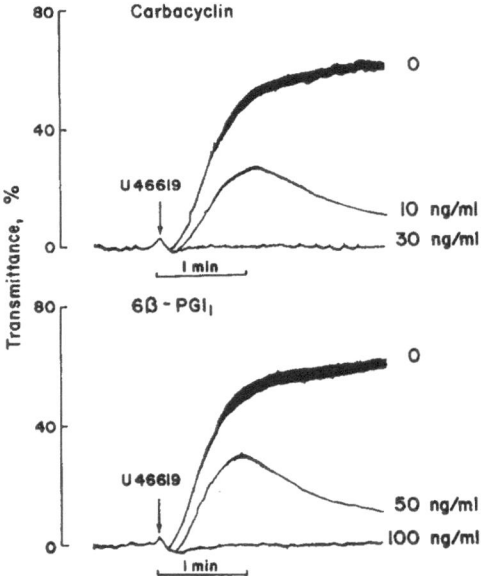

Fig. 15. Inhibition of U46619-induced platelet aggregation in
          suspension by stable prostacyclin analogues. First
          U46619 (1 μM) and then (after 1 min) the above mentioned
          doses of carbacyclin and 6β - PGI$_I$ were added to the
          platelet-rich human plasma, and platelet aggregation was
          measured in a Payton aggregometer.

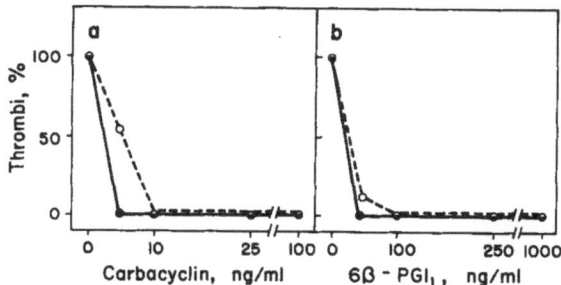

Fig. 16.   Inhibition of adherent thrombi-like aggregate formation
by stable prostacyclin analogues. Different doses of
carbacyclin (a) or 6β – PGI$_I$ (b) were added into CSC-
covered wells; 3-5 min after they were followed by
platelets and, finally, after the same interval – by
1 μM U46619 (o——o) or 200 μm arachidonic acid
(●——●). Thrombi-like aggregates were measured by
SEM.

induced by arachidonic acid and U46619 has been studied. It was
demonstrated that both analogues fully inhibit thrombi formation on
collagen substrate, but to produce the effect a 10-fold lower concentration of carbacyclin is needed in comparison with 6β – PGI$_I$
(Figure 16).

GENERAL CONCLUSIONS

    The study suggests a simple model system, which makes it poss-
ible to study thrombogenesis on collagen-coated surfaces, namely:

1) to quantitate adherent thrombi-like platelet aggregates;
2) to study platelet spreading and their role in thrombogenesis;
3) to study the contribution of various collagen types to platelet-
   vessel wall interaction;
4) to study the modulation of adhesion and thrombi formation by
   humoral factors;
5) to perform the screening of antithrombotic and thrombolytic drugs.

Acknowledgements

    We wish to acknowledge valuable criticism and support of Dr. V.
N. Smirnov, Dr. V. S. Repin, and Dr. E. V. Lyubimova (USSR Cardiology
Research Center). We are also grateful to Dr. S. Moncada (Wellcome
Laboratories, U.K.) for his generous gift of stable prostacyclin
analogues.

IMPAIRMENT OF FIBRINOLYSIS AS A RISK FACTOR FOR THROMBOSIS

D. Collen

Center for Thrombosis and Vascular Research
Department of Medical Research
University of Leuven, Belgium

PATHOGENESIS OF ARTERIAL AND VENOUS THROMBOSIS

The factors generally accepted to be important in thrombus formation are known as Virchow's triad:[1] the vessel wall, the composition of the blood and the flow of the blood in the vessel. The components in the blood which play a role in the pathogenesis of thrombosis are the blood platelets, the coagulation system and the fibrinolytic system.

The contribution of the three factors of Virchow's triad to the pathogenesis of thrombosis is different in arterial as compared to venous thrombosis. The main cause of arterial thrombosis appears to be intimal atheroma. However, other factors also interfere since severe atheromatosis may exist without thrombosis while thrombosis may occur in the presence of minimal vessel lesions. There is a considerable overlap in the extent of atherosclerosis between patients who died from myocardial infarction and patients who died from other causes, although the myocardial infarction group as a whole, showed more coronary artery disease.[2] Atheroma may lead to platelet adherence to the exposed subintimal layer, leading to formation of a platelet plug which is then covered by fibrin (white thrombus). Platelet aggregation on a diseased vessel wall appears to be the primary event in arterial thrombosis; the formation of fibrin is secondary although it may largely contribute to the occlusion of the artery.

Astrup[3] suggested that impaired fibrinolysis may lead to the persistence of fibrin deposits at sites of luminal injury, the incorporation of the fibrin into the vessel wall, and ultimately, the further development of degenerative atherosclerotic changes.

The key event in myocardial or cerebral infarction is not the
development of the arterial lesions themselves, but the occlusion
of an artery by a thrombus. There is indeed little correlation between infarction and the severity of atherosclerotic plaques in the
brain or coronary vessels, but a close correlation between infarction
and thrombosis of a major supply vessel.

Venous thrombosis mainly occurs in areas with stasis and acccumu-
lation of procoagulants. Venous thrombi essentially consist of
fibrin and entrapped red cells (red thrombus). "Hypercoagulability"
of the blood, such as encountered in the postoperative period, during
pregnancy or in women on oral contraceptives greatly increases the
frequency of venous thromboembolism. Deficient fibrinolysis may
result in delayed clearance of fibrin and thus predispose to overt
thrombosis.

Thus all three commonly encountered vascular lesions, namely
cardiac infarction, cerebral infarction and venous thromboembolism
have as their underlying pathological process thrombosis of critically
situated vascular segments.

REGULATION AND CONTROL OF FIBRINOLYSIS

The blood fibrinolytic system consists of three main components:
the pro-enzyme plasminogen, which can be activated by limited proteolysis to plasmin; plasminogen activators which may be of different
origin; and inhibitors which rapidly neutralize plasmin or which
may interfere with the activation of plasminogen.

During the past few years, specific molecular interactions between plasminogen activator and fibrin, between plasminogen and
fibrin and between plasmin and α_2-antiplasmin have been described,
on the basis of which a molecular model for the regulation of fibrinolysis in vivo was proposed.[4,5]

Extrinsic plasminogen activator has a weak affinity for plasminogen in the absence of fibrin (K_M = 65 μM) but a much higher affinity in the presence of fibrin (K_M between 0.15 and 1.5 μM).[6,7]
This increased affinity appears to be the result of a "surface
assembly" of plasminogen activator and plasminogen on the fibrin
surface. In this reaction plasminogen binds to fibrin primarily
via specific structures called the "lysine-binding site". Thus one
way of regulating fibrinolysis is at the level of plasminogen activation localized at the fibrin surface.

Plasmin is extremely rapidly inactivated by α_2-antiplasmin
($k_1 \approx 10^7$ $M^{-1}s^{-1}$ [8]; the half-life of free plasmin in the blood is
therefore estimated to be approximately 0.1s. Plasmin with an oc-
cupied lysine-binding site is however inactivated 50 times slower

by α_2-antiplasmin. Reversible blocking of the active site of plasmin with substrate also markedly reduces the rate of inactivation by α_2-antiplasmin. From these findings one can extrapolate that plasmin molecules generated on the fibrin surface, which are bound to fibrin through their lysine-binding sites and involved in fibrin degradation, are protected from rapid inactivation by α_2-antiplasmin. Plasmin released from the fibrin surface would however be rapidly inactivated by α_2-antiplasmin.

IMPAIRMENT OF FIBRINOLYSIS AS A RISK FACTOR FOR THROMBOSIS

Impairment of fibrinolysis at several levels has been identified and shown to be associated with an increased tendency to thrombosis.

Deficient Synthesis and/or Release of Plasminogen Activator from the Vessel Wall

Isaacson and Nilsson[9] found a defective release of plasminogen activator from the vessel walls during venous occlusion and/or a decreased plasminogen activator content in walls in superficial veins in about 70% of a large series of patients with idiopathic venous thrombosis. This association between non-acute venous thrombosis and a defect in the fibrinolytic system is closer than that between the former and any other known disturbance of the hemostatic balance.

Phenformin combined with ethylestrenol stimulated the release of the fibrinolytic activity in the vessel wall in these patients and was found to be associated with a diminished frequency of thrombotic episodes.[10]

Johansson et al.,[11] found a defective release but a normal content of plasminogen activator in the vessel wall in members of a large family with a high incidence (37 percent) of deep vein thrombosis. Thus, this family appeared to suffer from a hereditary thrombotic tendency in association with a defective release of plasminogen activator; the pattern of heredity was however not clear.

Clayton and coworkers[12] determined several clinical and laboratory parameters preoperatively in women undergoing gynecological surgery and measured the occurrence of postoperative deep vein thrombosis. On the basis of three clinical parameters (age, percentage overweight for height, presence of varicose veins) and two laboratory tests (the euglobulin clot lysis time and the level of fibrin(ogen) related antigen in serum) they could construct a preoperative index which allowed to make a clinically useful separation between patients subsequently developing deep vein thrombosis or not. Of these parameters, a prolongation of the euglobulin clot lysis time was the most discriminating to identify patients who would develop thrombosis.

Rákóczi and coworkers[13] have applied Clayton's index to a comparable group of gynecological patients and confirmed that a low level of plasma plasminogen activator preoperatively is associated with an increased risk of developing postoperative deep vein thrombosis.

Deficiency or Functional Defects of the Plasminogen Molecule

Congenital plasminogen deficiencies have so far not been described and may be incompatible with life. Plasminogen production is however delayed in the human fetus; an infant will reach adult levels at the age of 7-10 months. Ambrus et al.,[14] have therefore performed a double-blind, randomized study in which 500 premature infants were treated with plasminogen or placebo intravenously within 60 minutes of birth. They found a substantial decrease in severe clinical respiratory distress, death caused by hyaline membrane disease, and total mortality in the plasminogen-treated infants as compared to the controls. This study may attest to a vital function of the fibrinolytic system, at least during the first hours after birth.

Abnormalities in the plasminogen molecule resulting in defective activation to plasmin have been described by several authors.[15,16] Some of the affected individuals presented with thromboembolic disease, which became prominent only during their adult life.

Increased Levels of Inhibitors

Some reports suggest that impaired fibrinolytic activity due to the presence of increased levels of inhibitors of fibrinolysis is associated with a thrombotic tendency. In these studies the identity of the inhibitors was not established.

CONCLUSION

It appears that thrombosis is a disease of mosaic etiology, caused by multiple interacting factors such as lesions of the vascular wall, stasis of blood, hypercoagulability and deficient fibrinolysis.

Although the role of deficient fibrinolysis in the pathogenesis of arterial thrombosis and of atherosclerosis is not firmly established, there is ample evidence that impairment of the fibrinolytic system which may be localized at the level of deficient synthesis or release of plasminogen activator from the vessel wall, abnormalities in the plasminogen molecule or increased levels of inhibitors predisposes to venous thromboembolic disease.

REFERENCES

1. R. Virchow, Gesammelte Abhandlungen zur wissenschaftlichen
    Medizin, Meidinger Sohn und Comp., Frankfurt (1856).
2. J. R. A. Mitchell and C. J. Schwartz, in: "Arterial disease,"
    Blackwell, Oxford, (1965).
3. T. Astrup, Biological significance of fibrinolysis, Lancet
    2:565 (1956).
4. D. Collen, On the regulation and control of fibrinolysis,
    Thrombos.Haemostas. 43:77 (1980).
5. B. Wiman and D. Collen, Molecular mechanism of physiological
    fibrinolysis, Nature 272:549 (1978).
6. M. Hoylaerts, D. C. Rijken, H. R. Lijnen, and D. Collen, Kinetics
    of the activation of plasminogen by human tissue plasminogen
    activator. Role of fibrin, J.Biol.Chem. 257:2912 (1982).
7. D. C. Rijken, M. Hoylaerts, and D. Collen, Fibrinolytic proper-
    ties of one-chain and two-chain human extrinsic (tissue-type)
    plasminogen activator, J.Biol.Chem. 257:2920 (1982).
8. B. Wiman and D. Collen, On the kinetics of the reaction between
    human antiplasmin and plasmin, Eur.J.Biochem. 84:573 (1978).
9. S. Isacson and I. M. Nilsson, Defective fibrinolysis in blood
    and vein walls in recurrent "idiopathic" venous thrombosis,
    Acta Chir.Scand. 138:313 (1972).
10. I. M. Nilsson, U. Hedner, and S. Isacson, Phenformin and ethylo-
    estrenol in recurrent venous thrombosis, Acta Med.Scand.
    198:107 (1975).
11. L. Johansson, U. Hedner, and I. M. Nilsson, A family with
    thromboembolic disease associated with deficient fibrinolytic
    activity in vessel wall, Acta Med.Scand. 203:477 (1978).
12. J. K. Clayton, J. A. Anderson, and G. P. McNicol, Preoperative
    prediction of postoperative deep vein thrombosis, Brit.Med.J.
    2:910 (1976).
13. I. Rákóczi, D. Chamone, D. Collen, and M. Verstraete, Prediction
    of postoperative leg vein thrombosis in gynaecological
    patients, Lancet 1:509 (1978).
14. C. M. Ambrus, T. S. Choi, and E. Cunnanan, Prevention of hyaline
    membrane disease with plasminogen. A cooperative study,
    JAMA 237:1837 (1977).
15. N. Aoki, M. Moroi, Y. Sakata, N. Yoshida, and M. Matsuda, Ab-
    normal plasminogen. A hereditary molecular abnormality found
    in a patient with recurrent thrombosis, J.Clin.Invest. 61:1186
    (1978).
16. R. C. Wohl, L. Summaria, and K. C. Robbins, Physiological acti-
    vation of the human plasminogen variants. Chicago I and
    Chicago II, J.Biol.Chem. 254:9063 (1979).

BLOOD TESTS FOR THE DIAGNOSIS OF THROMBOEMBOLISM

A. G. G. Turpie

Department of Medicine, McMaster University
Hamilton, Ontario
Canada L8L 2X2

In the past ten years, there has been an explosion of knowledge in the field of hemostasis and thrombosis. During this time, there has been a great deal of interest both for the clinician and the investigator in finding blood tests that can be used to predict thrombosis in high-risk patients or to confirm or exclude the diagnosis of thrombosis when it is clinically suspected. In addition, attempts have been made to find tests that can be applied in the investigation of the role of thromboembolism in the genesis and the complications of ischaemic heart disease, peripheral and cerebrovascular disease and in the vascular complications of diabetes.

Numerous reports of the relationship between blood tests and thrombosis have appeared in the world literature and have been the subject of a number of recent reviews.[1-6] The interpretation of the reports has been fraught with many difficulties because the tests have lacked sensitivity and specificity and because the experimental design of the studies has been adequate. For the most part they have provided a stimulus to perform more rigorously designed studies.

The methodology is now available to carry out properly designed and controlled trials. Firstly, sensitive and specific biochemical and immunochemical tests have been developed which have allowed the detection of very small concentrations of the products of intravascular thrombin generation, intravascular fibrin formation and products of platelet activation and release. In addition, methods to detect circulating activated clotting factors and complexes of activated clotting factors with their inhibitors have been developed. The second major advance has been the development of readily available objective techniques to diagnose thrombosis, both arterial and venous. Finally, advances in the field of epidemiology and in the

design of clinical trials have enabled more definitive studies on
the laboratory diagnosis of thrombosis to be carried out.

There are a number of criteria that should be fulfilled to
provide evidence of a relationship between an abnormal blood test
and a clinical thrombotic event. These criteria include an adequate
study design, consistency, biologic gradient and biologic plausi-
bility.

The relationship between an abnormal test and thrombosis might
be either causal or incidental and in practice, it may be difficult
to differentiate between these. In addition, it may be difficult
to determine whether an abnormal test precedes or occurs as a consequence of the thromboembolic event. However, if a relationship
can be demonstrated, it is of practical importance because it may be
used as a marker or predictor of a thrombotic event and may provide
valuable information on the pathogenesis of thrombosis.

Although the pathogenesis of arterial and venous thrombosis is
similar, there are a number of important differences. In arterial
thrombosis, the interaction between platelets and damaged blood
vessel wall may be the initiating event whereas in venous thrombosis,
activation of blood coagulation and the formation of a mass of intravascular fibrin is the predominant feature. It is likely therefore,
that these differences will be reflected in changes in different
blood tests. In addition, arterial thrombosis frequently complicates
arteriosclerosis and changes in the blood may be secondary to the
arteriosclerotic process itself, whereas in the case of venous
thromboembolism, the blood changes are probably more directly related to the occurrence of the thrombotic event.

In venous thromboembolism, transient abnormalities in blood may
occur in association with tissue injury which predisposes to thrombosis. The systemic response to injury includes a non-specific acute
phase reaction and a more specific response of activation of blood
coagulation. The non-specific acute phase reaction includes elevation of a number of plasma proteins including fibrinogen, factor
VII, alpha 1-antitrypsin and other alpha globulins, leukocytosis,
thrombocytosis and fever. Increase of fibrinogen and factor VIII
results in a shortening of coagulation tests such as the activated
partial thromboplastin time although there is no evidence that this
change predisposes to thrombosis. An increase in alpha 1-antitrypsin
concentration is associated with an increase in antiplasmin activity
which results in a decrease in blood fibrinolytic activity which
may be causally related to the development of thrombosis. Tissue
injury is also associated with systemic activation of blood coagulation. This may be caused by release of tissue thromboplastin or
in the interaction of plasma coagulation factors and platelets with
injured vessel walls. When thrombin is generated changes in peripheral blood which can be detected by laboratory tests may occur.

Thrombin releases fibrinopeptide A and B (FpA, FpB) from fibrinogen
and through a feedback mechanism which activates factor V and VIII.
Thrombin also stimulates prostaglandin synthesis (Thromboxane A_2,
TXA_2) by platelets and stimulates the platelet release reaction
(Betathromboglobulin, BTG; Platelet factor 4, PF4). These products
of thrombin action can be detected by sensitive radioimmunoassays
in blood. The fibrinolytic enzyme system may also be activated
which produces soluble fibrin degradation products (FDP) from fibrin
which can be detected in plasma or in serum.

Many of these tests have been applied for the diagnosis of venous
thromboembolism but none has been found to be sufficiently sensitive
or specific.

In deep vein thrombosis (DVT), the core peptide of fibrinogen,
Fragment E, has been found to be useful to exclude a diagnosis of
deep vein thrombosis in high risk patients.[7] Betathromboglobulin
was originally introduced as a new blood test for the diagnosis of
deep vein thrombosis and has been critically evaluated and found to
be of no diagnostic value although increased urine BTG concentration
may predict occurrence of DVT in high risk patients.[8]

In arterial thrombosis, which usually occurs as a complication
to arteriosclerosis or in the presence of prosthetic surfaces, the
initial process involves the reaction of platelets with damaged
vessel walls or arterial surfaces whereupon they adhere, release the
contents of their granules and aggregate. Thus, tests that reflect
platelet activation, aggregation or release may be abnormal in arterial thromboembolism. These include measurement of platelet release proteins, betathromboglobulin and platelet factor 4, or
measurement of products of prostaglandin synthesis including thromboxane B_2. If the process is extensive or continuous, platelet
survival measured by isotope techniques may be used. If occlusive
thrombi occur in the arterial circulation, blood changes may also
occur as a consequence of tissue infarction which includes typical
acute phase reaction response. The process of blood coagulation
may be activated both locally and systemically leading to changes
similar to those described for venous thrombosis.

The use of blood tests for the diagnosis of acute arterial
thrombosis has been of limited value but they have given useful
information on the pathogenesis of the process.[9]

A number of abnormal blood tests have been shown to be associated with an increased risk of thrombosis and some of these have
been reported to be predictive of thrombosis.

The best documented of these is antithrombin III deficiency.
Antithrombin III is a protein that inhibits activated factors XII,
XI, X and IX and thrombin and there are a number of reports of

idiopathic and secondary venous thrombosis occurring in families
with Antithrombin III deficiency, which is transmitted as an autosomal
dominant trait. Secondary Antithrombin III deficiency occurs in
patients with liver disease, patients on estrogen therapy and in
premature infants. In some cases of Antithrombin III deficiency,
unusual episodes of arterial thrombosis occur.

Dysfibrinogenemia is a disorder which results in a prolonged
thrombin clotting and reptil times in the presence of normal or decreased levels of plasma fibrinogen and is associated, paradoxically,
with reports of recurrent venous thrombosis. There is one specific
fibrinogen abnormality Fibrin Oslo in which there is a familial
incidence of recurrent venous thrombosis.

There are anecdotal reports that patients with persistent
thrombocytosis associated with myeloproliferative disorders or after
splenectomy have an increased risk of thrombosis but moderate post-
operative thrombocytosis and in most patients with splenectomy, there
is no increased risk. Patients with polycythemia have an increased
risk of arterial and venous thrombosis which is contributed to by
increased plasma viscosity and thrombocytosis.

These is one report of recurrent venous thrombosis in a patient
with reduced functional but normal immunological levels of plasminogen.

A number of studies have reported an association between defective fibrinolysis and thrombosis. Defective fibrinolytic activity
has been reported in patients on oral contraceptives, during the last
trimester of pregnancy, in patients with malignant disease and in
obese patients. There is, however, no conclusive evidence that the
predisposition to thrombosis in these clinical states is associated
with a decrease in fibrinolysis. There is a specific condition of
recurrent superficial or deep vein thrombosis which has been shown
to be associated with reduced fibrinolytic activity measured by
vessel wall plasminogen activator activity or as circulating plasminogen activator.

Increased levels of coagulation factors such as factor VIII
accelerate blood coagulation in vitro but there is no evidence that
increased levels lead to increased rate of in vivo fibrin formation.
There have been several reports of increased concentrations of
factors VII, VIII and V and accelerated thromboplastin generation
in patients with a history of thrombosis. There is, however, no
evidence that these changes have a causal role. Levels of coagulation
factors are increased in pregnancy and in patients on oral contraceptives but there is no evidence that these changes are associated
with an increased risk of thrombosis.

Platelet survival has been reported to be reduced in patients with arterial thromboembolism, vasculitis, homocystinemia, chronic valvular heart disease, prosthetic heart valve replacement, prosthetic arterial grafts, arteriovenous shunt, recurrent venous thrombosis and ischaemic heart disease. However, the reports are inconsistent and often conflicting. This may be related to differences in the experimental technique used to perform the test and in the method used to calculate the results. Abnormalities in platelet adhesion, aggregation and coagulant activity have been reported in various thrombotic disorders but the results are variable and the tests are insufficiently sensitive or specific to be of clinical value. Circulating platelet aggregates are measured either by a screen filtration method or by platelet aggregate ratios which have been reported in patients with ischaemic heart disease, transient cerebral ischaemia, recurrent venous thrombosis and myocardial infarction, but it is uncertain whether these techniques actually measure aggregates in vivo or whether it is an in vitro artefact.[9]

The development and application of specific tests for thrombin generation, fibrin formation and its dissolution, and for activation of platelets have provided valuable information about the pathogenesis of thrombosis. However they have only a limited role in the management of patients with thromboembolic disease. There are currently no blood tests which are appropriate for use as predictors of post-operative deep vein thrombosis. High-risk patients can be recognized by well-established clinical criteria although there is some evidence that measurement of fibrinolytic activity may improve the predictive power but the benefit is marginal and does not justify its routine use. As far as the investigation of patients with proven thrombosis is concerned, the measurement of Antithrombin III concentration is the only test that should be performed routinely. On the arterial side of the circulation, increased platelet turnover has been reported with arterial thromboembolism but there is considerable overlap of patients and controls and the results cannot be used in clinical practice. Elevated levels of platelet specific proteins have been reported in arterial thromboembolism but the significance of these findings is as yet uncertain.

REFERENCES

1. J. A. Penner, Hypercoagulation and Thrombosis, Med.Clinics of N.America 64:743 (1980).
2. J. J. Sixma, Annotation. The prethrombotic state, Br.J. Haematol 46:515 (1980).
3. J. Hirsh, Blood Tests for the Diagnosis of Venous and Arterial Thrombosis, J.Am.Soc.Hematol 57:1 (1981).
4. G. D. O. Lowe, Laboratory Evaluation of Hypercoagulability, Clin.Haematol 10(2):407 (1981).

5. J. Hirsh, Laboratory Diagnosis of Thrombosis, in: "Haemostasis
    and Thrombosis. Basic Principles and Clinical Practice,"
    Robert W. Colman, Jack Hirsh, Victor J. Marder, Edwin W.
    Salzman, eds., J. B. Lippincott Co., Philadelphia, (1982).

6. J. A. Davies and G. P. McNicol, Detection of a Prethrombotic
    State, in: "Haemostasis and Thrombosis," Duncan P. Thomas,
    ed., Churchill Livingstone, Edinburgh, London, Melbourne,
    and New York, (1981).

7. A. C. deBoer, P. Han, A. G. G. Turpie, R. Butt, A. Zielinsky,
    and E. Genton, Plasma and urine betathromboglobulin concen-
    tration in patients with deep vein thrombosis, Blood 58:693
    (1981).

8. A. Zielinsky, J. Hirsh, A. Straummanis, C. Carter, M. Gent,
    D. L. Sackett, R. Hull, J. G. Kelton, P. Powers, and A. G.
    G. Turpie, The diagnostic value of fibrinogen/fibrin fragment
    E assay in clinically suspected deep vein thrombosis, Blood
    59:346 (1982).

9. A. G. G. Turpie, A. C. deBoer, and E. Genton, Platelet consump-
    tion in cardiovascular disease, Semin Thromb.Hemostas. 8:157
    (1982).

HEART MICROCIRCULATION

A. M. Chernukh

Institute of General Pathology and Pathological
Physiology
USSR Academy of Medical Sciences
Moscow, USSR

It is not by chance that our Symposium is dedicated to the
peculiarities of the macro- and microcirculation in the heart work
in normal and pathological conditions. The heart blood supply is a
complex of mechanisms and it is provided by the coronary vessels,
though the heart microcirculation is a subsystem of the general
heart circulation. It is important to note, that the epicardium
layers and the myocardium middle layers are supplied with the blood
by other branches, as compared with the endocardium layers. The
branches of the coronary vessels, entering the endocardium,
ramify and form the anastomosing arcades, which interlace above the
endocardium. Smaller arteries continue into the arterioles and
capillaries and then venules, which gather in the veins. About
85% of the blood from the left coronary artery outflows from the
myocardium into the coronary sinus and then into the right auricle.
About 15% of the blood enters the right ventricle via Tebesia's
veins. The rest small portion of the blood outflows into the left
ventricle. The blood outflowing from the right coronary artery
and flowing through the capillaries, enters the right auricle and
ventricle via the anterior cardiac veins. The blood filling rate
in the vascular bed makes up 6-14 ml per 100 g. of the myocardium
and it comes for the account of the venous vessels. The microcirculatory part of the coronary circulation begins from the small
arteries (150÷250 mkm) and continues by the collecting venules.
Thus, the microcirculatory bed is organically involved in the
coronary (regional) circulation of the heart and represents its
integral part, reflecting the functional and morphological
peculiarities of the heart circulation. This corresponds to the
general proposition, that the organ microcirculatory unit - the
so-called modules (W. Fransher and H. Wayland, 1972; V. V. Kuprianov

et al., 1975) - composing the microcirculatory bed, are intimately
connected with the organ surrounding tissues. They organize
peculiar "quantums" of the organs and tissues, therefore we have
called them "functional elements" of organs. The functional
elements of the organs and tissues are intermediate in their transition from the cellular level of the organism integration to the
organ-tissue one. Our investigations have shown, that in the
primary lesions of the nervous system (neuritis, cutting), significant disturbances were developed not only in the muscular tissue,
but in the capillaries and venules, in which the direct (synaptic)
connections with the nervous system were not visible. Due to the
functional elements the heart microhemocirculatory system is closely
connected with the organ-tissue physiology and pathology. The myocardial tissues have the functional elements, consisting of the
formations specific for these tissues. The microcirculatory unit,
finely adapted by its architectonics to the heart function, is the
center of such an element. The blood vessel capillaries form a
complicated network, passing via the fissure-like spaces between
the heart muscular cells. Thus, the latter are oriented around
the microcirculatory unit. The myocardial cells (fibers) are known
to be represented by two types: muscular cells and specialized cells
of the conductive system. Therefore there are two types of the
heart functional elements. The fibrous formations and cells of the
connective tissue (mast cells included) are oriented around the
microvessels in the space between the myocardial cells. They play
equally a supporting and exchange-physiological role. The lymphatic
capillaries are related hereto. The nerve formations (parasympathetic
and sympathetic efferent and afferent nerve endings) are interlaced
with the architectonics of the heart functional element. So, the
structure of the heart functional element is optimally adapted to its
activity. The heart function, in its turn, is realized by participating of physiologically active substances (first of all, bioamines -
catecholamines as well as prostaglandins, metabolites a.o.), which
are organically involved in the microcirculation regulatory
mechanisms.

As a part of the whole blood circulation system, the heart
microhemocirculation has numerous and significant connections with
the general hemodynamics. The state of all the parts of the microcirculatory bed may affect, in any case, on the main homeostatic
parameters of the general hemodynamics and, first of all, on the
arterial pressure.

The blood flow in the cardiac muscle, which is necessary for
its effective metabolism, is regulated, in the end, at the microcirculatory level. Of a particular significance is the unity of
metabolism, blood supply, regulation and activity, which is realized
at the level of the heart functional element. Hence, we may conclude,
that the heart microcirculatory system plays the important role as

in the myocardium physiological conditions (i.e. in the healthy
state) and in the ischemic lesions. In this case, of a great importance in the normal heart activity is the oprimal correlation
between the lumen size, blood pressure and blood flow velocity in
the microvessels in the cardiac cycles, when the perfusion of the
exchange part of the heart microcirculatory bed is realized.

For a long time, all these peculiarities of the heart microcirculation had been rather difficult for being studied. However,
for the recent years, it has become possible to elaborate principally
new methods for studying the heart microcirculation in the normal
and pathological conditions. There appeared the techniques for
measuring the microhemodynamics by using the isotopic technics,
radioactive microspheres. The methods of the heart biomicroscopy
have been considerably developed. The electromicroscopic examinations, including the cardiac muscle biopsy during the heart
surgery, became of a great value. Though there is much to be
clarified, the ways have been outlined and the valuable data
obtained in the following trends of investigations:

1. The myocardial blood flow, its regulation at the microcirculatory level, transmural blood distribution and optimal
perfusion of the heart microvessels, including blood rheological
properties.

2. The capillary-cellular metabolism in the cardiac muscle,
role of the capillary-venular departments, ways and mechanisms of
the transcapillary transport.

3. The optimal coronary circulation and its correlation with
the dynamics of the myocardial metabolic processes.

A great attention is also paid to the study of the heart
microcirculation disturbances.

The work in these directions have been made in many countries,
and some results were summarized at the 1st Symposium held in
September 1980 in Garmisch-Partenkirchen (FRG) at the X1 European
Conference for Microcirculation (see Biblioteca anatomica, N. 20,
1981).

I would like to cite some examples from our data. The regulation of the myocardial blood flow at the microcirculation level,
is realized mainly by changing the tonus and, hence, the size of
the muscle arterioles lumen. It is disputable, whether the microvessels contractile endothelial cells (particularly in the
capillary wall) are involved in this process. Although in our
laboratory there are available some data, evidencing such a possibility. In the heart vessels the precapillary sphincters are less
pronounced (or absent) and they do not regulate the myocardial

blood flow. It was shown by us, that under the effect of histamine, EDTA and the denervation, produced in the cytoplasma, the formed fascicles, consisting of the actin-like microfibrils (by diameter not more than 8 mm), appeared in the exchange vessels endotheliocytes. Using cytochalasin B — a specific polymerization blockator of the actin proteins — it is possible not only to prevent the formation of the fibrillar actin, but to dissolve the early formed actin gel. However, it was observed, that the "endothelial contraction" was fragmentary and differently pronounced. In this case, there takes place, without fail, the structuralization of the contractile apparatus in the endothelial apparatus, in distinct from the contraction of the muscles cells. The nervous system and local physiologically active substances are involved in the regulatory mechanisms of the myocardial blood flow.

We have specially studied the myocardial microvessels in the adult intact rats and mice by the electronmicroscopic method. Due to the use of serial sections, we have convinced in a number of cases, of the presence of the nerve endings not only at the arterioles, but also on the capillary wall. We have revealed some variants of the interrelation between the nerve terminals and effectory structures: similar terminals were observed directly at the endothelium and pericytes; at the myocardial cells; sometimes they "contacted" simultaneously with the capillary and muscular cell; however, more often they were disposed in the interstitial space at some distance from the vessels and muscle cells, reminding the "free endings". Both, the cholinergic and adrenergic endings were found. It appeared, that the microvessels regulation of a capillary type, was realized, most likely, by their innervation, according to the dissynaptic type, with the neuromediators free diffusion towards these microvessels. Depending on the distance, passed by the neuromediators, the nervous regulation of the capillary wall may be the "direct and fast", "direct and delayed" and conjugated with the myocardium cells regulation. It is clear, that the mediator, releasing from free terminals, diffuses in all sides and effects on the whole "microregion" with its cellular and non-cellular elements. For the account of such terminals, the indirect regulation of the microvessels function may be realized immediately the vasoactive substances, if, under the neuromediators action, these terminals are liberated from the connective tissue cells, particularly from the mast cells. Thus, our data and those of other authors evidence that the significance of the nervous, in particular, adrenergic regulation of the heart microvessels, was under-valued. The use of such powerful blockators as α or β adrenoreceptors allowed to give a favourable value in this respect.

The coronary blood flow is directly connected with the oxygen consumption and, therefore, such factors as the oxygen tension (P_{O2}), carbonate gas (P_{CO2}), hydrogens (H+), kalium (K+), osmotic pressure, lactate, prostaglandins, serotonin and adenosin are under

the special intensive study. Adenosin is known to provide the
metabolic dilatation of the coronary vessels and to easily penetrate
through the myocardial cells membrane. Its concentration rapidly
increases at any stage of the sensitivity to the hypoxia (for
instance, in ischemia), thus promoting the vessels dilatation.

However, it should be taken into account, that the coronary
vessels perfusion depends on many other factors and, first of all,
on the aorta blood pressure and then on the difference in the
arterio-venous pressure, peculiarities of the heart muscle contraction,
metabolic processes, myocardium intramural pressure and blood
rheological properties (viscosity, erythrocytes aggregability and
other blood elements). It is especially important with regard, that
the size of the heart capillaries lumen makes up 3-5 mkm. It is
generally known, that the difficulty in the myocardium vessels
perfusion by the ventrical contractions, is a complicating factor
of the blood flow in the heart microvessels. Due to the microcirculation peculiarities during the cardiac cycle, the study of
the myocardial regional blood flow with the aim to elucidate the
transmural blood distribution in different parts of the myocardium,
has become an important advance of the recent years. With this
purpose, we have widely used the mobile radioactive microspheres
(10 mkm), which being administered in the left auricle, mixed up
with the blood and then penetrated into the coronary vessels. In
the left ventricle, the intramyocardial pressure was found to be
higher in the subcardial layers and it fell almost up to zero in
the subepicardial layers. Due to such an unequal distribution of
the pressure in the left ventricular wall, the blood flow in the
subcardial layers was realized only during the diastole, and in the
subepicardial layers - during the systole and diastole.

In this respect, the study on the interrelation of such blood
flow values as : pressure-diameter-velocity in the heart microvessels is of a great interest.

We have studied the ways and mechanisms of the capillary-
cellular exchange in the cardiac muscle as in the experiment and
in the clinic. These experiments allowed us to reveal a significant
role of the microcirculation capillary-venular department in this
exchange. It should be taken into account that there are two
barriers between the blood and myocardial cell: capillary wall and
sarcolemma. The exchange is realized via the capillary and venular
walls by several ways, depending on the molecule size and lipo-
solubility degree of the penetrating substance. These are the
diffusion, filtration, microbubbling and passage of substances via
the interendothelial intervals. The penetration is easy for the
liposoluble substances and limited for the water soluble and large
molecules. The electromicroscopic equivalents of small and large
pores have been already studied. The substances passage via the
sarcolemma is supposed to be more complicated.

Now briefly about the generally-pathological characteristics of the heart microcirculation disturbances. In my opinion, they may be divided into three groups:

1. Vascular wall disturbances. They include the destructions and deformations of the endothelial cells, changes of the wall permeability, adhesion of the blood elements, cells diapedesis via the microvessel walls and, finally, microhemorrhages. By the frequency, the disturbances of the vascular wall permeability are to be put in the first place.

11. Intravascular disturbances. Hereto should be related three processes, playing an important role in the heart pathology - blood rheology disorders, coagulation and thromboembolism disturbances, changes of the blood flow velocity, connected with the difficulties in the blood perfusion (up to a complete microvessel occlusion).

111. Intravascular changes. They include the injuries of the perivascular components of the functional element, and, first of all, the mast cells activation, microlymphatic circulation disorders and, finally, the microvascular bed involvement in the tissue dystrophic process.

A particular emphasis should be made on the important role of the blood rheological disturbances, which impede the perfusion through the microvessels lumen. In this case, two parameters are of a large importance: blood viscosity and critical radius value of the vessel lumen, both depending on the following factors: the appearance of thrombi in the blood liquid part, aggregation of thrombocytes and erythrocytes; deformation and changes of the erythrocytes rheological properties, hematocrit, blood plasma viscosity. The factors, resulting in the erythrocytes aggregation, may be divided into two groups: 1) influence of the environment, i.e. the shift rate and tension, concentration of the plasma proteins, plasma ion composition and cells concentration; 2) the erythrocytes tendancy to aggregate (deformability of cells, affinity of cellular surfaces to the macromolecules, surfaces electrical potentials).

As it was shown in our experiments, the erythrocyte aggregates might be of a different form and structure in the pathological conditions, depending on the organism state and peculiarities of the pathological process (shock, hypoxia, trauma etc).

The development of some forms of the cardiovascular diseases (heart coronary disease, hypertension, kidney failure, artherosclerosis, thrombosis, peripheric vascular diseases, diabetes) is known to depend not only on the environmental factors, but on the genetic ones, which, in their turn, are likely to influence on the peculiarities of the intravascular changes of the blood rheology and, hence, on the degree of its perfusion via the microvessels lumen.

Finally, some words about the correlation between the coronary blood flow and myocardial metabolism. This is an important, but, at the same time, difficult problem. In the healthy heart, the blood flow rate in the microcirculatory bed is proportional to the oxygen consumption. Hence, the vasomotor processes are dependent directly on the myocardial metabolism. It is also likely, that there exists a direct interdependence between the rich in energy phosphatides and the liberation velocity of the vasoactive metabolites. It should be noted, that the mechanisms of this interconnection have not been yet clarified even for the norm. The matter is that a lot of factors, which act simultaneously and cooperatively, participate in these processes. Between these factors there is not a direct (linear), but probabilistic (cybernetic) interconnection. The interaction processes between these factors should be determined quantitatively, and not qualitatively.

We have made special comparative studies on the myocardium metabolic and functional changes in connection with the microcirculation disturbances. These disturbances have been produced by a simultaneous administration of high-molecular dextran and vasopressin in the rabbits and rats. The heart ischemia and hypoxia, caused by such a way, resulted in a change of the mitochondria oxidative metabolism, a decrease of the respiration and phosphorylation, and of the ATP concentration under an increase of the creatine-phosphate level. The glycogen content and phosphorylase "a" activity were unchanged.

Of a great importance are our data evidencing that the disturbances of the myocardial microcirculatory bed in hypercholesterinemia represent an initial link of the coronary atherosclerosis. Hence, the microcirculation disturbances of a dystrophic nature may be the starting points in the further development of disturbances in the microvessels lipoid metabolism.

Further studies on the heart microcirculation will promote a successful development of this important field of the modern cardiology.

DYNAMIC CORONARY STENOSIS: THE ELUSIVE LINK BETWEEN CORONARY ATHEROSCLEROSIS AND CLINICAL MANIFESTATIONS OF ISCHAEMIC HEART DISEASE

Attilio Maseri

Sir John McMichael Professor of Cardiovascular Medicine
Director of the Cardiovascular Unit
Royal Postgraduate Medical School, Hammersmith Hospital
Ducane Road, London W12 OHS, United Kingdom

SUMMARY

Recent concepts on the roles of dynamic coronary stenosis in ischaemic heart disease are reviewed, with particular reference to episodes of transient myocardial ischaemia and their implications for patient management and therapy. The possible contribution of spasm and other obstructive mechanisms, such as platelet aggregation and thrombosis, to the various forms of angina pectoris, to myocardial infarction and sudden death are analysed in the light of clinical experience and clinical investigations. Based on these conceptual and clinical considerations, guidelines are suggested for future research and therapy. Long-term treatment with nitrates and calcium antagonists, which appear to be effective in preventing dynamic stenoses, resulted in low mortality and infarction rates over a period of two to four years, in a group of patients with ischaemic heart disease at high risk.

INTRODUCTION

Our understanding of coronary artery disease is rapidly expanding as a result of a major revision of traditional concepts. This revision is based on new observations which have disproven the deeply endowed theory that increased myocardial demand in the presence of critical coronary atherosclerotic stenosis was the only respectable cause of angina pectoris.[1-2]

Objective measurements[3-5] have convincingly proven the hypothesis that coronary vasoconstriction, or other factors interfering with coronary blood supply, are usually responsible for nocturnal angina,[6]

431

for angina at rest,[3-10] for cold-induced angina,[11] for "variant"
angina caused by exertion,[12-13] and for the variable threshold of
exertional angina, frequently observed in some patients.[14] It is
important to stress the fact that "variant" angina is by no means
the only electrocardiographic manifestation of coronary vasospasm
but rather it represents only the most striking electrocardiographic
change.[15] Indeed S-T segment depression or T wave changes can be
caused by coronary vasospasm when ischaemia is not transmural.[3,5,]
[16-18] It was also objectively demonstrated that coronary vasospasm
may occur in vessels with an extremely variable degree of coronary
atherosclerotic obstructions.[5,15] In those patients with severe
critical atherosclerotic obstructions angina from vasoconstriction
occurring at rest or on cold exposure or for variable levels of
exertion may be associated with the traditional form of exertional
angina occurring any time the patient exercises beyond a rather fixed,
critical level of effort.[15] These views seem to be gaining acceptance[19,20] and find experimental confirmation.[21,22,23,24]

Furthermore the studies of patients with frequent anginal attacks
at rest have shown that coronary vasospasm may cause sudden death[15,25]
and, probably in association with platelet aggregation and thrombosis
may be one of the causes of myocardial infarction.[26,27]

In this lecture I wish to discuss the role of coronary spasm
and vasoconstriction in ischaemic heart disease with particular reference to episodes of transient myocardial ischaemia and its implications for patient management and for research

THE NEW UNDERSTANDING OF ANGINA PECTORIS

It is now well established that angina may be caused by different
pathogenetic mechanisms even in the same patient: it can be secondary
to increased demand beyond supply according to the traditional textbook theory, or it can be primary*: i.e. caused by other mechanisms
not directly related to the presence of a coronary atherosclerotic
stenosis which, in this case, is the by-stander or a favouring element
rather than the culprit.[1,2,28] Coronary vasoconstriction is the only

---

* The term "primary" borrowed from other fields of medicine is only
  meant to provide an immediate clear-cut separation between "secondary" angina, for which the diagnostic and therapeutic approaches
  are well established, from all other types of angina which will require specific diagnostic and therapeutic approaches. It is ex-
  pressly used to emphasize that this differentiation, rather than
  the proof of the existence of coronary spasm, is the most important
  message of the new understanding of angina: thus, rather than bask
  in the now accepted concept of spasm, we will keep our minds open
  to the possible existence of other causes of angina.

cause of "primary" angina identified so far, possibly because it was more carefully searched for than other mechanisms such as transient platelet aggregation,[29] inappropriate vasodilatation,[30] small vessel disease[31] and alterations of myocardial metabolism.[32]

Furthermore, systematic study of angina patients has demonstrated that angina pectoris should be now considered only one of the possible manifestations of acute transient myocardial ischaemia,[1,2,15] which can be caused by different pathogenetic mechanisms. Indeed, acute transient myocardial ischaemia might manifest itself with typical chest pain (which usually follows minutes after its onset) or only with signs of left ventricular failure and/or with arrhythmias or it may remain completely asymptomatic (in spite of severe left ventricular function impairment and, often, of arrhythmias.[3,9,16,17]

The myth of coronary stenosis and of excessive increase of myocardial demand

The concept that an excessive increase of demand in the presence of atherosclerotic obstructions of the large coronary branches is the only respectable cause of angina has conditioned our diagnostic and therapeutic management of patients during the past three decades. By extrapolation, without objective evidence, it was commonly accepted that rest angina was caused by a sudden increase of heart rate and/or blood pressure, decubitus angina by an increased venous return, nocturnal angina by increased heart activity associated with dreaming. The common observation that these same patients sometimes had a good exercise tolerance was totally overlooked. Accordingly, cold-induced angina and the variable threshold of exertional angina so often observed, were attributed to variable levels of demand for the same external work of the heart.

Again by extrapolation, the identification of a coronary obstruction was automatically accepted as proof of the patients' symptoms. Conversely, in the absence of this proof, the ischaemic symptoms of the patient or the coronary arteriogram was questioned.[33] The attitude was similar to that of the police officer who incriminates an individual found on the scene of the crime just because he is well known for his previous crimes. Monitoring of the variables that control myocardial oxygen demand has clearly disproven this hypothesis.

Coronary Flow Reserve

According to the traditional mechanism, angina occurs because the possibilities of coronary flow reserve are transiently exceeded by myocardial demand. Although this is certainly a frequent event in patients with critical coronary obstruction, now it must be ob-

jectively proved in order to be accepted as the actual cause of the
ischaemic episodes.

Animal experiments indicate that an acute reduction of the
lumen of a major coronary branch by 85% still allows a three fold
increase of myocardial flow[34] sufficient to allow a physical exercise
of about one half the maximum working capacity. In chronic condition
the stenosis, being compensated at least in part by collaterals, will
cause an even smaller impairment of flow. These data are consistent
with the rather frequent observation of patients with severe, proximal triple vessel disease and remarkably good exercise tolerance.
Thus, even when acute ischaemia ensues during increased heart activity it should be considered "primary" unless it is proven that
it occurs because coronary flow reserve has been exceeded and often
the role of organic stenosis, per se, may be more important prognostically than pathogenetically.

Since organic stenosis, per se, are directly responsible for
ischaemic attacks only when they reduce coronary flow reserve below
the levels required by the patient, it becomes essential to evaluate
practically the coronary flow reserve of the patient. Stress testing should establish the level of exertion that the patient can
never exceed without signs of symptoms of ischaemia (as a percentage
of his theoretical maximal working capacity): this gives an indication of the limitation to the increase of coronary flow caused by
organic stenosis. The reproduction of the test may be a reasonable
guarantee that the limitation is caused by organic rather functional
transient obstructions.[2] Indeed, the positivity of the test, per se,
may not give us a clue as to the actual cause of the patients'
symptoms:

1.   if the test is positive, but only at a maximal or submaximal
     level of work (which he may never reach in his ordinary daily
     life) it fails to explain anginal attacks occurring at much
     lower levels of cardiac work.
2.   When the threshold is variable or the patient presents the
     phenomenon of walk through angina, ischaemia can be caused by
     a transient, dynamic stenosis which causes a reversible reduction
     of blood supply. This case is described by a recent typical
     case report of a patient with a variable threshold of exertional
     angina documented by stress testing: coronary arteriography
     performed during exercise revealed a transient increase of the
     severity of a stenosis in the LAD from 75% to over 90%.[14] A
     recent report[36] indicates that ischaemic changes occurring in
     walk through angina may be caused by coronary vasospasm. Tran-
     sient ischaemia during ordinary activity occurring well below
     the maximal heart rate tolerated during exertion was documented
     by Holter monitoring.[37,38]

Reduction of coronary blood supply

Continuous haemodynamic monitoring has shown that the attacks
of angina occurring at rest during the day, the early or late part
of the night or after meals are not caused by increased demands.[3],
[6-10] Furthermore, they usually occur at much lower levels of heart
rate-blood pressure product than achieved without symptoms during
exertion or during a pacing test.[39],[40] In the majority of the cases
the temporal sequence of events is remarkably similar to that observed in dogs following ligation of a coronary artery.[41] Thallium[201]
myocardial scintigraphy consistently shows a reduction of tracer uptake during angina at rest, transmural when the S-T segment is elevated[4] and diffuse when it is depressed.[18] Continuous monitoring of
coronary sinus oxygen saturation has shown that the onset of the
attacks is preceded by a pronounced drop of saturation thus providing
the missing link for the demonstration that a reduction in flow preceded, and hence caused, the ischaemic episodes.[16],[17] A reduction
of coronary flow has been also shown by thermodilution during cold
pressor test induced anginal episodes,[11] and following ergonovine.[42]
Thus, dynamic transient coronary stenoses appear to play an important
role in causing angina.

Role of coronary vasospasm and of platelet aggregation

In this era of transience of our understanding of the mechanism
of ischaemia, reduction of coronary flow caused by vasoconstriction
can be provisionally grouped together under the broad term of "spasm".
As soon as we can identify different mechanisms for vasoconstriction
in larger branches free from organic stenosis and in branches with
severe stenosis, or as soon as we can identify constriction of smaller
vessels, it will become appropriate to develop an appropriate nomenclature. In the present discussion we use "spasm" as a broad equivalent of vasoconstriction of epicardial coronary arteries.

Several pieces of evidence converge to indicate that vasospasm
of the large epicardial coronaries is responsible for the transient
reduction of myocardial blood supply in the presence of an extremely
variable degree of atherosclerotic narrowing.

1. The angiographic demonstration of transient obstruction reversible by sublingual or intracoronary nitrates.
2. The reproducibility of the spasm by drugs such as ergonovine.[5],
   [43,44]
3. The prevention of anginal attacks by nitrates.[45]

These elements, although indicative of the role of vasospasm,
do not allow any inferences on the role of platelet aggregation as
a triggering factor or as a possible consequence of the blood stagnation and intimal damage caused by coronary spasm. Nor do they

allow us to exclude that transient aggregation of platelets may sometimes, per se, be responsible for a reduction of flow. The conflicting interpretation of the cyclic coronary flow variations across an experimental stenosis[46,47] confirms the complexity of the factors responsible for transient reduction of coronary flow. The demonstration that prostacyclin and thromboxane A_2 affect both platelets and smooth muscle, provides the ground for the possible causal role of both intravascular and of vascular wall obstruction in large arterial branches in the genesis of transient ischaemia.

Angiographic demonstrations of coronary vasospasm, once limited to "variant" angina at rest and to angina at rest in general, have now extended to "variant" angina during exertion,[12,13] to angina occurring in the post-exercise period[36] or with a variable threshold.[14] Ischaemia caused by reduced myocardial blood flow was demonstrated with the cold pressor test and attributed to increased alpha tone.[11]

Continuing investigations on a large scale will contribute to clarify the relative role of exhaustion of coronary reserve, limited by fixed organic lesions, and of transient dynamic stenoses, suddenly and transiently interfering with myocardial blood supply in the genesis of angina pectoris. Our experience indicates that the role of transient dynamic stenoses plays a large contributory role in the genesis of angina, together with atheroslcerotic obstructions. When carefully questioned angina occurring only and exactly for the same level of exercise is not common.

Is typical angina pectoris only the tip of the iceberg?

The traditional definition of angina as of "characteristic chest pain brought about by exertion and relieved by rest"[48] is certainly far too restrictive to be still acceptable. This conclusion is derived from a series of studies where the presence of transient myocardial ischaemia could be objectively assessed by electrocardiography, continuous haemodynamic monitoring and myocardial perfusion studies.[3-18]

This proposition demands a redefinition of angina pectoris, and the study of the natural history and epidemiology of the disease in this new, broader conception. We believe that the following points deserve careful consideration and further investigation.

Angina with preserved exercise tolerance

It was reported some years ago for patients with "variant" angina[49] but according to our experience, it can be observed quite frequently if electrocardiographic recordings are taken at the time

when patients experience the episodes of chest pain. Since these
recordings may be difficult to obtain, these patients are usually
dismissed with the assurance that their pain is not of cardiac origin.
Indeed, the diagnostic problem in these patients is not an easy one.
Unless they had some previous objective demonstration of ischaemia,
such as unequivocal electrocardiographic ischaemic changes recorded
after one episode, which would alert the physician, the normality of
the stress test usually is considered a sufficient element to dis-
card the ischaemic nature of pain. Even when more modern approaches
are taken, it may be difficult to arrive at the diagnosis if no episodes occur during the Holter monitoring period or if the inappropriate leads were monitored. Accordingly, provocative tests[41,42] may
be negative if the patient is in a relatively "cool" phase of the
disease.[50]

Thus a careful follow up of the patient and a prolonged observation during the waxing phase of his symptoms may often be the only
means to arrive at the diagnosis.

Painless myocardial ischaemia Continuous electrocardiographic
and haemodynamic monitoring showed that pain is quite a late marker
of ischaemia occurring well after obvious signs of left ventricular
function and electrocardiographic abnormalities.[51] Furthermore, it
may be completely absent.[3,7-9,52] Not only episodes of ischaemia
may spontaneously resolve before the pain occurs, but sometimes, in
some patients, also prolonged episodes of ischaemia with severe
impairment of left ventricular function may remain completely asymptomatic or be accompanied only by dyspnoea, although often they may
cause severe arrhythmias, including ventricular tachycardia and
fibrillation.[15]

Painless episodes in patients with recurrent episodes of angina
at rest often find their equivalent in stress testing when diagnostic
S-T segment changes occur before, or in the absence of chest pain.

The observation of asymptomatic transient myocardial ischaemia
should not be surprising since it is known that even myocardial infarction may be asymptomatic in about 10% of cases.[53] Continuous
electrocardiographic ambulatory monitoring suggest that asymptomatic
myocardial ischaemia may be quite frequent in some individuals.[46,47]

Atypical pain Having been forced to accept that transient myocardial ischaemia can occur in patients with preserved exercise
tolerance and that it can sometimes be completely asymptomatic, we
began to explore the possibility that atypical pain, such as sharp,
inframammary or dull, localized, continuous precordial pain may be
in some patients occasionally caused by transient myocardial ischaemia. Once more continuous electrocardiographic monitoring
showed unequivocal changes indicative of myocardial ischaemia during
these atypical symptoms. In one of those patients who presented

repeatedly with dull, mild inframammary pain with transient electrocardiographic changes, during angiography we were able to document
repeatedly a transient complete spasm of the left anterior descending
coronary artery.[54]

Thus it seems reasonable that an electrocardiogram taken at the
moment of atypical pain, when clearly positive, may be useful for
the diagnosis of atypical chest pain.

Anginal pain without electrocardiographic changes   The absence
of transient electrocardiographic changes during angina in patients
with a history of ischaemic heart disease and with a grossly abnormal
resting tracing is rather common.   However, we were repeatedly unable to detect electrocardiographic changes in any of the 12 standard
leads during typical severe anginal pain at rest, even in patients
with normal resting electrocardiograms.

This puzzling observation poses two questions:

1.   the sensitivity of the electrocardiogram in detecting ischaemia
      on certain occasions;
2.   the possible extracardiac origin of typical anginal pain. Al-
      though the possibility of oesophageal spasm deserves consider-
      ation,[55] techniques capable of detecting ischaemia such as
      measurement of regional myocardial flow, metabolism or contrac-
      tile function are required for a correct diagnosis in these
      cases. Anginal pain without ECG changes was shown to be as-
      sociated with the appearance of transient impairment of ven-
      tricular function similar to those occurring during transient
      ischaemic episodes.[56]

CORONARY VASOSPASM AND MYOCARDIAL INFARCTION

One of the major difficulties in the study of the pathogenetic
mechanisms of myocardial infarction is the inability of the physician
to witness the onset of the event. The study and the close observation of patients who are under high risk of developing infarction
allowed us to make some interesting observations[26] that appear to
find support.[57]

The possible role of spasm

As recently reported[26] it appears remarkable that infarction
developed in all cases in the same territory previously undergoing
repeated transient episodes of acute myocardial ischaemia shown to
be caused by vasospasm. Furthermore, in the patients in whom the
infarction appeared to be small, transient episodes of ischaemia
often recurred in the same territory. These observations indicate

a remarkable analogy between the pathogenetic mechanisms of angina
at rest and of infarction.

In addition, in all patients the onset of the ischaemic episode
which evolved in infarction was indistinguishable from the previous
ones which were reversible, in particular it was not caused by any
increased heart activity.[26] Thus, the demonstration that anginal
attacks preceding the infarction were indeed caused by coronary
vasospasm and that myocardial infarction clearly followed the development of spasm in one patient,[26] suggest that coronary spasm appears
to be an initiating mechanism of myocardial infarction and perhaps
of reinfarction in patients with recurrent anginal episodes. Since
often myocardial infarction occurs at rest and since premonitory
episodes of chest pain are frequently reported in carefully collected
histories, it is conceivable that spasm may be frequently involved
in the genesis of infarction. The recent observations of coronary
spasm in some patients with acute myocardial infarction[60] supports
this hypothesis.

Prolonged vascular occlusion

We were able to document a prolonged vascular occlusion at the
onset of acute infarction in all the three patients in whom we performed coronary arteriography within a short time of the onset of
pain. The occlusion could not be reversed by repeated intracoronary
injection of nitrates in any of the cases. The first case has been
described already.[26,27] Two other patients were investigated following the report of vessel reopening following intracoronary nitroglycerin injection in the early phase of acute infarction.[60]

A protocol was approved for emergency coronary artery injection
of nitrates within one hour of the onset of an irreversible episode
of myocardial ischaemia. Contrast injections were performed into
the right coronary of two patients with persisting inferior ST-segment elevation and intractable pain, 30 and 40 minutes after the
onset of symptoms and repeated after intracoronary administration
of isosorbide dinitrate up to 5 mg. The vessel was occluded without
distal filling respectively at the origin of the posterior descending
and at the proximal third of the right coronary and remained occluded
also after nitrates. According to the established protocol, after
heparine infusion, on the next day a single contrast injection was
repeated: the previous occlusion appeared partially reopened with
the aspect of recanalized vessel and with good distal filling. Unfortunately, we have no information as to whether this aspect of
recanalized thrombus was already present before the onset of MI
(which was documented by typical electrocardiographic changes and
serum enzymes elevation in both cases). At present it is impossible
to tell to what extent the prolonged occlusion documented in these
two patients and in the patient previously reported[26] was sustained

by an irreversible spasm, by platelet aggregation and/or by thrombosis
which subsequently underwent a process of lysis. The temporal sequence of events observed in the patient previously described[26]
indicates that spasm may lead to platelet aggregation of initiate
thrombus formation. In this patient spasm was documented during an
anginal attack shortly before the irreversible episode and also at
its onset; at post mortem a mural platelet thrombus was observed
distal to the site of the occlusive spasm. Reopening of coronary
arteries after MI was previously reported in 3 patients following
angiographically documented occlusion attributed, without clear
proof, to embolus.[58,59] Accordingly the recurrence of episodes of
angina in patients in whom the infarction was small, with the same
location of transient electrocardiographic changes and with the same
characteristics of the episodes preceding the infarction, indicates
that the vessel was not permanently occluded and that vasospasm may
recur in the same vessel.[26,27] A similar finding was recently reported.[61]

   Conversely, in patients who sustained a large infarction, we
observed a permanent vascular occlusion with an organized thrombus
documented at post mortem in one case.[26]

An unifying hypothesis

   The thrombotic hypothesis has been challenged by several path-
ologists[62,65] on the basis of the inconsistent relationship between
thrombotic occlusion and infarction, in particular, small infarctions
coming to autopsy were much less frequently associated with occlusive
thrombosis than large infarctions coming to autopsy relatively late.
Accordingly, data with labelled fibrinogen suggest late or progressive
thrombus formation occurs in acute myocardial infarction.[66]

   Our observations suggest that a combination of spasm and platelet
aggregation and thrombosis rather than coronary spasm by itself,[67]
may result in a vicious circle leading to prolonged vascular occlusion. The subsequent balance between positive and negative feed-
back mechanisms controlling the duration of vasospasm and the dynamic
equilibrium between thrombotic and fibrinolytic processes which is
likely to be influenced by the size of infarction,[64] may be responsible for the reopening, permanent closure or recanalization of the
vessel.

   The occlusive role of spasm which usually involves a long
segment of the vessel, and therefore may prevent also flow from
collaterals, may explain the occurrence of large infarctions distal
to thrombotic occlusion occurring in vessels with old stenoses greater
than 90% in the presence of well developed collaterals which cannot
be explained only by the small further reduction of the lumen caused
by thrombus alone.[64]

The hypothesis of spasm as a possible mechanism of infarction is consistent with the frequent finding of plaque haemorrhage and explosion of plaque debris into the lumen sometimes observed at post mortem. These events, associated with blood stagnation caused by spasm, are likely to greatly enhance local thrombosis with thromboxane A_2 liberation from platelets and potentiation of vasospasm. This hypothesis is also consistent with the observation of radio-fibrinogen presence in the thrombus, early after the onset of symptoms.[68]

Following vascular occlusion the final infarct size is probably determined by a complex combination of humoral, nervous and haemodynamic factors and by the basic anatomic alterations of the coronary bed and of the ventricle. The different types of cellular damage observed by Baroldi[69] suggest that differences in metabolic response of the myocardium may play a major role in determining the final size of the infarction. The recent demonstration that fibrinolytic agents directly infused into the occluded coronary artery may reopen the vessel adds conclusive proof to the role of thrombosis in infarction.[70,71] However, the frequent occurrence of reversible ischaemic episodes prior to the onset of irreversible ones suggest that spasm may play the initiating role.[26,27]

SUDDEN DEATH

The epidemiological definition of sudden death is too broad to allow a pathogenetic classification. Thus, we prefer to adopt a clinical definition: death resulting from ventricular fibrillation or asystole. These fatal arrhythmias may occur apparently as primary rhythm disturbances or they may develop during clinically recognizable episodes of acute myocardial ischaemia. Since coronary spasm may be responsible for acute aschaemia, it obviously may be one of the causes of sudden death resulting from ischaemia-induced arrhythmias.

Ventricular fibrillation was often observed during "variant" angina, a reasonable hallmark of vasospastic angina and in our series it was much more frequent than asystole.[15] It showed the tendency to recur in the same patient during the central phase of the ischaemic attack (independent of the presence of pain) or at its end.[15,25]

We have yet no clue as to why potentially fatal arrhythmias during transient ischaemic attacks are frequent in some patients and rare in others.

In our patients arrhythmias could not be prevented by antiarrhythmic therapy with lidocaine, procainamide, disopyramide but were not observed when attacks were prevented by antianginal drugs.

INDICATIONS FOR FUTURE RESEARCH AND THERAPY

These expanding views on ischaemic heart disease, based on a
series of objective demonstrations, offer new lines of research and
indicate new therapeutic approaches.

Historical perspectives

In the process of trying to outline research lines it is quite
instructive to look back and find that most of the conclusions that
we are arriving at now are mere rediscoveries. H. Huchard in 1889
noted that attacks of spontaneous angina were less frequent than
those for which a provocative cause could be identified, and suggested
that spasm superimposed on organic lesions could explain the paroxysmal nature of anginal attacks. He also admitted that angina could
occur in the absence of organic stenosis, in particular, in smokers.[72]
W. Osler in 1910 suggested the existence of a circulating, perverted
internal secretion which favors spasm of the (coronary) arteries.
He also described sudden death during angina with normal coronary
arteries at autopsy.[73] But the most clear and comprehensive report
is that of Gallavardin who concluded that spontaneous angina at rest
was much more rare than typical exertional angina, however, he was
unable to separate all angina patients into two distinct categories
because both syndromes so frequently occurred in the same patient.
He believed that a variety of angiospasmodic perturbations, reflexes,
and coronary spasmogenic influences superimposed their effects on
the coronary stenotic lesions to produce the variety of clinical
anginal syndromes he saw.[74]

The "scientific" approach, according to which only "demonstrated"
hypotheses can be accepted, lead to the simplistic dismissal of
careful observation and deduction, simply because it could not (yet!)
be proved. This sequence of events must be kept in mind.

Lines of Research

A major effort should be directed towards the development of
methods for the objective detection of myocardial ischaemia since it
appears to be much more polimorphic than traditionally thought and
since the presence or absence of coronary stenosis cannot be any
longer considered at all a diagnostic criterium.

It is also necessary to define the natural history and epidemiology of I.H.D. in the new broader conception where myocardial
ischaemia is not only caused by increased demand, can present itself
also with varied symptoms or remain asymptomatic.

The awareness of the relevant role of spasm and platelets in the genesis of myocardial ischaemia must stimulate investigations on the predisposing and precipitating mechanisms of coronary spasm as well as the feed-back mechanisms which control its duration and reversibilities.

The observation of anginal pain in patients with myocardiopathy cannot be induced by ergonovine prompt the search for the pathogenetic mechanisms of these clinical syndromes.

Indication for Therapy

Since often ischaemia is not caused by excessive increase of demands, reduction of myocardial oxygen consumption cannot be considered any longer the basic therapeutic approach would require the identification of the pathogenetic mechanisms responsible for the ischaemic attacks. Unfortunately, these mechanisms are probably varied, complex and still largely speculative. Therefore, our treatment remains empirical. The hypothesis of alpha-sympathetic and mediated spasm[75,76,77,78] lead to the reappraisal of plexectomy[79] with some encouraging results.[80] However, medical treatment is usually adequate for management of these patients. Drugs that are known to raise the threshold for smooth muscle stimulation, like nitrates and calcium antagonists, are so far the only medication that, in controlled clinical trials, were consistently effective in reducing drastically the number of ischaemic episodes.[45,81,82,83,84]

In preliminary trials we were unable to obtain comparably consistent responses with the use of atropine,[50] phentolamine,[85] aspirin (140 mg every 72 hours)[86] and prostacyclin.[87] Finally, the common clinical observation that onset and waxing of anginal symptoms often coincide with psychological problems and breakdown in adaptation should not be understressed.[88]

For the evaluation of the response to treatment the frequent spontaneous waning and waxing of symptoms and the quite frequent presence of asymptomatic ischaemic episodes suggests:

1. the design of trials preferably according to a double cross-over scheme[45,81] or with interruption of treatment to check the reappearance of symptoms when off the drug.
2. the continuous monitoring of at least two ECG leads for an objective detection of the ischaemic episodes, preferably lead III and V3.[89]

In our hands, long term treatment with nitrates and calcium antagonists resulted in a low mortality (1.7% per year) and infarction rate (0.8% per year) over a two to four year period in a group of 120 patients who presented with severe angina at rest.[90]

REFERENCES

1. A. Maseri, Expanding views on coronary artery disease: Role of vasospasm and other modulatory factors, in: "Atherosclerosis Reviews," R. Hegyeli, ed., Raven Press, New York p.271 (1980).

2. A. Maseri, Pathogenetic mechanisms of angina pectoris: expanding views, Thomas Lewis Lecture, London, November 24, 1977. Br.Heart J. 43:648 (1980).

3. A. Maseri, R. Mimmo, S. Chierchia, C. Marchesi, A. Pesola, and A. L'Abbate, Coronary artery spasm as a cause of acute myocardial ischaemia in man, Chest 68:625 (1975).

4. A. Maseri, O. Parodi, S. Severi, and A. Pesola, Transient transmural reduction of myocardial blood flow, demonstrated by thallium-201 scintigraphy, as a cause of variant angina, Circulation 56:280 (1976).

5. A. Maseri, A. L'Abbate, A. Pesola, A. M. Ballestra, M. Marzilli, S. Severi, G. Maltini, M. De Nes, O. Parodi, and A. Biagini, Coronary vasospasm in angina pectoris, Lancet 1:713 (1977).

6. S. Chierchia, M. Guazzelli, C. Maggini, and A. Maseri, Absence of correlation of nocturnal angina with sleep stages, Circulation 57 & 58 (Suppl.II):753 (1978).

7. M. Guazzi, A. Polese, C. Fiorentina, F. Magrini, M. T. Olivari, and C. Bartorelli, Left ventricular performance and related haemodynamic changes in Prinzmetal's variant angina pectoris, Br.Heart J. 33:84 (1971).

8. M. Guazzi, A. Polese, C. Fiorentini, F. Magrini, M. T. Olivari, and C. Bartorelli, Left and right heart haemodynamics during spontaneous angina pectoris. Comparison between angina with S-T segment depression and angina with S-T segment elevation, Br.Heart J. 37:401 (1975).

9. S. Chierchia, C. Marchesi, and A. Maseri, Evidence of angina not caused by increased myocardial metabolic demand and patterns of electrocardiographic and haemodynamic alterations during "primary" angina, in: "Primary and Secondary Angina Pectoris," A. Maseri, G. A. Klassen, and M. Lesch, eds., Grune & Stratton, New York, p.145 (1978).

10. L. Tavazzi, J. A. Salerno, M. Ray, G. Specchia, M. Chimienti, L. Angoli, S. De Servi, A. Mussini, and P. Bobba, Acute myocardial ischaemia induced by ergonovine maleate in patients with "primary" angina, in: "Primary and Secondary Angina Pectoris," A. Maseri, G. A. Klassen, M. Lesch, eds., Grune & Stratton, New York, p.247 (1978).

11. G. H. Mudge Jr., W. Grossman, R. Millis, M. Lesch, and E. Braunwald, Reflex increase in coronary vascular resistance in patients with ischaemic heart disease, N.Engl.J.Med. 295: 1333 (1976).

12. H. Yasuc, S. Omote, A. Takazawa, and S. Tanaka, Circadian variation of exercise capacity in patients with Prinzmetal's variant angina: role of exercise-induced coronary arterial spasm, Circulation 59:938 (1979).

13. G. Specchia, S. De Servi, C. Falcone, E. Bramucci, L. Angolie,
     A. Mussini, G. P. Marinoni, C. Montemartini, and P. Bobba,
     Coronary arterial spasm as a cause of exercise induced ST-
     segment elevation in patients with variant angina, Circulation
     59:948 (1979).

14. C. Brunelli, M. Lazzari, I. Simonetti, A. L'Abbate, and A.
     Maseri, Variable threshold of exertional angina: a clue to
     a vasospastic component, European Heart J. Vol. II, p.155
     (1981).

15. A. Maseri, S. Severi, M. De Nes, A. L'Abbate, S. Chierchia,
     M. Marzilli, A. M. Ballestra, O. Parodi, A. Biagini, and A.
     Distante, "Variant" angina: One aspect of a continuous
     spectrum of vasospastic myocardial ischaemia. Pathogenetic
     mechanisms, estimated incidence and clinical and coronary
     arteriographic findings in 138 patients, Am.J.Cardiol. 42:
     1019 (1978).

16. S. Chierchia, A. Maseri, I. Simonetti, and C. Brunelli, O_2
     myocardial extraction in angina at rest. Evidence of a
     primary reduction of blood supply, Circulation 55,56 (Suppl.
     III):37 (1977).

17. S. Chierchia, C. Brunelli, I. Simonetti, M. Lazzari, and A.
     Maseri, Sequence of events in angina at rest: primary re-
     duction in coronary flow, Circulation April (1980).

18. O. Parodi, N. Uthurralt, S. Severi, W. Bencivelli, C. Michelassi,
     and A. Maseri, Transient reduction of regional myocardial
     perfusion during angina at rest with ST segment depression
     or normalization of negative T waves (Submitted for publi-
     cation).

19. J. Mellor, A. Pichard, and S. Dack, Coronary arterial spasm in
     Prinzmetal's angina: a proved hypothesis, Am.J.Cardiol. 37:
     938 (1976).

20. L. D. Hillis and E. Braunwald, Coronary artery spasm, N.Engl.
     J.Med. 299:695 (1978).

21. J. Figueras, B. N. Singh, W. Ganz, Y. Charuzi, and H. J. C.
     Swan, Mechanisms of rest and nocturnal angina: observations
     during continuous haemodynamic and electrocardiographic
     monitoring, Circulation 59:955 (1979).

22. M. E. Bertrand, C. Laisne, J. M. Lefebvre, A. Carre, H.
     Warembourg, and J. Lekieffre, Le spasme des arteres
     coronaires, Arch.Mal Coeur 70,1233 (1977).

23. M. Bory, M. Benichou, P. Dijiane, A. Egre, and A. Serradimigni,
     Angor de Prinzmetal et spasme arteriel coronarien, Arch.
     Mal Coeur 73,7 p.825 (1980).

24. J. P. Delahaye and Ph. Gaspard, Le spasme coronarien, Revue
     generale et etude critique a propos de 87 observations
     personnelles d'angine de Prinzmetal, Lyon Medical 245 p.123
     (1981).

25. A. Maseri, Variant angina and coronary vasospasm: clues to a
     broader understanding of angina pectoris, Cardiovasc.Med.
     4, p.647 (1979).

26. A. Maseri, A. L'Abbate, G. Baroldi, S. Chierchia, M. Marzilli,
    A. M. Ballestra, S. Severi, O. Parodi, A. Biagini, A. Distante
    and A. Pesola, Coronary vasospasm as a possible cause of
    myocardial infarction. A conclusion derived from the study
    of "preinfarction" angina, N.Engl.J.Med. 299:1271 (1978).

27. A. Maseri, S. Chierchia, and A. L'Abbate, Pathogenetic mechan-
    isms underlying the clinical events associated with athero-
    sclerotic heart disease, Circulation 62 (Suppl.V)3-13 (1980).

28. A. Maseri, Preface, "Primary and Secondary Angina Pectoris,"
    eds., G. A. Klassen, A. Maseri, and M. Lesch, Grune &
    Stratton, New York, p.xiii (1978).

29. J. F. Mustard, Reversible platelet aggregation and myocardial
    ischaemia, Circulation 29 (Suppl.III)111-130 (1964).

30. W. Kubler, D. Opherk, H. Mehmel, D. Zebe, and W. Maurer, Sig-
    nificance of coronary reserve in patients with different
    forms of "ischaemic heart disease". VIII World Congress of
    Cardiology, Tokyo, Abstract Book 1, p.124 (1978).

31. T. N. James, Pathology of small coronary arteries, Am.J.Cardiol.
    30:679 (1967).

32. P. J. Richardson, G. Jackson, E. G. J. Olsen, and S. Oram,
    Angina pectoris with normal coronary arteriograms: a meta-
    bolic problem? in: "Primary and Secondary Angina Pectoris,"
    A. Maseri, G. A. Klassen, and M. Lesch, eds., Grune &
    Stratton, New York, p.3 (1978).

33. T. N. James, Angina without coronary disease (sic), Circulation
    42:18y (1970).

34. D. E. Gregg and J. L. Bedynec, Compensatory changes in the
    heart during progressive coronary artery stenosis, in:
    "Primary and Secondary Angina Pectoris," A. Maseri, G. A.
    Klassen, and M. Lesch, eds., Grune & Stratton, New York,
    p.3 (1978).

35. R. Lambert, D. S. Hess, and R. J. Bache, Effect of exercise on
    perfusion of collateral-dependent myocardium in dogs with
    chronic coronary artery occlusion, J.Clin.Invest. 59:1 (1977).

36. P. K. Sturzenhofecker, P. Peters, L. Gornandt, and H. Roskam,
    Coronary artery spasm combined with walk-through phenomenon.
    A special type of Prinzmetal angina. Symposium on Coronary
    Arterial Spasm, Lille, November (1979).

37. S. J. Schang Jnr., and C. J. Pepine, Transient asymptomatic
    S-T segment depression during daily activity, Am.J.Cardiol.
    38:396 (1977).

38. A. P. Selwyn, K. M. Fox, D. Oakley, H. J. Dargie, and J. P.
    Shillingford, Myocardial ischaemia in patients with angina
    pectoris, Br.Med.J. 2:1594-1596 (1979).

39. T. B. Berndt, J. Fitzgerald, D. C. Harrison, and J. S. Schroeder,
    Hemodynamic changes at the onset of spontaneous versus
    pacing-induced angina, Am.J.Cardiol. 39:784 (1977).

40. A. Biagini, D. Rovai, A. Maseri, G. Mazzei, C. Carpeggiani, F.
    Aghini-Lombardi, and M. Lazzari, Comparison of the double
    product determined during angina at rest and during atrial

pacing. Diagnostic significance, Trans.Eur.Soc.Cardiol. 1:51 (1978).

41. M. Pagani, S. F. Vatner, B. R. Gain, and E. Braunwald, Initial myocardial adjustments to a brief period of ischaemia and reperfusion in the conscious dog, Circ.Res. 43:83 (1978).

42. D. R. Ricci, A. E. Orlick, P. W. Doherty, P. R. Cipriano, and D. C. Harrison, Reduction of coronary blood flow during coronary artery spasm occurring spontaneously and after provocation by ergonovine maleate, Circulation 57:392 (1978).

43. J. S. Schroeder, J. L. Bolen, R. A. Quint, D. A. Clark, W. G. Hyden, C. B. Higgins, and L. Wesler, Provocation of coronary spasm with ergonovine maleate, Am.J.Cardiol. 40:487 (1977).

44. R. C. Curry, C. J. Pepine, M. B. Sabom, R. L. Feldman, L. G. Christie, and C. R. Conti, Effects of ergonovine in patients with or without coronary artery disease, Circulation 56:803 (1977).

45. A. Distante, A. Maseri, S. Severi, A. Biagini, and S. Chierchia, Management of vasospastic angina at rest with continuous infusion of isosorbide dinitrate, Am.J.Cardiol. 44:533 (1979).

46. Y. Uchida, N. Yoshimoto, and S. Murao, Cyclic fluctuations in coronary blood pressure and flow induced by coronary artery constriction, Jap.Heart J. 454-464 (1975).

47. J. D. Folts, E. B. Crowell Jnr., and G. G. Rowe, Platelet aggregation in partially obstructed vessels and its elimination with aspirin, Circulation 54:365-370 (1976).

48. C. K. Friedberg, Diseases of the Heart, 3rd Edition, Saunders, New York (1966).

49. R. N. MacAlpin, A. A. Kattus, and A. B. Alvaro, Angina pectoris at rest with preservation of exercise capacity: Prinzmetal's variant angina, Circulation 47:946 (1973).

50. A. Maseri, S. Severi, S. Chierchia, O. Parodi, and A. Biagini, Characteristics and pathogenetic mechanism of "primary" angina at rest, in: "Primary and Secondary Angina Pectoris," A. Maseri, G. A. Klassen, and M. Lesch, eds., Grune & Stratton New York, p.265 (1978).

51. A. Distante, A. L'Abbate, A. Maseri, L. Londini, and C. Michelassi, Echocardiographic changes in vasospastic angina, in: "Echocardiography," Ch. T. Lancce, ed., Martinus Nijoff Publishers, The Hague, p.119 (1979).

52. L. S. Gettes, Painless myocardial ischaemia, Chest 66:612 (1975).

53. J. W. Hurst, and R. B. Logue, Arteries and veins, in: "The Heart," McGraw-Hill, New York, p.904 (1966).

54. A. Biagini, C. Carpeggiani, M. G. Mazzei, R. Antonelli, C. Michelassi, A. L'Abbate, and A. Maseri, Transient coronary spasm as a cause of asymptomatic S-T segment and T wave changes during Holter monitoring, (Submitted for publication).

55. A. M. Dart, H. Alban-Davies, R. H. Lowndes, J. Dalal, M. Ruttley, and A. H. Henderson, Oesophageal spasm and angina: diagnostic value of ergometrine provocation, Eur.Heart J. (in press).

56. G. J. Davies, S. Chierchia, M. Myers, A. Maseri, and R. E.
    Steiner, Transient changes in left ventricular volume in
    acute myocardial ischaemia, Clinical Science 60:13 (1981).
57. J. E. Madias, The syndrome of variant angina culminating in
    acute myocardial infarction, Circulation 59:297-306 (1979).
58. P. M. Richardson and M. S. Gotsman, Angiographic evidence of
    coronary embolism and resolution, S.Afr.Med.J. 45:805 (1971).
59. R. J. O'Reilly and R. D. Spellberg, Rapid resolution of coronary
    arterial emboli: myocardial infarction and subsequent normal
    coronary arteriograms, Ann.Int.Med. 81:348 (1974).
60. Ph. B. Oliva and J. C. Breckenridge, Arteriographic evidence
    of coronary arterial spasm in acute myocardial infarction,
    Circulation 56:366 (1977).
61. J. A. Trigano, G. Chiesa, and C. Diard, Alterations electro-
    cardiographiques de type angor de Prinzmental en phase aigue
    d'infarctus du myocarde, Arch.Mal Coeur 70:901 (1977).
62. A. W. Branwood and G. L. Montgomery, Observations on the morbid
    anatomy of coronary artery disease, Scot.Med.J. 1:367 (1956).
63. D. M. Spain, V. A. Brades, A. Matero, and R. Tarter, Sudden
    death due to coronary atherosclerotic heart disease: age,
    smoking habits and recent thrombi, J.Am.Med.Ass. 207:1347
    (1969).
64. G. Baroldi, Acute coronary occlusion as a cause of myocardial
    infarct and sudden coronary heart death, Am.J.Cardiol. 16:
    859 (1965).
65. W. C. Roberts, Coronary thrombosis and fatal myocardial
    ischaemia, Circulation 49:1 (1974).
66. L. R. Erhardt, T. Lundman, and H. Mellstedt, Incorporation of
    ^{125}I-labelled fibrinogen into coronary arterial thrombi in
    acute myocardial infarction in man, Lancet 1:387 (1973).
67. W. H. Sewell, Coronary spasm as a primary cause of myocardial
    infarction: a preliminary report, Angiology 17:1 (1966).
68. W. F. M. Fulton, Does coronary thrombosis cause myocardial
    infarction or vice versa? in: "Advanced Medicine," 14:
    138-147, J. Weatherall ed., Royal Coll.Phys.London, Pitman
    Medical.
69. G. Baroldi, Different types of myocardial necrosis in coronary
    heart disease: a pathophysiologic review of the functional
    significance, Am.Heart J. 89:742 (1975).
70. K. P. Rentrop, H. Blanke, and K. R. Karsch, Acute myocardial
    infarction intracoronary application of nitroglycerin and
    streptokinase, Clin.Cardiol. 2:354-363 (1979).
71. W. Ganz, N. Buchbinder, M. S. Marcus, A. Mondkar, J. Maddahi,
    Y. Charusi, M. C. Fishbein, R. Kass, A. Miyamoto, W. Shell,
    and H. J. C. Swan, Intracoronary thrombolysis in evolving
    myocardial infarction, Am.Heart J.(in press) (1981).
72. H. Huchard, Traite des maladies du coeur et des vaisseaux
    arteriosclerose, aortites, cardiopathies arterielles, angines
    de poitrine, Paris, p.466 (1889).

73. W. Osler, The Lumlcian lectures on angina pectoris II, Lancet
    839-844 (1910).
74. L. Gallavardin, Les angines de poitrine, Paris, p.45 (1925).
75. H. Yasue, M. Youyama, H. Kato, S. Tanaka, and F. Akiyama,
    Prinzmetal's variant form of angina as a manifestation of
    alpha-adrenergic receptor mediated coronary artery spasm:
    documentation by coronary arteriography, Am.Heart J. 91:148
    (1976).
76. D. L. Levene and M. R. Freeman, Alpha adrenoceptor-mediated
    coronary artery spasm, JAMA 236:1018-1022 (1976).
77. D. R. Ricci, A. E. Orlick, P. R. Cipriano, D. F. Guthaner, and
    D. C. Harrison, Altered adrenergic activity in coronary
    arterial spasm: insight into mechanism based on study of
    coronary haemodynamics and the electrocardiogram, Am.J.Cardiol.
    43:1073 (1979).
78. D. Robertson, R. Robertson, A. Nies, J. Oates, and G. Friesinger,
    Variant angina pectoris: investigation of indexes of sym-
    pathetic nervous system function, Am.J.Cardiol. 43:1080 (1979).
79. G. Arnulf, De la section du plexus pre-aortique: justification
    et technique, Press Med. 47:94 (1939).
80. M. E. Bertrand, J. M. Lablanche, M. Rousseau, H. Warenbourg,
    C. Stankowiak, and G. Loots, Surgical treatment of
    Prinzmetal's variant angina. Utility of plexectomy associ-
    ated with aortocoronary bypass, Circulation 61:877-882 (1980).
81. O. Parodi, A. Maseri, and I. Simonetti, Management of unstable
    angina at rest by verapamil: a double blind cross-over
    study in CCU, Br.Heart J. 41:167 (1979).
82. J. E. Muller and S. J. Gunter, Nifedipine therapy for
    Prinzmetal's angina, Circulation 57:137 (1978).
83. M. Previtali, J. A. Salerno, and L. Tavazzi, Treatment of angina
    at rest with nifedipine: a short term controlled study,
    Am.J.Cardiol. 45:825-830 (1980).
84. P. Maurice, B. Lancelin, and J. L. Guermonprez, Traitment de
    l'anger de Prinzmetal par le diltiazem, 8th Congres Europeen
    de Cardiologie, Paris, p.127 abstract, (1980).
85. S. Chierchia, F. Crea, G. Gasperetti, R. De Caterina, and A.
    Maseri, Effects of alpha-adrenergic blockade with phen-
    tolamine in vasospastic angina, in: "Alpha Blocking Agents:
    Experimental and Clinical Pharmacology," Masson, Paris
    (in press).
86. S. Chierchia, R. De Caterina, C. Brunelli, F. Crea, C. Patrono,
    and A. Maseri, Low dose aspirin prevents thromboxane A_2
    synthesis by platelets but not attacks of Prinzmetal's
    angina, Circulation (abstract) 62 (Suppl.)III-215 (1980).
87. S. Chierchia, F. Crea, W. Bernini, R. De Caterina, and A. Maseri,
    Results of prostacyclin (PG_{12}) continuous infusion in angina
    at rest (abstract) Circulation 62 (Suppl.III):310 (1980).
88. A. Jouve, La place de la Medecine Psychosomatique en cardiologie,
    Coeur et Med.Int. VII:327-331 (1968).

89. R. N. MacAlpin, Correlation of the location of coronary arterial
       spasm with the lead distribution of ST segment elevation
       during varian angina, Am.Heart J. 99:555-564 (1980).
90. S. Severi, G. J. Davies, A. Maseri, P. Marzullo, and A. L'Abbate,
       Long term prognosis of variant angina with medical treatment,
       Am.J.Cardiol. 46:226-232 (1980).

FATE OF THE CORONARY MICROVASCULATURE IN INFARCTING CANINE

MYOCARDIUM: ROLE OF COLLATERAL BLOOD FLOW

Jutta Schaper

Max-Planck-Institute
Department Experimental Cardiology
Benekestrasse 2, D-6350 Bad Nauheim

It has been shown in many studies (for review see[1]) that occlusion of a left coronary descending artery in an initial phase produces ultrastructural symptoms of myocardial ischemia that finally pass the phase from reversible to irreversible injury, i.e. infarction. Duration of coronary artery occlusion, actual oxygen consumption of the left ventricle, and absence or presence of collateral perfusion have been shown[2] to be factors modifying the speed of development of infarction, but after 24-48 hrs the final infarct size of 80% of the area at risk will, nevertheless, be present. Collateral blood vessels apparently do not influence very significantly final infarct size, but they greatly modify the process of infarction, as will be described in the following text. All data relate to ultrastructural observations made on cardiac tissue from dog hearts subjected to experimental myocardial infarction by occlusion of a coronary artery.

Electron microscopic investigation of needle biopsies taken from the center of the infarcted area or from a normally perfused part of the left ventricle revealed the following changes in the myocardial microvessels:

1. Microvessels from nonischemic myocardium contained an abnormally large number of neutrophil granulocytes even after a relatively short occlusion time such as 90 min (Figure 1). The fact that the surrounding myocardial cells were of normal appearance lead to the conclusion that these leucocytes were "on their way" to the ischemic zone. It is well known from histologic pathology that leucocytes accumulate between the 6th and 24th hour of infarction in afflicted tissue to form the characteristic demarcation line between infarcted and noninfarcted tissue.

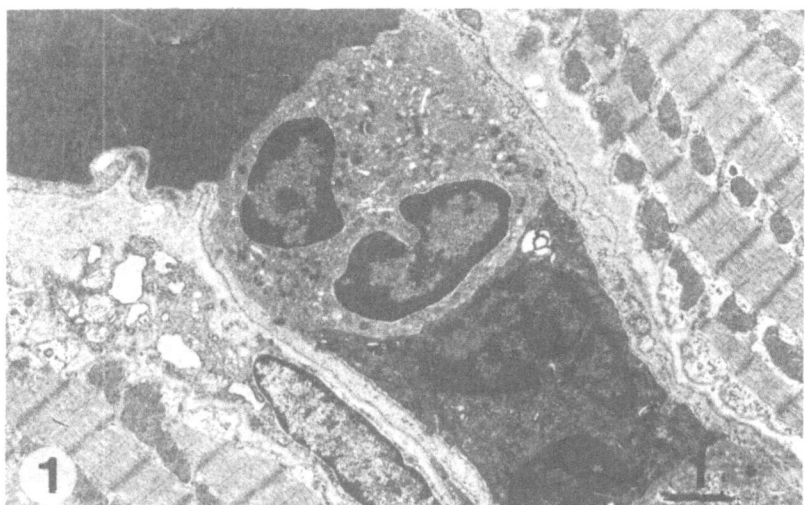

Fig. 1.   Nonischemic myocardium.   Intact microvessels containing
          neutrophils and erythrocytes.

2.   On the other hand neutrophil granulocytes were already observed
     in microvessels of ischemic or already infarcted myocardium
     (Figure 2) as early as 45-90 min after occlusion. They fre-
     quently showed close adhesion to endothelial cells, i.e. the
     early inflammatory phenomenon of "stickiness", was observed.
     The endothelium in this case may either be intact (Figure 2)
     or it may show extensive cellular swelling (Figure 3). These
     granulocytes most probably leave the microvessels because they
     frequently showed adhesion to irreversibly injured myocardial
     cells (Figures 4, 5, 6). Accumulation of neutrophils in intact
     or damaged microvessels of ischemic myocardium and their im-
     migration into the injured tissue were observed at early stages
     of infarction and without any reperfusion of the tissue by
     loosening of the arterial ligature. Since by numerous careful
     measurements the collateral perfusion rate has been shown to
     vary between 5-20% of preischemic coronary blood flow,[2] it has
     been assumed that these blood cells entered the ischemic myo-
     cardium via this route but not by capillary proliferation. It
     may be possible that ischemic myocardial cells provoke neutro-
     philic movements by releasing a potent chemotactic agent, such
     as histamine or other substances.
3.   Some microvessels with either intact or slightly injured endo-
     thelium showed an accumulation of erythrocytes, neutrophils
     and especially of platelets (Figure 7) indicative of formation
     of microthrombi during ischemia.

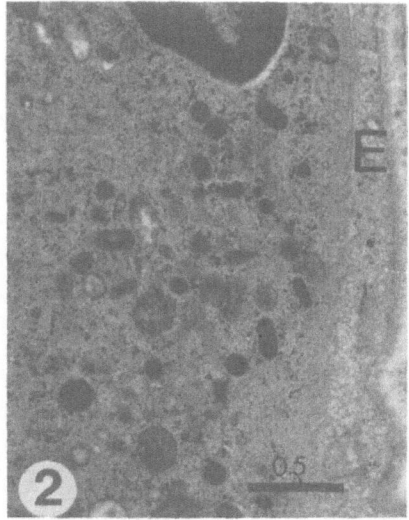

Fig. 2. Part of a neutrophil adheres closely to endothelial cell
(E) of microvessel from ischemic zone.

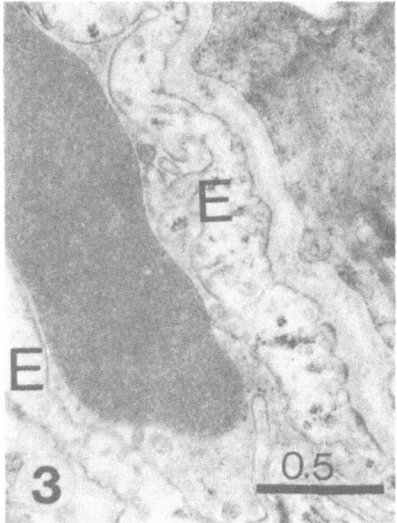

Fig. 3. Capillary endothelial cells (E) from ischemic myocardium.

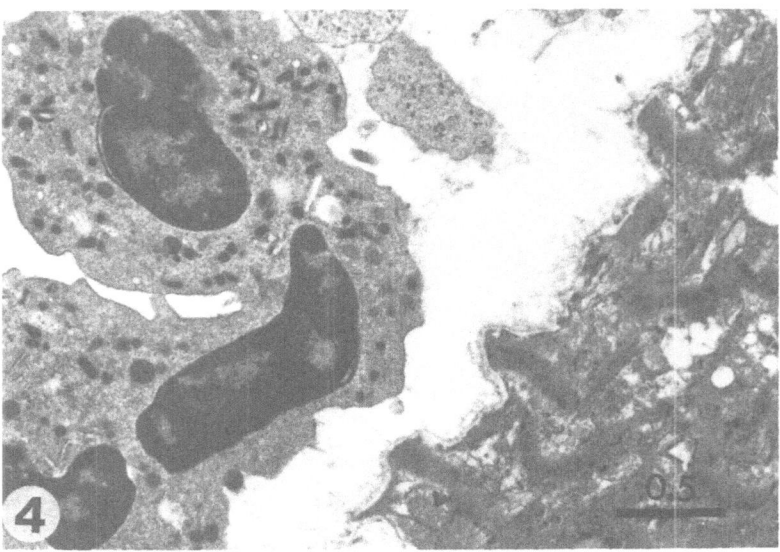

Fig. 4. Neutrophil in the interstitial space next to an irreversibly
         injured myocardial cell (left).

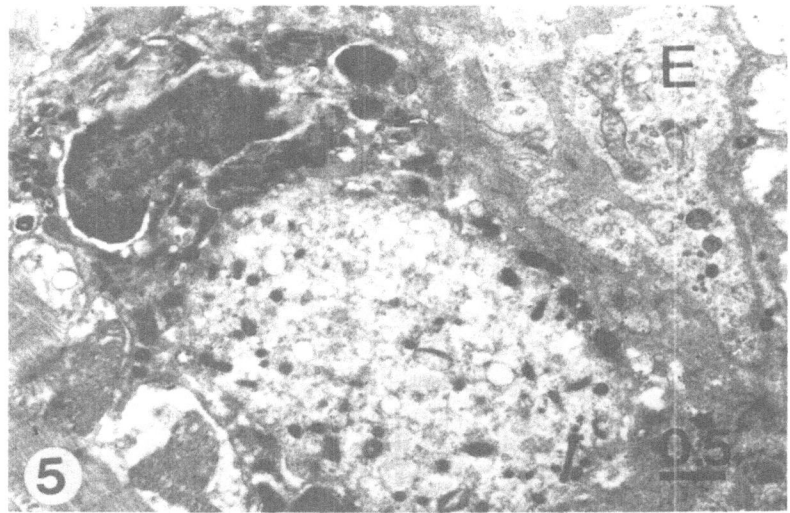

Fig. 5. Extravasation of neutrophils from capillary with swollen
         endothelium (E).

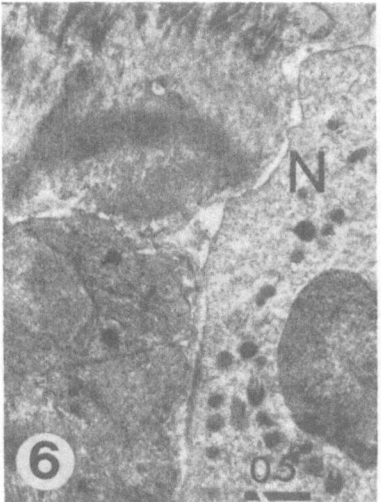

Fig. 6.   Neutrophil (N) closely adhering to irreversibly injured
          myocardial cell.

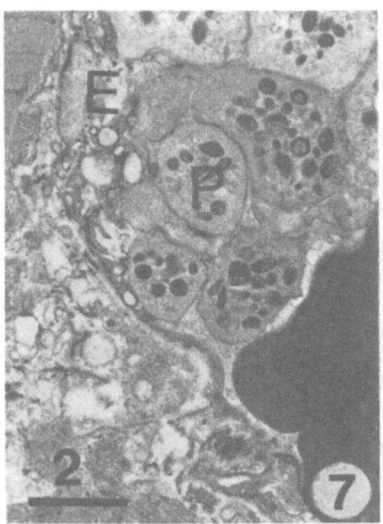

Fig. 7.   Intact venule from ischemic zone (E) containing platelets
          (P) and erythrocytes.

4.   Microvessels in ischemic myocardium that did not receive any
     collateral blood flow contained "old" erythrocytes (ghosts)
     and cellular debris (Figure 8). Destroyed microvessels were
     numerous even in hearts with high collateral blood flow, a fact
     indicative of inhomogeneous distribution of persisting coronary
     flow and thereby also indicative of an insufficient total blood
     supply.
5.   First symptoms of tissue reparation were observed already
     during the first 6 hrs of the infarction process. Ultrastruc-
     turally, this was evidenced by the occurrence of monocytes be-
     sides erythrocytes and neutrophils, within as well as outside
     of the microvessels, and by the presence of macrophages (origi-
     nated from blood monocytes), fibroblasts and histiocytes in the
     extracellular space (Figures 9, 10).

     Large parts of the cardiac microvasculature are destructed by
ischemic injury leading to infarction of the myocardium. Numerous
small vessels, however, that were supplied by collateral blood flow,
usually stay intact from a morphological point of view. These contain neutrophil granulocytes, erythrocytes, occasionally platelets,
and later on monocytes. These blood cells most probably are contributing to an early unspecific inflammatory reaction that may accelerate the destruction process of irreversibly injured myocardial
cells. In later stages of ischemia, these blood vessels facilitate
scar formation by providing blood cells and substances for proliferation of interstitial cells.

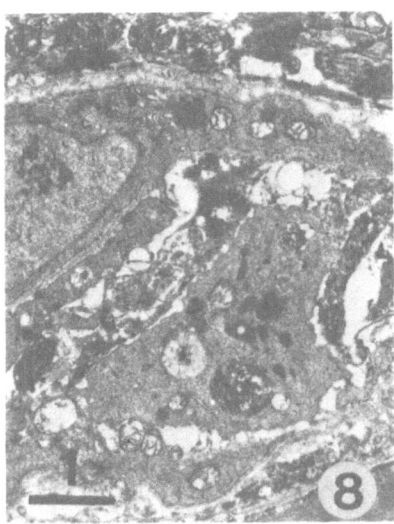

Fig. 8.   Completely destroyed microvessel from ischemic zone
          without collateral flow.

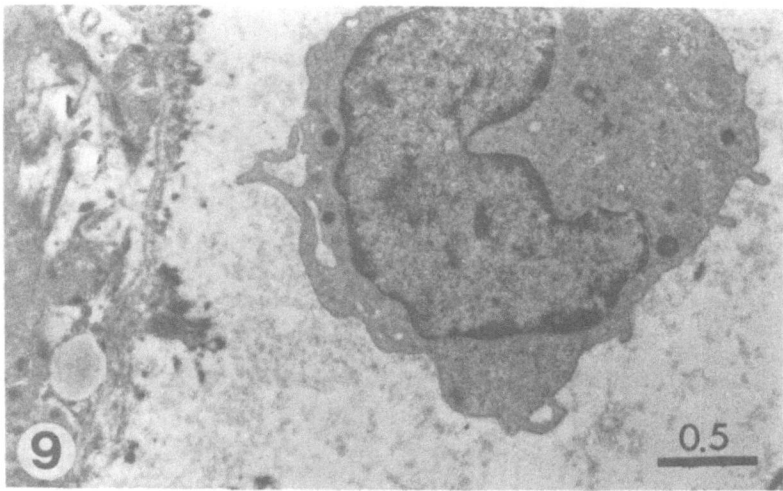

Fig. 9.   Monocyte transforming into a macrophagic cell is situated
          next to irreversibly injured myocardial cell (left).

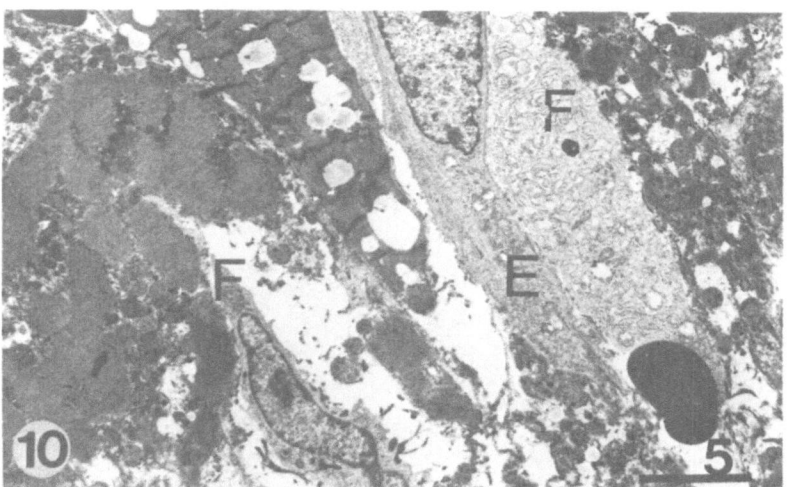

Fig. 10. Destruction of injured myocytes is accompanied by
          simultaneous proliferation of fibroblasts (F) and new
          microvessel (E).

     In the absence of collateral blood flow, on the other hand, an
inflammatory reaction is absent, destruction of myocytes occurs by
processes resembling autolysis, and scar formation, an essential

prerequisite for the survival of the heart as an intact entity, is an extremely slow process. The presence or absence of collateral perfusion of ischemic myocardium may therefore be regarded as an important factor contributing to the process of ischemic injury but also to scar formation and therefore to survival of the whole heart.

REFERENCES

1. Schaper, Jutta, Ultrastructural changes of the myocardium in regional ischemia and infarction, in: "Experimental Myocardial Ischemia and Infarction," W. Schaper, ed., Marcel Dekker, New York, in press (1982).
2. W. Schaper, The Pathophysiology of Myocardial Infarction, Elsevier/North-Holland Biomedical Press, Amsterdam, New York, Oxford (1979).

EPIDEMIOLOGY OF SUDDEN CARDIAC DEATH

William Ruberman and Eve Weinblatt

Health Insurance Plan
of
Greater New York

Although deaths due to coronary heart disease (CHD) have declined in the United States in the past decade, they still constitute
about one third of all deaths. Further, of all CHD deaths, one
third occur in persons under age 65, and about 60% occur outside the
hospital. Sudden cardiac death remains one of the major problems
facing medicine today.

In 1970 Lown and Ruberman[1] suggested that sudden death outside
the hospital was in large measure due to ventricular fibrillation.
They noted that such deaths occurred in persons with variable amounts
of acute ischemic damage and constituted a public health problem
requiring a broad range of strategies. But because such deaths for
the most part occurred shortly after onset of symptoms – or without
any overt symptoms – they concluded that early identification of
potential victims offered the best hope for prevention. Drawing
from experience in coronary care units,[2] they reasoned that evidence
of electrical instability of the myocardium in patients with CHD
might identify those at relatively high risk for sudden death.

In 1972 we began a study focused on this issue at the Health
Insurance Plan of Greater New York, a large prepaid group-practice
plan offering comprehensive medical care. From a population of
120,000 men aged 35-74, those with recent myocardial infarction (MI)
or effort angina were offered a special examination which included
one hour of single-lead ECG monitoring for ventricular arrhythmia,
as well as a standard ECG, clinical and laboratory observations.
Over a period of almost four years, 2155 men who met study criteria[3]
for MI (1739 men) or angina without prior MI (416 men) were examined
and monitored for ventricular premature beats (VPB). Patients were
followed for mortality for periods up to $5\frac{1}{2}$ years, with a minimum

observation of 2 years. Mortality status as of the cut-off date of
April 1, 1978 was known for all patients. There were 411 deaths
from all causes during this period, with 167 meeting study definition
of sudden cardiac death - occurring within minutes of the patient's
usual state of health in the absence of symptoms or findings suggesting acute MI. Non-sudden cardiac deaths were predominantly due
to recurrent infarction, but also included some ascribed to congestive heart failure.

Of the 1739 MI survivors monitored at baseline, 50% had experienced acute MI within the preceding 3 months and 30% within 4
to 8 months, while 9 or more months had elapsed in the remaining 20%.
Slightly over half of these patients showed one or more VPB during
the baseline monitoring hour, and these cases were in turn divided
about evenly between men with simple VPB only and those who had one
or more of the qualitative features defined as complex VPB - R on T,
runs of two or more, bigeminal or multiform beats. There is a
strong association between VPB of high frequency and the presence
of these complex features.[4] Of men with simple VPB only, less than
one fourth demonstrated 10 or more VPB in the hour, compared with
over three fourths of men with complex VPB.

Cumulative probability of death over a 5-year period is shown
in Figure 1 for men with and without complex VPB in the baseline
monitoring hour. Among the patients with complex VPB, 5-year mortality risk from any cause is almost twice (35% vs 20%) and risk of
sudden cardiac death is more than twice that of the men free of
such forms (18% vs 8%, Figure 2). For non-sudden cardiac deaths,
the corresponding rates are 15% and 7%. Figure 3 examines differ-
entials in cardiac death with respect to the presence of ventricular
arrhythmia in greater detail. In the upper half of the figure, we
see a very large risk for sudden cardiac death associated with the
presence of runs of 2 or more VPB or R on T during the monitoring
hour. Five years after baseline, the age-adjusted probability of
sudden death in these men was 25%, compared with 13% in men with
other forms of complex VPB, 12% in men with simple VPB only, and
6% in men with no VPB in the monitoring hour. In contrast, the
curves for non-sudden cardiac death (lower half of Figure 3) show no
difference between men with runs or early VPB and those with other
complex forms; nor is there any difference associated with the
presence of simple VPB in comparison with men free of any ventricular
ectopic activity. The age-adjusted relative risk for sudden cardiac
death over the 5-year period in the men with runs or R-on-T forms
is 4 to 5 times the risk of the men without VPB in the hour. But
the corresponding relative risk for non-sudden cardiac death in the
men with runs or early beats (or with other complex forms) is only
twice that of the men without any ventricular arrhythmia during
monitoring.

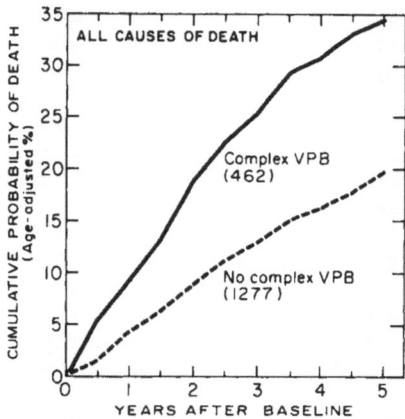

Fig. 1.   Mortality over a 5-year period among male survivors of
          myocardial infarction, in relation to presence of complex
          ventricular premature beats (VPB) during 1 hour of base-
          line monitoring.

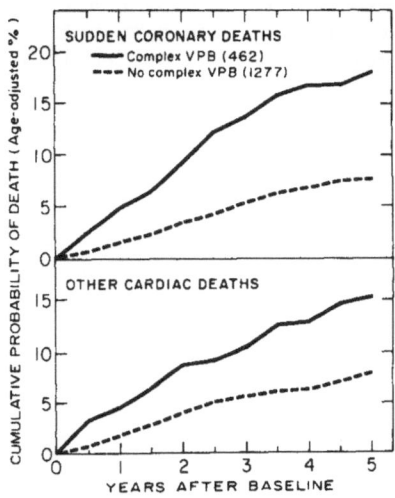

Fig. 2.   Sudden and non-sudden cardiac death over 5 years among
          male MI survivors, in relation to presence of complex
          ventricular premature beats (VPB) during 1 hour of base-
          line monitoring.

        Cross-classification of our data with respect to three strong
prognostic variables in this study - VPB, ST depression, and ex-

perience of congestive heart failure - and performance of age-
adjusted survival analyses reveal important mortality differences
in relation to how many of the three factors are positive. Table 1
shows that in moving from patients free of ST depression, congestive
heart failure and VPB during the monitoring hour to patients with
all three of these characteristics present, the 5-year cumulative
probability of death from any cause increases almost fivefold, from
11% to 52%. The gradient in risk in relation to the number of
positive characteristics suggests that each of these factors contributes independently to mortality risk. Although complex VPB are
indeed more likely to be encountered in the presence of other factors
associated with severe myocardial damage, multivariate analyses
establish that the presence of such beats makes a contribution to
poor prognosis that is independent of these other features.[5,6]

     In developing our first mortality data for the HIP studies on
VPB and sudden death, we examined the influence of social and personal characteristics on prognosis of the 1739 male MI survivors
over a period of three years after baseline examination.[7] Estimates
were developed, controlled for age, with respect to color, religion,
marital status, place of birth, work status, education, occupation,
alcohol and coffee consumption, smoking habits, and weight/height
ratio. With one important exception - educational attainment -
none of these characteristics showed any ability to identify men at

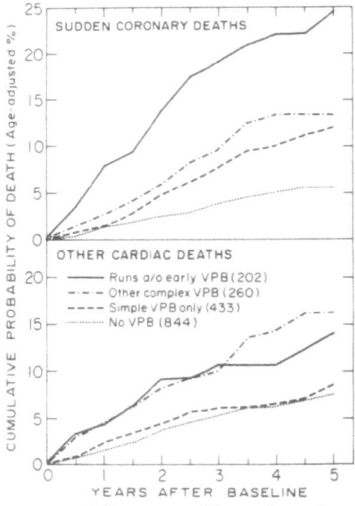

Fig. 3. Sudden and non-sudden cardiac death over 5 years among
         male MI survivors, in relation to type of ventricular
         premature beats (VPB) during 1 hour of baseline monitoring.

Table 1. Five-year mortality among male MI survivors in relation
to combinations of ST depression (STD), congestive heart
failure (CHF), and presence of one or more ventricular
premature beats (VPB) in one hour of baseline monitoring

No. of positive factors	STD	CHF	≥ 1 VPB	No. of patients	5-yr cumulative probability of death (age-adjusted %)	
					All causes	Sudden coronary
None	−	−	−	421	11.1	4.5
One only	+	−	−	178	20.2	6.1
	−	+	−	145	18.6	4.2
	−	−	+	327	18.5	10.1
Two	+	+	−	100	35.6	11.6
	+	−	+	224	30.3	16.5
	−	+	+	177	31.0	16.3
Three	+	+	+	166	51.9	28.4

relatively high, or low, risk of death. But among men who had completed only 8 years of schooling or less, a large disadvantage became apparent in comparison with the better educated men. Men in
the low education group who showed complex VPB in the monitoring
hour showed a far higher risk of sudden death than comparable men
in the high-education group. But in the absence of complex beats,
almost identical survival curves were found for the two education
categories (see Figure 4). Extending the follow-up period to produce
5-year mortality estimates did not change these relationships. The
excess risk for sudden death among low-education men demonstrating
complex VPB in the baseline monitoring hour persists in multivariate
analyses that control for other factors of importance. We are
currently exploring the hypothesis that low education may be a
marker for relatively high levels of psychosocial stress that favor
conversion of a chronic stable arrhythmia – complex VPB – to lethal
ventricular fibrillation.

Identification of ventricular ectopic activity in one hour of
ECG monitoring of men with effort angina but no antecedent MI also
served to select a group at elevated risk of death over the ensuing
5 years.[8] Among the 416 men with angina in the absence of prior
MI, those with VPB in the hour of monitoring showed a 5-year mortality risk of 28% compared with 12% for the men free of VPB. Thus,
among men with ischemic heart disease, ventricular ectopic activity
detected in one hour of monitoring serves to mark a group at elevated
risk of death, especially sudden death. Among patients with prior
MI, our findings with respect to sudden death define a gradient of
risk, from patients with no VPB in the hour, through those with
simple VPB only, to those at higher risk – men with complex VPB.
Among the latter, the subgroup with runs and/or early VPB is at

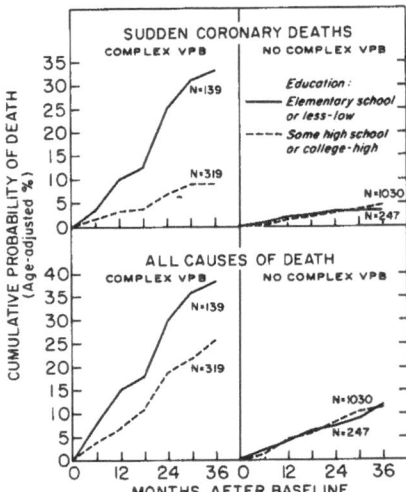

Fig. 4. Mortality over a 3-year period among MI survivors, according
to educational level and presence of complex ventricular
premature beats (VPB) in the baseline monitoring hour.

extremely high risk for sudden death, and this finding is consistent
with the hypothesis that such ectopic forms are uniquely related to
ventricular fibrillation. These findings emphasize the importance
of continued controlled trials of antiarrhythmic drugs in patients
with CHD to determine whether such use reduces the risk of sudden
cardiac death. Such an effect has recently been documented in two
large, controlled trials of beta-blockers.[9,10] Additional trials
of antiarrhythmic drugs in subsets of CHD patients could potentially
increase our ability to protect against the threat of sudden death.

REFERENCES

1. B. Lown and W. Ruberman, The concept of precoronary care,
    Mod.Con.Cardiovas.Dis. 39: (1970).
2. B. Lown, M. D. Klein, and P. I. Hershberg, Coronary and pre-
    coronary care, Am.J.Med. 46:705 (1969).
3. C. W. Frank, E. Weinblatt, S. Shapiro, G. E. Seiden, and R. V.
    Sager, The HIP study of incidence and prognosis of coronary
    heart disease: criteria for diagnosis, J.Chronic Dis. 16:
    1293 (1963).
4. W. Ruberman, E. Weinblatt, C. W. Frank, J. D. Goldberg, S.
    Shapiro, and C. L. Feldman, Prognostic value of one hour of
    ECG monitoring of men with coronary heart disease, J.Chronic
    Dis. 29:497 (1976).

5. W. Ruberman, E. Weinblatt, J. D. Goldberg, C. W. Frank, and
    S. Shapiro, Ventricular premature beats and mortality after
    myocardial infarction, N.Engl.J.Med. 297:750 (1977).
6. W. Ruberman, E. Weinblatt, J. D. Goldberg, C. W. Frank, B. S.
    Chaudhary, and S. Shapiro, Ventricular premature complexes
    and sudden death after myocardial infarction, Circulation
    64:297 (1981).
7. E. Weinblatt, W. Ruberman, J. D. Goldberg, C. W. Frank, S.
    Shapiro, and B. S. Chaudhary, Relation of education to
    sudden death after myocardial infarction, N.Engl.J.Med.
    299:60 (1978).
8. W. Ruberman, E. Weinblatt, J. D. Goldberg, C. W. Frank, S.
    Shapiro, and B. S. Chaudhary, Ventricular premature complexes
    in prognosis of angina, Circulation 61:1172 (1980).
9. The Norwegian Multicenter Study Group, Timolol-induced reduction
    in mortality and reinfarction in patients surviving acute
    myocardial infarction, N.Engl.J.Med. 304:801 (1981).
10. Beta-blocker Heart Attack Trial Research Group, A randomized
    trial of propranolol in patients with acute myocardial in-
    farction. I. Mortality results, JAMA 247:1707 (1982).

NEURAL FACTORS IN SUDDEN DEATH

Peter J. Schwartz

Centro di Fisiologia Clinica e Ipertensione
Ospedale Maggiore and University of Milan
Via F. Sforza, 35, 20122 - Milan, Italy

To understand the relationship between the nervous system and ventricular fibrillation, the leading cause of sudden death, is a key factor to comprehend the underlying pathophysiologic mechanisms, to establish rational preventive measures, and to improve the early identification of high risk patients. Considerable progress has been made during the last decade[1,2,3] and some of the main points will be mentioned here, including the problem of adequate animal models for sudden death, the role of psychologic stress, of the cardiac sympathetic nerves and of the vagi, and the potential for autonomic reflexes to be used for the identification of high risk subgroups.

A recent realization is the need for appropriate animal models for sudden cardiac death; this is important both for understanding the different roles of the main factors involved and for a meaningful assessment of antiarrhythmic interventions. Too often drugs are claimed to have a major antiarrhythmic effect on the basis of results obtained in conditions too different from those relevant to the clinical problem. The following is a model specifically designed to explore the role and interaction of a few factors, all clinically relevant, in the genesis of sudden cardiac death, with special care for the autonomic nervous system. Briefly, dogs undergo implantation for chronic measurement of various hemodynamic variables and balloon occluders are placed around the left descending and left circumflex coronary arteries. The dogs are subjected to submaximal exercise on a motor-driven treadmill for 18 minutes. At the 17th minute a balloon occluder is inflated for 2 minutes and acute myocardial ischemia is produced. Thus, this short-lasting ischemia episode affects the last minute of exercise and the first minute after exercise, and this sequence of events allows separation between

467

arrhythmias dependent on cessation of exercise or on release of occlusion. This protocol begins 3 weeks after initial surgery and is repeated after production of an anterior or inferior myocardial infarction.[4] Grossly, this model resembles what may happen to a patient with a prior myocardial infarction who engages in physical activity and has a brief reduction in coronary flow (spasm?) leading to acute myocardial ischemia, cardiac pain and arrest of exercise. A critical point is represented by the fact that such a brief myocardial ischemia does not induce ventricular arrhythmias at rest; however, when it is coupled with exercise, it results in a high incidence of life-threatening arrhythmias, which are particularly frequent immediately after cessation of exercise. In this new model, the ventricular tachyarrhythmias depend on the interaction between acute myocardial ischemia, level of heart rate, exercise and its cessation, and vagal and sympathetic reflexes. Using this protocol, ventricular tachyarrhythmias occurred in 8 of 15 control dogs (53%) culminating in ventricular fibrillation in 6 (40%). Ten dogs were studied 3 weeks after production of an anterior myocardial infarction and in this group the incidence of ventricular arrhythmias and of ventricular fibrillation was higher (70% and 60%, respectively). It is noteworthy that most instances of ventricular fibrillation occurred immediately after cessation of exercise. The underlying mechanism for this still unexplained specific temporal relationship is under investigation; in any case, it bears a striking similarity with what happens in most sudden deaths in athletes. Do autonomic interventions affect the susceptibility to ventricular fibrillation in this setting? Preliminary data suggest an affirmative answer, because in 10 dogs with an anterior myocardial infarction that were studied after left stellectomy, ventricular arrhythmias occurred in only two cases (20%) and ventricular fibrillation in none, despite the fact that heart rate was even higher compared with that of control animals.

Psychologic stress has been shown to precipitate life-threatening arrhythmias, both experimentally and clinically. Lown, Verrier and their associates have demonstrated that the exposure to a stressful environment is sufficient to induce ventricular tachyarrhythmias in a dog with a recent myocardial infarction.[5] Very recently they have shown that psychologic stress can increase coronary artery resistance and lower the threshold for repetitive extrasystole, an index of vulnerability to fibrillation.[6] These changes are mediated by increases in sympathetic activity and can be prevented by antiadrenergic interventions. The idiopathic long QT syndrome is a clinical entity in which ventricular fibrillation frequently occurs following a psychologic stress and unquestionably represents the most provocative example of neurally mediated non-coronary sudden death. Experimental and clinical evidence supports the concept that it depends on a congenital imbalance in cardiac sympathetic innervation with a dominance of left sided nerves, secondary to a lower-than-normal right cardiac sympathetic activity.[7]

Our data on almost 600 patients with the idiopathic long QT syndrome indicate that mortality in untreated patients is 78% and with beta-adrenergic blockade is reduced to 7%; 41 patients, who continued to have syncopal episodes despite full dose beta-blockers, thus constituting a subgroup at a even higher risk, underwent left stellectomy and only 3 of them (7%) died subsequently. If these patients had not received this surgical treatment the mortality figure for beta-adrenergic blocking agents would undoubtedly be higher. Thus, anti-adrenergic interventions seem to have radically modified the prognosis of these patients.

A new and important concept is that right and left cardiac sympathetic nerves exert a different influence on cardiac arrhythmias and, more specifically, that left sided nerves have a particularly high arrhythmogenic potential.[8] This is partially due to their quantitative dominance at ventricular level. Stimulation of the left stellate ganglion may induce ventricular tachyarrhythmias, even in the absence of acute myocardial ischemia, in dogs and in man. In conjunction with myocardial ischemia activation of the sympathetic nervous system, or of the left sided nerves alone, easily induces ventricular fibrillation.

The high arrhythmogenic potential of left sided cardiac sympathetic nerves, discussed earlier, has unavoidably led to the realization of the antiarrhythmic effect of their removal. We have indeed shown that left stellectomy has several effects which, directly or indirectly, increase the electrical stability of the heart.[9] It reduces the ventricular arrhythmias associated with acute myocardial ischemia and increases the threshold for ventricular fibrillation. It lengthens the ventricular refractory period, thus decreasing cardiac excitability. It halves the incidence of ventricular fibrillation in conscious dogs undergoing an episode of acute myocardial ischemia one month after an anterior myocardial infarction. It reduces to zero (0 out of 10) from 60% (6 out of 10) the incidence of ventricular fibrillation in dogs subjected to a brief episode of acute myocardial ischemia superimposed at the end of an exercise stress test, also in this case one month after an anterior myocardial infarction. Also, left stellectomy by increasing the capability of coronary bed to dilate, both at rest and during exercise, may limit the ischemic area by improving the perfusion of the border zone and contribute to the preservation of ventricular function.

It is noteworthy that the antiarrhythmic effect of left stellectomy, at variance with the most of antiarrhythmic drugs, is not accompanied by a negative inotropic effect. Thus, myocardial contractility is not reduced by left stellectomy neither at rest nor during an exercise stress test. Of particular clinical relevance is the fact that this lack of negative effects on the contractility of the left ventricle is present also in dogs with a prior myo-

cardial infarction performing an exercise stress test. Also in man
left stellectomy does not induce the appearance of dyspnea on effort
during an exercise stress test at variance with what happens with
bilateral stellectomy, which indicates the opportunity of not entirely
depriving the heart of adrenergic support.

These data have led to a multicenter trial, ongoing in Northern
Italy since 1979, in which a subgroup of patients with an anterior
myocardial infarction at high risk for sudden death is randomized
between placebo, the beta-blocker oxprenolol and high thoracic left
stellectomy.

A growing body of evidence, largely obtained by Lown and Verrier,
suggests that enhancement in vagal efferent activity, when is not
excessive, has a salutary effect in protecting from sympathetically
induced decreases in cardiac electrical stability. This effect
partly depends on the maintenance of an optimal heart rate, preventing
excessive tachycardia, which preserves underperfused tissue from
advancing ischemia and partly depends on an electrophysiologic effect
which seems to be mediated by a cholinergic antagonism of adrenergic
effects.

The knowledge of both the arrhythmogenic potential of high sympathetic activity and of the protective action of increased vagal
activity led us to investigate the possibility that the analysis of
autonomic reflexes could identify subgroups at high risk for sudden
death.[10] Baroreceptor reflex mediated changes in heart rate can
provide a meaningful way to assess autonomic neural control of the
heart. Seventeen dogs were chronically instrumented and studied
four weeks after an anterior myocardial infarction. The animals
were given i.v. injections of phenylephrine and nitroprusside to
raise or lower systolic arterial pressure by 30-55 mmHg. The R-R
intervals versus the systolic pressure of the preceding beats were
plotted and the baroreflex slope was determined. On a subsequent
day a 2 min. occlusion of the left circumflex coronary artery was
initiated at the beginning of the last minute of an exercise stress
test and was continued for 1 min. after the cessation of exercise,
as discussed above. The animals were divided into two groups on
the basis of their response to this test; 11 animals had ventricular
fibrillation (65%, susceptible), whereas 6 dogs (35%) did not and
survived (resistant). When the baroreflex slopes of the two groups
were compared it was evident that they were strikingly different
because the slopes of the resistant dogs were much steeper (11±4.5
vs 4.5±2 msec/mmHg); also the heart rate reduction for a 30 mmHg
increase in arterial pressure was significantly different for the
resistant (-40±12 b/min) and for the susceptible dogs (-13±5 b/min).
This indicates that the resistant animals have a greater capability
to react with strong vagal reflexes, which has been shown to reduce
vulnerability to ventricular fibrillation. Also, among dogs with
a prior myocardial infarction, an almost flat baroreceptive slope

identifies a subgroup at very high risk for ventricular fibrillation. The possibility that these results may be applied to man and that may help in identifying high risk patients after a myocardial infarction is currently under investigation. This study stresses further the tight relationship between the autonomic nervous system and the susceptibility to sudden death.

REFERENCES

1. P. J. Schwartz, A. M. Brown, A. Malliani, and A. Zanchetti, "Neural Mechanisms in Cardiac Arrhythmias," Raven Press, New York (1978).
2. B. Lown, Cardiovascular collapse and sudden cardiac death, in: "Heart Disease," E. Braunwald, ed., W. B. Saunders, Philadelphia (1980).
3. P. J. Schwartz and H. L. Stone, The role of the autonomic nervous system in sudden coronary death, Ann.NY.Acad.Sci. 382:162 (1982).
4. P. J. Schwartz, G. E. Billman, and H. L. Stone, Autonomic interventions in a new animal model for sudden death, Circulation Suppl.IV 64:289 (1981).
5. B. Lown, R. L. Verrier, and R. Corbalan, Psychologic stress and threshold for repetitive ventricular response, Science 182:834 (1973).
6. R. L. Verrier, F. Lombardi, and B. Lown, Effects of different types of behavioral stress on coronary hemodynamics, Fed. Proc. 41:1599 (1982).
7. P. J. Schwartz, The long Q-T syndrome, in: "Sudden Death," M. E. Kulbertus and H. J. J. Wellens, eds., M. Nijhoff, The Hague (1980).
8. P. J. Schwartz, Sympathetic imbalance and cardiac arrhythmias, in: "Nervous control of Cardiovascular Function," W. C. Randall, ed., Oxford University Press, in press (1982).
9. P. J. Schwartz and H. L. Stone, Left stellectomy in the prevention of ventricular fibrillation caused by acute myocardial ischemia in conscious dogs with anterior myocardial infarction, Circulation 62:1256 (1980).
10. G. E. Billman, P. J. Schwartz, and H. L. Stone, Baroreceptor reflex control of heart rate: a predictor of sudden cardiac death, Circulation 66: in press (1982).

MANAGEMENT OF THE PATIENT AT HIGH RISK

FOR SUDDEN CARDIAC DEATH

Bernard Lown, Thomas B. Graboys
Philip J. Podrid, and Steven Lampert

Cardiovascular Research Laboratories, Dept. of Nutrition
Harvard School of Public Health and The Cardiovascular
Division, Dept. of Medicine Brigham & Women's Hospital
Boston, MA

Can one protect the subject at high risk for sudden cardiac death? To be able to answer this question requires identification of the specific pathologic derangement contributing to the sudden fatality. However, in most victims of sudden cardiac death (SCD) no acute lesions are demonstrable. Autopsy studies document severe occlusive atherosclerotic disease of major epicardial coronary arteries.[1,2] But acute arterial events such as thrombosis of diseased vessels, hemorrhage into a plaque, fracture of atherosclerotic lesion are observed in a minority of cases.[3] Even if coronary occlusion is not demonstrable, this does not preclude the occurrence of myocardial infarction. But even with sensitive stains, a majority of patients dying suddenly exhibit no evidence of myocardial infarction. Reichenback and coworkers[4] noted such findings in only 5% of sudden death victims.

How then is one to identify the subject at risk; and once identified, how is the potential victim to be protected? It is this latter question that we want to concern ourselves with, namely, management of the patient at high risk. The incidence of sudden cardiac death in a population with coronary heart disease is about 1% to 2% annually. It is therefore difficult to determine efficacy of any particular measure except as a multicenter trial involving many thousands of participants. While the use of beta-adrenergic blocking drugs is associated with a substantial reduction of mortality in the immediate period following acute myocardial infarction, treatment with antiarrhythmic drugs, as yet, has not been proven efficacious in such a population.

We have attempted to determine drug effectiveness somewhat differently, namely, by focusing on the patient who is exhibiting life threatening ventricular arrhythmias. Increasing numbers of patients are now presenting who have been resuscitated from sudden death. In fact they present an explicit syndrome (see Table 1). Such resuscitated patients are at high risk for having recurrence.[5] Thus, the mortality was 26% at 1 year and 36% at 2 years. Most of those dying had a second episode of ventricular fibrillation. The high risk for recurrence indicates that only modest numbers of patients are required to ascertain drug effectiveness.

Another group of patients that can be profitably studied involve those who have potentially malignant ventricular arrhythmia. The availability of cardioversion and lidocaine have contributed to the survival of many patients with recurrent episodes of hemodynamically compromising ventricular tachycardia. We have designated as malignant arrhythmia, those patients who have experienced either ventricular fibrillation or have had repeated episodes of sustained ventricular tachycardia with either syncope or hemodynamic decompensation.

The essential hypotheses actuating our work is that sudden cardiac death is due to ventricular fibrillation. The putative background condition is electrical instability of the myocardium. By that, we mean a predisposition of the myocardium to respond to stimuli of threshold intensity with repetitive reentrant arrhythmia. Furthermore, we believe that the presence of certain ventricular premature beats (VPBs) constitute markers for electrical instability of the myocardium. These concepts have been extensively reviewed.[6,7]

VPBs AS RISK FACTORS

Coronary risk factors, either individually or in combination, do not select patients predisposed to sudden cardiac death. Other identifying factors need to be found. It has been our view that the electrical instability of the myocardium long antedates the terminal event which results from an electrical accident. Because the mechanism of sudden death is invariably ventricular fibrillation, it is logical to regard arrhythmias as potential harbingers.[8] We have therefore hypothesized that advanced grades of ventricular premature beats in patients with ischemic heart disease constitute markers of susceptibility to ventricular fibrillation.[9,10] Numerous reports associate the presence of ventricular ectopic activity during longer monitoring intervals with increased occurrence of out-of-hospital sudden cardiac death.[11-17]

The mere presence of VPBs in a single hour of monitoring, however, has limited prognostic significance. The fact that ventricular premature beats are noted in a majority of patients with ischemic

Table 1. Syndrome of Sudden Cardiac Death

Sex	Male (4:1)
CHD	75%
Acute Myocardial Infarction	Unusual
Prodromes	None
Death	Instantaneous
Mechanism	V.F.
VPBs	Present and of advanced grade
Recurrence after resuscitation	30% annually

heart disease argues that if ectopic beats augment the risk for sudden death, this property must be ascribed to some special attributes rather than mere occurrence. While VPBs are prevalent in a population without evident heart disease, complex forms are noted in less than 2% of such patients.

The grading of VPBs is compelled by some of the consideration discussed below and is presented in Table 2.

EARLY CYCLE VPBs

Patients in whom an extrasystole interrupts the T wave, the so-called R-on-T phenomenon, are predisposed to major ventricular arrhythmias. This conclusion finds support in animal work as well as in clinical observations. In early days, when pacemakers were not synchronized, but discharged randomly, a number of reports documented the occurrence of ventricular fibrillation when the pacer pulse accidentally discharged during the vulnerable period occurring at the apex of the T wave. Recently the significance of R-on-T VPBs has been questioned, this is based on several misunderstandings:[18]

1. Ventricular tachycardia and ventricular fibrillation are two distinct electrophysiologic disorders. T-wave interruption is of significance in the genesis of ventricular fibrillation but not in ventricular tachycardia. Campbell and coworkers[19] have demonstrated that R-on-T VPBs triggered ventricular fibrillation in 16 of 17 episodes. Such early ectopics initiated arrhythmia in only 4 of 250 odd patients with ventricular tachycardia.
2. Early cycle VPBs are rarely encountered except in the presence of acute myocardial ischemia or infarction or in patients with severe heart disease, these are the very subjects with increased susceptibility to sudden death. The study by Campbell[19] indeed confirmed that the incidence of early VPBs was highest in the first 3 hours after onset of myocardial infarction. Thereafter, mid and late cycle VPBs were preeminent.

Table 2. VPB Grading System

Grade	Characteristics
0	No ventricular beats
1A	Occasional, isolated VPBs (less than 30 per hour) less than 1 per minute
1B	Occasional, isolated VPBs (less than 30 per hour) more than 1 per minute
2	Frequent VPBs (more than 30 per hour)
3	Multiform VPBs
4A	Repetitive VPBs Couplets
4B	Repetitive VPBs Salvos (ventricular tachycardia)
5	Early VPBs (i.e. abbutting or interrupting the T-wave)

This grading system is applied to a 24-hour monitoring period and indicates the number of hours within that period that a patient has VPBs of a particular grade, which is expressed in the resulting "equation" as a superscript. Subscripts are used to indicate particular aspects of the VPBs of a given grade. In the equation below, for example, the subscript of grade 2 indicates the approximate total number of grade 2 VPBs over the 24-hour period; for grade 3 it denotes the number of different forms observed in any single hour; for grade 4B the two subscripts indicate first the largest number of paroxysms of tachycardia in a single hour and the second denotes the maximum number of successive cycles; for grade 5 the subscript represents the largest number of early ectopic beats in any single hour. A complete translation is given below for this particular equation:

$$0^3 \quad 1A^0 \quad 1B^4 \quad 2^6_{760} \quad 3^6_2 \quad 4A^2_3 \quad 4B^2_{4-7} \quad 5^1_3$$

Grade	
0	Occurred during 3 hours
1A	No infrequent VPBs
1B	Infrequent VPBs but greater than 1 per minute observed during 4 hours
2	Occurred during 6 hours (with a total of 760 VPBs)
3	Occurred during 6 hours and exhibited two forms
4A	Occurred during 2 hours and their greatest frequency in any 1 hour was 3
4B	Occurred during 2 hours, there were 4 paroxysms, the longest duration was 7 cycles
5	An early VPB was observed 3 times during a single hour in the 24-hour monitoring session

3. The prolonged QT interval has been recognized over many years as predisposing to sudden death, especially in patients who have frequent VPBs. This combination increases the likelihood of an ectopic beat discharging during the vulnerable period of the T wave and thereby triggering ventricular fibrillation.

4. When a late cycle ectopic beat initiates a paroxysm of tachyarrhythmia there is no certainty that the succeeding early cycle VPB was not the culprit. Several decades ago, Smirk[20,21] called attention to this phenomenon and designated it V-V' in which V is the late extrasystole and V' is the early one which interrupts the T wave of the preceding ectopic cycle and launches the tachyarrhythmia.

REPETITIVE VENTRICULAR PREMATURE BEATS

Animal studies have shown that discharging a stimulus during the vulnerable period does not provoke ventricular fibrillation unless a large electric current is delivered. Since extrasystoles carry but miniscule electric charges, how is ventricular fibrillation provoked? Significant is the fact that when extrasystoles are repetitive, the threshold of the vulnerable period is progressively reduced. Thus, in the ischemic heart a sequence of 3 early cycle extrasystoles lower the vulnerable period threshold to the point wherein fibrillation can be induced by current just sufficient for mid-diastolic depolarization.[22] Clinicians have long been aware of this physiologic relationship that salvos of ventricular ectopic beats, especially if they occur in accelerating sequences, are harbingers of ventricular fibrillation.

It has been our view that these categories of VPBs, namely, early ectopics interrupting T waves and those that fire in salvos, constitute the essential attributes which impart risk for ventricular fibrillation. These advanced grades of VPBs therefore help in identifying those predisposed to sudden cardiac death.

SEVERITY OF HEART DISEASE WITH VPBs IN RELATION TO THE RISK OF SUDDEN DEATH

It may be that the VPB is not an indicator of risk for SCD, but merely an expression of the type and severity of the underlying heart disease which is the decisive variable. A number of studies have shown an association between the severity of heart disease and the prevalence as well as grade of ventricular ectopic beats. Calvert et al.,[23] reported that the presence of advanced grades of VPBs correlated with the extent of coronary artery involvement, with elevation of left ventricular end-diastolic pressure and with the occurrence of assynergy. Schulze and coworkers,[24] who studied patients with myocardial infarction in the late convalescence phase, found that advanced grades of VPBs occurred predominantly among those having an ejection fraction of less than 40%. However, in a later follow-up, sudden death afflicted only those who had advanced grades of ectopic activity and spared those who had a low ejection fraction, but were free of such complex VPBs. Ruberman and co-workers[25] noted that men with congestive heart failure who did not exhibit advanced grades of VPBs during a one hour period of monitoring showed a lesser risk of sudden cardiac death compared to men who had exhibited congestive heart failure. The poor prognosis among those with advanced grades of VPBs was largely due to sudden cardiac death. Graboys and coworkers[26] studied a small exceptional group of patients who had no heart disease but experienced ventricular fibrillation. These patients showed the same constellation of VPB grade distribution as those with coronary heart disease who had experienced sudden death. The pattern of advanced grade was quite dissimilar among patients merely having ischemic heart disease. The VPB of advanced grade thus emerges as a predictor of mortality independent of a host of hemodynamic variables.

WHO NEEDS TO BE TREATED?

     At the present time predisposition to sudden death is indicated in the following subsets of patients: (1) among those resuscitated from ventricular fibrillation in the absence of myocardial infarction; (2) when potentially malignant ventricular tachycardia recurs frequently; (3) when ventricular tachycardia and multiple ventricular responses are precipitated by intracardiac electrophysiologic techniques; (4) when certain advanced grades of VPBs are exposed by monitoring and exercise testing in patients with ischemic heart disease (see Table 3).

     The vast majority of patients with VPBs require no therapy other than reassurance about the benignity and ubiquity of their disorder. Therapy is prescribed for a minority in whom arrhythmias prove symptomatically disabling. It needs to be emphasized that patients are generally unaware of irregular heart beats. This is true even when ectopic activity is abundant and renders the underlying rhythm seemingly chaotic.

HOW TO TREAT

     The physician confronts a number of clinical questions. How does one select a drug that is both effective and safe? How is an appropriate antiarrhythmic program to be instituted with economy of time and effort? How is one to know that a drug selected will be effective long range? How can one be certain that a particular dosing schedule will not result in chronic toxicity? Neither

Table 3.   Indications for Treatment of VPBs

---

1. Primary ventricular fibrillation in the absence of acute myocardial infarction.
2. Postmyocardial infarction < 6 months and grade 4 or 5 VPBs.
3. New onset of angina pectoris and grade 4 or 5 VPBs.
4. In patients with coronary heart disease accelerating salvos of ventricular tachycardia on 24-hour monitoring or exercise stress testing.
5. Peak exercise > 1 mm ST ↓ with grade 4 or 5 VPBs.
6. Advanced grades of VPBs during angina pectoris.
7. Prolonged QT syndrome with syncope and VPBs.
8. Flail mitral leaflet with symptomatic paroxysms of ventricular tachycardia.
9. Symptomatic arrhythmia.

---

electrophysiologic classification of drugs into categories based on attributes determined in isolated Purkinje fibers nor pharmokinetic concepts relating to the so-called therapeutic blood level have helped the clinician in selecting a drug for the individual patient. In effect present day therapy is largely pragmatic.

If pragmatism is to be the order of the day, there is need to admit this honestly and to systematize the approach. To accomplish a systematic approach, we have developed a strategy consisting of 4 phases: Phase 0 involves data acquisition, Phase 1 is based on acute drug testing, Phase 2 consists short-term drug maintenance and Phase 3 includes long-term chronic therapy.

PHASE 0 - DATA ACQUISITION

The objective of this Phase is to define the patient's level of spontaneous dysrhythmia. This constitutes a control period against which drug action is compared. When the patient enters the hospital, all cardioactive drugs including beta-adrenergic blocking agents, unless being employed for unstable angina, are discontinued. This has been mandated by our finding that life-threatening arrhythmias may result from the very agents used for their suppression.[27] We have not encountered rebound accentuation of an arrhythmia by abruptly stopping any drug. Digitalis drugs are maintained only if overt cardiac decompensation is present. During the drug-free period of 48 hours, continuous Holter monitoring and maximal symptom-limited exercise testing is carried out. Two 24 hour monitoring sessions provide adequate data relating to VPB variability and to the reproducibility of advanced grades. An exercise test is maximal, fatigue-limited and is accomplished on a motorized treadmill accord-

ing to a Bruce protocol. Phase O, in addition to providing baseline
data relating to the frequency and grade of VPBs, also permits
acquisition of insight as to psychologic and social factors which
may have contributed to the genesis of arrhythmia.

PHASE 1 - ACUTE DRUG TESTING

Crucial to the effectiveness of many antiarrhythmic drugs is
the establishment of a significant so-called therapeutic blood concentration.[31] This can be achieved by the oral administration of a
single large dose. The purpose of acute drug testing is to induce
a therapeutic blood level during a brief period to observe the
course of drug action and the extent of VPB suppression, and to
determine promptly whether any toxic complications ensue. Since
only a single dose is used, side effects, if any, are short-lived
and risk to the patient is brief (Table 4). Moreover, highly
trained personnel are in attendance at all times and are well
equipped to deal with threatening arrhythmias. By a series of such
tests with different drugs during phase 1 studies, one establishes
in a relatively short period of time which drugs are most effective.
The therapeutic objective is to eliminate grade 4 and 5 VPBs. When
a patient has been experiencing malignant ventricular arrhythmias,
the aim of phase 1 studies is to test efficacy of several antiarrhythmic drugs. If untoward effects emerge during long range
maintenance therapy, another effective agent can then be substituted
immediately without requiring costly hospitalization for retesting
and without exposing the patient to the hazard of interrupted therapy.

Acute drug testing involves four essential elements:

1. Administration of a single large oral dose of a selected anti-
    arrhythmic drug.
2. The use of programmed trendscription to display the time course
    of drug action.
3. Exercise on a bicycle ergometer to help define drug action and
    reproducibility.
4. Sampling of blood for drug concentration to permit correlation
    with the onset and dissipation of antiarrhythmic or toxic
    effects.[7]

Testing for Digitalis Effect

During this phase, the effect of digitalis drugs on VPB frequency and grade is determined as well. This is accomplished by
using acetyl strophanthidin, an ultra rapid acting digitalis-like
drug. We have found that acetyl strophanthidin will ameliorate
ventricular arrhythmia in nearly half the patients who have ectopic
activity.[28] If the patient's response is favorable, digitalization

Table 4. Antiarrhythmic Drugs and Dosages during Phase 1
and Phase 2 Studies

Drug	Phase 1 Acute Drug Test (Single oral dose, mg)	Phase 2 Short-term maintenance (mg/day)
Quinidine	600	1200-1600
Procainamide	1500	3000
Disopyramide	300	400-600
Propranolol	80	120-160
Metoprolol	100	100-200
Mexiletine	400	600-1200
Tocainide	---	1200-2400
Aprindine	200-300 (i.v.)	100-200
Pindolol	20	40-80

with digoxin is carried out. In 142 patients with VPBs who underwent testing with acetyl strophanthidin, the frequency and grade
were diminished in 65 or 46%. In this group, VPBs were reduced by
82% and in nearly half, all ectopic activity was abolished. The
antiarrhythmic action of acetyl strophanthidin did not appear to
depend on its positive inotropic effect. In 30 patients without
demonstrable heart disease, but with frequent VPBs, acetyl strophanthidin reduced or eliminated arrhythmia in 60%. It has been suggested that the action of digitalis glycosides to diminish or abolish
VPBs is due to an indirect reduction in Purkinje fiber automaticity
resulting from augmented vagus nerve tone. Such vagal enhancement
induces a lessening in adrenergic effects on the myocardium.

Electrophysiologic Studies

In about 20% of patients who have experienced malignant arrhythmias, ventricular ectopic activity is either scanty or non-repro-
ducible. In such patients invasive techniques are required to expose the presence of myocardial electrical instability and assess
its response to antiarrhythmic drugs. These techniques utilize
programmed electrical stimulation (see Podrid & Lown paper presented at this Congress).

Two approaches have been pursued: one involves the provocation
of ventricular tachycardia as an endpoint and was developed independently by Durrer et al.,[29] and Coumel et al.[30] The second approach is based on the induction of multiple ectopic beats following single, dual and triple pulses, and have been termed the multiple
repetitive response or (MRVR) or nonsustained ventricular tachycardia.

When sustained ventricular tachycardia is the endpoint employed,
complications are frequent. Ventricular fibrillation is provoked
in 10-15% of such studies. Not uncommonly the ventricular tachycardia does not respond to burst pacing and the arrhythmia results
in hemodynamic impairment, one has to resort then to cardioversion.
Our approach using nonsustained VT or MRVR as a marker of electrical
instability has significantly reduced the risk of provoking sustained
ventricular tachycardia or ventricular fibrillation.

PHASE 2 STUDIES

Short Term Drug Maintenance

After completion of phase 1 testing during which one or more
drugs have been shown to suppress advanced grades of arrhythmia, the
patient enters phase 2. In the minority of patients who require
electrophysiologic studies, the 2 phases are amalgamated. The aim
of this phase is to determine efficacy of antiarrhythmic drugs with
a dosing program simulating chronic drug administration. A further
aim is to assess patient tolerance of the antiarrhythmic agent with
chronic therapy. Antiarrhythmic drug efficacy is evaluated by means
of 24 hour Holter monitoring and maximal exercise testing.

In monitoring and exercise the criteria for therapeutic response involve:

1. Total abolition of grade 4B and 5 VPBs
2. Reduction of more than 90% in grade 4A VPBs
3. Greater than 50% reduction in the number of VPBs per 24 hours
   and/or a reduction of more than 50% in the number of hours
   during which grade 2 VPBs occurred compared to monitoring
   during phase 0 and during exercise a 50% reduction compared to
   the control preexercise stage.

If the underlying arrhythmia has been ventricular fibrillation,
more than one drug is employed. The use of drug combinations is the
rule - "a fail-safe" system of drug protection is mandated by the
high risk of recurrence.[32] Unlike other disorders wherein the physician may have opportunity to remedy a therapeutic error, this is
rarely the case with ventricular fibrillation. In addition to the
use of drugs, proper management of the patient requires attention
to the psychologic problems that abound in nearly every patient afflicted with malignant ventricular arrhythmias. The use of relaxation technique as well as other psychologic support has proven invaluable in contributing to amelioration of the refractory rhythm
disorder.

PHASE 3 - CHRONIC THERAPY

This is post hospital follow-up phase and defines long range drug efficacy. Furthermore, information is provided concerning the prevalence of complications with chronic use. In the majority of patients tested as indicated above, adverse reaction can generally be overcome by minor adjustments in daily dose. The type of screening we have outlined here prevents serious toxicity from surprising the physician and upsetting the sensitive apple cart of therapeutic management. At 3 to 6 month intervals, Holter monitoring and exercise stress testing is repeated to determine whether the arrhythmia remains under adequate control.

Drug-induced Arrhythmic Complications

The methods of management outlined here, especially phase 1 and phase 2 studies, alert the physician to drug-induced complications before serious injury has been incurred. We have encountered signigicant aggravation of arrhythmia with nearly all the drugs in current use.[27] A systematic examination of this problem has been conducted in 155 patients who were subjected to 722 drug studies. In 53 patients having 80 drug tests, aggravation of arrhythmia was observed in 11%. The criteria used to judge aggravation of the arrhythmic disorder included a four fold increase in VPB frequency, a ten fold increase in grade 4 and the first occurrence of ventricular tachycardia. In all cases blood drug levels were within the established therapeutic range. Thus, antiarrhythmic drugs in a substantial number of patients aggravate ventricular arrhythmias. Phase 1 and Phase 2 studies permit early detection of such susceptibility.

Long Range Therapeutic Results

If advanced grades of VPBs are indicators of electrical instability, their suppression should afford protection against sudden cardiac death. Our studies now encompass nearly 300 patients having malignant ventricular arrhythmias. When advanced grades of VPBs were controlled, the annual occurrence of sudden death was less than 3%. In 20% of patients in whom such an objective could not be achieved, sudden death exceeded 40% during the follow-up period.[32] Even when patients were matched for extent of hemodynamic deficit, survival was far better for those in whom evidence of myocardial electrical instability had been eliminated.

CONCLUSIONS

The present studies extending for more than 10 years indicate that the VPB hypothesis has been validated and is of practical significance. Advanced grades of ventricular ectopic beats, namely those of grade 4B and 5 are the targets of therapy. In 20% of patients recourse to invasive electrophysiologic techniques are required. There is need for multiple drug screening. Therapy must be individualized. A systematic approach involving acute drug testing as well as phase 2 studies facilitate identification of these drugs which are effective as well as those which are potentially hazardous. Ventricular fibrillation can be prevented by currently available antiarrhythmic drugs.

The problem now on the frontier of research is to identify more precisely the patient at risk for sudden death so as to justify interventions with antiarrhythmic agents.

Acknowledgements

Supported in part by Grant No. HL-07776, 24456 and 28387 from the National Heart, Lung and Blood Institute, National Institutes of Health, US Public Health Service, Bethesda, Maryland.

REFERENCES

1. J. A. Perper, L. H. Juller, and M. Cooper, Atherosclerosis of coronary arteries in sudden unexpected deaths, Circulation 52:111 (1973).
2. W. C. Roberts, Coronary arteries in fatal acute myocardial infarction, Circulation 45:215 (1972).
3. W. C. Roberts, Relationship between coronary thrombosis and myocardial infarction, Mod.Conc.Cardiovasc.Dis. 41:7 (1972).
4. D. D. Reichenback, N. S. Moss, and E. Meyer, Pathology of the heart in sudden cardiac death, Am.J.Cardiol. 39:865 (1977).
5. L. A. Cobb, A. P. Hallstrom, D. W. Weaver, M. K. Copass, and R. E. Haynes, Clinical predictors and characteristics of the sudden cardiac death syndrome, in Proceedings of the First U.S. - U.S.S.R. Symposium on Sudden Death, Yalta, October 3-5, 1977 (U.S. Department of Health, Education and Welfare, Public Health Service, National Institutes of Health, DHEW Publication No.(NIH) 78-1470 (1978).
6   B. Lown, Cardiovascular collapse and sudden cardiac death, in: "Heart Disease. A textbook of Cardiovascular Medicine," E. Braunwald, ed., W. B. Saunders, p.778 (1980).
7. B. Lown and P. J. Podrid, Ventricular premature beats: Why, when and how to treat, in: "Harrison Update II Principles of Internal Medicine," McGraw-Hill Co., p.131 (1982).
8. B. Lown and W. Ruberman, The concept of precoronary care, Mod. Concepts Cardiovasc.Dis. 39:97 (1970).
9. B. Lown and M. Wolf, Approaches to sudden death from coronary heart disease, Circulation 44:130 (1971).

10. B. Lown, Sudden death from coronary artery disease, in: "Early Phases of Coronary Heart Disease: The Possibility of Prediction," J. Waldenstrom, T. Larsson, and N. Ljungestedt, eds., (Skandia Internation symposia) Stockholm, Nordiska Bokhandelns Forlag, p.255 (1973).

11. L. A. Vismara, E. A. Amsterdam, and D. T. Mason, Relation of ventricular arrhythmias in the late hospital phase of acute myocardial infarction to sudden death after hospital discharge, Am.J.Med. 59:6 (1975).

12. L. E. Hinkle Jnr., S. T. Carver, and D. C. Argyros, The prognostic significance of ventricular premature beats in healthy people and in people with coronary heart disease, Acta Cardiol. (Brux.)Suppl.18:5 (1974).

13. W. Ruberman, E. Weinblatt, C. W. Frank, J. D. Goldberg, S. Shapiro, and C. L. Felman, Prognostic value of one hour of ECG monitoring of men with coronary heart disease, J.Chron. Dis. 29:497 (1976).

14. M. Kotler, B. Tabatznik, M. M. Mower, and S. Tominaga, Prognostic significance of ventricular ectopic activity with respect to sudden death in late post-infarction period, Circulation 47:959 (1973).

15. G. C. Oliver, Ventricular arrhythmias in coronary artery disease and their relationship to sudden death, in Proceedings of the First U.S. - U.S.S.R. symposium on Sudden Death, Yalta, October 3-5, 1977 (Bethesda, Maryland, U.S. Department of Health, Education and Welfare, U.S. Public Health Service, National Institutes of Health, Publication No.(NIH) 78-1470, p.171 (1978).

16. R. A. Schultze, H. W. Strauss, and B. Pitt, Sudden death in the year following myocardial infarction, Am.J.Med. 62:192 (1977).

17. A. Moss, R. Schnitzler, R. Green, and J. DeCamilla, Ventricular arrhythmias three weeks after acute myocardial infarction, Ann.Intern.Med. 75:837 (1971).

18. T. R. Engel, S. G. Meister, and W. S. Frankl, The "R on T" phenomenon. An update and critical review, Ann.Int.Med. 88:221 (1978).

19. R. W. F. Campbell, A. Murray, D. G. Julian, Ventricular arrhythmias in first 12 hours of acute myocardial infarction. Natural History Study, Br.Heart J. 46:351 (1981).

20. F. H. Smirk, R waves interrupting T waves, Brit.Heart J. 11: 23 (1949).

21. F. H. Smirk and D. G. Palmer, A myocardial syndrome with particular reference to the occurrence of sudden death and of premature systoles interrupting antecedent T waves, Am.J. Cardiol. 6:20 (1960).

22. P. J. Axelrod, R. L. Verrier, and B. Lown, Vulnerability to ventricular fibrillation during acute coronary arterial occlusion and release, Am.J.Cardiol. 36:776-782 (1975).

23. A. Calvert, B. Lown, and R. Gorlin, Ventricular premature beats
    and anatomically defined coronary heart disease, Am.J.
    Cardiol. 39:627 (1977).

24. R. A. Schultze, H. W. Strauss, and B. Pitt, Sudden death in the
    year following myocardial infarction, Am.J.Med. 62:192 (1977).

25. W. Ruberman, Ventricular premature complexes and sudden death
    after myocardial infarction, Circulation 64:297 (1981).

26. T. B. Graboys, M. B. Stockman, B. Lown, and P. Reich, "Lone"
    ventricular fibrillation, Circulation 58:195 (1978).

27. V. Velebit, P. J. Podrid, B. Lown, B.H. Cohen, and T. B. Graboys,
    Aggravation and provocation of ventricular arrhythmias by
    antiarrhythmic drugs, Circulation 65:5 (1982).

28. B. Lown, T. B. Graboys, P. J. Podrid, B. H. Cohen, M. B.
    Stockman, and C. E. Gaughan, Effect of a digitalis drug on
    ventricular premature beats (VPBs), N.Engl.J.Med. 296:301
    (1977).

29. D. Durrer, L. Schoo, R. M. Schulenbrug, and H. J. J. Wellens,
    The role of premature termination of supraventricular
    tachycardia in the WPN syndrome, Circulation 36:655 (1967).

30. P. H. Coumel, C. Cabral, A. Fabioto, R. Gourgon, and R. Slama,
    Tachycardia permanente per rhythm reciproque, Arch.Mal Coner.
    60:1830 (1967).

31. B. Lown, Ventricular premature beats in the recognition and
    management of the patient susceptible to sudden death, in
    Proceedings of the First U.S. - U.S.S.R. Symposium on Sudden
    Death, Yalta, October 3-5, 1977 (U.S. Department of Health,
    Education and Walfare, Public Health Service, National
    Institutes of Health, DHEW Publication No.(NIH) 78-1470
    p.79 (1978).

32. B. Lown and T. B. Graboys, Management of patients with malignant
    ventricular arrhythmia, Am.J.Cardiol. 39:910 (1977).

STROKE AND CARDIAC DISORDERS

E. V. Schmidt

Moscow

Combined lesions of the heart and the brain with circulatory
disorders in them are observed very often due to their common
etiology (atherosclerosis, hypotensive disease, other arterial
hypertensions) and frequent interdependence. The relations between
circulatory disorders in the both organs may be various.

Cardiocerebral pathology in which heart lesions produce disorders of cerebral circulation frequently with the development of
infarct in the brain occurs most often and is studied better than
other pathology. Copious literature deals with infarcts. I'd like
to mention two Symposia "Infarcts of Heart and Brain" held in
Cologne. Prof. Zülch who is present here was the chairman of these
Symposia.

Sharp fluctuations of coagulative and rheological properties
of the blood in the presence of changed vessels of the heart and
the brain can lead to simultaneous circulatory disorders in them
with the development of infarcts.

Another possibility when brain stroke produces disorders of
the coronary circulation and metabolism in the myocardium is
studied to a less extent. It is these cerebrocardial changes that
are the subject of the present communication.

The possibility of cerebrogenic disorders of the coronary
circulation and cardiac activity leaves no doubts although the
question about the possibility of cerebrogenic infarct remains to
be discussible.

Numerous experiments and observations of neurosurgeons demonstrated that actions on some areas of the brain cause disorders of the coronary circulation and cardiac activity. The limbico-hypothalamo-reticular complex and the hypophysial-adrenal system related to it are of primary importance.

Clinical manifestations of the cerebrocardiac syndrome in an acute stage of stroke are usually little pronounced and do not differ greatly depending on the character of stroke. They show up mainly as rhythm disturbances (tachycardia, transient arrhythmias). Pains in the region of the heart as a rule do not occur. Pronounced manifestations of cardiac or cardiovascular insufficiency are observed only when stroke is associated with myocardial infarction, pneumonia or when the terminal state develops.

Much has been already written about very common ECG changes in stroke but they still attract attention of investigators.

According to our data, 76.5% of patients in an acute stage of stroke exhibited in addition to ECG changes which are usual for ischemic heart disease and arterial hypertension other changes in ECG of the cerebrogenic character.

The most characteristic changes of these are sinus tachycardia, an increase of P wave, an elongation of Q-T interval, a displacement of S-T segment downward of the isoelectrical line, an inversion of T wave, presence or absence of U wave.

The most dynamic cerebrogenic changes in the ECG were disorders of cardiac rhythm and T wave which could rapidly change their form, disappear for some time and appear again, sometimes within several hours. On improvement of the patient's condition in most cases first of all heart rate became normal, arrhythmias disappeared, then displacements of S-T segment disappeared. Changes in T and U waves and an elongation of Q-T interval could be recorded for a longer period.

Individual cerebrogenic changes in the ECG as a rule are found in various combinations that enabled us to identify three variants of them depending on the degree of severity.

Variant I is characterized by cardiac rhythm disturbances, a moderate elongation (by 10-20%) of Q-T interval. Insignificant changes of T wave, presence of U wave can take place.

Variant II is characterized by a displacement below the iso-electrical line of S-T segment, an elongation of Q-T interval, changes of T wave up to inversion. There can be disturbances of cardiac rhythm and present of U wave.

Variant III observed in severe strokes is characterized by
an increase of T wave in the right or right and medial chest leads,
often in its combination with an inversion in the left chest leads;
T wave is not infrequently wide, U wave is often increased.

The cerebrogenic character of the above described changes in
the ECG is confirmed by their dynamics related to the course of the
process in the brain. They occur in the first days following stroke,
sometimes later - during deterioration of the patient's condition,
in the terminal state they become particularly pronounced. In a
favourable course of stroke they disappear already within the first
week but more often they persist for several weeks.

Also, we could often observe cases when the ECG recorded not
long before stroke was normal and following stroke it changed according to the type described above.

Cerebrogenic changes in the ECG were seen in hemorrhagic
strokes more frequently than in ischemic strokes (in 96.5% and 68.5%,
respectively) and were more pronounced- variants II and III were
encountered twice more often than in brain infarct.

In an acute stage of brain stroke the ECG changes are very
similar to those in subendocardial myocardial infarction.

The ECG changes in stroke reflect disorders of the coronary
circulation and metabolism of the cardiac muscle resulting from
direct, neurogenic, and indirect, humoral influences which we shall
dwell on later.

Recently Dimant and Grob (1977) and then Norris et al., having
carried out very thorough investigations found an increased content
of cardiac enzymes in the blood of stroke patients, in particular -
a significant elevation of the level of cardiac fraction of creatine
phosphokinase (CPK). Creatine phosphokinase was found already in the
initial phase of stroke and its level gradually increased. Thus
lesion of the myocardium is caused by stroke. We also noted a
considerable rise of CPK activity in an acute stage of stroke. These
studies show that organic changes in the heart in brain stroke
occur much more frequently than it has been considered until recently.

Post-stroke disorders of systemic hemodynamics show up as
changes in the cardiac output value and a reduction of the myocardial contractile function.

In most cases marked changes were found in hearts of patients
who had died from stroke. Light and electron miscroscopy showed
scattered dystrophic changes of myocytes in the form of eosinophylia
of plasma, disappearance of cross striation, fragmentation, vacuo-

lization and globular disintegration as well as disseminated foci
of myolysis and coagulative necrosis. Uneven and focal character
of damage of myocytes is combined with dystonia of vessels of the
microcirculatory bed. In some areas capillaries were paralytically
dilated with stases from erythrocytes and "coin columns"; in other
areas – thickened capillaries. There were plasmorrhagias, hemorrhages,
infiltrates from lymphoid elements and monocytes around some vessels.
Microvascular aneurysms observed so often in the brain in arterial
hypertension were not found.

Such changes which can be considered as "cerebrogenic" were
noted by us in 20.5% of stroke patients who had no pronounced atherosclerosis of the coronary arteries.

Recent myocardial infarctions in an acute period of stroke occur
usually on the background of already existing atherosclerotic changes
of the cardiac arteries. In such situations it is difficult to
establish cause and effect relations. However it is possible to
determine according to morphological signs which focus (in the
brain or in the heart) developed earlier.

The possibility of the development of extensive myocardial
infarction following stroke in the absence of pronounced atherosclerosis of the coronary arteries is in doubt and continues to be
discussed.

We recognize such possibility. I shall present two observations
to illustrate this. The both patients were elderly (aged 60 and
58) and suffered from hypertensive disease. They both developed
extensive hemorrhage into deep areas of the hemispheres, the blood
gradually went inside and eventually rushed into the ventricles.
In the first days the ECG showed only slight changes indicating
slowing of intraventricular conduction. Sudden death occurred
some days after stroke. Recent infarctions were found in the heart.
The coronary arteries proved to be unchanged: their ostia were wide,
there were no plaques in the intima along the course of the arteries.

One can suppose that in these patients myocardial infarction
resulted from spasm of the coronary arteries (like in subarachnoid
hemorrhage extensive infarcts develop in the brain due to spasm of
the arteries supplying the brain). But such cases are encountered
rarely. Among our 600 autopsy cases of stroke myocardial infarction
which can be considered as cerebrogenic occurred only in 3% of them.
Although in these cases (apart from the observations mentioned above)
atherosclerotic changes were found in the cardiac coronary arteries,
they did not cause stenosis of their lumina.

In all cases of cerebrogenic myocardial infarctions there
were either extensive brain infarcts damaging the hypothalamus or
the brain stem directly or as a result of edema and dislocation, or

deep hemorrhages. Cardiac infarction developed simultaneously or
several days after stroke if the volume of the focus in the brain
gradually increased.

Pathogenetic mechanisms responsible for disorders of the
coronary circulation and myocardial metabolism in stroke are very
complicated and have not yet completely been understood. By the
present the following conception is the most common.

Damage of the brain, mainly of the limbico-hypothalamo-
reticular region, leads to cardiac disorders in two ways: the
direct one through the cardiac nerves, and the indirect one -
through changes in the adrenal glands' functions.

The direct neurogenic action produces both neurotrophic and
vasomotor changes.

Recently V. Golubykh (1981) showed in experiments on dogs that
destruction of the hypothalamus in the region of the lateral
mamillary nucleus caused sympathetic constrictory reactions of the
coronary vessels. Earlier Melvill et al. by stimulating the hypothalamus in cats produced lesions of the myocardium including the
development of infarction; interruption of sympathetic tracts in
the spinal cord eliminated this effect.

Stress in the form of stroke leads to hyperfunction of the
sympathetico-adrenal system with an increase of serum level of
catecholamines whose "cardionecrotic effect" is well known. Excretion of catecholamines by nervous elements located in the heart
increases. Greenhoot and Reichenback (1969) demonstrated that the
most pronounced changes in the heart are found just near the endings
of the adrenergic nerve fibers excreting noradrenalin into the
extracellular space. An increased corticosteroid content in the
blood leads to a loss of intracellular potassium and thereby enhances the damaging action of catecholamines. Catecholamines also
increase platelet aggregation that worsens microcirculation and
contributes to formation of ischemic foci of necrosis.

Products of lipid peroxidation also have the damaging action
on the myocardium. In an acute period of stroke we found a sharp
rise of the content of the final product of peroxidation - malondialdehyde.

The data on disturbances of electrolyte balance in stroke are
extremely contrary and it is yet difficult to determine what concrete
role these shifts play in disorders of cerebral circulation.

During recent decade the attention of investigators was focused
on such highly active substances as prostaglandins and cyclic
nucleotides. Their role in disorders of cerebral circulation began
to be studied as well (Welch, Fukuda et al.).

The influence of prostaglandins (PG) on the frequency and rhythm of cardiac contractions, value of stroke volume, permeability of myocardial cell membranes, contractility of the cardiac muscle and on the coronary blood flow.

An important role in the mechanism of cerebrocardial interaction belongs also to the system of cyclic nucleotides responsible for realization of intracellular effects of catecholamines, serotonin, prostaglandins and other neurohumoral substances.

Our workers studied the contents of some prostaglandins and cyclic nucleotides in the blood and cerebrospinal fluid of patients with stroke. It turned out that concentrations both of prostaglandins and cyclic nucleotides elevated in the blood and CSF particularly in the first days of stroke, irrespective of its character. In the peripheral blood an increase of PG of E series was greater than that of $F_2\alpha$. A considerable elevation of PG level as well as some increase of cGMP took place in strokes with damage of the brain stem. In these patients the PGE level was three times increased and the level of PG $F_2\alpha$ was almost twice increased. These changes were much less pronounced in lesions of cerebral hemispheres. Only in two very severe cases of stem stroke causing death of the patients a predomination of PG $F_2\alpha$ was noted on the background of low general content of PG.

Concentration of both cyclic nucleotides (cAMP and cGMP) in the first days of stroke also increased, the cAMP concentration being greater so that their ratio noticeably changed. Subsequently dysbalance between individual fractions of PG and cyclic nucleotides reduced.

It should be noted that the content of cyclic nucleotides (especially cAMP) in the venous blood flowing off the brain was significantly greater than in the arterial blood that confirms their cerebral genesis.

The available data on the influence of prostaglandins and cyclic nucleotides on the cardiac activity and circulation make it possible to conclude that the change of their quantitative composition in the blood and cerebrospinal fluid of stroke patients exerts a certain influence on formation of cerebrocardial disorders. Dysbalance in ratio of pressor and depressor prostaglandins and their "mediators" - cGMP and cAMP, which in particularly severe cases of stroke manifests itself in predomination of vasoconstricting prostaglandins can lead to myocardial ischemia.

Activation of the prostaglandin and cyclic nucleotide systems in stroke patients can probably be of the compensatory and adaptative character; however in some cases as a result of hypercompensation shifts in these systems can turn into a pathologic factor exerting an unfavourable effect on myocardial blood supply and metabolism.

Summing up, it should be stressed first of all that cerebrogenic pathology of the cardiac activity and the coronary circulation in brain stroke is observed often and can be very serious up to the development of myocardial infarction. It aggravates the course of stroke and sometimes determines its outcome. Its presence should be taken into consideration by a therapeutist and a neurologist during elaboration of the programme of treatment.

The intimate mechanisms responsible for the development of this pathology are not quite understood and their further investigation is of great importance. The new methods of research - study of myocardial blood supply by using isotopes, ultrasound, echography, computed tomography, etc. will permit to evaluate more objectively and precisely cerebrogenic pathology of the heart and this can exert a significant influence on the character of therapeutic measures.

THE PATHOGENESIS OF VASCULAR DISORDERS OF BRAIN AND HEART –

ARE THERE SIMILARITIES OR DISSIMILARITIES?

K.J. Zülch* and V. Hossmann**

* Max-Planck-Institut für Hirnforschung, Köln-Merheim
**Lehrstuhl für Innere Medizin II
   Universität Köln

INTRODUCTION

This review is based on the discussion of two international symposia in Köln/Cologne 1976 and 1978 and our own experience. It will be understood that only a few problems of the discussion can be pointed out, particularly since the proceedings of both symposia are extensively published with Springer, Heidelberg–New York 1977/ 1979,[1,2] and summarized later.[3]

I. Terminology

First some semantic misunderstandings in the nomenclature have to be clarified: the angloamerican term "atherosclerosis" corresponds to "arterioclerosis" in German. "Arteriosclerosis" in English apparently sums up atherosclerosis and "small vessel disease" which corresponds in German pathology to "arteriolosclerosis" or "hyalinosis". The latter is subsequent to long-standing hypertension and responsible for mass hemorrhage in the brain and granular nephrosclerosis in the kidney.

II. Risk Factors

It seems of importance to distinguish between two sets of different risk factors, namely 1) for the causation of stenosing atherosclerosis and 2) for the acute promotion of the clinical events of stroke and myocardial infarction. Although most risk factors involve the whole arterial system, there are differences in the grade of arteriosclerotic manifestation in the different

body organs, either on the base of constitutional or environmental
factors, disregarding the fact that normally cerebral atherosclerosis
follows the coronary disease with a delay of one decade. One co-
incidental observation could be that risk factors for atherosclerosis
have a different rank order in brain and heart.

For instance, in brain infarcts hypertension is accused particularly on epidemiological grounds to be the risk factor number
one, although certain morphological observations do not always support such a concept.

In myocardial infarction the most important risk factor is
hypercholesterolemia followed by cigarette smoking, while hypertension is only on third place. Interesting to remember that in
peripheral vascular arterial disease the most important risk factor
is undoubtedly cigarette smoking.

On the other hand, the cholesterol level is only weakly related
to atherothrombotic brain infarct (ABI) as is also cigarette smoking.

Diabetes is an important factor in both disorders.

For the clinical manifestation the risk factor hypertension is
certainly of prime importance for both types of stroke, namely (a)
cerebral mass hemorrhage (via hyalinosis in the striatal arteries
etc.) and (b) cerebral infarct.

Meanwhile it is undoubtedly proven that by a strict regime with
antihypertensive treatment both the number of strokes and of myocardial infarctions have decreased remarkably. This has been proven
by several multi-center-studies, e.g. the project of the National
Heart, Lung, and Blood Institute Bethesda, and the Finland project.

III. Predilection site of atherosclerosis

Cerebral atherosclerosis has a pronounced local predilection
and follows here the local factors of increased wall stress as at
bifurcations, branchings, curves, bony fixations, and outer strangu-
lations of the artery. The first atherosclerotic plaque is observed
at the bifurcation of the basilar artery already sometimes as early
as 25 years of age, yet it is hardly impeding. In contrast marked
stenosis in the coronaries has been observed in the same age group
already during World War I and later in the Korean War. Decisive
stenoses usually occur in the brain at the origin of the middle
cerebral arteries and less commonly in the posterior cerebral arteries and in the third place only in the anterior and basilar
arteries. The vertebral arteries are liable to total occlusion
particularly at the point of penetration of the dura.

The predilection sites of stenoses for the heart are the following:

a)   the left descending artery 2 cm after its origin
b)   the right main artery 2-3 cm distally to its origin, however, also in 8-10 cm distance, and
c)   the left circumflex artery again 2-3 cm from the ostium.

Where do we find the total occlusions and what is their pathogenesis? Most frequently they develop on and occlude a highly stenosed vessel segment in the brain; only rarely the thrombosis of a youthful vessel occurs.

Since early coronary angiography is now more often performed in acute myocardial infarction for subsequent intracoronary fibrinolysis it has become clear that in almost 80% of acute infarctions a complete thrombotic occlusion is demonstrable: following lysis of the occluding clots atherosclerotic stenoses of less than 50% are found in only about 6% of patients, 75-90% stenoses in around 50% of patients, and sub-total stenoses in 30%.

Clinical important investigations of 1000 stroke patients of our unit have proven that in more than 80% the very cause of cerebral infarction was stenosing atherosclerosis. Only in 60% macroembolism was the cause.

From the patient group with complete occlusion, whereby those with macroembolism were disregarded, 4/5 of these cases showed a very pronounced atherosclerosis with a final thrombosis on top, whereas a totally occlusing primary thrombosis comprised only 20% of the cerebral arteries.

IV. Anastomoses and collaterals

In the brain the possibility of a collateral supply in emergency is favorable, because of a great number of preexisting anastomoses:

1.   Transverse anastomoses between the two carotid arteries and between the two vertebral arteries.
2.   Anastomoses between the external carotid and (a) the internal carotid via ophthalmic artery and (b) the vertebral artery via its occipital branch.
3.   Circle of Willis.
4.   Intracranial meningeal anastomoses of Heubner from 200 up to 1000 micra(!) in diameter. This proves that the general pattern of the vascular supply of the brain has an almost web-like net, allowing collateral pathways at any level.

Of these the role of the meningeal anastomoses may be so effective that in proximal occlusion of the middle cerebral artery the
defect can be completely compensated for by retrograde flux through
the meningeal anastomoses from the anterior and posterior arteries.
Clinically up to 20% of middle cerebral artery occlusions are free
from neurological symptoms. Most of these anastomoses are usually
sufficiently developed as to be able to operate <u>immediately</u> in
emergency. They can be further dilated during increasing functional
demand, however, a new-growth of functional vessels occurs in the
brain only on the capillary level and will hardly be of any advantage
for a defected circulation.

The significance of the functional role of the collateral network of the heart is controversial, although there exists a vast
network of precapillary collaterals especially in the subendocardium
and the middle layers of the myocardium: these are small vessels
with a diameter of approximately 50 micra which are not able to
restore a sufficient coronary blood flow following an acute occlusion
of a coronary artery. In acute myocardial infarction collaterals
seem to be of minor importance, yet a smaller action of collaterals -
if present - may be operative and the actual territory of infarction
is then smaller than the real distribution area of the artery. No
convincing explanation has so far been found for the considerable
variability of development of collaterals in the heart. It may be
secondary to a different genetic disposition or due to different
responses to the various stimuli capable to increase the anastomotic
network. The pressure gradient is the decisive stimulus for the
development of efficient collaterals by increasing of the diameter.
A close correlation is therefore found between the extent of the
collateral network and the severity of coronary disease (degree of
stenosis and number of involved vessels). To illustrate the extraordinary importance of existing collaterals we want to point to the
survival times of the various organs. Cerebral tissue in man has
a survival time still oscillating at about 5-8 minutes and only in
animal experiments, this can be prolonged to 1 hour. This limited
survival time inhibits any successful action due to a growth of
collaterals.

The same is true for the heart although there the survival time
may be higher up to 30-45 minutes.

However, for the brain we have to point out to two facts which
allow to understand the process of infarction in man better. The
human brain has normally already a reserve circulation of 200% of
the demand. Loss of function follows only after decrease to 50% of
the normal circulation. However, necrosis is only caused by a
further fall beneath 15-20%. There is a safety mantle then of 30%
between the 50 and 20% borders. Here function is lost yet tissue
can recover. While in the center of an infarcted area the brain
may already be necrotic, the surroundings may be functionless, yet

recoverable. This afunctional tissue is liable to recovery by
further improvements of circulation and metabolism which can be
achieved either by conservative treatment or even by surgical means
such as extraintracranial anastomoses etc. Although it has been
shown that local cerebral blood flow may increase markedly according
to the local demand, overall cerebral blood flow is rather stable.
On the other hand, overall coronary blood flow has to increase extensively on exercise. The so-called "coronary reserve" corresponds
to 300-400% of coronary blood flow at rest. However, since wall
stress is higher in the subendocardium the reserve for vasodilation
is also less in these layers and overall limitation of perfusion
pressure and augmentation of extrinsic compressive factors comprises
the subendocardial tissue first.

V. Metabolic changes leading to brain edema

We now know from many hundreds of experiments of microembol-
ization in the cat that a pericapillary edema in the cortex arises
already after a few minutes due to blood brain barrier damage. However, this damage disappears already after four hours and then the
barrier will be tight again.

Thereafter a second form of edema occurs extracellularly.
Pathogenetically this is a transudation through the larger veins.
This extracellular edema may be volume taking and has a detrimental
action on the myelin. This form of edema is mainly located in the
white matter and may diffusely propagate from the perivenous base
through the whole white substance, leading to necrobiosis of the
myelin sheaths in the course of weeks, causing both an acute impairment of the tissue oxygenation and finally by secondary uptake
of the protein-rich edema into the myelin sheaths a necrosis. Only
sometimes, particularly in the hemorrhagic forms of infarcts the
increase of volume can be so enormous as to lead to remarkable mass
shifts and a fatal symptomatology.

Experimental work is only rarely focussed on the problem of
edema in myocardial infarction, since the pericardial sac is large
enough not to counteract the minor expansion of the myocardium by
edema. The role of edema should, however, not be underestimated.
Ischemic edema first adds to the extrinsic factors increasing coronary
resistance such as the systolic compressive effects and secondly increases the distance of oxygen diffusion in the tissue.

VI. Pathogenesis of infarction

Cerebral infarction is widely dependent upon two factors, first
the general systemic circulation, e.g. "vis a tergo" and secondly
local impediments to the blood flow in the arteries.

For the clinical promotion of stroke hypertension may participate 1) by acute elevation of blood pressure, the "hypertensive
crisis" inducing a "break-through" of autoregulation and blood brain
barrier damage, the vessels assuming a pseudospastic image which is
only the highest degree of autoregulation according to the Bayliss
principle. 2) By the acute fall of chronic hypertensive pressure
values to "normal" or even "hypotensive" levels with subsequent impairment of local circulation.

It seems to be proven now that at least during the "hypertensive crisis" real spasm "sensu strictu" does not follow the cerebral
arterial tree. That spasm may occur in the brain by mechanic
causes is undoubted.

In the heart coronary spasm is widely accepted to be the cause
of Prinzmetal angina and may even lead to myocardial infarction.

VII. Transient ischemic attacks and angina pectoris

To pass over from the more morphological phenomena to the
functional processes a comparison between the transient ischemic
attacks (TIA) in the brain and angina pectoris in the heart will be
tried. The most favored explanation of TIAs is now a speculated
microembolism from ulcerated arteriosclerotic plaques either at the
carotid bifurcation or at any other proximal point of the arterial
tree. We admit that such emboli have been photographed in the retina
in amaurosis fugax, e.g. transient blindness. Yet, 1) a statistical
proof that these retinal microemboli do occur also in TIAs is still
lacking. 2) In Toole's series of carotid endarterectomies of patients
with TIAs only 13 of the 123 surgical specimens showed such an ulcerated thrombotic surface, however, the patients were cured after
removal of the obstacle in the arterial wall. 3) According to the
symptoms of TIA the emboli should always go to a particular circum-
scribed clear-cut vessel territory. Yet, in the experiment smaller
microemboli of less than 80 micron, injected into the carotid artery,
are spread evenly over the total distribution area. Only emboli of
1 mm - 10-15 times larger - remain in the central blood stream,
when injected into the carotid artery, and have therefore a local
predilection for the middle cerebral artery. 4) Another important
observation is that in patients with retinal emboli neurological
symptoms never occur which would have been expected if the microemboli would be evenly distributed over the whole carotid artery.
We personally favor therefore the hemodynamic theory, e.g. a local
stenosis in an artery and a temporary decrease of flow as the two
promotors of a local disorder and triggered by circadian blood pressure fall, heart arrhythmias, orthostasis, etc.

VIII. Therapy

Most interesting would be a discussion of implications for therapy. This may be only introduced by one statement: The interpretation of an "ideal" blood pressure for the patient in a given situation may be different for the cardiologist and neurologist. The brain specialist will keep the blood pressure as high as possible emphasizing that this organ may secondarily suffer an irreversible infarct following lowering of the blood pressure distal to a vascular stenosis. The internist on the other hand tries to protect the heart from any unnecessary demand by maintaining a low systemic blood pressure. Many other implications of this kind are worthy of a serious discussion. Symposia of this kind, where neurologists and cardiologists are discussing these problems together, may intensify our knowledge for the benefit of the patients.

Acknowledgement

This paper is supported by a grant of Frau Andrea Möller, Hamburg.

REFERENCES

1. K. J. Zülch, W. Kaufmann, K. -A. Hossmann, and V. Hossmann, Brain and Heart Infarct, Springer, Berlin-Heidelberg-New York (1977).
2. K. J. Zülch, W. Kaufmann, K. -A. Hossmann, and V. Hossmann, Brain and Heart Infarct II, Springer, Berlin-Heidelberg-New York (1979).
3. K. J. Zülch, and V. Hossmann, The pathogenesis of vascular disorders of brain and heart: are there similarities or dissimilarities? in: "Studies in Cerebrovascular Disease," C. Loeb, ed., Masson Italia Editori, Milano (1981).

ATHEROSCLEROSIS AND THROMBOSIS OF THE

CEREBRAL AND CORONARY ARTERIES

Kenzo Tanaka and Junichi Masuda

Department of Pathology, Faculty of Medicine
Kyushu University
Fukuoka, Japan

An association between cerebrovascular diseases and cardiac diseases has been recognised.[1,2] Three mechanisms are considered to contribute to the relation between them:

1. Cardiac diseases and cerebrovascular diseases are linked through common risk factors, e.g. hypertension, serum lipids and cigarette smoking.
2. Cerebral hypoperfusion due to impaired cardiac function contributes to the development of cerebral infarction and cerebral ischemia.
3. Thromboembolization from the heart associated with myocardial infarction, rheumatic heart disease, etc.

Prevalence of cerebrovascular diseases associated with organic heart diseases and the cases with abnormal ECG findings was investigated by reviewing 1162 autopsy cases (20 or over 20 years of age) at Department of Pathology, Kyushu University from Nov. 1971 to Oct. 1981. Forty-eight cases with cerebral infarction (CI) were found among 86 cases with myocardial infarction (MI) and its prevalence was higher than that of the control group (the cases without organic heart diseases, collagen disease, amyloidosis or chronic renal failure) according to sex and age adjusted statistical analysis (Table 1). Eighteen out of 40 cases with rheumatic heart disease (RHD) were associated with CI, which was higher in prevalence than the control group. It was considered that cerebral embolism contributed to these CI in some cases (Figure 1). Ten cases of CI seemed to be embolic cerebral infarction. Intracardiac thrombi and atrial fibrillation (af) were frequently found in these cases. Eleven out of 18 cases with RHD and CI were believed to be embolic. Eight cases were associated with af and intracardiac thrombi and

503

Table 1.   Cerebrovascular Diseases among the cases with
Cardiac Diseases

	No. of cases	Cerebral infarction	Non-embolic cerebral infarction	Cerebral hemorrhage
Myocardial infarction	86	48**	38*	1
relative risk		2.83	2.10	0.27
Rheumatic heart disease	40	18**	9	1
relative risk		3.38	1.16	0.52
Control	994	238	231	41

* $p < 0.05$
** $p < 0.01$ vs. control group (the cases without organic heart
diseases) by Mantel-Haenszel χ^2

one case with af only. It was further studied whether the cases
with MI were frequently associated with non-embolic cerebral infarction (Table 1). Prevalence of non-embolic CI among the MI group
was significantly higher than the control group. But there was no
difference in the prevalence of non-embolic CI in the RHD group and
the control group. The cases with abnormal ECG findings (af, left
ventricular hypertrophy, non-specific ST-T change) showed higher
prevalence of CI than the cases without each abnormal ECG findings
(Table 2).

The results of autopsy studies in Hisayama town in Japan[3] revealed that the severity of atherosclerosis showed variety in each
case and each organ. Cerebral atherosclerosis was usually less
severe than atherosclerosis of the aorta and coronary arteries. The
severity of cerebral atherosclerosis was promoted statistically
significantly by hypertension, but it showed less dramatic increase
by serum cholesterol level.

Hypertension not only promoted cerebral atherosclerosis but
also affected the pathogenesis of cerebral artery thrombosis.
Thirty-nine cases of occluded cerebral arterial segments and 54
cases of occluded coronary arteries were investigated histopatho-
logically by serial sections (Table 3).[4,5] The most conspicuous
and frequently observed finding in the thrombosed segments of the
cerebral arteries was intramural hemorrhage, which was present in
28 out of 39 segments. Hypertension was associated with 76.0% of
the cases with intramural hemorrhage. Five cases showed fibrinoid
necrosis of the small blood vessels in the atheroma. On the other
hand, it was found that major cause of thrombus precipitation in

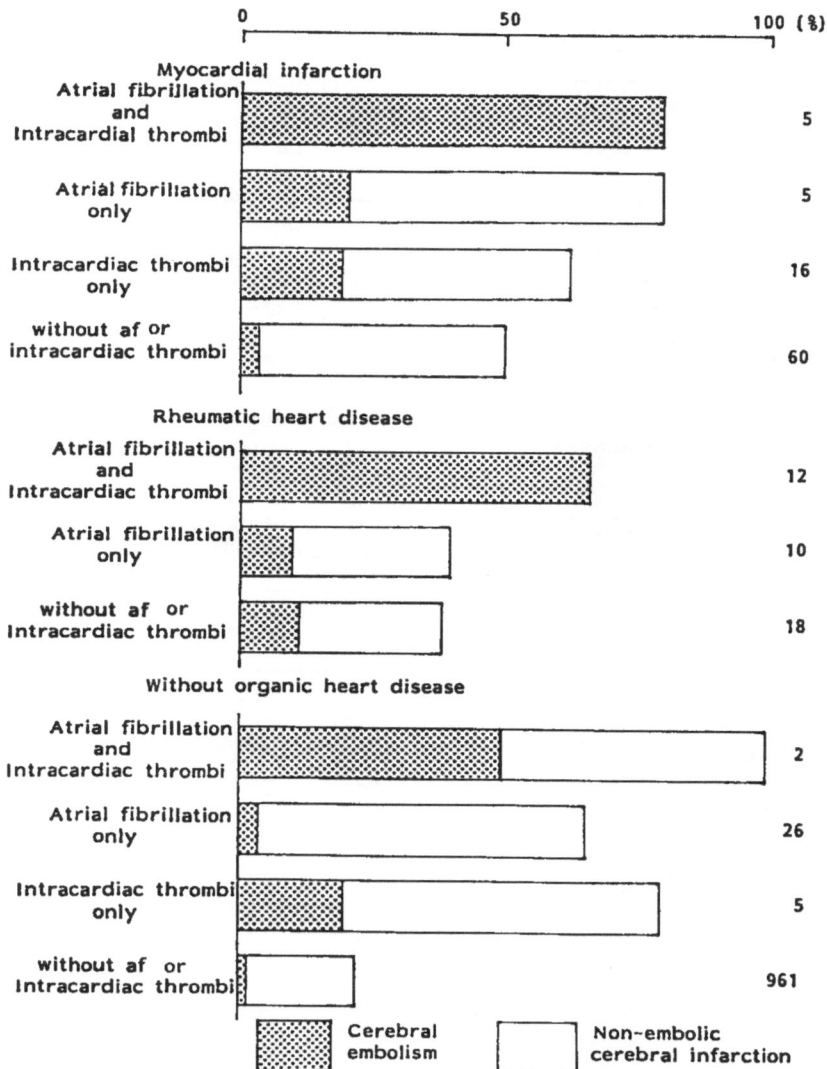

Fig. 1.   Cerebral infarction among the cases with atrial
          fibrillation and intracardiac thrombi

the pathogenesis of coronary artery thrombosis was rupture or fissure
formation of atherosclerotic plaque occupying 55.6% (30 cases).
These characteristics in the pathogenesis of the cerebral atherosclerosis and the cerebral artery thrombosis are important in considering the relationship between cerebrovascular diseases and
cardiac diseases.

Table 2. Cerebral Infarction among the cases with
Abnormal ECG Findings

	No. of cases	Cerebral infarction No.	Cerebral infarction relative risk
in the cases without organic heart diseases			
Atrial fibrillation	28	19**	4.36
Left ventricular hypertrophy	170	82**	2.25
Non-specific · ST-T change	248	123**	3.41

** p<0.01 vs. the cases without each abnormal ECG findings
by Mantel-Haenszel χ^2

Table 3. Histological Characteristics of Coronary and
Cerebral Arteries with Occluding Thrombus

	Cerebral arteries	Coronary arteries
Hemorrhage in plaque	28 (71.2%)	20 (37.0%)
Rupture of plaque	1 (2.6%)	30 (55.6%)
Edema of plaque	4 (10.3%)	0
Liquefaction of intimal surface	0	1 (1.8%)
Plaque alone	6 (15.4%)	3 (5.6%)
Total	39	54

REFERENCES

1. T. Omae, M. Takeshita, and Y. Hirota, The Hisayama study and
joint study on cerebrovascular diseases in Japan, in:
"Cerebrovascular diseases, 10th Princeton conference,"
P. Scheinberg, ed., Raven Press, New York (1976).
2. P. A. Wolf, T. R. Dawber, and W. B. Kannel, Heart disease as
a precursor of stroke, in: "Advances in Neurology Vol.19,
Neurological epidemiology: Principles and clinical applications," B. S. Schoenberg, ed., Raven Press, New York (1978).

3. S. Sadoshima, T. Kurozumi, K. Tanaka, K. Ueda, M. Takeshita,
    Y. Hirota, T. Omae, H. Uzawa, and S. Katsuki, Cerebral and
    aortic atherosclerosis in Hisayama, Japan, <u>Atherosclerosis</u>
    36:117 (1980).
4. S. Sadoshima, T. Fukushima, and K. Tanaka, Cerebral artery
    thrombosis and intramural hemorrhage, <u>Stroke</u> 10:411 (1979).
5. K. Nakagaki, Coronary thrombosis and its role in the develop-
    ment of myocardial infarction, <u>Fukuoka Acta Medica</u> 68:541
    (1977).

MANIFESTATIONS OF CORONARY DISEASE PREDISPOSING TO STROKE:

THE FRAMINGHAM STUDY

W. B. Kannel, P. A. Wolf, and J. Verter

Chief Section of Preventative Medicine and
Epidemiology
Boston University School of Medicine

The relation of coronary heart disease to development of strokes in general and brain infarction in particular has been examined prospectively over 24 years of follow-up in the Framingham Study cohort. In the course of 24 years of biennial surveillance, there were 169 strokes in men and 175 in women aged 45-84; brain infarctions occurred in 100 men and 107 women, comprising 60% of strokes. Routine ECG's chest X-rays coronary heart disease and cardiac failure status were ascertained biennially on regular examinations and risk of strokes determined in relation to these. Age and other stroke risk factors (including blood pressure, diabetes, cigarettes and lipids were also routinely measured and were taken into account in multivariate analysis of the net and joint effects of CHD manifestations as precursors of strokes. The incidence of stroke was lower and stroke occurred later in life than coronary heart disease. Stroke incidence in men lagged that of myocardial infarction by more than 10 years. In women, the incidence of brain and myocardial infarction was similar. In men the average annual incidence of myocardial infarction (8.5/1000) was three times that for brain infarction (2.7/1000).[1] In both sexes, stroke incidence rose with age, more than doubling each successive decade above age 45 (Table 1). In contrast to myocardial infarction, where there is a striking male predominance, the incidence rate for brain infarction is only about 30% greater in men than women, and even this small sex differential is seen chiefly below age 65. Some 20% of brain infarctions occurred below age 65.

Since the underlying pathological features of atherosclerosis in the cerebral, cardiac and peripheral circulation are virtually identical, it is not unexpected that they share precursors. Atherosclerosis commonly affects all three areas simultaneously, and

Table 1. Occurrence of Stroke vs. Myocardial Infarction
          by Age and Sex. 24 yr. follow-up. Framingham
          Study. Average Annual Incidence per 10,000

Age	Brain Infarction		Stroke All Types		Myocardial Infarction	
	Men	Women	Men	Women	Men	Women
45–54	10	7	20	11	54	8
55–64	23	16	40	27	95	25
65–74	55	48	90	83	122	52
75–84	139	94	176	127	192	98
All Ages	26	21	44	34	83	25

persons with one clinical manifestation are at increased risk of
the others. Also, asymptomatic carotid bruits predicted myocardial
infarction as well as a brain infarction (Figure 1).[2] Brain and
myocardial infarction often coexist, particularly in advanced age
and coronary heart disease is the chief cause of death in stroke
and brain infarction survivors. This is also the case in patients
with transient ischemic attacks or carotid bruits.[1,2]

Coronary heart disease frequently occurs in persons who appear
well. Strokes and brain infarctions more often occur on a background of illness: coronary heart disease (30%), occlusive peripheral arterial disease (30%), cardiac failure (15%), and diabetes
(15%). Established hypertension is present in 70%.[1]

CARDIOVASCULAR RISK FACTORS

Although some non-trivial differences exist in their impacts
on the incidence of each disease, blood pressure, serum cholesterol,
ECG-LVH, glucose intolerance and cigarette smoking are precursors
common to brain infarction and myocardial infarction. When all
five major CHD risk factors are considered jointly, they are actually
more highly predictive of brain infarction than coronary heart
disease. Blood pressure and ECG-LVH are the chief determinants of
this predictive capacity. Hyperlipidemia and the cigarette habit
are less important than for coronary heart disease. Nevertheless,
the coronary risk profile predicts stroke risk over a wide range,
identifying in the upper decile of risk a tenth of the population
from which half the strokes evolved compared to only 25% of CHD
events (Table 2).

The dominant predisposing risk factors for brain infarction
are hypertension and various cardiac impairments, including clinical

(a)

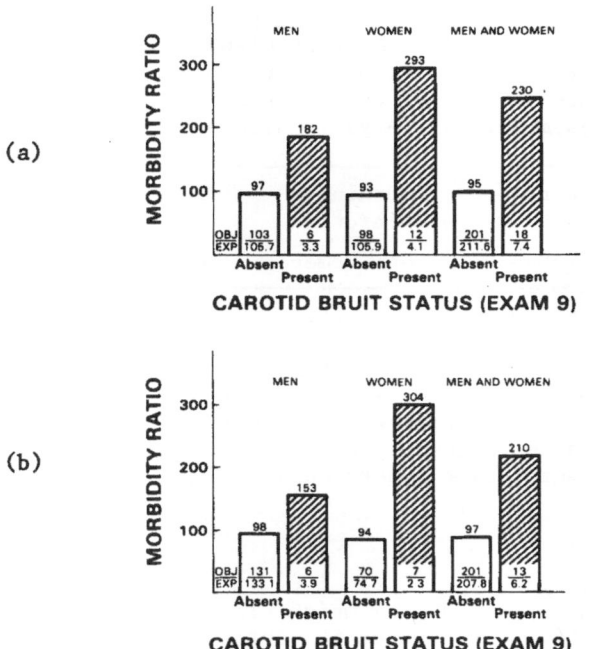

CAROTID BRUIT STATUS (EXAM 9)

(b)

CAROTID BRUIT STATUS (EXAM 9)

Fig. 1.   (a) Age adjusted 2-year incidence of stroke by carotid
             bruit. Men and women 50-79 years. Framingham Study.
          (b) Age adjusted 2-year incidence of myocardial infarction.

manifestations of coronary heart disease, cardiac failure, atrial
fibrillation and preclinical evidence of a compromised coronary
circulation. In candidates for coronary heart disease with an
ominous cardiovascular risk profile, suggesting accelerated atherogenesis, the appearance of ECG abnormalities and X-ray evidence of
cardiac enlargement not otherwise explained were hallmarks of a
compromised coronary circulation, associated with an increased risk
of myocardial infarction.[3]

CARDIAC IMPAIRMENTS

For stroke in general, an abnormal ECG indicated a greater
than 3-fold increased risk of an event in men and 4-fold in women;
the excess risk persisting on adjustment for age and other risk
factors including blood pressure. ECG-LVH was the strongest ECG
precursor with an associated 5 to 6-fold increased risk (Table 3).
Chronic atrial fibrillation carried a 6-fold excess risk, persisting
at 3-fold after adjusting for coexistent risk factors.[4] X-ray
cardiac enlargement was not as powerful as ECG abnormalities,

Table 2. Percentage of cases of Coronary Disease, Brain
          Infarction, and Intermittent Claudication in the
          Upper Decile of Multivariate Risk* among Men and
          Women 45-74 years of age who participated in the
          Framingham Study: 16-year follow-up

Age	Coronary Disease		Brain Infarction		Intermittent Claudication	
	Men	Women	Men	Women	Men	Women
45-54	25.9	20.0	54.5	44.4	30.0	60.0
54-64	26.7	25.7	52.3	42.9	46.7	42.9
65-74	21.3	40.9	57.1	45.5	26.7	50.0

* Based upon systolic blood pressure, serum cholesterol,
  number of cigarettes smoked, electrocardiographic evidence of left-ventricular hypertrophy, and glucose
  tolerance.

carrying only a 2-fold increased risk which also increased uniformly
with heart size. For brain infarction in particular, ECG-LVH was
also the most powerful ECG predictor (greater than 4-fold) and was
more ominous when there were associated ST-T wave repolarization
abnormalities. Again, X-ray left ventricular hypertrophy was a
less powerful predictor, but more important than generalized enlargement (Table 3). In men, there was no independent contribution
of X-ray enlargement when ECG-LVH and hypertension were taken into
account. Nonspecific ST-T wave abnormalities carried an increased
risk in both sexes, independent of age and associated risk factors.
Intraventricular block was a significant contributor to brain infarction risk only in women.

Thus, even asymptomatic cardiac impairments associated with a
compromised coronary circulation were clearly associated with an
increased risk of stroke. Cardiac impairments ranked third, following age and hypertension, as risk factors for stroke in general
and for brain infarction in particular. At any age, in either sex,
and at any level of blood pressure, persons with cardiac disease,
whether overt or subclinical, have more than a doubled risk of a
stroke (Figure 2). These predisposing cardiac impairments include
not only overt coronary heart disease, but occult diseases such as
left ventricular hypertrophy by ECG or X-ray and atrial fibrillation.

OVERT CARDIAC DISEASE

Subjects with overt cardiac disease had almost a tripled risk
of a stroke (Table 4). This applied equally in both sexes. As

Table 3. Risk of Stroke according to Left Ventricular Hypertrophy by ECG vs. X-Ray. Subjects 45-84. The Framingham Study. 24-year follow-up. Age-adjusted average annual incidence per 10,000

	Stroke (all types)				Brain Infarction			
	ECG-LVH		X-Ray LVH		ECG-LVH		X-Ray LVH	
Abnormality	Men	Women	Men	Women	Men	Women	Men	Women
None	39	28	41	28	23	17	24	15
Possible	68	86	54	29	62	39	34	18
Definite	206	182	68	54	102	133	42	41
Risk Ratio	5.3	6.5	1.7	1.9	4.4	7.8	1.8	2.7
Multivariate Z-Value	3.57	5.09	0.90	2.39	2.39	3.72	0.78	3.21

might be expected, the risk associated with a myocardial infarction (5-fold) was substantially greater than that associated with angina (2-fold).

Cardiac failure which is predominantly due to hypertension and coronary heart disease, increased the risk of stroke 5 to 6-fold for strokes in general and 2 to 4-fold for brain infarction in

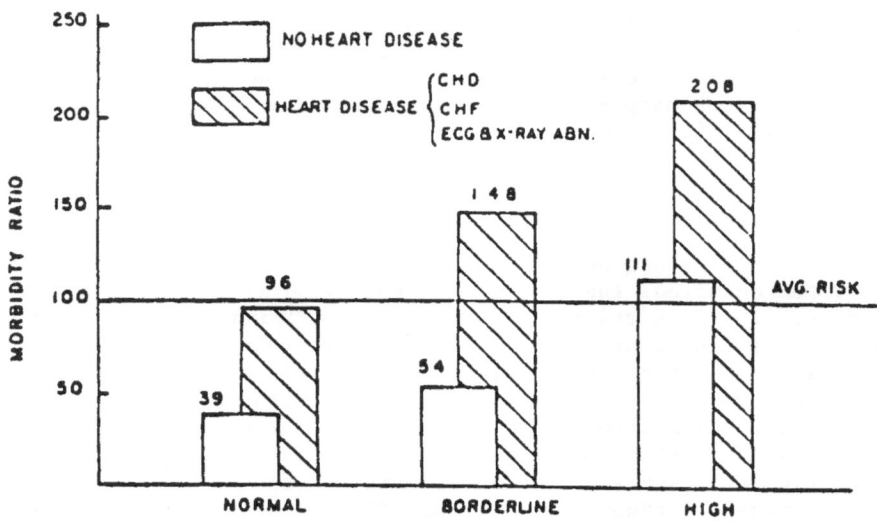

Fig. 2. Risk of stroke according to blood pressure and cardiac impairment. 24-year follow-up. Framingham Study.

Table 4.   Risk of Stroke comparing ECG-LVH, Cardiac
Failure and Coronary Disease.   24-year follow-
up.   Framingham Study.   Subjects 45-84.   Age-
adjusted average annual incidence per 10,000

Abnormality	CHF		CHD		ECG-LVH	
	Men	Women	Men	Women	Men	Women
Negative	41	31	37	28	39	28
Definite	221	192	102	78	206	182
Risk Ratio	5.4	6.2	2.8	2.8	5.3	6.5
Multivariate Z-Value	5.13	3.59	4.04	3.59	3.87	5.09

particular (Table 4).   The risk appears to be greater in women than
men.   Both for congestive heart failure and coronary heart disease
the excess risk, particularly for men, persists on taking associated
risk factors, including hypertension, into account.   Coronary disease,
when associated with hypertension or cardiac failure, carried a
greater risk than when not complicated by these features (Figure 2).

Thus, strokes are a part of a larger problem of cardiovascular
disease and once coronary heart disease, congestive heart failure
appear, or even asymptomatic evidence of a compromised coronary
circulation appears, risk of stroke is greatly escalated (Figure 2).
Also, survival and recurrences following a stroke are greatly influenced by comorbidity; notably by the coexisting coronary heart
disease and congestive heart failure (Figure 3).   Prevention of
strokes requires not only control of hypertension, but prevention
and relief of coronary heart disease, congestive heart failure and
atrial fibrillation.

SUMMARY

Based on 24 years of biennial examinations, during which time
344 strokes occurred, the role of CHD was examined as a precursor
of stroke.   The five major risk factors for CHD were jointly even
more predictive of brain infarction than myocardial infarction,
identifying a tenth of the asymptomatic population from which half
the strokes evolved.   The dominant stroke risk factors were hypertension, clinical manifestations of CHD, cardiac failure and preclinical evidence of a compromised coronary circulation.   CHD more
than doubled the risk and cardiac failure was associated with a
5-fold increased incidence of stroke.   Chronic atrial fibrillation
increased the stroke risk 6-fold and ECG-LVH was the most powerful
ECG predictor.   All cardiac impairments added to the stroke risk
associated with hypertension.

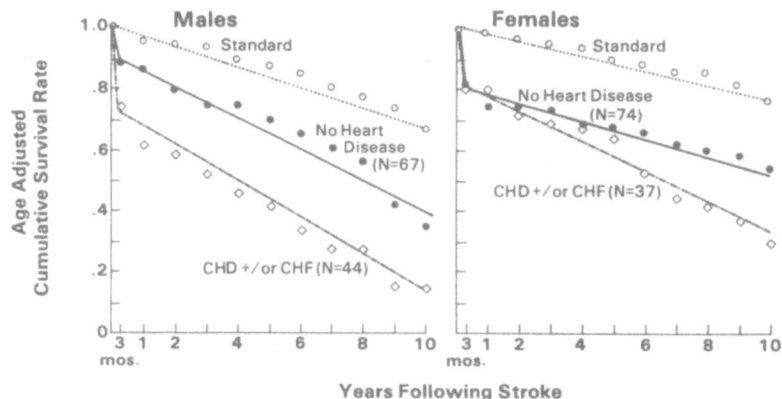

Fig. 3.   Survival following ABI, effect of prior Cardiac Comorbidity.
Framingham Study.   26-year follow-up.

REFERENCES

1. P. A. Wolf, and W. B. Kannel, Controllable risk factors for
    stroke: Preventive implications of trends in stroke mor-
    tality, in: "Diagnosis and Management of Stroke and TIA's,"
    J. S. Meyer and T. Shaw, eds., Addison-Wesley Publishing
    Company, p.26-61 (1981).

2. P. A. Wolf, W. B. Kannel, P. Sorlie, and P. McNamara, Asympto-
    matic carotid bruit and risk of stroke, JAMA 245:1442-1445
    (1981).

3. W. B. Kannel, T. Gordon, and W. P. Castelli, Electrocardio-
    graphic left ventricular hypertrophy and risk of coronary
    heart disease, The Framingham Study, Ann.Intern.Med. 72:
    813 (1970).

4. P. A. Wolf, T. R. Dawber, H. E. Thomas Jr., and W. B. Kannel,
    Epidemiological assessment of chronic atrial fibrillation
    and risk of stroke: The Framingham Study, Neurology 28:
    973-977 (1978).

LIMITATION OF INFARCT SIZE: THEORETICAL ASPECTS

G. Baroldi

Institute of Clinical Physiology, C. N. R.
University of Pisa and Institute of Pathological Anatomy
Medical School, University of Milan, Italy

The basic postulate is that cardiac infarct size is directly related to clinical complications and death. The consequent therapeutical implication is to reduce the "theoretical" size and/or to prevent its progression (or expansion) in the surrounding myocardium. The latter is considered more prone to ischaemia and therefore at high risk of necrosis ("jeopardized border zone").

In the present controversy on both the existence of such a border zone and the possibility to limit the infarct size, the definition of infarct necrosis and its natural history as well as the definition of the type of changes in the normal myocardium at the periphery of the infarct in man seem opportune.

Human infarct necrosis

The first functional disorder is the loss of contraction. The myocardial cells are dying in relaxation phase ("atonic death"). Thinning of the dead cells, elongation of sarcomeres and nuclei are the earliest histologic signs which reflect the passive distension of the irreversibly relaxed elements by the intraventricular pressure (systolic paradoxical bulging). Centripetal infiltration of polymorphonuclear leukocytes, secondary wall degeneration and thrombosis of the vascular structures, removal by macrophages and fibrous replacement are the main progressive changes of the repair process. A regular, periodic order of the myofibrils is maintained even in the last remnants of necrotic tissue.

This necrosis is usually termed "coagulation necrosis" and represents the pathognomonic postmortem finding in patients dying from typical clinical pattern of cardiac infarct.

Table 1. Infarct size and age in 200 consecutive acute cases

Age in Days	Infarct Size (%)						Total
	less 10	11-20	21-30	31-40	41-50	50	
2	34	11	11	9	1	4	70
3-10	17	9	24	10	9	5	74
11-30	9	17	9	8	8	5	56
Total	60	37	44	27	18	14	200

In the majority of the cases the lesion is monofocal. In 200 consecutive and selected (no other cardiac and non cardiac disease, no surgery) patients its size ranged from less than 10 per cent to more than 50 per cent of the left ventricular mass[1,2]. The survival time (from clinical onset to death) varied from less than two to 30 days and was not related to the infarct size (Table 1). In no one instance of these 200 acute infarct cases progression (or expansion) of the primitive coagulation necrosis was documented. In other words the association of an earlier phase of the coagulation necrosis external to an older one was never observed.

Little is known on the time relation between reversible and irreversible infarct damage in man. The only available data are from experimental coronary occlusion models. In dog it has been calculated that after an occlusion lasting 20 minutes there is a total recovery, while after one hour most of the involved myocardial cells are dead. Due to the obvious differences among various species and overall between experimental models and human pathology, we may only induce that approximately in a similar period of time coagulation necrosis is also settled in man.

Structural changes in the "normal" myocardium around the infarct

More precisely by normal myocardium we should intend the myocardium preserved by the coagulation necrosis. In fact in most of the fatal cases two other types of myocardial necrosis can be detected[3].

From the morpho-functional standpoint the first one is the opposite pattern of the coagulation necrosis. The myocardial cells are contracted, or better hypercontracted, with rhexis of the myofibrils and anomalous cross-band formation. These structural changes suggest that the myocells die in irreversible contraction state ("tetanic death"). The subsequent fragmentation is likely due to the mechanical action of the normal acting myocardium on the rigid, hypercontracted elements. This type of lesion is present around an

infarct in about 80 percent of the cases. It may involve single
elements or foci formed by few myocells or may become massive by
confluence of several foci. Apparently is not related to infarct
size and coronary damage, and is mainly located at the lateral-
external sites of the infarct. This necrosis never shows specific
inflammatory infiltration or vessel degeneration and its repair
process progresses again by macrophagic phagocytosis, followed by
collagenization of the empty salcolemmal tubes ("alveolar pattern").
Present in many other conditions (pheochromocytoma, stone heart,
transplanted human heart etc.) is reproduced experimentally by
catecholamine infusion. Variously called (contraction band necrosis,
myofibrillar degeneration, coagulative myocytolysis) may be simply
defined as "Zenker necrosis". The first structural changes can be
detected within few minutes and consist in alteration of the myofibrillar system.

The other type of necrosis is still a primary damage of the
myofibrils, but with a completely different pattern from the previous
one. This process is characterized by a progressive "edematous"
vacuolization with disappearance of the myofibrils. Histologically
the myocardial cell appears as an "Empty" clear element with an apparently normal nucleus. Found in any cardiomyopathy with low output
syndrome, has been variously named (sarcolysis, colliquative myocytolysis) and may be called "myocytolysis", using this term for this
specific lesion without confusion with the previously described
Zenker necrosis. The histologic findings associated with cardiac
failure suggest a progressive diminution in strength and velocity of
contraction as basic morpho-functional disorder ("failing death").
In more than 40 percent of the 200 acute infarcts this lesion was
seen in the preserved myocardium around the survived vessels and
beneath the endocardium mainly in cases with longer survival and
extensive myocardial fibrosis (Table 2).

Table 2. Myocytolysis in Relation to Survival Time and Myocardial
Fibrosis.

200 AMI	Survival time - days		
	2	3-10	11
Total	70	74	56
With myocytolysis	20 (28.5%)	28 (37.8%)	28 (50%)

	Myocardial fibrosis	
	no or minimal	extensive
Total	145	55
With myocytolysis	46 (31.7%)	30 (54.5%)

A last observation has to be mentioned to complete the whole
histologic pattern seen in the acute myocardial infarct. Practically
in all earliest cases a rim formed by a thin layer of hypercontracted
myocardial cells with anomalous cross band, at the lateral and external surface of the coagulation necrosis is visible. Already
described in the first reports as part of the latter, such a well
distinct rim may vary in depth and extension. Furthermore, since
the polymorphonuclear infiltration originates in the outer site where
blood flow is present, this rim of Zenker necrosis is associated with
leukocytes, and may be easily confused with the coagulation necrosis.

Finally it should be mentioned that in 208 selected cases of
sudden coronary death (apparently healthy people who died out-of-
hospital without any medical intervention and resuscitation attempts)
in 72 per cent Zenker necrosis was the only documented acute lesion,
while coagulation necrosis associated with Zenker necrosis was demonstrable in 15 per cent and myocytolysis was practically absent.
In 97 "controls" (normal subjects dying suddenly by accidental death)
no one showed coagulation necrosis and myocytolysis while 19 presented
minimal foci of Zenker necrosis.[4,5]

Theoretical aspects in relation to the morpho-functional findings

From the previous findings several aspects should be considered.
First the clear-cut morpho-functional difference indicates that the
three types of myocardial necrosis are distinct entities and not
stages of the same damage. Human and experimental data show that
each type represents a specific metabolic disorder. This implies
different pathogenesis in accordance with the general rule that each
pathogenic mechanism determines pathogonomic dysfunctional and
structural changes. The assumption that the three types of damage
may correspond to different degrees of ischaemia should imply that
any focus of infarct necrosis is a "mixed" lesion since topographical
and chronological gradients of ischaemia exist in the evolution of
the damage (total reversibility within 20 min, dyshomogeneous
irreversibility before one hour). Again Zenker necrosis is experimentally established in a few minutes and increasing doses of catecholamines produce a larger, but not different type of lesion.
Finally, according to the structural changes it is unlikely that a
fragmented, hypercontracted myocell may revert in a normal distended
cell or vice versa.

At present etiology and pathogenesis of each single myocardial
necrosis in man is controversial. Infarct necrosis (coagulation
necrosis) is likely due to reduction of the nutrient flow, even if
the cause-effect relation for many, if not all, the proposed causes
is still questionable. On the other hand Zenker necrosis and myocytolysis appear to be non ischaemic, primary "metabolic" myocellular
disorders in which excess or depletion of catecholamines or catechol-

amine-like substances seem to have an important role in determining
the specific cellular dysionism. However what seems not to be overlooked is the presence and the frequent association of these different
types of damage in the natural history of the so-called ischaemic
heart disease. In the latter complications and death seem more
linked with metabolic disorders at myocellular level than to blood
flow reduction. In particular in people predisposed by congenital
and/or acquired factors, sympathetic overstimulation leading to
malignant arrhythmias may occur as primary event (sudden death in
absence of an infarct); or following an infarct. In this condition
at a critical point of myocardial mass with loss of contraction
(infarct), the normal myocardium is stimulated to compensatory
hyperfunction mediated by the sympathetic nervous system, particularly
at the border of the infarct where there is maximal mechanical tension.

From the other site exhaustion or depletion of catecholamines
may be responsible for cardiac failure secondary to an acute infarct.
The histologic hallmark of this dysfunction (myocytolysis) is mainly
found in cases with longer survival and with associated myocardial
fibrosis.

The infarct size concept

A correct determination of the infarct size should be limited
to the measurement of the tridimensional extension of the coagulation
necrosis. Contradictory results, some misunderstanding and "delayed"
necrosis concept are likely due to the lack of discrimination between
the primitive coagulation necrosis and the other subsequent necrotic
processes by the various methods in vivo and by post-mortem enzymatic
tissue stain.

With this in mind, the first question is whether or not the
infarct size is related to the various clinical courses characterizing
this nosologic entity (uneventful recovery or recovery after more or
less severe complications or death both sudden during a regular
course or after complication). At present the only way to establish
the infarct size is a direct measurement of the necrotic tissue
controlling by microscope the exact type of necrosis. In turn this
means that our information is confined to the small percentage
of patients who die; and therefore they may not be representative
of the whole population of infarcted patients. Nevertheless the
finding that death, as end result of major complications, does
not correlate with the infarct size, strongly suggests that the latter
may, in general, not correlate with the different clinical courses.
In other words the clinical course may be benign or malignant independently of the size of coagulation necrosis (in thirty per cent
of the fatal acute infarcts the size is less than ten per cent and
about half of these patients had a size less than twenty per cent;
while only in 16 per cent the size was greater than 40 per cent).

In these circumstances one may argue if any attempt to reduce the size of the coagulation necrosis is appropriate. The establishment of infarct necrosis requires from 20 to 60 minutes. There is little time for any intervention to restore the nutrient flow in the ischaemic area. Last but not least reflow after 20-40 minutes aggravates the myocardial damage and lowers the threshold for ventricular fibrillation. Therefore any attempt to reduce the extension of the coagulation necrosis may be ineffective (small infarct) or unrealistic (too late) if not harmful (reflow damage); keeping in mind that there is no evidence that expansion of the primitive coagulation necrosis may occur in man. Since other non ischaemic types of irreversible damage linked with complications are present, the concept of limitation of infarct size should be substitutive by the concept of protection of the normal myocardium from damaging mechanisms other than blood flow reduction. For instance, betablockade before experimental coronary occlusion protects against ventricular fibrillation and Zenker necrosis[6]. Many therapeutical interventions thought to be effective in reducing the infarct size, are likely acting in this direction, and patients with uneventful recovery are self-protected by this damage.

In accordance therapeutical interventions and preventive actions should be related to etiology and pathogenesis of the metabolic damage, discovering effective signals capable of discriminating the patients at risk of complications.

ACKNOWLEDGEMENT

Special grants of the National Research Council on Preventive Medicine and Cardiopulmonary Diseases - "Atherosclerosis" and "Clinical Morphology" projects, Rome, Italy.

REFERENCES

1. G. Baroldi, F. Radice, C. Schmid and A. Leone, Morphology of acute myocardial infarction in relation to coronary thrombosis. Am. Heart J., 87:65 (1974).
2. M. D. Silver, G. Baroldi and F. Mariani, The relationship between acute occlusive coronary thrombi and myocardial infarction studies in 100 consecutive patients. Circulation, 61:219 (1980).
3. G. Baroldi, Different types of myocardial necrosis in coronary heart disease: a pathophysiological review of their functional significance. Am. Heart J., 89:742 (1975).
4. G. Baroldi, G. Falzi and F. Mariani, Sudden coronary death. A postmortem study in 208 selected cases compared to 97 "control" subjects. Am. Heart J., 98:20 (1979).

5. G. Baroldi, Pathology and Mechanisms of Sudden Death, in "The Heart" J. W. Hurst ed., McGraw-Hill Book Co., New York, 5th Edition, p. 393 (1982).

6. G. Baroldi, M. D. Silver, W. Lixfeld and D. C. McGregor, Irreversible myocardial damage resembling catecholamine necrosis secondary to acute coronary occlusion in dogs: its prevention by propranolol. J. Molec. Cell. Cardiol., 9:687 (1977).

QUANTITATIVE ASSESSMENT OF INFARCT SIZE AND ITS INFLUENCE

BY THROMBOLYSIS

Burton E. Sobel, Edward M. Geltman and
Steven R. Bergmann

Cardiovascular Division
Washington University School of Medicine
660 South Euclid Avenue
St. Louis, Missouri 63110 U.S.A.

INTRODUCTION

Conventional nuclear cardiology employs gamma-emitting tracers such as technetium-99 (^{99m}Tc) or thallium-201 (^{201}Tl). Such tracers are not physiological metabolites and accordingly behave somewhat differently from the physiological constituents being traced. Single-photon emitters decay by liberating energy in the form of photons characteristic of the parent radio-nuclide, much of which is absorbed (attenuated) before it reaches the detector. Because of the variability of attenuation it is difficult, if not impossible, to accurately define both the amount of radiation emitted and its location. Thus, even though the reconstructed images may be aesthetically satisfying, quantitative limitations preclude definitive correspondence between the reconstructed image and the actual distribution of tracer in the organ of interest in absolute terms.[1]

Tracers employed in positron emission tomography (PET) such as carbon-11 (^{11}C), nitrogen-13 (^{13}N), oxygen-15 (^{15}O), and others decay by emitting positively charged particles, positrons, which traverse only a short distance before encountering a negatively charged electron and undergoing annihilation with liberation of two 511 kev photons directed approximately 180° apart. Accordingly, coincidence counting provides electronic collimation and spatial localization of the emitted positron with attenuation compensated regardless of the locus of the source with respect to each member of each detector pair. [2]

Instrumentation employed at Washington University, developed by Dr. Michel M. Ter-Pogossian and his colleagues, permits reconstruction of seven 16 mm thick transaxial sections of the heart with an inter-section distance of 10 mm from apex to base. Repeat imaging after the patient has been shifted 9.5 mm provides a total of 14 tomographic reconstructions after a single injection of tracer. Since most positron-emitting radionuclides have short half-lives (for example, 20.4 min for ^{11}C), they can be utilized sequentially without imposing excessive radiation burdens on the patient.

Regional Myocardial Metabolism

During the past several years, we have demonstrated that regional myocardial metabolism can be defined in vivo with the use of positron-emitting radionuclides despite influences of residence time and altered extraction fractions as a function of flow.[3-11]

Because fatty acid is the primary substrate for energy production by myocardium in vivo, we have utilized carbon-11 labeled palmitate. Time-activity curves permitted calculation of extraction fraction and the monoexponential rate of metabolism of ^{11}C-palmitate incorporated into cellular lipids in isolated perfused rabbit hearts, verified by chemical and radio-chemical analyses. Subsequently, normal canine myocardium was shown to accumulate the tracer homogeneously in vivo. Tissue rendered ischemic exhibited markedly decreased uptake demonstrated tomographically correlating closely (r=.97) with regions of necrosis verified histologically and enzymatically at autopsy. When imaging was performed prior to the development of irreversible injury but in the face of ischemia, an analogous "cold-spot" was evident. However, under these conditions reflow led to accumulation of intravenously administered ^{11}C-palmitate in the previously ischemic zones.[3] With a multi-slice system (PETT 1V) and delineation of the intracardiac blood pool and the endocardial border of the heart in patients with the use of inhaled [11]CO-labeled hemoglobin, close correspondence between the electro-cardiographic locus of infarction and persistent impairment of fatty acid metabolism was well demonstrated and infarct size estimated by PET correlated closedly (r=.92) with infarct size estimated by the serial creatine kinase method.

Others have utilized agents such as glucose labeled with fluorine-18 and obtained qualitatively similar images. On the other hand, the introduction of a halogen alters the metabolism of glucose. Thus, it is difficult to interpret such images unequivocally since analysis of carbohydrate metabolism in normal and ischemic tissue cannot be extrapolated directly to metabolism of congeners with altered affinity for enzymes involved.

The present study was performed to determine whether PET with ^{11}C-palmitate provides a potentially useful approach for assessment of the efficacy of thrombolysis in restoring myocardial metabolism and to delineate the temporal dependence of its efficacy.

METHODS

Conditioned dogs anesthetized with sodium thiopental (12.5 mg/kg) and α-chloralose (60 mg/kg) were studied after left femoral artery and vein cannulation and administration of lidocaine. Coronary thrombus was induced with a copper coil (5 to 7.5 mm in length) inserted into the left anterior descending coronary artery.[12] An occlusive thrombus developed within 5 to 15 minutes, heralded by typical electrocardiographic signs of ischemia including ST elevation and ventricular dysrhythmia and confirmed angiographically. Thirty minutes after induction of thrombus, and at selected intervals from 1 to 14 hours after occlusion each dog was given 15 to 20 mCi of ^{11}C-palmitate ($t_{1/2}=20.4$) intravenously and studied tomographically.

Immediately after tomography had been completed, streptokinase (4000 U/min) dissolved in saline (2000 U/min) or saline alone was administered through the intracoronary catheter. In control and treated dogs, positron emission tomography was performed again after a second intravenous injection of ^{11}C-palmitate 1.5 hr after the initial tomographic study, coronary arteriography was repeated, and a catheter was advanced into the left ventricle for injection of approximately 4 million [85]Sr microspheres (50 μCi, 15 μm diameter spheres) for measurement of myocardial blood flow.

RESULTS

Coronary thrombi was lysed successfully, judging from sequential angiograms, in approximately 85% of all attempts. Approximately 30 minutes after the initiation of thrombolysis, reperfusion arrhythmia occurred (ectopic ventricular beats often progressing to accelerated idioventricular rhythm).[13] All dogs with induced coronary thrombus exhibited tomographic defects of ^{11}C-palmitate accumulation in initial transverse tomograms. In the absence of lysis, tomographic defects were stable (Table 1). After reperfusion tomographic changes indicative of restored metabolism in these previously identified zones were markedly dependent on the duration of the preceding occlusion (Figure 1). Longer intervals of occlusion were associated with persistence, rather than of the defects.[14]

Occlusion for one to two hours followed by reperfusion led to a 51.1± 6.3% <u>decrease</u> in the overall extent of metabolically

Table 1. Tomographically Estimated Infarct Size in Dogs with and
          without Coronary Thrombolysis

Experimental Group and Interval After Occlusion	n	Tomographically Estimated Jeopardized Zones[a]	
		Tomogram I	Tomogram II [b]
Controls; 1 to 6 hours	6	24.7 ± 1.5	25.6 ± 2.7
Thrombolysis; 1 to 2 hours	4	24.6 ± 3.8*	12.0 ± 2.3*
Thrombolysis; 2 to 4 hours	6	25.7 ± 2.8*	20.3 ± 2.3*
Thrombolysis; 4 to 6 hours	4	24.7 ± 3.2	21.6 ± 4.0
Thrombolysis; 12 to 14 hours	3	23.9 ± 3.1	24.5 ± 3.7

* $p < .01$ within the same experimental group.
a)   Values are means ± SE of the number of pixels exhibiting less
     than 50% of the maximum count rate/total left ventricular wall
     pixels (thus expressed as % of left ventricle).
b)   The second tomographic study was initiated 1.5 hours after the
     first scan. In each case in experimentally treated animals,
     thrombolysis was initiated after tomogram I had been obtained.

Table 2 Tomographically Estimated Metabolic Activity in the
         Jeopardized Zone Before and After Coronary Thrombolysis

Experimental Group and Interval After Occlusion	n	Metabolic Activity in the Initial Tomographically Defined Jeopardized Zone[a]	
		Tomogram I	Tomogram II [b]
Controls; 1 to 3 hours	6	31.0 ± 2.5	33.6 ± 3.5
Thrombolysis; 1 to 2 hours	4	30.1 ± 2.6*	61.8 ± 4.6*
Thrombolysis; 2 to 4 hours	6	39.1 ± 2.8*	55.6 ± 5.0*
Thrombolysis; 4 to 6 hours	4	28.2 ± 2.8	37.6 ± 6.2
Thrombolysis; 12 to 14 hours	3	31.3 ± 3.9	33.8 ± 1.6

* $p < .01$ within the same experimental group.
a)   Values are means ± SE of ^{11}C-radioactivity/pixel in the initial
     jeopardized zone (defined as the region in which count rate was
     less than 50% of maximum normal left ventricular wall count rate
     in the initial tomogram) normalized by expressing the values as
     % of average counts/pixel in the normal zone.
b)   The second tomographic study was initiated 1.5 hours after the
     first scan. In each case in experimentally treated animals,
     thrombolysis was initiated after tomogram I had been obtained.

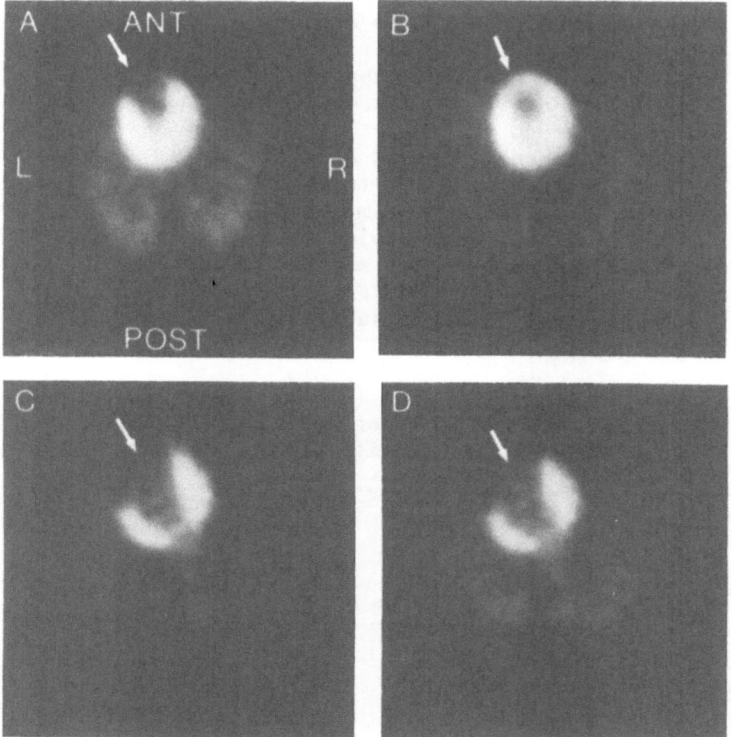

Fig.1 Transverse cardiac positron emission tomographic recon-
       structions obtained after intravenous administration of
       ^{11}C-palmitate in dogs. Reconstructions depicted are those
       obtained 1 hour after experimentally induced left anterior
       descending coronary artery thrombosis (A) and again after
       thrombolysis in the same dog (B). Normal myocardium
       extracts palmitate uniformly, whereas the ischemic zone
       exhibits diminished accumulation of tracer (arrow). The
       tomogram in panel B demonstrates substantial restoration
       of metabolism in the previously compromised anterior
       myocardium. In the lower panel, a tomogram 6 hours after
       onset of thrombosis and prior to the administration of
       streptokinase (C) is shown with a repeat tomogram (D) from
       the same dog 1 hour after intracoronary thrombolysis with
       streptokinase (confirmed angiographically). In contrast
       to the restoration of metabolism observed in dogs in which
       reperfusion was induced early after thrombosis, animals
       subjected to thrombolysis later than 6 hours after occlusion
       exhibited no significant restoration of metabolism despite
       angiographically documented lysis of coronary thrombi.
       (After Sobel et al, reprinted with permission from the Am.
       J. Med.)

compromised zones (p < .01) (Table 2). Occlusion for two to four hours prior to thrombolysis led to a more modest decrease in the overall extent of the metabolically compromised zone (by 21 ± 1.8%) and to a more modest increase in apparent metabolic activity (by 51.8 ± 12.6%) (p < .01). With occlusion of longer duration prior to thrombolysis no statistically significant change in the distribution of impaired metabolic activity was evident and dogs with twelve hour occlusions prior to thrombolysis showed no alteration in the distribution or magnitude of metabolic compromise (Table 3). Hearts of all dogs subjected to reperfusion exhibited transmural myocardial hemorrhage, contraction bands, and interstitial edema. After both early (≤ 6 hours) and late (6 to 14 hours) reperfusion, transmural flow was substantial in previously ischemic zones (>80% and >60% of normal).

Table 3   Percentage Change in Tomographically Estimated Jeopardized Zone and Metabolic Activity After Coronary Thrombolysis

Experimental Group and Interval After Occlusion	n	Changes as a Function of Time With and Without Thrombolysis	
		Jeopardized Zone[a]	Metabolic Activity[a]
Controls; 1 to 6 hours	6	2.5 ± 7.0%	9.5 ± 10.1%
Thrombolysis; 1 to 2 hours	4	−51.1± 6.3%	111.0 ± 24.3%*
Thrombolysis; 2 to 4 hours	6	−21.0± 1.8%	61.8 ± 12.6%*
Thrombolysis; 4 to 6 hours	4	−13.9± 7.5%	40.1 ± 30.2%
Thrombolysis; 12 to 14 hours	3	1.0 ± 10.0%	10.1 ± 9.0%

*   p < .01 within the same experimental group.
a)   Values represent means ± SE expressed as the percentage change in comparisons between results of the two tomographic studies for each of the parameters expressed in absolute terms in Tables 1 and 2.

Tables 1, 2 and 3 are from S. R. Bergmann, R. A. Lerch, K. A. A. Fox, P. A. Ludbrook, M. J. Welch, M. M. Ter-Pogossian, and B. E. Sobel, The temporal dependence of beneficial effects of coronary thrombolysis characterized by positron tomography, published with permission of the American Journal of Medicine.

DISCUSSION

These results indicate that the metabolic status of jeopardized ischemic myocardium can be assessed objectively by sequential positron emission tomography after administration of ^{11}C-palmitate —— a modality already employed successfully for other purposes in patients.[8,11,15]. When reperfusion was initiated within four hours after coronary occlusion, restoration of myocardial metabolism was substantial. However, with longer intervals of occlusion prior to reperfusion, salutary effects on metabolism were less pronounced.

Thus, the interval during which reperfusion will be beneficial to myocardium appears to be limited sharply. Its boundaries will obviously depend on the extent of the collateral circulation, the completeness of occlusion, hemodynamic and metabolic demands, and other factors.

Although intracoronary thrombolytic therapy early after the onset of apparent infarction and as late as 18 hours after the onset of infarction in patients has been reported to be helpful, conventionally available criteria of efficacy may be misleading. When thrombolytic therapy is initiated prior to evolution of unequivocal signs of infarction and ST-segment elevation is present with prolonged chest pain but plasma CK values are still normal, results are difficult to interpret.[16] Infarction does not occur invariably in this setting, as shown in a large, well controlled multi-center study of preinfarction angina which demonstrated that documented infarction accompanies such episodes in the absence of thrombolysis only infrequently.[17] Thrombolysis initiated as late as 18 hours after the onset of infarction may be accompanied by amelioration of chest pain and ST-segment changes; accelerated evolution of Q waves; elevated plasma CK activity; and improved left ventricular ejection fraction analogous to changes reported after early thrombolysis. However, reperfusion may fail to restor viability or exacerbate injury after such prolonged intervals.[18,19]

This study demonstrates the potential value of positron emission tomography as a tool for objectively assessing effects of thrombolysis on myocardial viability in patients. Results indicate that salvage of jeopardized myocardium by early coronary thrombolysis in experimental animals _in vivo_ is detectable readily. They underscore the dependence of its efficacy on the interval available for effective reperfusion and may be of particular relevance to the design of longitudinal, clinical trials employing objective endpoints which can be interpreted unambiguously in the continuing effort to elucidate this potentially promising intervention.

Acknowledgment

We gratefully acknowledge preparation of the typescript by Ms. Carolyn Lohman.

REFERENCES

1.   M. M. Ter-Pogossian, Limitations of present radionuclide methods in the evaluation of myocardial ischemia and infarction, Circulation 53:Suppl. 1:119 (1976).

2. E. S. Weiss, B. A. Siegal, B. E. Sobel, M. J. Welch, and M. M. Ter-Pogossian, Evaluation of myocardial metabolism and perfusion with positron-emitting radionuclides, Prog. Cardiovasc. Dis. 20:191 (1977).

3. R. A. Lerch, H. D. Ambros, S. R. Bergmann, M. J. Welch, M. M. Ter-Pogossian, and B. E. Sobel, Localization of viable, ischemic myocardium by positron emission tomography (PET) with ^{11}C-palmitate, Circulation 64:689 (1981).

4. E. S. Weiss, E. J. Hoffman, M. E. Phelps, M. J. Welch, P. D. Henry, M. M. Ter-Pogossian, and B. E. Sobel, External detection and visualization of myocardial ischemia with ^{11}C-subtrates in vitro and in vivo, Circ. Res. 39:24 (1976).

5. M. S. Klein, R. A. Goldstein, M. J. Welch, and B. E. Sobel, External assessment of myocardial metabolism with (^{11}C) palmitate in rabbit hearts, Am J Physiol: Heart Circ. Physiol. 237:H51 (1979).

6. R. A. Lerch, S. R. Bergmann, H. D. Ambos, M. J. Welch, M. M. Ter-Pogossian, and B. E. Sobel, Effect of flow independent reduction of metabolism on regional myocardial clearance of ^{11}C-palmitate, Circulation 65:731 (1982).

7. E. S. Weiss, S. A. Ahmed, M. J. Welch, J. R. Williamson, M. M. Ter-Pogossian, and B. E. Sobel, Quantification of infarction in cross sections of canine myocardium in vivo with positron emission transaxial tomography and ^{11}C-palmitate, Circulation 55:66 (1977).

8. B. E. Sobel, E. S. Weiss, M. J. Welch, B. A. Siegel, and M. M. Ter-Pogossian, Detection of remote myocardial infarction in patients with positron emission transaxial tomography and intravenous ^{11}C-palmitate, Circulation 55-853 (1977).

9. K. A. A. Fox, H. Nomura, B. E. Sobel, and S. R. Bergmann, Constant radiolabeled palmitate consumption despite reduced flow in isolated hearts performing constant work, Clin Res 30:186A (1982)(abstract).

10. R. A. Goldstein, M. S. Klein, M. J. Welch, and B. E. Sobel, External assessment of myocardial metabolism with C-11 palmitate in vivo. J. Nucl. Med. 21:342 (1980).

11. M. M. Ter-Pogossian, M. S. Klein, J. Markham, R. Roberts, and B. E. Sobel, Regional assessment of myocardial metabolic integrity in vivo by positron emission tomography with ^{11}C-labelled palmitate, Circulation 61:242 (1980).

12. R. K. Kordenat, and P. Kezdi, Experimental intracoronary thrombosis and selective in situ lysis by catheter technique, Am J. Cardiol. 30:640 (1972).

13. P. B. Corr, J. A. Shayman, J. B. Kramer, and R. J. Kipnis, Increased β-adrenergic receptors in ischemic cat myocardium: A potential mediator of electro-physiological derangements, J. Clin. Invest. 67:1232 (1981).

14. S. R. Bergmann, R. A. Lerch, K. A. A. Fox, P. A. Ludbrook, M. J. Welch, M. M. Ter-Pogossian, and B. E. Sobel, The temporal dependence of beneficial effects of coronary thrombolysis characterized by positron tomography, Am. J. Med. (in press).

15. E. M. Geltman, D. Biello, M. J. Welch, M. M. Ter-Pogossian, and B. E. Sobel, Characterization of nontransmural myocardial infarction by positron emission tomography, Circulation 65:747 (1982).

16. B. E. Sobel, and S. R. Bergmann, Coronary thrombolysis: Some unresolved issues, Am J. Med. 72:1 (1982).

17. Unstable angina pectoris: National cooperative study group to compare surgical and medical therapy. II In-hospital experience and initial follow-up results in patients with one, two and three vessel disease, Am J. Cardiol. 42:839 (1978)

18. G. F. Bresnahan, R. Roberts, W. E. Shell, J. Ross, Jr. and B. E. Sobel, Deleterious effects due to hemorrhage after myocardial reperfusion, Am J. Cardiol. 33:82 (1974).

19. V. S. Mathur, G. A. Guinn, and W. H. Burris, Maximal revascularization (reperfusion) in intact conscious dogs after 2 to 5 hours of coronary occlusion, Am J. Cardiol. 36:252 (1975)

LIMITATION OF INFARCT SIZE BY PHARMACOLOGICAL INTERVENTIONS

A. Waldenström, J. Herlitz
F. Waggstein and Å. Hjalmarson

Department of Medicine I
Sahlgren's Hospital
University of Göteborg
Göteborg, Sweden

By the introduction of coronary care units the mortality in acute myocardial infarction decreased from about 40% to about 15-20%. This was mainly due to:

(1) good monitoring of patients with early detection of arrhythmias,
(2) effective antiarrhythmic drugs (e.g. lidocaine),
(3) well trained staff with early and skilled handling of cardiac standstills.

For these reasons a further gain in mortality reduction due to arrhythmias could not be expected. The other main cause of death is left ventricular failure, which is correlated to myocardial infarct size. To further reduce mortality in acute myocardial infarction, it seems logical to try to limit infarct size.

A number of experimental studies show that if therapy is started early enough infarct size may be limited. Many clinical studies have demonstrated the correlation between infarct size and mortality (Table 1).[1-12] In 9 out of 10 studies there is a good correlation between peak enzyme values and hospital mortality. In 3 out of 5 studies where the patients were followed for 3 to 5 years high serum enzyme values were positively correlated to high mortality. It can thus be assumed that limitation of infarct size would decrease mortality after a myocardial infarction. Very few data on this subject have been available hitherto.

535

Table 1. Correlation Between Peak-enzyme Value and Mortality

Authors	Numbers of pat	Percentage of 1st infarction	Enzyme	Hospital mortality	1-5 years mortality
Kibe and Nilsson 1967	155	Not given	LD, GOT	+	+
Kluge 1969	84	Not given	CK	+	
Chapman 1971	376	Not given	LD,GOT	+	
Hofvendahl 1971	271	70%	GOT	-	-
Sobel et al. 1972	33	Not given	CK	+	
Scheinman and Abbot 1973	230	60%	LD, GOT	+	
Helmers 1973	606	74%	GOT	+	-
Henning et al. 1975	2008	63%	GOT	+	
Vedin et al. 1977	292	100%	GOT	+	+
Nordlander and Nyguist 1979	194	67%	CK, GOT	+	
Thompson et al. 1979	560	72%	CK, ASAT		+
Thanavaro et al. 1980	745	100%	GOT	+	

+ peak enzyme value and mortality correlated

- not correlated

METHODS FOR ESTIMATION OF INFARCT SIZE

There has been an intensive debate on the accuracy of the clinical methods for infarct size measurements. It is obvious that no existing method is ideal. The most widely used method is serum enzyme measurements, as introduced by Shell et al.[13] Using an enzyme with a flat disappearance curve, such as lactate dehydrogenase (LD), there is a good chance to hit the curve near its maximum. This means that LD_{max} could be used instead of enzyme curves. Creatine phosphokinase (CK) appears in serum and reaches maximum very early with a rapid disappearance rate. It is therefore more difficult to get a serum sample at the maximum serum concentration. Using this enzyme, serum concentration curves are more accurate.

Precordial ECG mapping, as described by Maroko et al,[14] using 24-28 electrodes, gives an estimate of infarct size in anterior and lateral wall infarctions.

Myocardial scintigraphy is a newly developed method for infarct imaging with very promising results. The best method in the future, however, will probably be the use of nuclear magnetic resonance (NMR) techniques.

CLINICAL STUDIES OF INFARCT SIZE LIMITATION

The prerequisite for effective limitation of infarct size is the concept that the acute phase of myocardial infarction is a dynamic process evolving over several hours (Figure 1).[15] Only then there is a chance that the patient can be treated before the completion of the infarction. This is confirmed by the results of the Swedish metoprolol trial[16,17] (Figure 2) where the best clinical effect was found among those patients who came into treatment early, i.e. within 12 hours.

The infarct evolves because of an imbalance between myocardial oxygen and substrate demand and metabolite production on one hand and oxygen and substrate supply and metabolic washout on the other. Different techniques have been used to restore this balance. This can be done either by optimizing the hemodynamic situation or by reducing heart work, optimizing coronary flow and increasing diffusion in the ischemic tissue. Utilization of glucose consumes less oxygen than that of free fatty acids (FFA) per mole ATP produced. It is thus advantageous in the ischemic situation to increase glucose and decrease FFA utilization. Moreover, intermediary metabolites of fatty acid metabolism are accumulated in the ischemic myocardium and will negatively influence adenine nucleotide metabolism.

Hyaluronidase was already tried in the 1950's to limit infarct size. This method was further studied by Dr Maroko both in dogs and

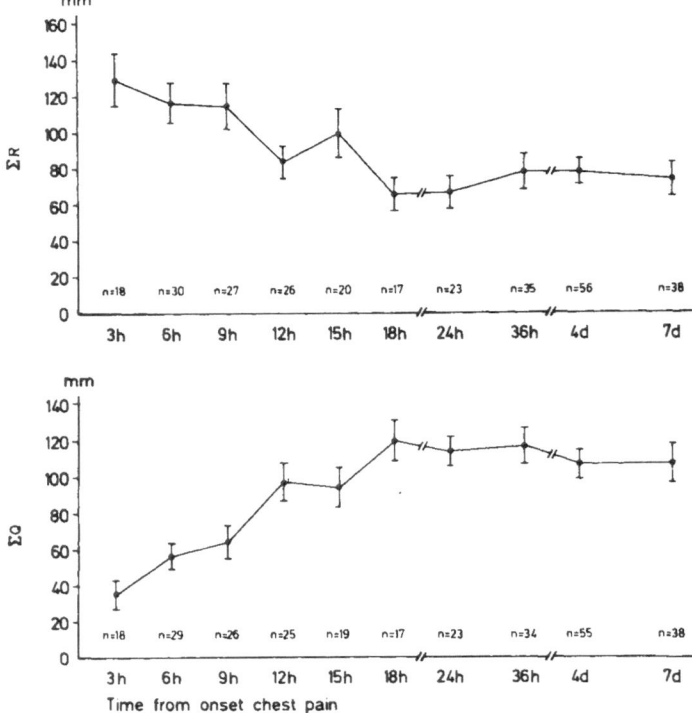

Fig. 1.   Time course for reduction of ΣR (above) and elevation of
          ΣQ (below) in anterior myocardial wall infarction.[15]

man.   In 1977 a randomized study of 91 patients with anterior infarction was presented.[18] Only patients with infarcts not older than 8
hours were included.   The patients were treated with hyaluronidase

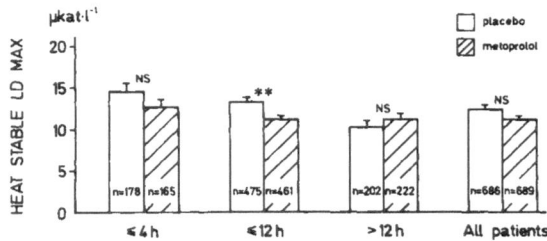

Fig. 2.   Mean max heat stable LD activities in all patients and in
          those given blind injections within different time inter-
          vals after onset of pain. Missing data in 15 of the
          patients in whom enzyme values were obtained. *P < 0.05;
          **P < 0.01. Mean ± SEM.[15]

i.v. for only 48 hours. The ECG changes consistent with myocardial necrosis were reduced in the treatment group when a 35-lead precordial ECG mapping was performed.[18] In 1982 three studies were published in the same issue of the Lancet.[19-21] In a study by Saltissi et al.,[19] 79 patients with suspected acute myocardial infarction were randomly treated with placebo or i.v. hyaluronidase within 6 hours after onset of chest pain. Precordial electrocardiographic indices of infarct size (R-wave loss and Q-wave appearance) were reduced in the treatment group.[19] Flint et al.[20] demonstrated a reduction in mortality in 483 patients (Figure 3) at 6 months when all patients irrespective of trial diagnosis were analyzed. Henderson et al.[21] randomized 192 consecutive patients arriving within 12 hours after onset of symptoms suspected of myocardial infarction. Patients with definite acute myocardial infarction in the treatment group had significantly less QRS changes and development of Q-waves than those in the placebo group.

Positive effects of infusion of glucose-insulin-potassium (GIK) was first reported by Sodi-Pallares in 1962.[22] Rogers et al.[23] reported lower CK-B leakage in 23 GIK-treated patients when compared to 27 controls. At this congress the same authors reported the results of a larger series comprising 190 patients admitted within 12 hours after onset of chest pain. No effect on infarct size could be confirmed but there was a trend towards lower hospital mortality. The data on GIK infusion are thus not conclusive.

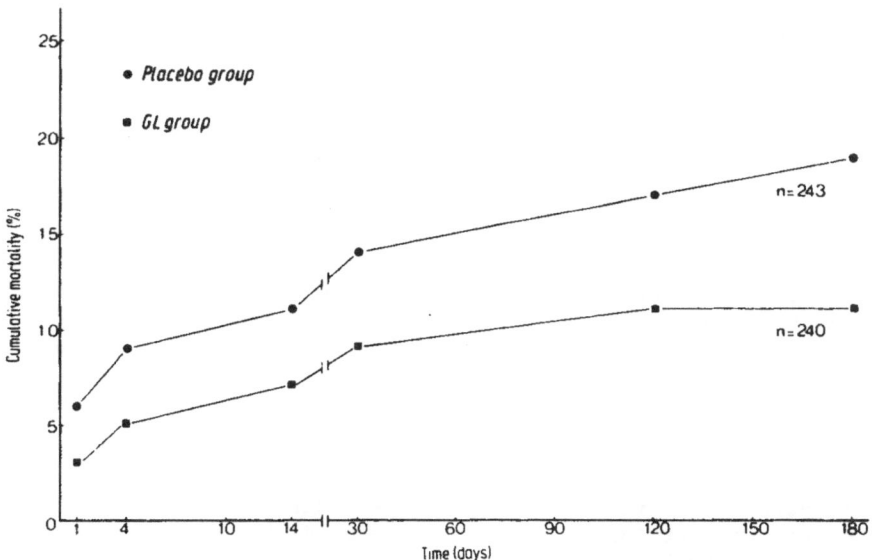

Fig. 3. Cumulative mortality over a 6-month period for all patients entered into the study.[20]

Table 2.   Effect of Beta-pyridylcarbinol in AMI.
           Treatment within 6 Hours of Clinical Onset
           Cumulated CK (ukat/1)

Hrs	-1	0	2	6	24	48
Control (9)	1.9	4.4	10.4	19.7	40.2	43.4
Drug (9)	1.0	1.9	5.2	12.9	46.8	54.1

Reduced evolution of QRS infarct vector during the 15
hours of betapyridylcarbinol infusion when FFA were
lowered. Overshoot after stop of infusion.

Kjekshus and Grøttum 1977

Methyprednisolone has proved effective in experimental myocardial infarction but when used in a clinical trial adverse effects
with higher mortality in the treatment group was reported by Roberts
and co-workers.[24]

During acute myocardial infarction serum levels of FFA are elevated. This might be deleterious for above mentioned reasons. In 1977
Kjekshus and Grøttum[25] published a study where patients were treated
within 6 hours of onset of symptoms (Table 2). Beta-pyridylcarbinol - a lipid-lowering drug - was infused for 15 hours. CK release
and ECG changes were reduced but after completion of infusion there
was an overshoot of CK release and more marked ECG changes. The
effect of this treatment thus seems to be controversial.

Lowering of myocardial work has also been done by nitroglycerine
infusion. Derrida et al.[26] used this treatment in a series of 74
patients with acute myocardial infarction. In the 39 treated
patients mortality was less than among the 35 controls. Also indices
of infarct size, such as Q and R-waves were favourable in the treatment group.

In 1979 Bussman et al.[27] presented another prospective randomized trial. When nitroglycerine infusion was started within 8 hours
after onset of chest pain a positive effect was shown. When treatment was started after 8 hours the signs of infarct size measured as
CK leakage were less marked. This was, however, a small trial with
only 15 patients.

In 1982 two trials were published in the same issue of New
England Journal of Medicine on effects of nitroprusside treatment in
acute myocardial infarction patients.[28,29] Durrer et al.[28] included
328 patients with ECG signs of acute myocardial infarction. One
hundred and sixty-three patients were randomly allocated to nitroprusside treatment. Myocardial infarct size was estimated by the
use of CK-MB levels and mortality was studied after one week.

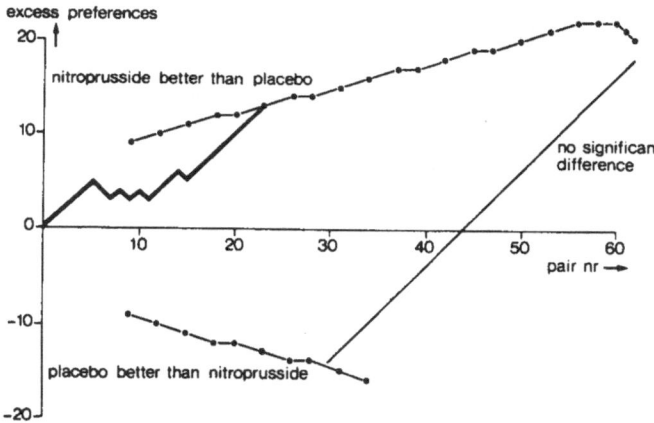

Fig. 4.   Sample path (thick line) and predesignated boundaries
          (thin line with dots) in armitage closed sequential plan.[28]

These authors could demonstrate smaller infarcts and lower death rate
(Figure 4)[28] in the treatment group. In a larger study by Cohn et
al.[29] no effect on mortality could be seen after 13 weeks in the 812
patients included in the trial. This was also a double-blind
placebo-controlled trial. Peak CK-B values indicated smaller infarcts in the treatment group irrespective of early or late treatment. The conflicting data of these trials are even more confusing
as nitroprusside appeared to have a deleterious effect on mortality
in patients treated early, although CK-B values tended to be lower in
this group. Both trials were prospectively randomized, placebo-
controlled and including appropriate trial number of patients. In
the study by Cohn et al.[29] all patients were male with elevated left
ventricular filling pressures and treatment was started later than in
the study by Durrer et al.[28] where both sexes were included, but
without any clinical signs of elevated filling pressures. As the two
trials are not totally comparable, no firm conclusion can be drawn.
Probably the treatment will not affect mortality when given late to
patients in failure but nitroprusside may reduce mortality when given
early to well compensated patients.

     Positive effects of beta-blockers in patients with acute myo-
cardial infarction was first reported by Snow in 1965.[30] Since then
four randomized trials with beta-blockers for infarct size limitation
have been published.[17,31-33].

     In a small trial by Peter et al.,[31] 18 patients were treated
with propranolol within 4 hours and compared to controls. CK-release
was smaller in the treatment group. In another group treated after
12 hours after onset of chest pain, no difference in CK could be seen

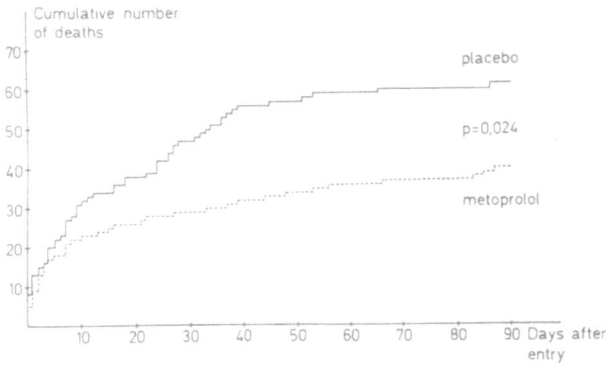

Fig. 5.   Cumulative number of deaths in all patients randomly
          allocated to treatment with metoprolol and placebo.
          P-value is calculated according to Mantel-Haenzel.[17]

between the two groups. Alprenolol was used in a study from
Copenhagen[32] where the patients were treated within 12 hours after
onset of symptoms. A lower CK leakage was noted in the treatment
group. One-year mortality was reported to be lower in the treatment
group among patients ≤ 65 years of age. In patients > 65 years there
was a trend towards a higher mortality in the treatment group[33] and
the study was stopped prematurely in this age group.

     In the Göteborg metoprolol trial,[17] 1395 patients were randomly
allocated to placebo or beta-blockade. The patients were followed
for 3 months. "Infarct size" was smaller when metoprolol was given
≤ 12 hours after onset of pain, as judged from enzyme curves and
from Q and R-wave changes. The reduction in mortality was significantly lower after 3 months (Figure 5). In this study, the number of
analgetic injections and need for furosemide were reduced among
patients treated ≤ 12 hours in whom "infarct size" was limited. In a
study by Sleight et al.,[34] including 504 patients with myocardial infarction, atenolol was found to limit "infarct size" measured as
cumulative CK-B.

CONCLUSION

     In Table 3 are listed regimes where a positive effect on infarct
size has been reported. For most of the drugs listed the results are
inconclusive. Beta-blockade seems to be the only drug today with reliable positive effects in acute myocardial infarction. Heart work is
reduced and thereby oxygen consumption, lactate production is decreased, and supraventricular and ventricular arrhythmias are re-
pressed. Even ventricular fibrillation is prevented by beta-blockade.

Table 3.   Drugs with Documented Positive
Effects on Infarct Size in Man.

o   Beta blockade
o   Hyaluronidase
o   Nitroglycerin
o   Nitroprusside
o   Trimethaphan (in hypertensive patients)

The important question today is whether infarct size can be
limited, and if so, which effects of beta-blockade are directly related to such limitations. Although there is a well documented reduction in mortality, the above mentioned question cannot be satisfactorily answered. There is good circumstantial evidence that
"infarct size" is limited as CK and LD leakage is decreased, and this
is true only for patients treated early. This should rule out the
possibility that beta-blockade per se due to changes in washout and
metabolism would alter the enzyme curve, which would otherwise be the
case also for patients treated late. Another support for this idea
is that less patients went into failure in the treatment group. It
is reasonable to believe that this was because of salvage of muscle
mass. ECG mapping also indicated smaller infarcts in treated
patients. However, many questions remain to be answered: How much
of the myocardium may maximally be jeopardized and therefore salvage-
able? Is this amount of tissue compatible with the clinical effects?
There is an old observation that noradrenaline in the "normal" myocardium is depressed also when a coronary artery is ligated in a
dog.[35] This situation will last for up to six weeks. Is this decrease of noradrenaline the reason for cardiac failure in acute myocardial infarction and is this loss of noradrenaline prevented by
beta-blockade?

Acknowledgements

This study was supported by grants from the National Association
against Heart and Chest Diseases, the Göteborg Medical Society, and
AB Hässle, subsidiary of AB Astra, Sweden.

REFERENCES

1. O. Kibe and N. J. Nilsson, Observations on the diagnostic and
    prognostic value of some enzyme tests in myocardial infarc-
    tion, Acta.Med.Scand. 182:597-610 (1967).
2. W. F. Kluge, Prognostic value of serum creatine phosphokinase
    levels in myocardial infarction, Northwest Med, Sept 1979,
    pp.847-853.

3. B. L. Chapman, Correlation of mortality rate and serum enzymes in myocardial infarction. Test of efficiency of coronary care, Br.Heart J. 33:643-646 (1971).

4. S. Hofvendahl, Influence of treatment in a coronary care unit on prognosis in acute myocardial infarction. A controlled study in 271 cases, Acta Med. Scand. Suppl 519:9-78 (1971).

5. B. E. Sobel, G. F. Bresnahan, W. E. Shell and R. D. Yoder, Estimation of infarct size in man and its relation to prognosis, Circulation 46:640-648 (1972).

6. M. M. Scheinman and J. A. Abbott, Clinical significance of transmural versus nontransmural electrocardiographic changes in patients with acute myocardial infarction, Am.J.Med. 55: 602-607 (1973).

7. C. Helmers, Short- and long-term prognostic indices in acute myocardial infarction. A study of 606 patients initially treated in a coronary care unit, Acta Med.Scand. Suppl 555: 1-86 (1973).

8. R. Henning, T. Lundman and R. Maasing, Prognostic evaluation by means of automatic interaction detector analysis, Acta Med. Scand. Suppl 578:11-31 (1975).

9. A. Vedin, L. Wilhelmsen, H. Wedel, B. Pettersson, C. Wilhelmsson, D. Elmfeldt and G. Tibblin, Prediction of cardiovascular deaths and non-fatal reinfarctions after myocardial infarction, Acta Med.Scand. 201:309-316 (1977).

10. R. Nordlander and O. Nyquist, Mortality, arrhythmias and pump failure in acute myocardial infarction in relation to estimated infarct size, Acta Med.Scand. 206:65-71 (1979).

11. P. L. Thompson, E. E. Fletcher and V. Katavatis, Enzymatic indices of myocardial necrosis: influence on short- and long-term prognosis after myocardial infarction, Circulation 59:113-119 (1979).

12. S. Thanavaro, R. J. Krone, R. E. Kleiger, M. A. Province, J. P. Miller, V. R. DeMello and G. C. Oliver, In-hospital prognosis of patients with first nontransmural and transmural infarctions, Circulation 61:29-33 (1980).

13. W. E. Shell and B. E. Sobel, Deleterious effects of increased heart rate on infarct size in the conscious dog, Am.J.Cardiol. 31:474-478 (1973).

14. P. R. Maroko, P. Libby, T. W. Dovell, B. E. Sobel, J. Ross Jr and E. Braunwald, Precordial S-T segment elevation mapping: An atraumatic method for assessing alterations in the extent of myocardial ischemic injury, Am.J.Cardiol. 29:223-230 (1972).

15. J. Herlitz, Bedömning och begränsning av hjärtinfarktens storlek. En interventionsstudie med metoprolol, Thesis, Göteborg (1982).

16. J. Herlitz, Å. Hjalmarson, K. Swedberg, F. Waagstein and A. Waldenstöm, A double-blind trial of metoprolol in acute myocardial infarction. Effect on infarct size, clinical findings and 1-year mortality, Abstr. (American Heart Association, 55th Sessions.) Circulation (in press).

17. Å. Hjalmarson, D. Elmfeldt, J. Herlitz, S. Holmberg, I, Málek, G. Nyberg, L. Rýden, K. Swedberg, A. Vedin, F. Waagstein, A. Waldenström, J. Waldenström, H. Wedel, L. Wilhelmsen and C. Wilhelmsson, Effect on mortality of metoprolol in acute myocardial infarction. A double-blind randomised trial, Lancet ii:823-828 (1981).

18. P. R. Maroko, L. D. Hillis, J. E. Muller, L. Tavazzi, G. R. Heyndrickx, M. Ray, M. Chiariello, A. Distante, J. Askenazi, J. Salerno, J. Carpentier, N. I. Reshetnaya, P. Radvany, P. Libby, D. S. Raabe, E. I. Chazov, P. Bobba and E. Braunwald, Favorable effects of hyaluronidase on electro-cardiographic evidence of necrosis in patients with acute myocardial infarction, New Engl.J.Med. 296:898-903 (1977).

19. S. Saltissi, P. S. Robinson, D. J. Coltart, M. M. Webb-Peploe and D. N. Croft, Effects of early administration of a highly purified hyaluronidase preparation (GL enzyme) on myocardial infarct size, Lancet i:867-870 (1982).

20. E. J. Flint, J. de Giovanni, P. J. Cadigan, P. Lamb and B. L. Pentecost, Effect of GL enzyme (a highly purified form of hyaluronidase) on mortality after myocardial infarction, Lancet i:871-874 (1982).

21. A. Henderson, R. W. F. Campbell and D. G. Julian, Effect of a highly purified hyaluronidase preparation (GL enzyme) on electrocardiographic changes in acute myocardial infarction, Lancet i:874-876 (1982).

22. D. Sodi-Pallares, M. R. Testelli, B. L. Fishleder, A. Bisteni, G. A. Medrano, C. Friedland and A. de Micheli, Effects of an intravenous infusion of a potassium-glucose-insulin solution on the electrocardiographic signs of myocardial infarction. A preliminary clinical report, Am.J.Cardiol. 9:166 (1962).

23. W. J. Rogers, P. H. Segall, H. G. McDaniel, J. A. Mantle, R. O. Russell and C. E. Rackley, Prospective randomized trial of glucose-insulin-potassium in acute myocardial infarction. Effects on myocardial hemodynamics, substrates and rhythm, Am.J.Cardiol. 43:801-809 (1979).

24. R. Roberts, V. deMello and B. E. Sobel, Deleterious effects of methylprednisolone in patients with myocardial infarction, Circulation 53, Suppl I:204-206 (1976).

25. J. K. Kjekshus and P. Grøttum, Effect of inhibition of lipolysis on infarct size in man, in:"Acute and Long-term Medical Management of Myocardial Ischaemia," A. Hjalmarson and L. Wilhelmsen, eds., AB Hässle, Mölndal, Sweden, pp.373-387 (1978).

26. J. P. Derrida, R. Sal and P. Chiche, Favorable effects of pro-longed nitroglycerin infusion in patients with acute myocar-dial infarction, Am.Heart J. 96:833-834 (1978).

27. W-D. Bussman, D. Passek, W. Seidel and M. Kaltenbach, Reduction of creatine kinase, creatine kinase-MB, and infarct size by intravenous nitroglycerin, Adv.Clin.Cardiol. 1:536-541 (1980).

28. J. D. Durrer, K. I. Lie, F. J. L. van Capelle and D. Durrer, Effect of sodium nitroprusside on mortality in acute myocardial infarction, New Engl.J.Med. 306:1121-1128 (1982).

29. J. N. Cohn, J. A. Franciosa, G. S. Francis, D. Archibald, F. Tristani, R. Fletcher, A. Montero, G. Cintron, J. Clarke, D. Hager, R. Saunders, F. Cobb, R. Smith, H. Loeb and H. Settle, Effect of short-term infusion of sodium nitroprusside on mortality rate in acute myocardial infarction complicated by left ventricular failure. Results of a Veterans Administration Cooperative Study, New Engl.J.Med. 306:1129-1135 (1982).

30. P. D. Snow, Effect of propranolol in myocardial infarction, Lancet ii:551-553 (1965).

31. T. Peter, R. M. Norris, E. D. Clarke, M. K. Heng, B. N. Singh, B. Williams, D. R. Howell and P. K. Ambler, Reduction of enzyme levels by propranolol after acute myocardial infarction, Circulation 57:1091-1095 (1978).

32. H. J. Jürgensen, J. Frederiksen, D. A. Hansen and O. Pedersen-Bjergaard, Effekten af alprenolol på myokardeinfarktstørrelsen bedømt ud fra seriebestemmelser af serumkreatinkinase, Ugeskrf.laeg. 141:3089-3091 (1979).

33. M. P. Andersen, P. Bechsgaard, J. Frederiksen, D. A. Hansen, H. J. Jürgensen, B. Nielsen, F. Pedersen, O. Pedersen-Bjergaard and S. L. Rasmussen, Effect of alprenolol on mortality among patients with definite or suspected acute myocardial infarction, Lancet ii:865-872 (1979).

34. P. Sleight, S. Yusuf, R. Peto, P. Rossi, D. Ramsale, D. Bennett, C. Bray and L. Furse, Early intravenous atenolol treatment in suspected acute myocardial infarction, Acta Med.Scand. Suppl 651:185-191 (1981).

35. P. Mathes, C. Cowan and S. Gudbjarnason, Storage and metabolism of norepinephrine after experimental myocardial infarction, Am.J.Physiol. 220:27 (1971).

SUBSTRATE EFFECTS IN MYOCARDIAL ISCHEMIA

Lionel H. Opie

MRC Ischemic Heart Disease Research Unit
Department of Medicine, Groote Schuur Hospital and
University of Cape Town, Observatory, 7925, South Africa

It is now just 20 years ago since Sodi-Pallares (1962) produced his provocative idea that myocardial ischemic damage could be minimized by replacing potassium loss from ischemic cells by a solution of glucose-insulin and potassium. Although his ideas are still being evaluated, it is interesting to see how even controversial concepts can lead to the evolution of new and important hypotheses.

EFFECTS OF EXTERNAL GLUCOSE

In the late 1960's and early 1970's two lines of reasoning linked substrate supply to the heart with the outcome of ischemia. First, the ideas of Sodi-Pallares were carried further by supposing that the critical factor was not replacement of potassium but the enhanced uptake of glucose. It was argued that, according to the Pasteur-effect, increased anaerobic energy provision should help protect the ischemic myocardium. In regional ischemia there tended to be a swing in the substrate metabolism of the ischemic zone from fatty acid to glucose; it is now known that such data were based on local venous sampling techniques which must have drained largely cells of only a modest severity of ischemia. The idea that increased glycolysis should benefit the ischemic myocardium received a major setback with the discovery of Neely's group (Rovetto et al., 1975) that glycolysis was inhibited at at least two levels (phosphofructokinase and glyceraldehyde-3-phosphate dehydrogenase activity) by the products of glycolytic flux, namely protons and lactate (Rovetto et al., 1975). It has even been thought that increase in glycolytic flux might damage the ischemic myocardium by accumulation of protons.

Yet the possible role of glycolysis in minimizing ischemic damage can by no means be ignored. There is, as yet, no true evi-

547

dence that increased glycolysis has worsened ischemia, and there is
increasing evidence that increasing glycolysis might decrease ischemic
damage in zones of less severe ischemia. Recently, Liedtke et al.,
(1982) have proposed that increased glycolytic flux might protect
the ischemic myocardium chiefly by acting on the non-ischemic zone.

Abnormalities of glucose metabolism have been linked to electro-
physical abnormalities early in myocardial infarction in an important
article by Russell and Oliver (1979). A proposed and still speculative mechanism of action is that glucose can in some way, perhaps
by provision of glycolytic ATP, help maintain action potential
duration.

Whatever the result of conflicting experimental studies might
be (compare for example Dalby et al., with Heng et al.,) two other
points deserve emphasis:

1.   In patients, administration of glucose-insulin potassium leads
     to decreased fatty acid levels, and on present evidence this
     can be seen as a beneficial effect on the myocardium in patients
     with acute myocardial infarction according to the randomized
     study of Rackley et al., (1979).
2.   Administration of glucose to isolated rat hearts with constant
     circulating free fatty acid levels and with experimental in-
     farction, can lessen fatty acid-induced damage (de Leiris et
     al., (1975).

FREE FATTY ACIDS AND ARRHYTHMIAS

Another very important and even more seminal idea was being
evolved towards the end of the 1960's. Oliver et al., (1968) in
Edinburgh showed that in patients with high blood-free fatty acids
and myocardial infarction, the survival of these patients was limited
when compared with controls. There are many explanations for the
finding, of which probably the simplest is that patients with more
severe infarctions have greater release of catecholamines with
higher blood-free fatty acids. The question of "toxicity" of free
fatty acids (Kurien et al., 1971) has been much debated with the
present consensus of opinion seeming to favor the view that elevated
free fatty acids in acute myocardial infarction are on the whole an
undesired phenomenon.

The possible mechanisms of free fatty acid toxicity are manifold
and include: (a) a direct damage of the cell membrane as suggested
for example by increased rates of enzyme release; (b) increased
intracellular metabolism with accumulation of acyl CoA and acyl
carnitine; (c) an as yet unspecified mechanism whereby free fatty
acids induce increased oxygen uptake and "oxygen wastage".

Recently, the focus has swung away from possible abnormalities induced by circulating free fatty acids to abnormalities in myocardial lipid metabolism induced even in isolated myocardial tissue by ischemia. The very stimulating and novel idea has been proposed that accumulation of certain specific lipids could induce electrophysiological abnormalities which in turn could promote arrhythmias. The work of Sobel and Corr (1978) is therefore the original Oliver-Kurien hypothesis updated.

PHOSPHOLIPIDS AND ARRHYTHMIAS

It now becomes necessary to evaluate whether the changes in myocardial phospholipids can actually cause arrhythmias. Katz (1982) has adopted a theoretical analysis suggesting that in certain specified circumstances, lysophospholipids can reverse some of the effects of membrane hydrolysis associated with ischemia. Katz's proposals, provocative as they be, are not necessarily in conflict with the proposals of Corr, Gross and Sobel (1982). Katz is essentially looking at the effects of ischemia on membrane structure and arguing that membranes may be better off with, than without, their liberated lysophospholipids. Corr et al., on the other hand are looking at the results of the liberated lysophospholipids on arrhythmogenesis.

COMMENT

The original concepts that circulating substrates could influence the outcome of myocardial ischemia have undergone considerable refining. Especially in the case of lipids, the focus is now on the myocardial cellular damage which is largely seen as the consequences of ischemia in altering lipid pathways in the ischemic zone. The early seminal ideas of Sodi-Pallares and Oliver have led to further investigations which are now focussing on the effect of myocardial ischemia on the cell membrane.

REFERENCES

Corr, P. B., Gross, R. W., Sobel, B. E., (in press), Arrhythmogenic amphiphilic lipids and the myocardial cell membrane, Editorial, J.Mol.Cell.Cardiol.
Dalby, A. J., Bricknell, O. L., and Opie, L. H., 1981, Effect of glucose-insulin-potassium infusions on epicardial ECG changes and on myocardial metabolic changes after coronary artery ligation in dogs, Cardiovasc.Res., 15:588-598.
de Leiris, J., Opie, L. H., and Lubbe, W. F., 1975, Effects of free fatty acid and glucose on enzyme release in experimental myocardial infarction, Nature 253:746-747.

Heng, M. K., Norris, R. M., Peter, T., Nisbet, H. D., and Singh,
        B. N., 1978, The effects of glucose-insulin-potassium on
        experimental myocardial infarction in the dog, Cardiovasc.
        Res. 12:429-435.
Katz, A. M., (in press), Membrane-derived lipids and the pathogenesis
        of ischemic myocardial damage, Editorial, J.Molec.Cell.
        Cardiol.
Kurien, V. A., Yates, P. A., and Oliver, M. F., 1971, The role of
        free fatty acids in the production of ventricular vulner-
        ability following acute coronary artery occlusion in the
        dog, J.Molec.Cell.Cardiol. 11:31-34.
Liedtke, A. J., Nellis, S. H., and Whitesell, L. H., 1982, Effects
        of regional ischemia on metabolic function in adjacent
        aerobic myocardium, J.Molec.Cell.Cardiol. 14:195-205.
Oliver, M. F., Kurien, V. A., and Greenwood, T. W., 1968, Relation
        between serum free fatty acids and arrhythmias and death
        after myocardial infarction, Lancet 1:710-715.
Rackley, C. E., Russell, R. O., Rogers, W. J., Mantle, J. A., and
        McDaniel, H. G., 1979, Glucose-insulin-potassium infusion
        in acute myocardial infarction. Review of clinical experi-
        ence, Postgrad.Med. 65:93-99.
Rovetto, M. J., Lamberton, W. F., and Neely, J. R., 1975, Mechanism
        of glycolytic inhibition in ischemic rat hearts, Circ.Res.
        37:742-751.
Russell, D. C., and Oliver, M. F., 1979, The effect of intravenous
        glucose on ventricular vulnerability following acute coronary
        artery occlusion in the dog, J.Molec.Cel.Cardiol. 11:31-44.
Sobel, B. E., Corr, P. B., Robison, A. K., Goldstein, R. A.,
        Witkowski, F. X., and Klein, M. S., 1978, Accumulation of
        lysophosphoglycerides with arrhythmogenic properties in
        ischemic myocardium, J.Clin.Invest. 62:546-553.
Sodi-Pallares, D., Testelli, M. R., Fishleder, F. L., Bisteni, A.,
        Medrano, G. A., Friedland, C., and De Micheli, A., 1962,
        Effects of an intravenous infusion of a potassium-glucose,
        insulin solution on the electro-cardiographic signs of myo-
        cardial infarction. A preliminary clinical report, Amer.J.
        Cardiol. 9:166-181.

PREVENTION OF CATECHOLAMINE-INDUCED MYOCARDIAL DAMAGE

A. Waldenström, A. Hjalmarson, and B. Jacobsson

Department of Medicine 1, Sahlgren's Hospital
University of Göteborg, Göteborg, Sweden

The improvement of prognosis of the acute myocardial infarction has mainly been due to detection and treatment of arrhythmias and congestive heart failure.

To further improve treatment of the acute stage of myocardial infarction we have to influence the myocardial infarction process. There is ample circumstantial evidence for this process being dynamic for at least 12 hours (Figure 1)[1]. which would be long enough for interventions to start. But to do this we have to know more about the factors of importance for this process. How important is platelet aggregation?[2] How important is the plaque per se? Is spasm important? This paper will deal with the possible role of catecholamines for initiation and expansion of the infarction process.

EXPERIMENTAL STUDIES

The cardiotoxic effects of catecholamines have been known since the beginning of this century[3,4], but it was not until the works of Raab[5] that this field was extensively investigated and the clinical relevance was discussed. In 1962 Raab and co-workers[5] could induce ST-changes of the ECG of anesthetized and vagotamized cats by stimulation of the sympathetic nervous system, or by intravenous injection of adrenaline or by anoxia. This could be only be demonstrated when a coronary artery dilatation was prevented by the use of a special restriction device. No ST-changes were shown when heart rate was increased by atrial pacing or blood pressure elevated by the use of angiotensin 11. Their theory was that ischemic attacks may start because certain areas of the myocardium with restricted coronary supply are made hypoxic by e.g. noradrenaline release.

551

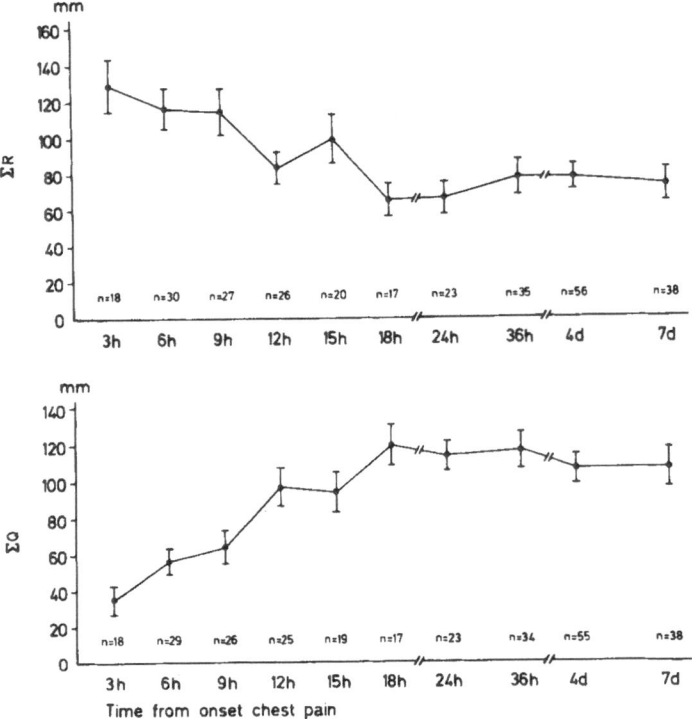

Fig. 1.   Time course for reduction of $\sum R$ (above) and increase of
$\sum Q$ (below) in anterior myocardial infarction.[1]

Rona et al[6] were able to demonstrate the cardiotoxic effects
of isoproterenol when it was injected into healthy rats.   In these
animals myocardial necrosis appeared without any restriction in coronary flow.   There are many possible explanations why catecholamines
exert this damage.   One possibility is that platelet aggregation is
enhanced with subsequent thrombosis formation in a coronary artery.[2,7]

When isoproterenol is given to turtles, the response is somewhat
different.   The epicardial layer of the myocardium is supplied by
vessels but the inner layer is spongy with lacunar supply.   Isoproterenol induces necrosis preferentially in the spongy part which
suggests that a vascular mechanism is most important.[8]   When large
doses are used ventricular aneurysms develop.   This could, however,
be prevented by keeping the animals at $+4^{\circ}C$.[9]

During the 1970's many studies were made in order to find factors that changed myocardial infarct size. Thus it was found that isoprenaline infused to a dog subjected to coronary ligation would increase the zone of ischemia (Figure 2)[10] whereas beta-blockade would decrease infarct size.[11,12]

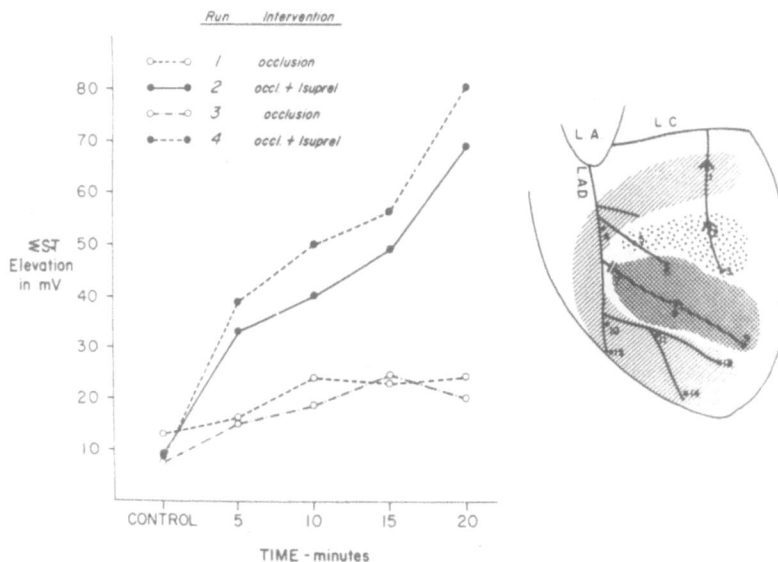

Fig. 2. Effects of occlusion alone and occlusion after the infusion of isoproterenol (0.25 ug/kg/min). Right panel: Schematic representation of the anterior surface of the heart. The coronary arteries and branches, and sites of epicardial electrograms are marked. LAD = left anterior descending coronary artery; LA = left atrial appendage; LC = left circumflex coronary artery; Cross-hatched area: area of injury after 15 minutes of occlusion. Stippled area: increase of area of injury when the occlusion was performed under the influence of isoproterenol. Lined area: area that showed no ST segment elevation under any circumstances. Left panel: $\sum$ST in the same experiment after three simple occlusions and after two occlusions under the influence of isoproterenol. Time = minutes after occlusion.[10]

The concept that acute myocardial infarction is caused by coronary artery thrombosis or occlusion has been debated lately.[13-17] Different types of cellular lesions in acute myocardial infarction

were described by Baroldi.[17] One type, coagulative myocytolysis, is
mainly seen in the border zone of an acute myocardial infarction but
also in patients with pheochromocytoma.[18] It is thus reasonable to
believe that this type of lesion is induced by catecholamines. In
the light of these observations we started our investigations in
isolated rat hearts. When the hearts were perfused with increasing
concentrations of adrenaline in the perfusion buffer, a myocardial
damage could be demonstrated (Figure 3) as a release of creatine
phosphokinase (CK) and aspartate aminotransferase (ASAT) to the
buffer and as typical histological changes.

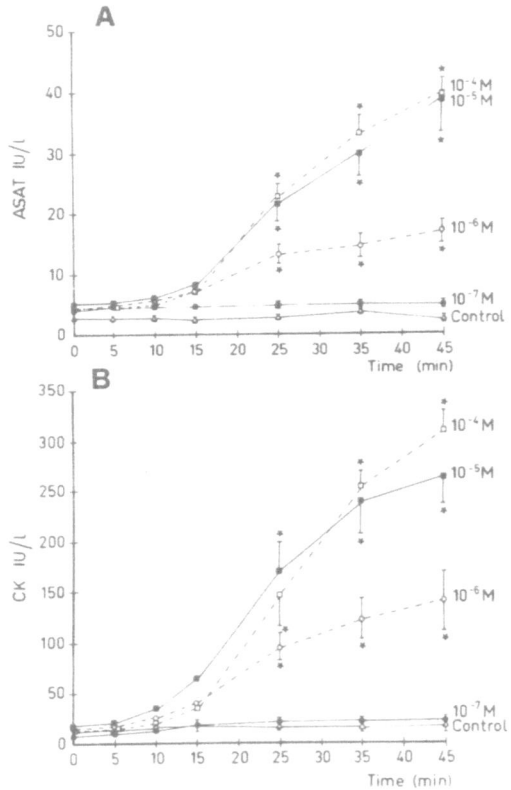

Fig. 3.   A (upper panel): Release of ASAT from the hearts to the
          perfusion medium when perfused with different concentrations
          of noradrenaline. After 15 minutes of anterograde perfusion
          30 minutes of retrograde perfusion followed.
          B (lower panel): Release of CK under the same conditions as
          in panel A. Each value represents the mean ± SE for 6-8
          hearts. x = significantly different from initial value
          (p<0.05).[19]

A concentration of noradrenaline of 10^{-6} M seemed to be needed to induce necrosis in this experimental model. And this is a concentration not unlikely to occur in real life. To test this hypothesis further, the noradrenaline stored in myocardial nerve endings was released by adding tyramine to isolated perfused hearts. Again a damage was induced with enzyme leakage and histological changes. This damage could be prevented by beta-blockade (Figure 4)[19] It could be shown that myocardial contents of noradrenaline, if extensively released, would induce infarct-like lesions and these lesions could be prevented by beta-blockade as well as by the calcium antagonist verapamil. More studies on the protective effects of calcium antagonists in ischemia have been performed by Nayler et al[20] where isolated perfused rabbit hearts were used. During ischemia ATP and CK levels were much better preserved in verapamil-treated animals.

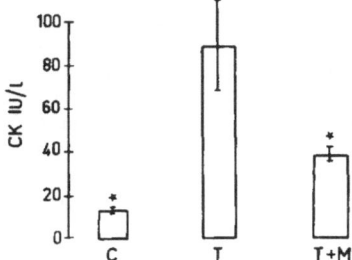

Fig. 4. Release of CK from hearts perfused anterogradely for 60 minutes with tyramine 250 ug/ml (T) with or without metoprolol 10^{-3}M (M). Controls are perfused without addition of tyramine or metoprolol. Each bar represents the mean ± SE for 6-8 hearts. x = significantly different from tyramine-treated hearts (p < 0.05).[19]

Locally released catecholamines may thus induce myocardial damage and under very special conditions, such as pheochromocytoma, circulating catecholamines may produce myocardial necrosis as well. Stress is also a "well known" important etiological factor for myocardial infarction but real proof is scarce. Some very interesting experiments were performed in the early 1960's by Melville and co-workers[21]. Based on the fact that patients with cerebrovascular accidents may show ECG changes indicative of myocardial ischemia or infarction they electrically stimulated hypothalamus of anesthetized cats. By doing so they could induce a rise in blood pressure, ST-T deviations on the ECG and ventricular arrhythmias including ventricular tachycardia.[21] The same authors could also show that injections of picrotoxin into the lateral cerebral ventricle of rabbits and cats evoked intense sympathetic cardiovascular effects. It is well known that domestic pigs sometimes die spontaneously during transport to the slaughter house. The hearts of such animals often show myo-

cardial damage from microscopical necrosis to macroscopical visible
areas of necrosis. And yet these animals are without signs of coronary
atherosclerosis or thrombosis. In some very interesting experiments,
Johansson et al[22,23] subjected pigs to restraint stress. This was
performed by i.v. infusion of succinylcholine chloride resulting in
paralysis for 12 minutes. Respiratory insufficiency was avoided.

The amygdaloid part of the limbic system is of importance in
eliciting emotions of fear and aggression. Stimulation of this area
can cause flight and fight behaviour whereas amygdalectomy suppresses
such behaviour. When restraint stress was induced in control pigs
as well as in amygdalectomized ones, myocardial degeneration was
found in all controls. No myocardial changes were found in the operated animals. These changes correlated to plasma catecholamines
so that amygdalectomized animals had significantly lower levels than
controls.[23] As this stress-induced myocardial necrosis seems to be
mediated via catecholamines, the same authors studied the protective
effect of propranolol. Interestingly, these authors find that low
i.v. doses of propranolol will not prevent from damage. A very high
dose of i.v. propranolol will protect the myocardium, but in this
case no increase in catecholamine release could be seen. Only with
oral treatment with clinical doses for a week stress-induced necrosis
could be totally prevented even though catecholamine concentrations
in blood were elevated (Table 1).[24] Maybe long-term treatment modifies
the myocardium and/or beta-receptors in a way that makes it more
efficient than acute beta-blockade! These mechanisms are complicated
and still obscure. We have some recent data on selective beta-
perfused rat hearts where contractility seems to be more sensitive
than chronotrophy.[25]

CLINICAL TRIALS

The cardiotoxic effects of catecholamines are now experimentally
well established. Possibly a clinical infarct could start by a
sudden release of noradrenaline in an area of restricted perfusion/
relative ischemia. A vicious circle may start ending up in myocardial
necrosis. During this stress, catecholamines are peripherally released accentuating the already compromised heart and the infarct
may increase. Following this hypothesis, the Göteborg metoprolol
trial[26] was designed in the mid 70's. Four well designed studies
have now been published with positive effects on mortality using
metoprolol[26], timolol[27], alprenolol[28] and propranolol.[29] It seems
clear that beta-blockers reduce mortality in acute myocardial infarction, and if used early data suggest that myocardial infarct
size is restricted as evidenced by ECG mapping and enzyme curves.
These findings have been found mainly in patients who were treated
within 12 hours after onset of chest pain.[30] It is very reasonable
to assume that the positive effect of beta-blockade in acute myocardial infarction is due to blockade of toxic effects of catecholamines.

Table 1. Effect of various pretreatments with propranolol on extent of heart lesions after stress

Different groups of pigs	Propranolol pretreatment	Total number of pigs	Number of pigs with myocardial cell necrosis graded according to point scale							Statistical sign*
			0	1	2	3	4	5	6	
Controls A	–	5	1				1	2	1	
Controls B	–	3				1	2			
acute — 1 mg/kg i.v., single dose		3				2	1			
3 mg/kg i.v., single dose		3				1	2			n.s.
10 mg/kg i.v., single dose		5	1	1	3					n.s.
long-term — 120 mg orally, 3x6 days		3	2	1						$p<0.02$
120 mg orally, 3x6 days		3	2	1						$p<0.005$

*The myocardial changes in the different groups were evaluated statistically versus those in the controls (A+B) by the Mann-Whitney U-test (n.s. = non-significant).

REFERENCES

1. J. Herlitz: Bedömning och begränsning av hjärtinfarktens storlek.
    En interventionsstudie med metoprolol. Thesis, Götenborg
    (1982).

2. J. I. Haft, P. D. Krantz, F. J. Albert and K. Fani: Intravas-
    cular platelet aggregation in the heart induced by nor-
    epinephrine. Microscopic studies. Circulation 46:698, (1972).

3. O. Josué: Hypertrophie cardiaque causée par l'adrénaline et la
    toxine typhique. C r Soc Bio (Paris) 63: 285, (1907).

4. K. Ziegler: Uber die Wirkung intravenöser Adrenalininjektion
    auf das Gefä β system und ihre Beziehung zur Arteriosklerose.
    Ziegler's Bietrage 38:229 (1905).

5. W. Raab, R. van Lith, E. Lepeschkin and H. C. Herrlich: Catechol-
    amine induced myocardial hypoxia in the presence of impaired
    coronary dilatability independent of external cardiac work.
    Am J Cardiol 9: 455, (1962).

6. G. Rona, C. I. Chappel, T. Balazs and R. Gaudry: An infarct-
    like myocardial lesion and other toxic manifestations pro-
    duced by isoproterenol in the rat. Arch Pathol 67: 443, (1959).

7. J. I. Haft: Cardiovascular injury induced by sympathetic cate-
    cholamines. Progr Cardiovasc Dis 17: 73, (1974).

8. B. Ostádal, V. Rychterová and O. Poupa: Isoproterenol-induced
    acute experimental cardiac necrosis in the turtle (Testudo
    Horsfieldi) Am Heart J 76: 645-649, (1968).

9. O. Poupa and A. Carlsten: Experimental cardiomyopathies in poi-
    kilotherms. In:"Recent Advances in Cardiac Structure and
    Metabolism, vol 2: Cardiomyopathies". Eds: E. Bajusz and
    G. Rona. University Park Press, Baltimore 1973, pp.321-351.

10. P. R. Maroko and E. Braunwald: Effects of metabolic and pharma-
    cologic interventions on myocardial infarct size following
    coronary occlusion. Acta Med Scand, Suppl 587: 125-136 (1975).

11. P. R. Maroko, J. K. Kjekshus, B. E. Sobel, T. Watanabe, J. W.
    Covell, J. Ross Jr. and E. Braunwald: Factors influencing
    infarct size following experimental coronary artery occlusions.
    Circulations 43: 67, (1971).

12. P. R. Maroko, P. Libby and E. Braunwald: Effect of pharmacologic
    agents on the function of the ischemic heart. Am J Cardiol
    32: 930, (1973).

13. I. Chapman: Relationships of recent coronary artery occlusion
    and acute myocardial infarction. J. Mt Sinai Hosp 35: 149,
    (1968).

14. C. J. Schwartz and J. R. A. Mitchell: The relation between myo-
    cardial lesions and coronary artery disease. 1: An unselected
    necropsy study. Br Heart J 24: 761, (1962).

15. D. Sinapius: Beziehungen zwischen Koronarthrombosen und Myo-
    kardinfarkten. Dtsch Med Wochenschr 97: 443, (1972).

16. W. C. Roberts and L. M. Buja: The frequency and significance
    of coronary arterial thrombi and other observations in fatal
    acute myocardial infarction. A study of 107 necropsy patients.
    Am J Med 52: 425, (1972).

17. G. Baroldi: Acute coronary occlusion as a cause of myocardial infarction and sudden coronary heart death. Am J. Cardiol 16: 859, (1965).
18. G. Baker, N. H. Zeller, S. Weitzner and J. K. Leach: Pheochromocytoma without hypertension presenting as cardiomyopathy. Am Heart J 83: 688-693 (1972).
19. A. P. Waldenström, A. C. Hjalmarson and L. Thornell: A possible role of noradrenaline in the development of myocardial infarction. Am Heart J 95: 43-52, (1978).
20. W. G. Nayler, R. Ferrari and A. M. Slade: Cardioprotective effect of calcium antagonists and beta-adrenergic blocking agents in myocardial ischaemia. In:"Calcium Antagonism in Cardiovascular Therapy. Experience with Verapamil".Eds.: A. Zanchetti and D. M. Krikler, Exerpta Medica, Amsterdam-Oxford Princeton 1981, pp. 74-88.
21. K. I. Melville, B. Blum, H. E. Shister and M. D. Silver: Cardiac ischemic changes and arrhythmias induced by hypothalamic stimulation. Am J. Cardiol 12: 781-791, (1963).
22. G. Johansson, K. Olsson, J. Häggendal, L. Jönsson and K. Thóren-Tolling: Effect of amygdalectomy of stress-induced myocardial necrosis and blood levels of catecholamines in pigs. Acta Physiol Scand 113: 553-555 (1981).
23. G. Johansson, K. Olsson, J. Häggendal, L. Jönsson and K. Thóren-Tolling: Effect of stress on myocardial cells and blood levels of catecholamines in normal and amygdalectomized pigs. Can J Comp Med 46: 176-182, (1982).
24. J. Häggendal, G. Johansson, L. Jönsson and K. Thorén-Tolling: Effect of propranolol on myocardial cell necroses and blood levels of catecholamines in pigs subjected to stress. Acta Pharmacol et Toxicol 50: 58-66 (1982).
25. A. Waldenström, B. Jacobsson and A. Hjalmarson: Heterogeneity of beta$_1$- receptors in the rat heart. J Mol Cell Cardiol 13 Suppl 1: 97., 1981 (Abstra.).
26. A. Hjalmarson, D. Elmfeldt, J. Herlitz, S. Holmberg, I. Málek, G. Nyberg, L. Rydén, K. Swedberg, A. Vedin, F. Waagstein, A. Waldenström, J. Waldenström, H. Wedel, L. Wilhelmsen and C. Wilhelmsson: Effect on mortality of metoprolol in acute myocardial infarction. A double-blind randomised trial. Lancet ii: 823-828, (1981).
27. The Norwegian Multicenter Study Group: Timolol-induced reduction in mortality and reinfarction in patients surviving acute myocardial infarction. N Engl J Med 304: 801-807, (1981).
28. M. P. Andersen. P. Bechsgaard, J. Frederiksen. D. A. Hansen, H. J. Jürgensen, B. Nielsen. F. Pedersen. O. Pedersen-Bjergaard, S. L. Rasmussen: Effect of alprenolol on mortality among patients with definite or suspected acute myocardial infarction. Lancet ii: 865-872, (1979).
29. Beta-Blocker Heart Attack Trial Research Group: A randomized trial of propranolol in patients with acute myocardial infarction. I. Mortality results. JAMA 247: 1707-1714, (1982).

30. J. Herlitz, A. Hjalmarson, K. Swedberg, F. Waagstein and A.
     Waldenström: A double-blind trial of metoprolol in acute
     myocardial infarction. Effect on infarct size, clinical
     findings and 1-year mortality. Abstr. (Am Heart Assoc, 55th
     Sessions). Circulation. In press.

MAINTENANCE OF Ca^{2+} HOMEOSTASIS IN THE MYOCARDIUM

Winifred G. Nayler

Department of Medicine
University of Melbourne
Austin Hospital
Heidelberg, Victoria
Australia

SUMMARY

Maintenance of intracellular homeostasis with respect to Ca^{++} during prolonged episodes of ischaemia and upon reperfusion is critical to the survival of the myocardium. Loss of Ca^{++} homeostasis results in massive ultrastructural damage, associated with excessive phospholipase and proteinase activation. Aggravating factors include hyperthermia, excessive cardiac work and hyperthyroidism. Conversely hypothermia, a reduction in sympathetic drive and a diminution in work load are all protective. Since the release of intracellular constituents, including enzymes and myoglobin, into the extracellular phase during post ischaemic reperfusion occurs as a secondary response to the Ca^{2+}-induced tissue damage the quantitation of protective procedures that are based simply on the measurement of serum enzymes may not provide an accurate assessment of the degree of protection that has been achieved. In some instances it is possible to dissociate the gain in tissue Ca^{2+} from the release of intracellular constituents into the extracellular phase.

Recently there has been a rapid growth of ideas concerning the involvement of Ca^{2+} in the progression of events that are precipitated by an ischemic episode and which become exacerbated upon reperfusion. Shen and Jennings (1972) first noted a possible association between the occurrence of the tissue damage which occurs under these conditions and the massive increase in Ca^{2+}. However measurements of total tissue Ca^{2+} provide little information as to why ischemic heart muscle loses its capacity to maintain ionic homeostasis with respect to Ca^{2+}. Loss

of ionic homeostasis with respect to Ca^{2+} is not the prerogative of
hearts that have been made ischemic and then reperfused. Thus, for
example, the administration of large doses of isoproterenol (Fleckenstein, 1971) and the re-introduction of Ca^{2+} after a relatively brief
period of Ca^{2+}-free perfusion (Zimmerman and Hulsman, 1966) both cause
mammalian heart muscle to become overloaded with Ca^{2+}. The consequences of a raised tissue Ca^{2+} are far reaching and include irreversible loss of mitochondrial function (Nayler, Ferrari and Williams,
1980; Nayler, 1982), massive ultrastructural damage, ATP wastage, a
raised end diastolic resting tension (Nayler, Poole-Wilson and Williams, 1979) and the development of membrane defects (Jennings and
Reimer, 1981). Possibly these membrane defects reflect the activation
of the phospholipases, some of which are under calmodulin-Ca^{2+} control.
Despite its importance comparatively little is known about the precise
sequence of events that ultimately results in the reperfused ischemic
heart becoming overloaded with Ca^{2+}. Probably several distinct phases
are involved.

Initially there may be a small modest gain in Ca^{2+} due, possibly
to an enhanced entry of Ca^{2+} in exchange for Na^+ (Figure 1). The
aetiology of this may be as follows:- as the result of an ATP-de-
pletion induced failure of the Na^+K^+ ATPase, the ischemic myocardium
fails to extrude Na^+ against the prevailing concentration gradient.
As a result the tissue Na^+ rises (Regan, Broisman, Haider, Eaddy and
Oldewurtel, 1980). Under these circumstances we can expect to see
a relatively short lived activation of the Na^+: Ca^{2+} exchange mechanism
so that Na^+ will leave the tissue in exchange for Ca^{2+} (Reuter, 1974).
However the amount of Ca^{2+} which can enter in this way will be limited
by at least two factors:-

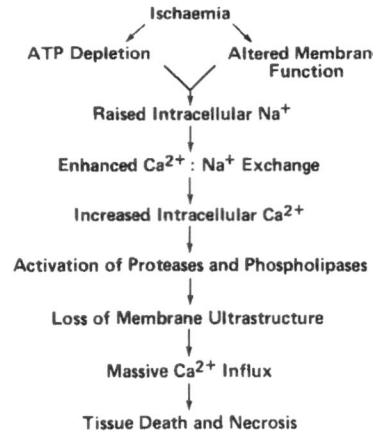

Fig. 1.   Schematic representation of the events involved in the post-
ischemic reperfusion-induced gain in tissue Ca^{2+}.

Table 1. Effect of H$^+$ accumulation on the Na$^+$-Ca^{2+}-exchange reaction in isolated cardiac sarcolemma.

pH	Ca^{2+} accumulated in exchange for Na$^+$ (nmoles/mg protein/min)
7.4	2.2
7.0	1.2
6.6	1.1

These results were obtained using isolated fragments of cardiac sarcolemma from normotensive Sprague Dawley rats.

(a) the amount of Na$^+$ available as an antiporter, and
(b) the inhibitory effect of the protons that accumulate under these conditions (Gevers, 1977, Table 1).

The early net gain in Ca^{2+} probably does not involve the entry of Ca^{2+} through sarcolemmal defects (Ashraf, White and Bloor, 1978) even although this may take place later (Jennings and Reimer, 1981). An excess entry of Ca^{2+} through the slow channels is also unlikely, because these channels require energy in the form of ATP for their maintenance (Sperelakis and Schneider, 1976).

Probably this early net gain in Ca^{2+} is accompanied, or even preceded, by another event - that is a redistribution of tissue Ca^{2+}. There are several reasons for believing that this may occur. Firstly energy (as ATP) is required for the correct functioning of the sarcoplasmic reticulum. Hence as the availability of ATP declines Ca^{2+} will remain in the cytosol where presumably it will remain free to activate the Ca^{2+}-dependent ATPases. Under these conditions, and because of the switch to anaerobic glycolysis, cytosol H$^+$ will rise. Tissue acidosis favours the process whereby Ca^{2+} induces a spontaneous release of Ca^{2+} from the sarcoplasmic reticulum (Fabiato and Fabiato. 1977; Dunnett and Nayler, 1978). Therefore, as the tissue becomes increasingly acidotic Ca^{2+} will tend to leave the sarcoplasmic reticulum, to remain in the cytosol. Some Ca^{2+} may also be displaced from the mitochondria, because a raised tissue Na$^+$ (Carafoli, Trozzo, Lugli, Grovetti and Kratzing, 1974) promoted a spontaneous release of Ca^{2+} from these organelles.

We may ask ourselves why this Ca^{2+} is not immediately extruded from the tissue. There are three possible explanations:-

(a) the prevailing concentration gradient will favour the entry and not the exit of Ca2+;

(b)   the Na^+: Ca^{2+} exchange mechanism will be functioning in the
      opposite direction; and

(c)   the Ca^{2+}-stimulated plasmalemmal-located Ca^{2+} pump will be failing,
      because of ATP depletion.

In summary, therefore, <u>early</u> during the ischemic event there may
be a modest gain in tissue Ca^{2+} and a large rise in cytosolic Ca^{2+}
due to the intracellular redistribution of these ions. The progression of events does not stop here, however, because as the duration
of the ischemia continues the cytosolic Ca^{2+} may reach the levels
needed to activate phospholipase A_2 (Chien, Reeves, Buja, Bonte,
Parkey and Willerson, 1981). Under these conditions membrane structure and function will be severely impaired, with large membrane
defects appearing (Jennings and Reimer, 1981). Consequently Ca^{2+}
will be free to flow along its concentration gradient, causing a
massive and explosive rise in tissue Ca^{2+} (Figure 1). Some of this
Ca^{2+} is rapidly accumulated by the mitochondria (Nayler, Ferrari and
Williams, 1980) which are then rendered incapable of rephosphorylating
adenosine diphosphate. Moreover, the large membrane defects permit
the loss of the precursors of adenosine triphosphate (adenosine and
its breakdown products, including hypoxanthine and inosine) from the
cell.

One of the problems encountered when trying to quantitate the
degree of protection that a particular regime provides involves the
problem of assessing the damage in a quantitative manner. Measurements of protein release (or intracellular enzymes, including creatine
kinase) have often been used but recent data indicates that this
technique may give misleading results. Thus agents which cause the
sarcolemma of heart muscle cells to remain intact may not prevent
Ca^{2+} ions from entering. Presumably a <u>small</u> membrane defect will
allow these ions to enter whereas a <u>large</u> hole may be needed for the
exit of these larger macromolecules. Possibly the recovery of mechanical function upon reperfusion provides a better assessment of the
effectiveness of a proposed protective regime, or of the deleterious
consequences of other interventions.

Using this approach we have begun to determine some of the factors that influence the sequence of events that are precipitated by
an ischemic episode. Pre-existing hypertension (Table 2) has been
found to cause an exacerbation of the gain in tissue Ca^{2+} that occurs
during post ischemic reperfusion, and this is accompanied by an excessive gain in Ca^{2+}.

That there is a positive correlation between the gain in tissue
Ca^{2+} that occurs upon reperfusion and the recovery of mechanical
function is shown by the data summarized in Table 3. Hyperthyroidism,
and hyperthermia cause an exacerbation of this gain in Ca^{2+}; hypothermia and the administration of the Ca^{2+} antagonists protect against it.

Another interesting correlation which emerged during these studies

Table 2. Effect of Hypertension on the Post-ischemic induced gain in tissue Ca^{2+}, and the recovery of mechanical function.

Rat Model	Mean BP (mm Hg)	% Recovery	Gain in Tissue Ca^{2+} (μmoles/gm dry wt)
Normotensive			
Sprague Dawley	112.3 ± 3.2	32.6 ± 3.2	34.3 ± 5.5
Wistar Kyoto	138.3 ± 6.12	29.8 ± 4.6	38.2 ± 4.8
Hypertensive			
S.H.R.	212.5 ± 6.1	15.8 ± 1.6	51.4 ± 3.6
Stroke prone	204.2 ± 5.4	12.9 ± 2.2	55.9 ± 6.8

Each result is mean ± S.E. of 6 experiments. Gain in tissue Ca^{2+} refers to the gain during 20 minute's reperfusion after 60 minutes normothermic global ischemia.

ated to the relationship between the recovery of mechanical function upon reperfusion and the increase in mitochondrial Ca^{2+}. Thus as Figure 2 shows there is a linear but inverse relationship between recovery of mechanical function and mitochondrial Ca^{2+} overload. If we remember, now, that cardiac mitochondria that are overloaded with Ca^{2+} fail to rephosphorylate ADP (Nayler, Ferrari and Williams, 1980) then we can begin to understand why, when we plot percentage recovery of mechanical function during post ischemic reperfusion and the ATP content of the heart after the required period of post ischemic reperfusion - in this case twenty minutes, a straight line relationship (Figure 3) is found.

In summary, therefore, these results show that conditions which favour the recovery of mammalian hearts upon post-ischemic reperfusion prevent the heart from accumulating large amounts of Ca^{2+}. Since the initial gain in Ca^{2+}, or rise in cytosolic Ca^{2+}, may reflect an ATP-induced failure to maintain ionic homeostasis with respect to Ca^{2+}, protective procedures should, perhaps, be aimed at preserving the tissue levels of ATP. Alternatively we should begin to explore the possibility of protecting the heart against the consequences of a raised Ca^{2+}, perhaps by searching for drugs which will decrease the Ca^{2+}-binding activity of calmodulin, for the activation of phospholipase A_2 by Ca^{2+} is modulated by calmodulin.

Table 3. Correlation between gain in tissue Ca^{2+} and percentage
          recovery of mechanical function upon reperfusion.

% Recovery of mechanical function	Gain in tissue Ca^{2+} (μmoles/gm dry wt)
92 ± 3	1.8 ± 0.6
44 ± 4	5.2 ± 1.3
10 ± 3	9.6 ± 2.1

These results were obtained from rabbit hearts that were made
globally ischemic for 60 minutes at 37°C and then reperfused
for 20 minutes. Each result is mean ± S.E. of 6 experiments.

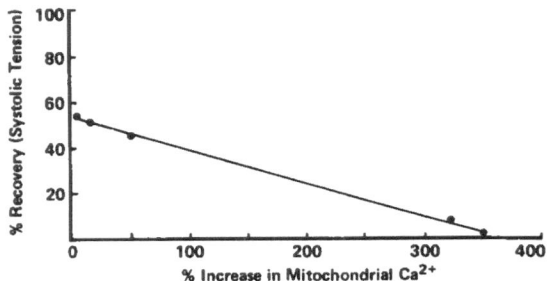

Fig. 2. Relationship between the recovery of mechanical function
         during post-ischemic reperfusion and the gain in mitochondrial
         Ca^{2+} expressed as a percentage change relative to the Ca^{2+}
         content of mitochondria from aerobically perfused hearts.
         Rabbit hearts: perfusion temp 37°C; perfusion buffer Krebs-
         Henseleit (Nayler, Ferrari and Williams, 1980).

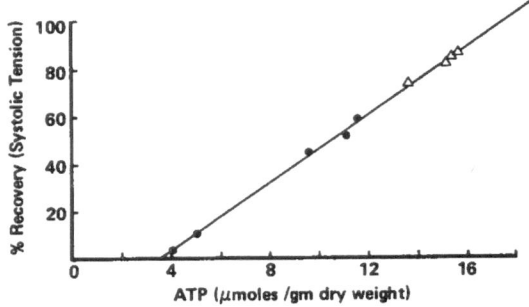

Fig. 3. Relationship between percentage recovery in mechanical func-
         tion and ATP content of left ventricular heart muscle in rab-
         bits made ischemic at 37°C for 60-90 minutes and then reper-
         fused for 15-20 minutes. For perfusion details see Nayler,
         Ferrari and Williams, 1980.

REFERENCES

Ashraf, M., White, F. and Bloor, C. M., 1978. Ultrastructural influences of reperfusing dog myocardium with calcium-free blood after coronary artery occlusion. Am. J. Path. 90: 423-434.

Carafoli, E., Tiozzo, R., Luggli, G., Crovetti, F. and Kratzing, C, 1974. The release of calcium from heart mitochondria by sodium. J. Mol. Cell. Cardiol. 6: 361-372.

Chien, K. E., Reeves, J. P., Buja, L. M., Bonte, F., Parkey, R. W. and Willeson, J. T., 1981. Phospholipid alterations in canine ischemic myocardium. Circ. Res. 48: 711-719.

Dunnett, J. S. and Nayler, W. G., 1978. Effect of pH on the uptake and efflux of calcium from cardiac sarcoplasmic reticulum vesicles. J. Physiol. 281: 16-17P.

Fabiato, A. and Fabiato, F., 1977. Calcium release from the sarcoplasmic reticulum. Circ. Res. 40: 119-129.

Fleckenstein, A., 1970/1971. Specific inhibitors and promoters of calcium action in the excitation-contraction coupling of heart muscle and their role in the prevention or production of myocardial lesions, Calcium and the Heart. Edited by P. Harris, L. Opie. London, New York, Academic Press, pp 135-188.

Gevers, W., 1977. Generation of protons by metabolic processes in heart cells. J. Mo. Cell. Cardiol. 9: 867-874.

Jennings, R. B. and Reimer, K. A., 1981. Lethal myocardial ischemic injury. Am. J. Path. 102: 241-255.

Nayler, W. G., 1982. "The role of calcium in myocardial ischemia and cell death". in "Calcium Channel Blocking Agents in the Treatment of Cardiovascular Disorders". ed. P. Stone and E. Antman. Futura Publishing Co., N. Y. In press.

Nayler, W. G., Ferrari, R. and Williams, A., 1980. The protective effect of pretreatment with verapamil, nifedipine and propranolol on mitochondrial function in the ischemic and reperfused myocardium. Am. J. Cardiol. 46: 242-248.

Nayler, W. G., Poole-Wilson and Williams, A., 1979. Hypoxia and calcium. J. Mol. Cell. Cardiol. 11: 683-706.

Regan, T. J., Broisman, L., Haider, B., Eaddy, C. and Olderwurtel, H. A., 1980. Dissociation of myocardial sodium and potassium alterations in mild versus severe ischemia. Am. J. Physiol. 238: H575-H580.

Reuter, H., 1974. Exchange of calcium ions in mammalian cardiology. Circ. Res. 34: 599-605.

Shen, A. C. and Jennings, R. B., 1972. Myocardial calcium and magnesium in acute ischemic injury. Am. J. Path. 67: 417-440.

Sperelakis, N. and Schneider, J. A., 1976. A metabolic control mechanism for calcium ion influx that may protect the ventricular myocardial cell. Am. J. Cardiol. 37: 1079-1084.

Zimmerman, A. N. E., Hulsmann, W. C., 1966. Paradoxical influence of calcium ions on the permeability of the cell membranes of the isolated rat heart. Nature. 211: 646-647.

THEORETICAL IMPLICATIONS OF THE USE OF ANTIOXIDANTS FOR HEART PROTECTION AGAINST STRESS-INDUCED AND ISCHEMIC DAMAGES

F. Z. Meerson and V. E. Kagan

Institute of General Pathology and Pathological Physiology
USSR Academy of Medical Sciences
School of Biology, Moscow State University
Moscow, USSR

Ischemia, stress-induced catecholamine excess and, most commonly, a combination of these two factors are the key links in the pathogenesis of the coronary disease and other damages of the heart muscle. The experimental data obtained independently on models of acute ischemia (Meerson, Kagan et al., 1982; Vasdev et al., 1979; Chien et al., 1979) and emotional-painful stress (Meerson, Kagan et al., 1980; Meerson, Arkhipenko et al., 1981) suggest that the crucial role in the damaging action of these factors, in particular in transition of reversible damages into irreversible ones, belongs to the events occurring at the level of the membrane lipid bilayer of cardiomyocytes. The excessive activation of at least three physiologically significant factors is of primary importance here, namely the activation of lipases and phospholipases, the activation of lipid peroxidation and the detergent-like action of lysophospholipids and free fatty acids (Katz and Messineo, 1981).

These three processes are closely interrelated both in a healthy organism and under ischemic and stress damage of the heart; therefore they have been termed by us as a "lipid triad" of modification or of damage of biomembranes (Meerson, Arkhipenko et al., 1981).

In the present paper our attention will mainly be focused on the role of lipid peroxidation. It will be demonstrated that excessive activation of this process is an essential link in the pathogenesis of stress-induced and ischemic damages of the heart and can be prevented or limited by lipid peroxidation inhibitors - antioxidants.

The scheme on Figure 1 shows that there exist two pathways of oxygen utilization in the organism. The first of them, the well-known oxidase pathway, is related with oxidation of energy substrates;

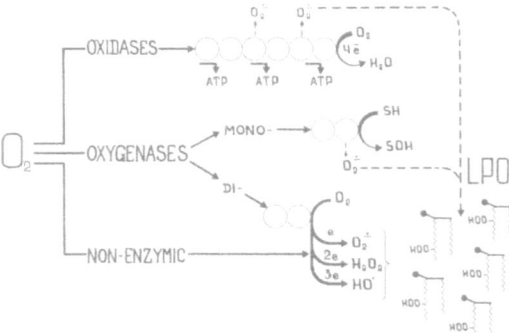

Fig. 1.   Two pathways of oxygen utilization and lipid peroxidation.
Explanation see in the text.

this pathway is realized by cytochrome oxidase, the terminal component
of the respiratory chain. In the course of the oxidase reaction
oxygen accepts four electrons; such a four-electron reduction of O_2
eventually results in a formation of a H_2O molecule. This pathway
does not involve oxygen incorporation into the oxidized substrate
molecule; under normal conditions it is coupled with a resynthesis of
ATP, thus being the main energy source in living systems.

The other, oxygenase pathway involves incorporation of one or
two oxygen atoms into the substrate molecule. The system of microsomal oxidation containing cytochrome P-450 can serve as a most
typical and common example of this pathway. Such oxygenase reactions
do not result in a complete reduction of O_2 to form water but give
rise to a formation of activated oxygen species, i.e. superoxide
anion radical, hydroperoxide, and hydroxyl radicals. It is essential
that the formation of these activated oxygen species can also take
place in the mitochondria by donating one electron to oxygen during
electron transport to cytochrome oxidase. The activated O_2 species
are capable of interacting with endogenous substrates, the structural
components of the cell and, in the first place, with biomembrane
phospholipids. The free radical oxidation of lipids gives rise to
the so-called peroxide compounds; therefore the overall process has
been termed lipid peroxidation, or LPO (Fridovich, 1974).

The results in Table 1 show that the heart muscle of intact
animals always contains intermediate products of lipid peroxidation,
such as lipid hydroperoxides, and LPO end products, namely Schiff's
bases. Simultaneously we can observe a rather high activity of the
antioxidant enzymatic systems, superoxide dismutase and catalase,
which restrict the LPO process. It is essential that the activity of
the antioxidant systems in the left ventricle myocardium is higher
and the content of LPO products is lower than in the right ventricle
myocardium.

Table 1. Activity of antioxidant systems and content of LPO products
          in heart ventricles.

	Right ventricle (10)	Left ventricle (10)
Superoxide dysmutase, conv. unit/mg.min	218±21	333±25
Catalase, nmol H_2O_2/mg.min	256±16	475±25
Fluorescence of Schiff's bases, rel. unit	1.64±0.12	1.00±0.15
Lipid hydroperoxides, opt. dens. unit/1 mg lipids in 1 ml.	1.49±0.2	1.03±0.13

Figures in parenthesis mean numbers of animals

Thus in normal heart muscle the lipid peroxidation process occurs continuously and its intensity is inversely dependent on the activity of natural antioxidant systems.

There are at least six factors known by now which can facilitate the switch-over of oxygen utilization from the oxidase pathway to the oxygenase one; they are the following:

1. Excess of catecholamines and products of their incomplete oxidation in stress (Kogan et al., 1976; Bors et al., 1978; Dilberto and Allen, 1981).

2. Excess of reduced pyridine nucleotides, the electrone donators in ischemia, hypoxia, and reoxygenation (Fridovich, 1974).

3. Increase in tension of oxygen, the electrone acceptor in hyperbaric oxygenation (Fridovich, 1974; Krachevskaya et al., 1980).

4. Inactivation of enzymic and non-enzymic antioxidant systems in avitaminosis E and other diseases (Arkhipenko et al., 1976).

5. Accumulation of unsaturated polyenic lipids attacked by activated oxygen species in obesity (Trostler et al., 1979).

6. Accumulation of metal-containing complexes with variable valency in hemolytic anemia and other diseases (Rachmilewitz et al., 1976).

Of primary interest here are the first four factors, namely the stress-induced catecholamine excess, ischemia and reoxygenation,

hyperbaric oxygenation and vitamin E deficiency, since in these
situations the activation of lipid peroxidation in heart muscle does
take place and the role of this activation in cardiomyocyte damage has
been proved.

The scheme on Figure 2 shows two possibilities responsible for
LPO activation by catecholamine excess and for the activation of its
biosynthesis in stress (Bors et al., 1978; Dilberto, 1981). First,
the activated oxygen species are formed at certain steps of catecholamine biosynthesis and second, epinephrine oxidation to adrenochrome
gives rise to a semiquinone radical which can donate electrons to
oxygen, thus generating the superoxide radical, an important LPO
inducer.

In full agreement with these assumptions is the finding that the
excitation of adrenergic regulation in emotional-painful stress
reproduced as an "neurosis of anxiety" causes LPO activation in heart
muscle and in other organs (Meerson, Kagan et al., 1980).

It can be seen from the Table 2 that in the myocardium of stress-
exposed animals the content of intermediate and end products of LPO
is increased more than 3-fold. It appears also that the stress-
induced activation of the lipid peroxidation can largely be prevented
by injecting ionol (2,6 ditertbutyl, 4 methyl phenol), a synthetic
antioxidant of a phenolic type prior to stress exposure (Meerson,
Golubeva et al., 1980). Further investigations have demonstrated that
beside LPO activation prevention ionol and other LPO inhibitors prevent the stress damages of the heart and other organs (Meerson, 1981).
The results obtained in our laboratory evidence that the stress-
induced disturbances of metabolism such as a decreased activity of
sarcoplasmic reticulum Ca-pump (Meerson, Arkhipenko et al., 1981) a
lowered content of glycogen (Meerson et al., 1978), uncoupling between
oxidation and phosphorylation in mitochondria (Meerson, Malyshev et

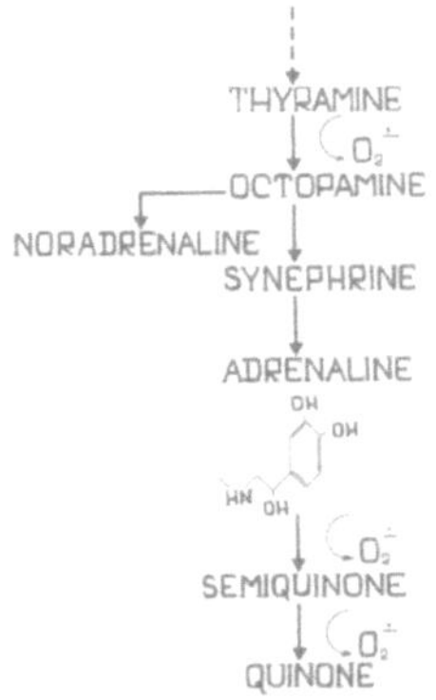

Fig. 2. Scheme of activation of lipid peroxidation by catecholamines.
         Explanation see in the text.

Table 2. Effect of ionol on LPO in myocardium in stress.

Series	Lipid hydroperoxides, opt. dens. unit/1 mg lipids in 1 ml.	Fluorescence of Schiff's bases, rel. units
1. Control (11)	1.08±0.13	1.00±0.33
2. Stress (10)	2.53±0.14	2.64±0.40
3. Ionol (10)	1.08±0.10	1.01±0.20
4. Ionol-stress (8)	1.71±0.14	1.26±0.17
Significance of differences, p.	P_{1-2} < 0.001 P_{1-3} non-significant P_{1-4} > 0.05	< 0.001 non-significant > 0.05

Figures in parenthesis mean number of animals

al., 1982), labilization of lysosomes (Meerson, 1981), and reversible damages of DNA (Meerson and Vasiliev, 1982) are partly or completely prevented by the LPO inhibitor ionol. In a similar way this antioxidant prevents other damaging effects caused by stress, namely the loss of enzymes by the myocardium (Meerson, Golubeva et al., 1980), an appearance of small-focal contractural and necrotic lesions (Meerson, 1981), a depression of the contractile function (Meerson and Trikhpoeva, 1980), and, finally the post-stress decrease of heart resistance to Ca^{2+} excess and hypoxia (Meerson, Golubeva et al., 1980).

Figure 3 shows the dynamics of the well-known event that is, hypoxic contracture of the myocardium. It can be seen that in the myocardium of rats exposed to stress the hypoxia-induced contracture is at least two times as high as in the control. A preliminary injection of ionol completely prevents the post-stress decrease of myocardium resistance to hypoxia.

It may thus be concluded that LPO activation which inevitably occurs in heart muscle upon stress is a key link in the stress damage of the heart and can therefore be prevented by antioxidants.

In terms of clinical cardiology it is essential that the observed changes in the metabolism and in the structure and function of the heart are not eliminated after cessation of the stress reaction. These relatively stable changes may be accumulated from one stress episode to another and become involved in a gradual development of cardiosclerosis and chronic heart insufficiency, which take place in aged individuals who have not suffered from the circulatory diseases before. The antioxidants prevent stress damages of the heart and, consequently, are cardioprotectors, the use of which can be a promising tool for prevention of cardiosclerosis and chronic heart insufficiency.

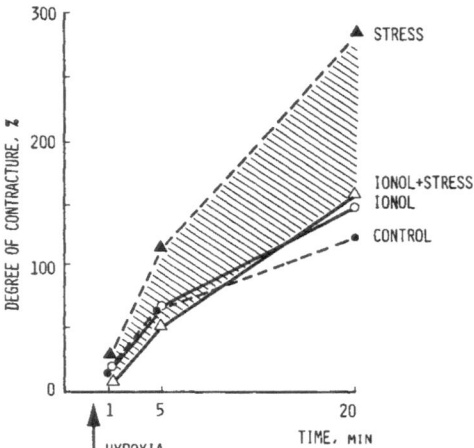

Fig. 3. Post-stress potentiation of the myocardium hypoxic contractur
and prevention of this phenomenon by the antioxidant ionol.

When studying the role of lipid peroxidation in the pathogenesis
of ischemic heart damage and the possibility of antioxidant protection
of the heart against such damage, the investigator is immediately face
with logical handicaps, since ischemic hypoxia is known to decrease
oxygen tension necessary for LPO activation. However, a more detailed
analysis shows that under "real organisms" conditions hypoxia and, in
a greater degree, reoxygenation may induce LPO activation.

The scheme on Figure 4 shows that the four-electron reduction of
oxygen on cytochrome oxidase can occur only upon continuous and well-
coordinated functioning of the respiratory chain, that is, under conditions of normal oxygen tension. When the respiratory chain is
blocked at its terminal component, i.e. in ischemic hypoxia, an
inevitable reduction of NAD to NADH and a reduction of the respiratory
chain carriers may cause a reduction of molecular oxygen dissolved in
the membrane lipid matrix. However, this will not be a four-electron
reduction to an end product, H_2O, but an incomplete reduction coupled
with generation of activated oxygen species. Naturally under oxygen
deficiency the accumulation of its activated species and LPO activatic
are considerably limited and occur at a slow rate. A far more intensive production of activated oxygen species and LPO products occurs
when the accumulation of reduced respiratory chain carriers, electron
donors, is accompanied by a sufficiently high oxygen tension. This
situation is observed during reoxygenation after hypoxia and ischemia
that is, in a situation apparently accompanying each coronary attack
under conditions of natural reperfusion of primarily ischemic zones
of the myocardium. A similar situation can be reproduced experimenta
by restoration of oxygen transport to anoxic heart.

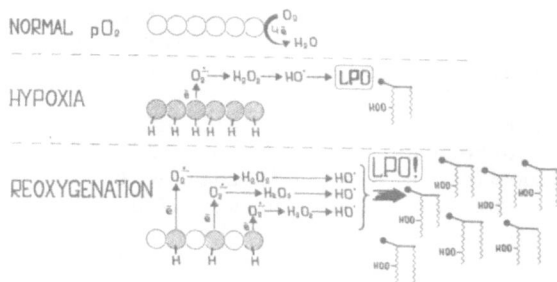

Fig. 4. Activation of lipid peroxidation in hypoxia and reoxygenation.
Explanation see in the text.

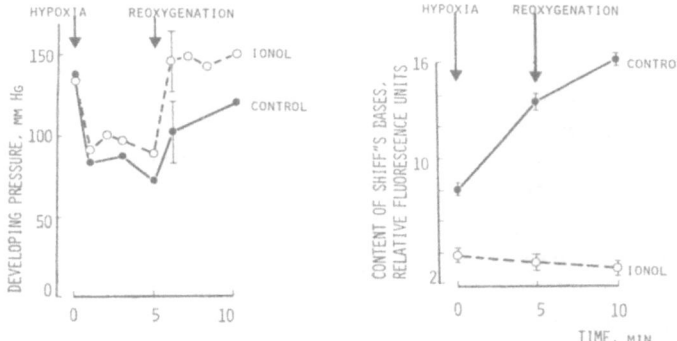

Fig. 5. Effect of preliminary ionol administration on the contractile
function of the heart muscle and content of Schiff's bases
in hypoxia and reoxygenation.

    The left part of Figure 5 shows the pressure developed by left
ventricle in the whole organism under hypoxia induced by a switch-off
of the respiratory apparatus and a subsequent reoxygenation. The right
half shows the concentration of end products of lipid peroxidation in
the ventricle myocardium under the same conditions. It can be seen
that a preliminary injection of the LPO inhibitor ionol prevents the
rise in the concentration of Schiff's bases in hypoxia and, even in a
greater degree, during reoxygenation. Ionol has no effect on the
hypoxic depression of the contractile function and effectively
prevents reoxygenational disturbances of this function. Thus, LPO
activation in the myocardium can be due to the effects of at least
three factors really existing in pathology namely to stress-induced

catecholamine excess, hypoxia and reoxygenation. All these factors
are inevitably associated with myocardial infarction; therefore a
considerable activation of LPO may be expected in this case.

It can be seen from the Table 3 that 24 hours after ligation of
the left coronary artery descending branch and the development of
experimental myocardial infarction in the rat the inactivation of
antioxidant enzymatic systems and the significant increase of the
intermediate and end products of LPO take place in the ischemic and,
which is most essential, in the non-ischemic zone of the myocardium.
This suggests a possibility of antioxidant use for protection of the
heart against ischemic damage. However, our preliminary results
were far from being encouraging.

Table 3. LPO activation and inactivation of antioxidant systems of
myocardium in experimental myocardial infarction.

| | | Infarction | |
	Control (10)	Ischemic zone (8)	Outside the ischemic zone (8)
Activity of enzymes:			
Superoxide dysmutase, conv. unit/1 g protein	344±25	283±18 $p < 0.05$	247±8 $p < 0.005$
Glutathion peroxidase I, nmol NADPH/1 mg protein in 1 min	315±18	134±22 $p < 0.01$	116±8 $p < 0.01$
Glutathion peroxidase II, nmol NADPH/1 mg protein in 1 min	218±11	74±13 $p < 0.01$	42±6 $p < 0.001$
Catalase, nmol H_2O_2/1 mg protein in 1 min	445±43	285±28 $p < 0.001$	178±8 $p < 0.005$
Lipid hydroperoxides, opt. dens. unit/1 mg lipids in 1 ml	1.08±0.13	3.71±0.42 $p < 0.005$	2.00±0.18 $p < 0.01$
Fluorescence of Schiff's bases, rel. unit	1.00±0.22	13.31±1.39 $p < 0.005$	5.11±0.60 $p < 0.005$

Figures in parenthesis mean number of animals

Data represented in Table 4 show that preliminary injection of
the antioxidant did not significantly affect the size of the infarction zone 48 hours after ligation of the left coronary artery
descending branch. Ionol only decreased the degree of fermentemia

Table 4. Effect of preliminary ionol administration on the necrosis
          size and fermentemia in experimental myocardial infarction

	Infarction (11)	Ionol-infarction (9)
Infarction area under epicardium, % of the total area of left ventricle	63.3±20	59.5±3.1 p < 0.05
Infarction area under endocardium, % of the total area of left ventricle	50.9±1.9	43.7±3.2 p > 0.5
Activity of aspartate transaminase, u/l	130.4±12.2	97.2±7.1 p < 0.05

Figures in parenthesis mean number of animals

associated with the infarction; the same effect of ionol was, however,
observed in the case of emotional-painful stress. It may therefore
be assumed that the fermentemia observed 48 hours after the onset of
myocardial infarction is mainly due to stress damage of various
tissues and its decrease is a result of the antistress effect of
ionol.

The curves shown in Figure 6 reflect the dynamics of the pressure
developed in the left ventricle during relative rest and at maximal
load caused by tension after 25 sec clamping of this pressure and the
velocity of its development are significantly decreased as compared
to the control. This depression caused by infarction is maximal at
the 25th second after aorta clamping when a fatigue of the safe zones
of the myocardium is developed. The most essential experimental
finding consists of the fact that a preliminary injection of the antioxidant considerably prevents the development of this contractile
function damage. The hatched area in the slide designates the protective effect.

Since the size of the ischemic necrotic zone is decreased by
the antioxidant only insignificantly, we have supposed that this effect may be due to the antioxidant protection of the safe, non-ischemic
zones of the myocardium against the stress-induced damages concomitant
with myocardial infarction. In other words, it seems probable that
in this case we deal with a protection of the intact divisions of
the myocardium against stress damage.

To test this assumption we studied the contractility of the
experimentally non-ischemic zones of the heart, namely the right
auricle of animals with experimental infarction of the left ventricle.

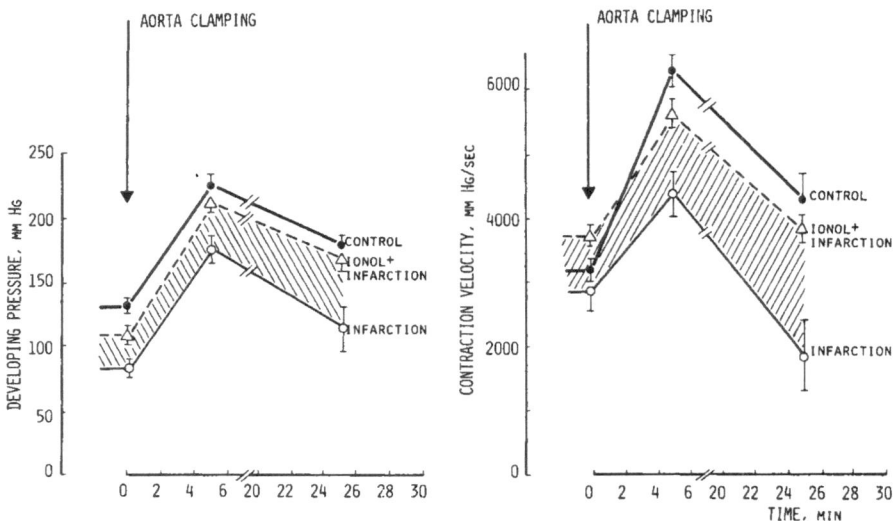

Fig. 6.   Effect of preliminary ionol administration on the contractile
function of the heart muscle at maximal load in control
animals and in those sustained experimental infarction.

    The Table 5 shows that 24 hours after the onset of experimental
infarction in rat left ventricle the contractile function of the right
auricle is strongly disturbed, showing in an almost 2-fold decrease
of the maximal pressure developed by the isolated auricle during iso-
metric contraction and of the intensity of its structure functioning
which was determined as auricle tension/mass ratio multiplied by the
contraction frequency. A preliminary injection of the β-blocker
inderal prevents this defect of the contractile function. Consequently the auricular damage is due to catecholamine excess, that is, to
adrenergic stress effect associated with infarction. The table also
demonstrates that ionol prevents the disturbed contractile function of
the auricle in the same degree as inderal. In this way the antioxidant prevents the depression of contractile function of the non-
ischemic part of the heart under acute period of myocardial infarction and the antioxidant protection of the heart is in this case an
antistressory one. Based on the facts given here it is purposeful
to come back to the very beginning of this paper to remind you that
the damages of the membrane lipid bilayer upon stress and ischemia
are due not to isolated activation of LPO but to the "lipid triad"
involving the activation of LPO and phospholipases and the detergent-
like action of excessive amounts of fatty acids and lysophosphatides.

Table 5. Effect of preliminary inderal and ional administration on
          the right auricle contractility in the infarction of left
          ventricle.

Series	Developed tension, mg	Intensity of structure functioning, g/mg.min
1. Control (10)	382±12.5	3.8±0.2
2. Infarction (15)	198.6±4.3	1.8±0.1
3. Inderal-infarction (11)	331±15	2.9±0.2
4. Ionol-infarction (10)	315.2±15	2.9±0.2
P_{1-2}	< 0.001	< 0.001
P_{1-3}	> 0.5	> 0.5
P_{1-4}	> 0.5	> 0.5

Figures in parenthesis mean number of animals

Based on this assumption we used, in addition to the antioxidants,
the phospholipase inhibitor chloroquene and the lipase inhibitor nicotinamide, for protection of the non-ischemic divisions of the myocardium.

Figure 7 shows that 24 hours after the producing of infarction
the contractile function of the non-ischemic division of the myocardium, that is, of the right auricle, is characterized by a marked
depression of the Sterling's curve, which is shifted downwards and
to the right. A preliminary injection of the above-mentioned membrano-
protectors prior to the infarction significantly prevents the disturbance of contractile function. The hatched area in the figure
designates the protective effects of ionol, nicotinamide and chloroquene.

When evaluating the fact that inhibitors of different components
of the lipid triade indirectly protect the safe divisions of myocardium one should keep in mind that in the whole organism conditions
the lipid triade components are inseparably linked with each other.
Really LPO activation results in labilization of lysosomes in which
a considerable part of cell phospholipases is concentrated. The
phospholipidases which are released from lysosomes and also the activated membrane-bound ones can play an important role in the destruction of the membranous lipid bilayer and in formation of lysophosphatides and free fatty acids (Katz and Messineo, 1981). Lysophosphatides
and high concentrations of fatty acids which are observed in blood
during stress and infarction, due to their detergent-like action,
disturb the regulary arrangement of phospholipids in membrane which,
in turn, may result in an additional LPO activation. This chain

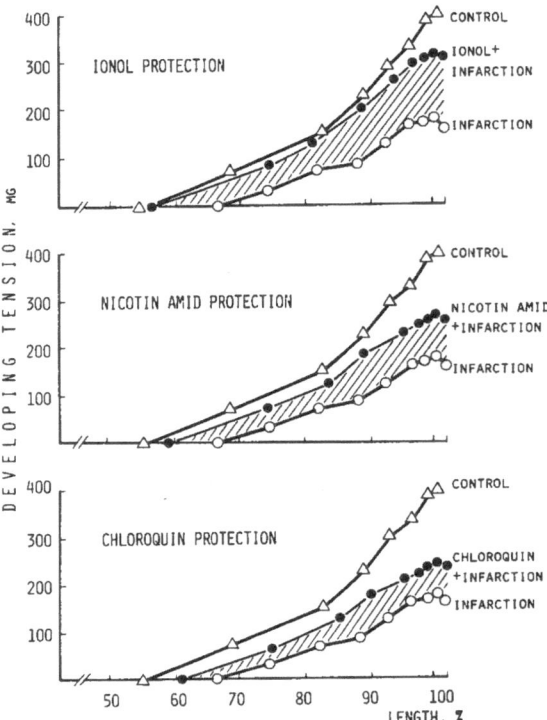

Fig. 7.   Prevention of the Starling's curve depression in the non-
           ischemized zone by membrane protectors ionol, nicotinamide,
           and chloroquene in the experimental myocardial infarction.

reaction enables an increase in the membrane permeability for Ca^{2+}
and the resultant excess of this cation, in turn, activates phospholipases (Vladimirov and Archakov, 1972). In the end the vicious circle
closes which plays an important role in cell membrane damage, in
transition of those damages to irreversible ones, and in myocyte death.

In this way one can imagine the process occurring in the ischemic
zone in infarction and foci of necrotic damages. Outside the ischemic zone in infarction and in the most part of myocardium in stress
the same cycle of events is less pronounced; it may be terminated at
one of its links by inhibiting any component of lipid triads. This
is precisely the point of view to understand the above-examined protective effect of the inhibitors of LPO, phospholipases, and lipases.

In conclusion we would like to emphasize that the contractile
function of the safe parts of the heart muscle largely predetermines

the fate of a myocardial infarction patient. These divisions are
damaged by stress which is always concomitant with infarction;
therefore their protection by antioxidants and other membrane protectors seems to be a promising one.

REFERENCES

Archipenko, Yu. V., Gazdarov, A. K., Kagan, V. E., and Spirichev, V.B.,
    1976, Lipid peroxidation and the direction of Ca^{2+} transport
    through sarcoplasmic reticulum membranes in E avitaminosis,
    Biokhimiya, 42: 1898. (in Russian).
Bors, W., Michel, C., Saran, M., and Lengfelder, E., 1978, The in-
    volvement of oxygen radicals during the autoxidation of adren-
    alin, Biochim. Biophys. Acta, 540: 162.
Chien, K.R., Pfaw, R.G., and Farber, J.L., 1979, Ischemic myocardial
    cell injury, Am. J. Pathol., 97: 505.
Diliberto, E.J., and Allen, P.L., 1981, Mechanism of β-hydroxylation.
    Semidehydroascorbate as the enzymic oxidation products of
    ascorbate, J. Biol. Chem., 256: 3385.
Fridovich, J., 1974, Superoxide and evolution, Horisons Biochem.
    Biophys., 1: 37.
Fridovich, I., 1975, Oxygen boon and bane, Amer. Sci., 63:54.
Katz, A.M., and Messineo, F., 1981, Lipid-membrane interactions and
    the pathogenesis of ischemic damage in the myocardium, Circul.
    Res., 48:1.
Kogan, A.Kh., Kudrin, A.N., and Nikolaev, S.M., 1976, On the role of
    lipid peroxidation in the mechanism of myocardial damage by
    epinephrine in: "Materialy simposiuma" Svobodnoradicalnoe
    okislenie lipidov v norme i patologii", "Nauka", Moscow (in
    Russian).
Krachevskaya, A.A., Lukash, A.I., and Bronovitzkaya, Z.G., 1980,
    "Biochemical mechanism of oxygen intoxication", Publ. Rostov
    University, Rostov (in Russian).
Meerson, F.Z., 1981, "Adaptation, stress and prophylaxis", "Nauka",
    Moscow (in Russian).
Meerson, F.Z., Arkhipenko, Yu.V., Rozhitzkaya, I.I., and Kagan, V.E.,
    1981, Damage of the Ca^{2-}-transport system of the heart sarco-
    plasmic reticulum in emotional-painful stress, Bull. exper.
    biol. med., 4:405 (in Russian).
Meerson, F.Z., and Vasiliev, V.K., 1982, Prevention of the structure
    damage of the heart muscle DNA caused by emotional-painful
    stress by blockade of β-adrenoceptors and lipid peroxidation,
    Voprosy med. khimii, 2:115 (in Russian).
Meerson, F.Z., Golubeva, L.Yu., Kagan, V.E., Shimkovich, M.V., and
    Ugolev, A.A., 1980, Activation of lipid peroxidation as the
    decisive link in the pathogenesis of stress damage of the heart
    and prevention of stress and hypoxic damage by the antioxidant
    ionol, in: "Fourth USA-USSR joint symposium on myocardial
    metabolism", Nat. Inst. Health Publication, Bethesda.

Meerson, F.Z., Kagan, V.E., Prilipko, L.L., and Rozhitzkaya, I.I., 1980, Inhibition of lipid peroxidation by ionol and gamma-hydroxybutyric acid in emotional-painful stress, Bull. exp. biol. med., 12:661.

Meerson, F.Z., Kagan, V.E., Kozlov, Yu.P., Belkina, L.M., and Arkhi-penko, Yu.V., 1982, Role of lipid peroxidation in the patho-genesis of ischemic damage and the heart antioxidant protection, Kardiologiya, 2:81.

Meerson, F.Z., Malyshev, V.V., Petrova, V.A., and Lifantiev, V.I., 1982, Prevention of activation of the hypophisial-adrenal system and heart damage by the antioxidant ionol in stress, Kardiologiya, 2:

Meerson, F.Z., Pavlova, V.I., Yakushev, V.S., and Kamilov, F.Kh., 1978, Disturbances of the heart energy metabolism in emotional-painful stress and prevention of this disturbance by sodium gamma-hydroxybutyrate, Kardiologiya, 3:52.

Meerson, F.Z., Trikhpoeva, A.M., 1980, Prevention by gamma-hydroxy-butyric acid and antioxidant ionol of disturbances of the heart muscle contractile function resulted from emotional-painful stress, Bull. exp. biol. med., 11:531.

Rachmilewitz, E.A., Lubin, B.H., and Shohet, S.B., 1976, Lipid mem-brane peroxidation in β-thalassemia major, Blood, 47:495.

Trostler, N., Brady, P., Romsos, D., and Leveille, G., 1979, Influence of dietary vitamin E on malondialdehyd levels in liver and adipose tissue and glatation peroxidase and reductase activity in liver and eritrocites of lean and obese mice, J. of Nutrition, 109:345.

Vasdev, S.C., Kako, K.J., and Biri, J.P., 1979, Phospholipid compo-sition of cardiac mitochondria and lysosomes in experimental myocardial ischemia in the dog, J. Mol. Cell. Cardiol. 11:1195.

Vladimirov, Yu.A., and Archakov, A.I., 1972, "Lipid peroxidation in biological membranes", "Meditzina", Moscow.

NUCLEAR MAGNETIC RESONANCE STUDIES OF INTRACELLULAR pH

AND MYOCARDIAL CONTRACTILITY DURING ISCHEMIA

William E. Jacobus*+, Clayton H. Kallman*,
Myron L. Weisfeldt*, and John T. Flaherty*

Peter Belfer Laboratory for Myocardial Research
*Department of Medicine
+Department of Physiological Chemistry
The John Hopkins University School of Medicine
Baltimore, Maryland 21205, USA

INTRODUCTION

Most investigators in the field of molecular cardiology define myocardial ischemia in terms of a metabolic supply demand imbalance. Normal cell function is observed when supply is equal to or greater than demand. However, if coronary flow is reduced such that oxygen supply cannot meet the metabolic demands for the aerobic production of ATP (and phosphocreatine), then there must be a reduction in cell function[1]. In other words, cell function is in a delicate balance between metabolic (energetic) supply and its physiological demands, as illustrated by Equation 1.

        Cell Function = Supply/Demand   Eq. 1

By this definition, ischemic dysfunction of the heart may occur from either a reduction in blood supply at a constant physiological work demand, or from an increase in demand at a constant but limited rate of supply (flow). In cardiology, the latter condition is the cause of the clinical syndrome of angina pectoris, whereas the former initiates acute myocardial infarction, the leading cause of death in the Western world. While almost universally accepted, this fundamental metabolic definition of myocardial ischemia raises an important basic question. Is the ischemia, or flow induced depression of ventricular function always associated with observable alterations in the cell metabolic supply/demand balance? If the above equation is valid under all cases, then the answer should be yes.

The experimental observations leading to this question are well known. In an isolated, perfused isovolumic heart model, when the perfusion line is clamped, coronary flow is abruptly halted. As a result, we see an almost instantaneous and progressive fall in performance. During this time several key metabolic events are occurring. These include the hydrolysis of ATP and phosphocreatine, the cessation of aerobic metabolism, and the onset of anaerobic glycolysis leading to the accumulation of lactate and ultimately to intracellular acidosis[2,3]. Tissue oxygen is severely reduced, and as a consequence of bicarbonate buffering and diminished wash-out, tissue carbon dioxide rises[4]. These well documented observations have become the metabolic hallmarks of ischemic tissue. They have also led to the following hypothesis: the fall in contractility associated with myocardial ischemia may result from a decline in the high energy phosphates, the development of intracellular acidosis, the lack of tissue oxygen, or some combination of all three. A more critical examination of this hypothesis using 31-P nuclear magnetic resonance and mass spectrometry methods forms the subject of this report.

EXPERIMENTAL METHODS

Nuclear Magnetic Resonance Methods

Heart perfusion techniques. Hearts (5-6g) from young female New Zealand white rabbits weighing less than 2.0 kg are routinely used in our experiments. The hearts are perfused retrograde in a modified Langendorff mode previously described in detail[5]. The perfusion canula is positioned well above the aortic valve, which is then competent. The Krebs Ringer bicarbonate buffer is phosphate-free and contains 117 mM NaCl, 6.0 mM KCl, 3.0 mM $CaCl_2$, 1.0 mM $MgSO_4$, 0.6 mM EDTA, 16.7 mM glucose, and 24 mM Na bicarbonate, and is vigorously bubbled with 95% O_2/5% CO_2 for a final buffer pH of 7.40. The perfusate temperature is 40°C in the reservoir. The temperature of the perfusate overflow from the heart is 35-37°C. Since the perfusate is phosphate-free, all 31-P NMR signals arise from endogenous tissue metabolites. The hearts are paced at a rate of 150-170 beats per minute. Isovolumic ventricular pressure is measured using a latex balloon positioned through the mitral valve into the left ventricular cavity and connected to a Statham P 23 Db transducer, which is calibrated with a mercury manometer. The control end diastolic pressure is set at 10 mm Hg. Care is taken to prevent balloon herniation into the left atrium. Figure 1 illustrates a heart positioned in the NMR sample tube. Perfusate overflow is removed by vacuum aspiration. The rest of the accessory apparatus required for our studies is shown in Figure 2.

Instrumental methods. 31-P NMR spectra are obtained from a wide-bore superconducting magnet (4.23 T) at 72.89 MHz, using a Bruker WH-180 spectrometer. The stability of the magnetic field is such that

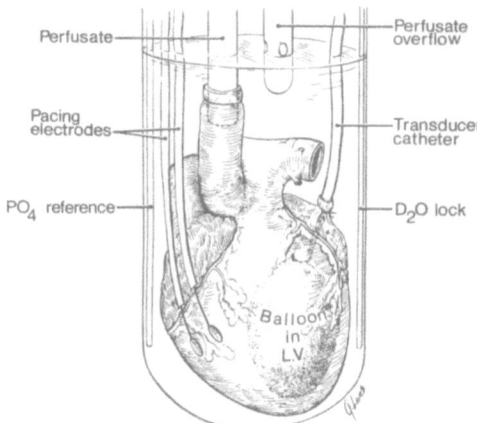

Fig. 1. A view of a perfused rabbit heart in the NMR sample tube.
         Tube diameter is 25 mm. Perfusate flows retrograde into the
         coronary arteries from the aortic perfusion cannula. The
         latex balloon in the left ventricle and the transducer cath-
         eter used for the measurement of isovolumic pressures are
         shown. Also illustrated are the pacing electrodes and the
         overflow line for removal of coronary flow. Reprinted with
         permission[5].

field/frequency D2O lock is not required; the probe diameter is 25 mm.
The instrument is operated in the pulsed, Fourier transform mode, and
is interfaced to a Bruker 1080 computer. Proton-decoupled spectra
are obtained from transients following 25 μsec (45°) pulses delivered
at 2-second intervals, conditions resulting in minimal spectral saturation. The data are collected at a 3,000 Hz width with a 2K data
table, or at a 5,000 Hz spectral width with a 4K table. A heart spectrum with each peak labeled is shown in Figure 3. Spectra required
200-400 transients. Estimates of intracellular pH (pHi) are determined from the chemical shift (δo) of the Pi peak according to
Equation 2.

$$pH = pK - \log (\delta_0 - \delta_b/\delta_a - \delta_0) \qquad \text{Eq. 2}$$

To minimize the effects of tissue inhomogenity, all chemical shift
values are determined relative to the phosphocreatine resonance, which
because of its low pK (4.6) is rather insensitive to pH changes above
6.0. Our best estimates of the constants for Equation 2 are as follows: pK = 6.90; δa = 3.290; δb = 5.805. The validity of these values
has been extensively discussed by us and others[5-7]. Using these constants, our current estimate of the heart's intracellular pH under
various conditions is presented in Table 1.

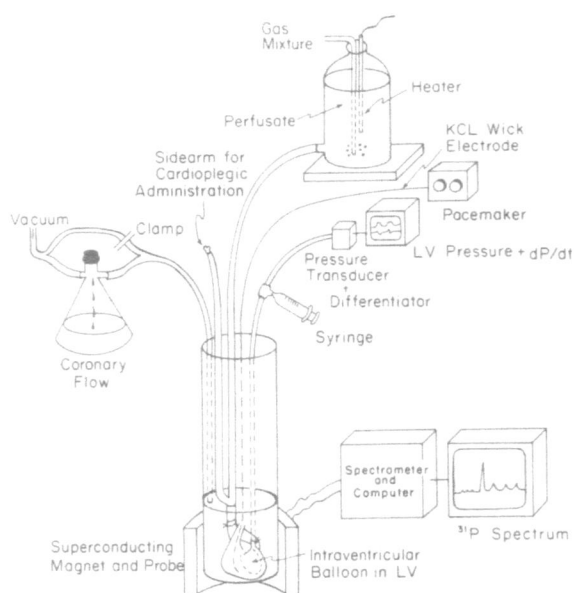

Fig. 2. A drawing of the accessory equipment required for physio-
         logical studies using NMR. LV is left ventricle; dP/dt is
         the first derivative of pressure. Reprinted with permission[5].

Table 1. Intracellular pH of perfused Rabbit Hearts.

Condition	Intracellular pH
Working (N = 15)	7.18 ± 0.02
KCL arrest (N = 4)	7.22 ± 0.02
Hypoxia (N = 7)	7.19 ± 0.01

Hearts were perfused with phosphate-free Krebs buffer. The working
heart was the normal isovolumic model. Hearts were arrested with
37 mM KCl added to the perfusate. Partial hypoxia was induced by
bubbling the perfusate with 65% O_2/30% N_2/5% CO_2. In all conditions,
buffer pH was 7.45 - 7.48. Intracellular pH values are given as mean
± S.E.

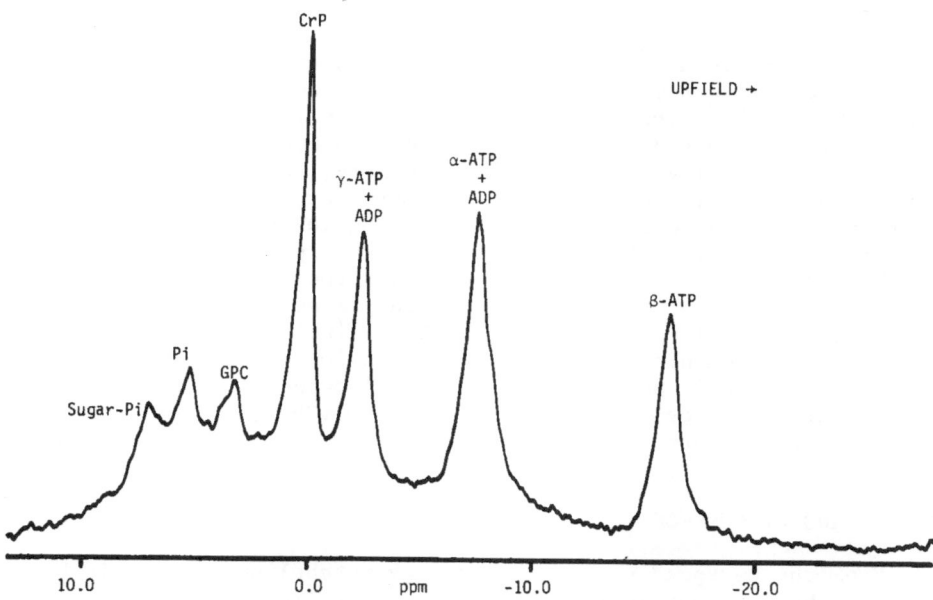

Fig. 3.   A 31-P NMR spectrum of a perfused rabbit heart. This is a
          9,000-pulse spectrum acquired at a 3,000-Hz spectral width.
          Peaks are observed for the glycolytic sugar phosphates (Sugar-
          Pi), inorganic phosphate (Pi), glycerol-3-phosphorylcholine
          (GPC), phosphocreatine (CrP), and ATP and ADP. The B-ATP
          peak is used to quantitate ATP. The abscissa scale is chemi-
          cal shift in parts per million (ppm) with 0.0 at the peak of
          the phosphocreatine resonance. Reprinted with permission[5].

Mass Spectrometry Methods

        The measurements of tissue gases were done by vacuum mass spec-
trometry methods standard in this laboratory. Briefly, a 22-gauge
Teflon-coated probe is inserted tangentially into the free wall of
the left ventricle and tightly sutured at the epicardial surface to
prevent contamination by room air. The tissue gas mixture is withdrawn across the Teflon membrane, through stainless steel tubing,
and into the mass spectrometer at a rate of 5×10^{-6} ml/sec. The
1/e response time of this system is 1.5 minutes for oxygen and 3
minutes for carbon dioxide, and the instrument is calibrated daily
using gases of known composition. Further details of the mass spectrometry method have been reported[8].

Protocols

Since ferrous metals cannot be placed in the NMR magnet, separate protocols were required for our NMR and mass spectrometry experiments. In our NMR studies perfusion pressure was stepwise lowered from control of 110 cm H_2O (80 mm Hg) to 80%, then to 60%, and then to 40% of control. At each level of perfusion pressure, functional stabilization required 5 minutes, and NMR data acquisition required an additional 15 minutes. At the end of the protocol function recovered to 90% of the initial control performance when perfusion pressure was restored to 100%. A slightly different protocol was employed in our parallel mass spectrometry experiments. Perfusion pressure was lowered stepwise from a control value of 80 mm Hg to a final value of 20 mm Hg, in 10 mm Hg increments. Myocardial gas tensions were recorded 10 min. after each change in perfusion pressure, allowing time for instrument stabilization. Rates of coronary blood flow (CBF), oxygen utilization (MVO_2) and left ventricular developed pressure (DP) were also measured.

RESULTS AND DISCUSSION

From the perspective of heart energy metabolism, oxygen is by far both the most necessary and also the most limited substrate in the myocardium, there being no major cytoplasmic reserve. It has been estimated that within less than 5 seconds after coronary artery ligation, the tissue concentration of oxygen falls below the Km for cytochrome oxidase, and the mitochondrial electron transport chain becomes reduced. Oxidative phosphorylation, the source of 90% of contractile ATP^9, stops under these conditions. Therefore, in addition to the considerations of high energy phosphate metabolism expressed by Equation 1, tissue oxygen content could also be an important cellular regulatory signal for the heart. Physiologically important oxygen chemoreceptors exist in the carotid bodies of the carotid arteries. These receptors monitor blood oxygen content and help ensure adequate oxygen delivery to the brain. In a similar manner, oxygen per se could directly exert a regulatory effect over myocardial contractility If such were the case, it is possible that the changes in contractility observed at the onset of ischemia might parallel the decline in tissue oxygen tension, or PmO_2. To examine the dynamics of these potential regulatory parameters (ATP, phosphocreatine, pHi, and oxygen during conditions of reduced coronary flow, we used the techniques of NMR and mass spectrometry to monitor changes in these metabolites (Figures 4 and 5). Hearts were initially perfused at a pressure of 80 mm Hg. In a stepwise manner, perfusion pressure was reduced in 10 mm Hg increments from 80 to 20 mm Hg, or expressed as a percentage reduction, to 25% of control pressure. In both Figures 4 and 5, the line of identity is indicated by the dashed line. In Figure 4 we see that three parameters closely parallel the line of identity. These are the rates of coronary blood flow (CBF), left ventricular developed pressure (DP), and the rates of myocardial oxygen utilization (MVO_2).

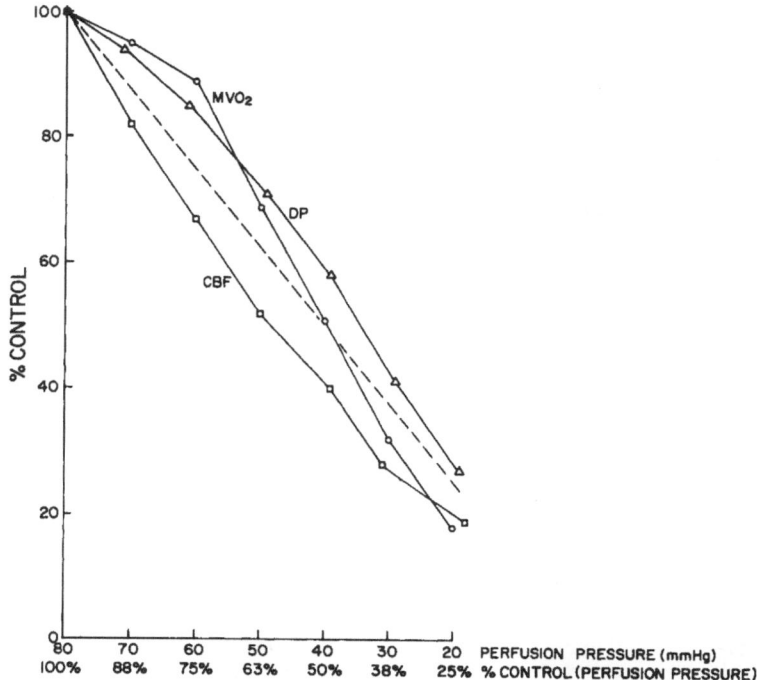

Fig. 4. Changes in coronary blood flow (CBF), developed pressure (DP),
         and the rate of oxygen utilization (MVO_2) as a function of
         decreased perfusion pressure in isolated, perfused rabbit
         hearts. Data were collected during a steady-state reduction
         in perfusion pressure, which was held constant at each point
         for at least 15 minutes. The dashed line is the line of
         identity. Reprinted with permission[5].

In other words, as perfusion pressure is diminished there is an almost
linear decline in coronary blood flow, indicating a lack of coronary
artery autoregulation. In conjunction, there is a similar decline in
developed pressure, which, because of the reduction in ventricular
work (ATP demand), leads to a parallel decline in oxygen utilization.
These results were neither new or surprising.

    In contrast, a rather striking and unanticipated set of results
are seen in the NMR and mass spectrometry data (Figure 5). If our
oxygen feed-back hypothesis had been correct, we would have predicted
an immediate fall in tissue PmO_2, a sharp rise in tissue $PmCO_2$, with
perhaps moderate changes in pHi and the high energy phosphate compounds.
This was not observed (Figure 5). Initially, as perfusion pressure
was decreased, PmO_2 increased while tissue $PmCO_2$ fell and pHi remained

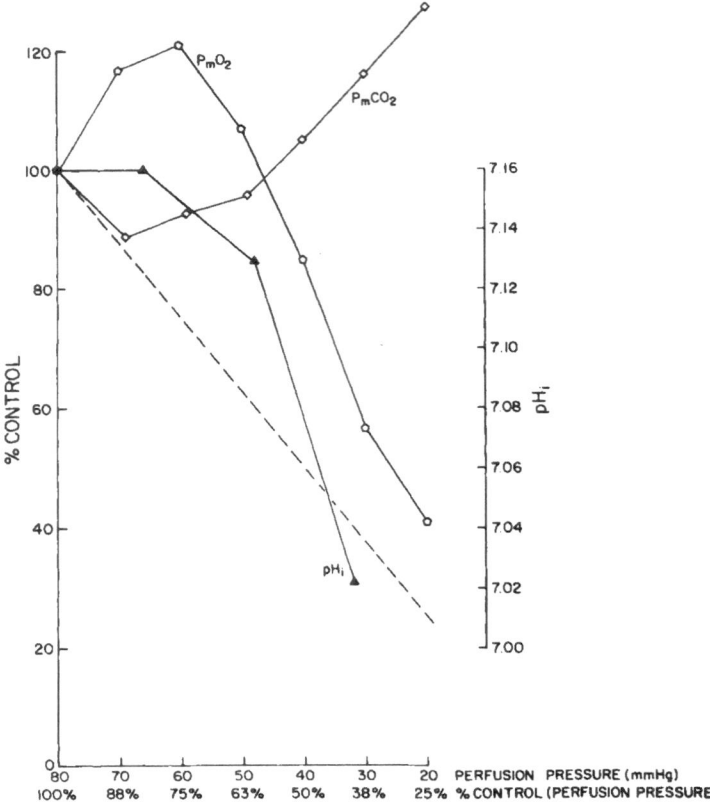

Fig. 5.   Changes in tissue oxygen content (PmO$_2$), carbon dioxide con-
          tent (PmCO$_2$), and intracellular pH (pHi) as a function of
          decreased perfusion pressure. Conditions were as described
          in Figure 4. Tissue gases were measured directly by mass
          spectrometry methods, and pH, was determined by NMR (see
          Experimental Methods). Reprinted with permission[5].

constant. As perfusion pressure was further decreased to about 75%
of control, PmO$_2$ then started to decline and PmCO$_2$ began to rise, still
at a rather constant pHi. The tissue gases continued to change until
a crossover point was reached, which occurred at about a 44% reduction
in perfusion pressure or a 52% reduction in flow (Table 2). Furthermore, at this point there was no change in the high energy phosphate
content of the heart. ATP and phosphocreatine were present in normal
amounts, up to the crossover point. Therefore, these hearts appear
to be metabolically in balance (Eq. 1) even though performance is decreased by 32% (Table 2). This condition appears to be a direct vio-
lation of Equation 1. These data clearly show that tissue oxygen tension is not a primary parameter regulating myocardial function.

Table 2.   Magnitude of the Changes Observed at the Crossover Point
for PmO_2 and $PmCO_2$.

Perfusion pressure	44% reduction
Coronary blood flow	52% reduction
Left ventricular developed pressure	32% reduction
Rate of O_2 utilization	˙38% reduction
Intracellular pH	0.04 pH unit acidification
High energy phosphate	No detectable changes
Myocardial PmO_2 and $PmCO_2$	Normal

Data were derived from Figures 5 and 6.

These data do provide a new insight into the flow dependent control of performance. They show that up to 50% reduction in flow, some
as yet undefined autoregulatory mechanism efficiently down-regulates
myocardial contractility and thereby reduces oxygen utilization. Despite decreasing coronary flow, oxygen supply apparently exceeds oxygen demand as evidenced by the PmO_2 being higher than control. This
level of tissue PmO_2 presumably allows aerobic metabolism to continue
and intracellular pH to remain in balance (Table 2). Beyond a 50%
reduction in flow, this mechanism apparently fails. Contractile demands then exceed supply and the classic metabolic indices of ischemia are expressed, including an elevated $PmCO_2$, and intracellular
acidosis. In other words, moderate reductions in coronary flow did
not result in a supply/demand imbalance (Equation 1), even though
left ventricular function was markedly diminished.

Since this mechanism also prevents the "ischemic" accumulation
of H^+ and Pi, agents known by themselves to induce cellular damage,[10,11]
it would appear that this functional autoregulation might well act
to protect the heart from "irreversible" damage during transient and
moderate reductions in flow. The idea that functional "down-regulation" might reduce myocardial oxygen demands and thereby prevent irreversible ischemic damage could be applied to several clinical settings.
In the case of myocardial infarction associated with thrombotic coronary
occlusion, functional down-regulation could reduce metabolic demands
such that in the presence of a sufficient degree of coronary collateral
flow, myocardium could remain viable until an intervention such as
thrombolysis could be employed to improve perfusion. In the case of
angina pectoris due to either reduced supply (e.g. coronary spasm)
or increased demand (e.g. exercise or atrial pacing) in the presence
of fixed coronary obstructive disease, left ventricular angiography
has demonstrated reversible segmental dyskinesis, akinesis, or hypo-
kinesis. Functional down regulation of segmental contractility would
be protective in any of these circumstances against irreversible

ischemic damage to cell membranes or enzyme systems. Segmental wall
motion abnormalities on preoperative catheterization in the absence
of symptoms suggesting angina pectoris have reversed or improved
following coronary artery bypass surgery. This observation could be
interpreted as suggesting the occurrence of functional down-regulation
of segmental function distal to significant coronary narrowing in the
absence of clinical or electrocardiographic signs of ischemia.

The results of this work leave us with a rather significant new
question: how do moderate changes in coronary flow induce a depression
in ventricular performance if there is no measurable decrease in tissue oxygen, intracellular pH, ATP or phosphocreatine? Certainly one
can evoke the concept of "microcompartmentation" of metabolites.
There is no current experimental methodology available to verify or
refute this notion. On the other hand, it is possible that these
effects are mediated by changes in wall tension[12]. The phenomenon
relating coronary perfusion pressure to the internal stretching of
the myocardial muscle fibers has been called the "garden hose" effect[13,15]. In brief, reductions in flow and perfusion pressure result
in a decrease in the distending pressure in the coronary arteries,
leading to a decrease in wall tension. By some intramural "internal
Starling Mechanism", reduced wall tension appears to decrease contractility.

When a viscous nonoxygenated, nonnutrient containing substance
was injected into the coronary arteries early after aortic occlusion
at a time when contractility was depressed, function transiently
returned toward normal[12]. These observations suggest that mechanical
distention of the coronaries was sufficient to improve function,
which supports the proposed "garden hose" effect. Although these
experiments and the so called "garden hose" effect are consistent
with our findings[12,16], whether or not this is the only major mechanism regulating myocardial function, during moderate ischemia, remains
unclear.

The importance of our observed "crossover point" remains uncertain. One could speculate that if coronary blood flow is reduced
by less than 50% that metabolic imbalance does not exist and therefore
myocardial cells should remain viable indefinitely, albeit with depressed function. In contrast, if coronary flow is reduced more than
50% (i.e., to the right of the crossover point) then metabolic evidence of ischemia is present. Thus, if the duration of exposure to
these conditions were sufficiently long, then myocardial necrosis
would result. Jugdutt et al[17] have suggested that myocardial preservation within an anatomic vascular risk region is seen when collateral
flow distal to a coronary ligation exceeds 50% of control. Regions
receiving less than 50% of control flow will ultimately undergo necrosis. Whether the crossover phenomenon seen in the isolated perfused
heart and this observation made in a conscious previously instrumented
canine model are casually related or, more importantly, are applicable
in the clinical setting remains open to further investigation.

SUMMARY

1. As coronary perfusion pressure was progressively reduced, coronary flow, left ventricular function, and oxygen utilization fell proportionately.
2. Under conditions of greater than 50% reduction in flow, energetic demands exceed supply, and the classic metabolic indices of is chemia were expressed, including decreased PmO2,: and intracellular acidosis.
3. However, with flow reductions of less than 50%, metabolic supply met or exceeded demands, and metabolic indices of ischemia were not observed. Under these conditions the heart was not in a metabolic supply/demand imbalance, even though function was reduced by 32%. These data show that the classic metabolic definition of ischemic cell dysfunction is not valid under all conditions of coronary flow reductions.
4. Therefore, some non-metabolic signal must be down-regulating contractility under the conditions of mild to moderate flow reduction. Although mechanical factors may play a role, the magnitude of its contribution along with other mechanisms responsible for this potentially protective, auto-regulation remain elusively undefined.

ACKNOWLEDGEMENT

Supported by United States Public Health Service grants HL-22080, HL-17655 and HL-19414, and by the resources of the Susan B. Clayton Fund of the Johns Hopkins University School of Medicine. W. E. J. is an Established Investigator of the American Heart Association.

REFERENCES

1. R. B. Jennings. Relationship of acute ischemia to functional defects and irreversibility, Circ. 53, Suppl I: I-26 (1976).
2. A. M. Katz. Effects of ischemia on the contractile processes of heart muscle, Am. J. Card. 32: 456 (1973).
3. W. Kubler and A. M. Katz. Mechanism of early "pump" failure of the ischemic heart. Possible role of adenosine triphosphate depletion and inorganic phosphate accumulation, Am. J. Card. 40:467 (1977).
4. S. F. Khuri, J. T. Flaherty, J. B. O'Riordan, B. Pitt, R. K. Brawley, J. S. Donahoo and V. L. Gott. Changes in intramyocardial ST segment voltage and gas tensions with regional myocardial ischemia in the dog, Circ. Res. 37:455 (1975).
5. W. E. Jacobus, I. H. Pores, S. K. Lucas, C. H. Kallman, M. L. Weisfeldt and J. T. Flaherty. The role of intracellular pH in the control of normal and ischemic myocardial contractility; a 31-P nuclear magnetic resonance and mass spectrometry study,

in: "Intracellular pH: Its measurement, regulation and utilization in cellular functions", R. Nuccitelli and D. W. Deamer,
eds., Alan R. Liss, New York, 537 (1982).

6. D. G. Gadian, G. K. Radda, M. J. Dawson and D. R. Wilkie. pHi
    measurements of cardiac and skeletal muscle using 31-P NMR,
    in: "Intracellular pH: Its measurement, regulation and utiliz-
    ation in cellular functions", R. Nuccitelli and D. W. Deamer,
    eds., Alan R. Liss, New York, 61 (1982).

7. R. J. Gillies, J. R. Alga, J. A. den Hollander and R. G. Shulman.
    Intracellular pH measured by NMR: Methods and results, in:
    "Intracellular pH: Its measurement, regulation and utilization
    in cellular functions", R. Nuccitelli and D. W. Deamer, eds.,
    Alan R. Liss, New York, 79 (1982).

8. S. F. Khuri, J. B. O'Riordan, J. T. Flaherty, R. K. Brawley,
    J. S. Donahoo and V. L. Gott. Mass spectrometry for the measure-
    ment of intramyocardial gas tensions: Methodology and applic-
    ation to the study of myocardial ischemia, in: "Recent Advances
    in Studies on Cardiac Structure and Metabolism, Vol. 10: Meta-
    bolism of Contraction", T. E. Roy and G. Rona, eds., University
    Park Press, Baltimore, 539 (1975).

9. J. R. Neely and H. E. Morgan. Relationship between carbohydrate
    and lipid metabolism and the energy balance of heart muscle,
    Ann. Rev. Physiol. 36: 413 (1974).

10. W. E. Jacobus, J. A. Bittl and M. L. Weisfeldt. Loss of mito-
    chondrial creatine kinase in vitro and in vivo. A sensitive
    index of ischemic cellular and functional damage, in: "Heart
    creatine kinase: The integration of isozymes for energy
    distribution", W. E. Jacobus and J. S. Ingwall, eds., Williams
    and Wilkins, Baltimore, 155 (1980).

11. A. Mukherjee, T. M. Wong, G. Templeton, L. M. Buja and J. T.
    Willerson. Influence of volume dilution, lactate, phosphate
    and calcium on mitochondrial functions, Am. J. Physiol. 237:
    H 224 (1979).

12. C. A. Apstein, J. Ahn, L. Briggs and H. M. Shapiro. Role of
    decrease in wall thickness in causing ischemic cardiac failure,
    Clin. Res. 27:436a (1979).

13. P. F. Salisburg, C. E. Cross and P. A. Rieben. Influence of
    coronary artery pressure upon myocardial elasticity, Circ. Res.
    8:794 (1960).

14. P. F. Salisburg, C. E. Cross and P. A. Rieben. Intramyocardial
    pressure and strength of left ventricular contraction, Circ.
    Res. 10:608 (1962).

15. G. Arnold, F. Kosche, E. Miessner, A. Neitzert and W. Lochner.
    The importance of CK perfusion pressure in the coronary arter-
    ies for the contractility and oxygen consumption of the heart,
    Pfluegers Archiv. 299:339 (1968).

16. B. N. Brent and C. S. Apstein. Kinetics of acute cardiac failure.
    Comparisons of ischemia, hypoxemia and cyanide, Clin. Res. 27:
    156a (1979)

17. B. I. Jugdutt, L. C. Becker and G. M. Hutchins. Early changes
     in collateral blood flow during myocardial infarction in
     conscious dogs, <u>Am. J. Physiol.</u> 237(3):H371 (1979).

INTERVENTION TRIALS - PROBLEMS OF INTERNATIONAL COORDINATION

AND EVALUATION

Geoffrey Rose

Department of Medical Statistics and Epidemiology
London School of Hygiene and Tropical Medicine
Keppel St., London WC1, England

THE SEARCH FOR PROOF

Does prevention really work? Until that question can be answered, inertia will persist; for it will continue to be said, "There is no proof".

How can the question be answered? If the demand is for proof (that is, for certainty) then that is and will remain beyond our reach. In clinical practice patients are not diagnosed and treated on the basis of certainties, but on a best clinical judgement of all the available evidence; and that is also how we have to manage populations.

Historically the great advances in public health have not been based on prior proof. The decision that sewage should be kept out of the water supply was taken before Pasteur had discovered bacteria. Recommendations on a healthy balanced diet preceded randomised controlled trials, and are still based on judgement rather than proof. Public health policy on control of air pollution and of cigarette smoking is based on an overall assessment of the epidemiological, laboratory and clinical evidence; where that evidence has been accepted, chronic bronchitis and lung cancer have declined - but that could not have been known until after the decisions had been taken.

Unfortunately a judgement based on indirect and circumstantial evidence may sometimes go wrong. Until recently it was thought that foods with high residue and high fibre content made a poor diet, especially in diverticular disease; and in my country at the end of the last century an unfortunate physician was banned from medical practice for life because he told the public that brown bread was

597

healthier than white. A controlled trial might have saved him!
Views on that issue have now changed. No doubt there are many items
of current medical practice and belief which are in fact mistaken.
They ought to work, but for some reason they may not: why continue
to guess, if you can perform the experiment?

WHAT DO CONTROLLED TRIALS OFFER?

     Thus it became widely believed that a properly controlled inter-
vention trial might at last offer certainty in public health decisions
That view is now giving way to a more moderate assessment: the controlled intervention trial provides one more piece of evidence -
uniquely important, because it is unbiased, quantitative and experimental - but yet providing neither unambiguous nor universal conclusions; and to be considered, not as the ultimate court of appeal,
but as contributing one part of the totality of evidence.

     There have been two reasons for this shift of opinion. The first
is the realisation that we must be cautious about the generalisation
of findings. Different trials may give different answers, and local
results can depend on local circumstances. The acceptance of health
advice varies. This has been the experience of the WHO European Multi
factorial Trial of CHD Prevention (whose results are to be reported
later in this Congress). In Britain we were less successful in gettin
men to change their diet than were our Belgian and Italian colleagues;
but we did rather better with cigarette smoking. Also, biological
response may vary. Thus results of hypertension control may be different in men and women, or in blacks and whites; or the effect of
reducing dietary fat in our trial could be different in well-fed Bel-
gians from what it is in Poland, where alternatives are less readily
available.

     There is another reason why today we are more moderate in our
expectations from controlled trials. This arises from the gap betweer
the size of effect which a trial can hope to detect and the size of
effect which would be of public health importance.

     In 1971, when we started our multifactorial CHD prevention trial
in Britain, our human and financial resources did not permit us to
recruit and to follow for 5 years more than about 20,000 men. Statistical calculations suggested that such a trial might fail to detect
any reduction in CHD incidence which was less than 25%. That was a
serious limitation. We were evaluating a relatively cheap preventive
program, operating largely through existing medical services. From
a public health point of view, the costs would have been justified
by a much smaller benefit: after all, a reduction of only 5% in CHD
deaths would be more than equivalent to preventing all our deaths fror
road accidents.

THE DEVELOPMENT OF INTERNATIONAL TRIALS

These same two concerns have prompted the important trend towards international collaborative trials. By involving a number of countries within a common protocol, they test the consistency of the findings in a variety of populations; and by combining the resources of several groups they increase the trial's size and statistical power.

The development of an international study is illustrated by the experience of our WHO European Collaborative Trial in the Multifactorial Prevention of CHD. The original UK centre was both too small, and also too narrow a base for generalizing the findings into international recommendations. Enlargement and diversification were clearly desirable, and the possibility of international extension was discussed among a small group of cardiovascular epidemiologists from Belgium, Italy, Poland and Spain. We already knew each other, and we welcomed the chance of working together. As a result the number of subjects grew to about 64,000.

I believe that these human relationships, which take time to develop, were vital; and they led directly to our efficient and pleasant working relationships. International studies cannot be initiated centrally according to some tidy plan: they have to grow out of existing scientific communications and dispositions. Thus their location cannot be freely determined.

In our trial, as in the WHO Clofibrate Trial and other collaborative studies, one center had already made a start before international collaboration was sought. This meant that our collaborators were faced with a predetermined protocol: they were asked to operate a study which they had not designed, and for highly experienced investigators this was not easy. To some extent the problem was reduced by our decision to standardize only a minimum core of protocol items that were essential to the pooling operation: each national center was free to extend the core study according to local interest. For example, the core protocol required electrocardiograms at entry to the control group in only a random 10% of subjects; in the Belgian center it was decided to extend this to 100% of control subjects, and as a result they are now able to test the effects of intervention according to whether or not there was early ischaemic injury.

The scientific status of individual centers was further strengthened by our agreement that each study was to be justified in its own right, with the pooled results of the whole collaborative group coming as a bonus. In each of the five countries it was necessary to know how much the intervention could change risk factors; and each study has been able to produce this important local information, together with estimates from the control group of naturally occurring changes in risk factors. There was also the possibility that the larger centers might (with some luck) see a significant change in incidence of intervention. It is unlikely that individual centers would have been funded if they had not been seen as justified in their own right.

PROBLEMS OF DATA QUALITY

International collaboration involves major problems of standardizing the methods of data acquisition. This issue was crucial in a number of WHO studies which set out to compare in different countries the absolute levels of disease (for example, the incidence of heart attacks, or the severity of atherosclerosis). It is not nearly so serious in trials, whose purpose is to study the differences in incidence observed between intervention and control groups within individual countries: inter-center differences in the level of ascertainment should affect both the intervention and the control groups equally.

This does not mean, of course, that external quality control of data can be ignored in a collaborative trial. Inter-center difference may not bias the overall estimate of intervention effect, but they do influence its interpretation. To understand the results one needs to have used a common language for critical events; and incidence finding need to be related to absolute levels and trends of major risk factors In our collaborative trial we therefore followed the WHO registry procedures for defining coronary events, and we set up external quality control systems for cholesterol (through the WHO reference laboratory in Prague) and blood pressure. Electrocardiograms were reported according to Minnesota Code criteria, and each center submitted samples for central checking every 6 months. Inter-center differences were much smaller than is usual in multicenter studies, reflecting the fact that all the principal investigators had already worked together in using the Minnesota Code. Here, as at so many points, successful collaboration requires more than a common protocol: it depends on an accumulated mutual understanding between investigators who know each other and who are used to working together.

THE WHO CONTRIBUTION

The WHO contribution in our trial was important in two ways. First of all, the name of WHO sets a scientific and ethical standard which influences the investigators, the subjects and the sponsors - and all this at no financial cost to WHO! The job is done better because it is done in part for a supranational purpose.

At a more practical level, it is difficult for national studies to get money for those regular meetings with other investigators which are vital to the successful pooling of international data. A further expense arises for the data processing of pooled results. The amount of money involved may not be large; but without help from WHO I do not see how our collaboration could have succeeded.

HYPERTENSION CONTROL IN POPULATIONS

T. Strasser and E. Dowd

World Health Organization, Geneva, Switzerland
on behalf of the WHO Cooperative Hypertension
Community Control Study Group*

In a masterly review of major developments and trends in health
care in the twentieth century Milton Roemer quotes 16 points, including health manpower growth, specialization, organization for team
work, population control, geriatrics and rehabilitation, health care
planning, medical humanization, internationalism in health and health
as a human right[1]. To this World Perspective on Health Care in the
Twentieth Century one more important point should be added: the development of the concept of community control of disease. According
to this concept, disease control rests on a defined community as a
socio-biological entity. All its strata and components are taken
into account and the community itself is being used to control and
combat its own disease or diseases. There is an important difference
between this participatory concept of community disease control and
the earlier, classical public health approaches to disease prevention
such as the draining of swamps as part of malaria prevention, or the
provision of safe community water supply, or vaccination. In the
classical situation, the community is rather the scene on which a
medical or public health action is taking place. On the contrary,
the community disease control programme of our days is like a happening
in which all those present are required to participate.

Hypertension control provides an important example of the il-
lustration of modern disease control programmes, if for no other
reason than because of its very high prevalence a considerable part
of the population has to be involved. With a prevalence of 15% in
adult populations, hypertension may occur in one out of 3 to 4 families.

*Principal investigators and co-authors: G. Ambrosio, C. Dal Palu.
De Padua, N. Dondog, A. Froment, I. Macias Castro, H. Milon, A. Nis-
sinen, T. Omae, J. M. Pereira Miguel, J. O. M. Pobee, P. Puska, J.
Richard, V. E. Smirnov, J. Tuomilehto.

In such a situation the only feasible solution is control through primary health care, backed by specialized services. Thus, blood pressure detection and treatment (in most cases) should be part of routine primary health care. For the diagnostic work-up of cases not responding to simple therapy, appropriate referral clinics should reinforce the primary health care services. In addition, for statistical (and clinical) surveillance of the great number of hypertensive subjects certain information systems are needed. These may be established in the form of various types of registers which, however, should be adapted to local circumstances. Such registers may range from simple manual card files in the offices of general practitioners to sophisticated and automated computer-based information systems, covering communities of several hundreds of thousands of people.

The real bases of hypertension community control programs consist, however, of a systematic education of both the population and the health workers. The two educational approaches should be initiated simultaneously, since they are complementary. A population aware of its hypertension problem should be backed up by its health corps motivated to spend time and effort on the control of this disease. Conversely, the health workers of a community should act in a population responsive to their efforts, or the community programs will remain barren. Such "formes frustes" of community programs have been observed. In fact, a community program triggers off an interplay between the population and its health workers: by creating, through health education, greater awareness and thus greater demand in the population, the health workers themselves will be stimulated; and conversely increasing offer from the part of the health services will in turn stimulate greater demand in the population. While in a number of health fields such a positive feedback mechanism may lead to an unwanted spiral of rising health consumption, in the field of hypertension it may result in adequate community control of hypertension, which was the original aim of the exercise. Whether this is invariably the best solution is, however, another question to which we shall come back somewhat later.

In 1972, the World Health Organization has started a multicenter international cooperative hypertension community control project with the aim of assessing whether such community programs are feasible and effective in various circumstances, such as socialized or private medical care, or developed and developing countries. Despite a number of difficulties, the project was carried to its end, and its final results are now being analyzed. It has been shown by the project that such community programs are, indeed, both feasible and effective.

In the following some findings from this study will be demonstrated on three simple graphs.

In a hypertension control program, blood pressure changes should be the most elementary indicator. Figure 1 shows the changes in blood

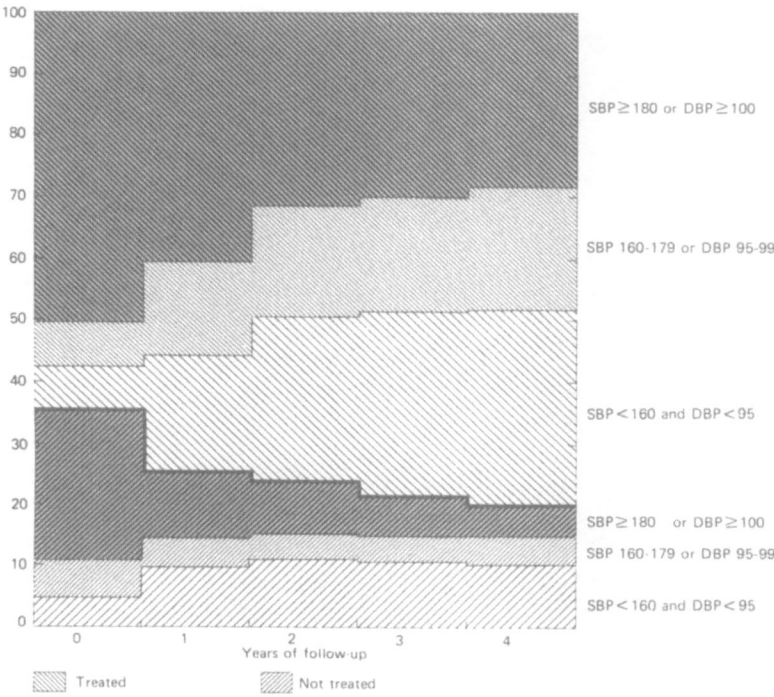

Fig. 1. Percentage of persons in various blood pressure categories
         in a cohort of 4,475 hypertensive subjects during a 5-year
         observation period; subjects without and with drug treatment.

pressure in a cohort of 4,475 hypertensive subjects, identified at
the outset of the study and followed up throughout the first four
years of the project. The graph shows that the proportion of non-
treated hypertensive subjects was constantly decreasing, but that
the most appreciable decrease occurred at the beginning of the project.
Conversely, the proportion of treated subjects increased particularly
at the beginning of the study, while in later years there was little
further increase. The conclusion is that the effect of diagnosing
hypertension is being immediately exploited for the starting of drug
treatment. The graph also shows that the proportion of hypertensive
subjects whose blood pressure had been brought under control (had
become normal) increased considerably during the project, accompanied
by an appropriate decrease in the group of severe blood pressure elevations. The proportion of mild hypertension, within the cohort of
diagnosed hypertensives, increased due to the fact that a number of
subjects with higher elevations of blood pressure moved down, due
to treatment, to the mild hypertension zone.

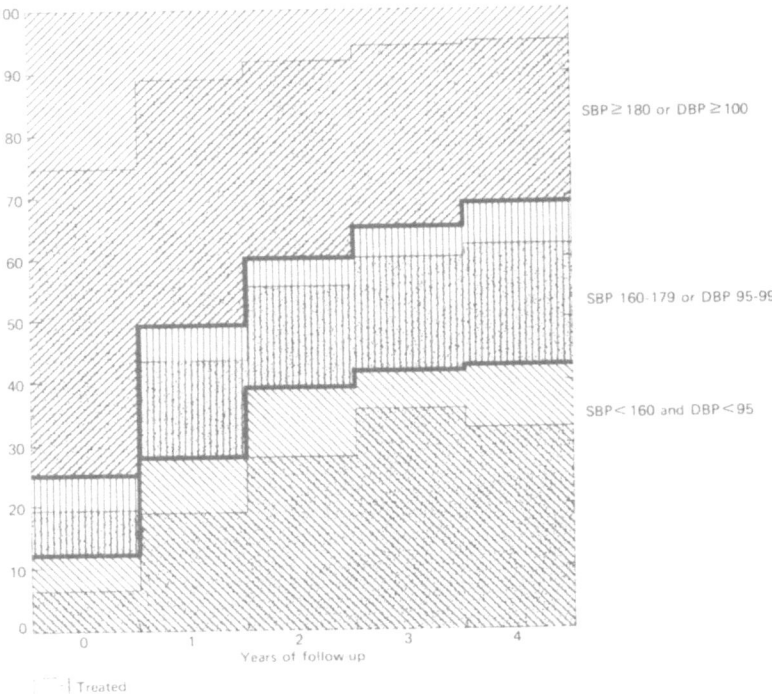

SBP ≥ 180 or DBP ≥ 100

SBP 160-179 or DBP 95-99

SBP < 160 and DBP < 95

Years of follow up

Treated

Fig. 2.   Percentage of persons in various blood pressure categories
          in a cohort of 4,475 hypertensive subjects during a 5-year
          observation period; decreasing proportion of blood pressure
          values and increasing proportion of normotensive subjects.

Figure 2 presents the same information in a slightly different
way. It shows more clearly the decreasing proportion of high values,
the increasing proportion of normotensive subjects within the hypertensive cohort, and the moderate increase of the proportion of subjects in the range of mild hypertension. It should be noted that
lowering of blood pressure to normal levels occurred also among the
non-treated hypertensives. This finding is in agreement with reports
from other studies, i.e. the Australian National Blood pressure Study[2].

It should be emphatically pointed out that the WHO Study was not
a controlled therapeutic trial. Therefore, treated and untreated
subjects may not be comparable. The WHO project was a community study
where the option for treatment or non-treatment was left both at the
discretion of the physicians and the patients. Figures 1 and 2 thus
show what happens in a cohort of identified hypertensives in the community under "natural" circumstances. Part of the changes is, no
doubt, due to the effect of regression to the mean. It is difficult,
however, to assess what proportion of the observed changes should be
interpreted in this way.

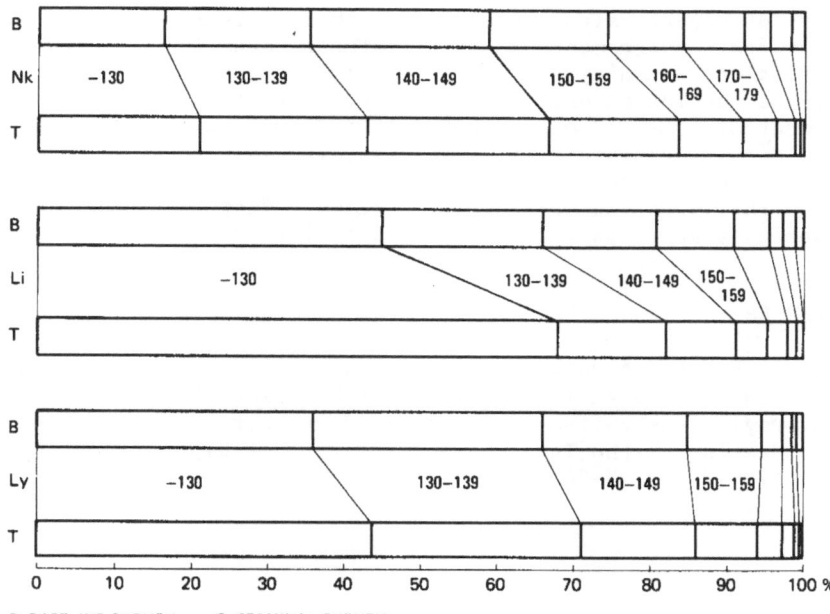

B: BASELINE SURVEY   T: TERMINAL SURVEY

Fig. 3. Percentage distribution of systolic blood pressure in the
         population, age 30-59.
         Blood pressure changes in all communities during a 5-year
         period, age group 30-59. Nk, Ly, Li: 3 communities where a
         blood pressure control program took place. The proportion
         of lower blood pressure classes is increasing; that of the
         higher classes diminishing (B: Baseline survey, T: Terminal
         survey).

     Unlike the previous graphs which presented the changes in a cohort
of hypertensive subjects, figure 3 demonstrates the blood pressure
changes in whole communities based on a comparison of representative
samples surveyed at the beginning and at the end of the project. In
the three communities, selected as examples, the lower blood pressure
classes were clearly expanding with an appropriate shrinking of the
upper blood pressure classes. Such a shift in the distribution of
blood pressure values in the entire community is, in fact, the ideal
goal at which any community program should be striving. The figures
on which graph 3 is based stem for a preliminary analysis of the study.
It is to be hoped that this finding will be confirmed by the forthcoming final analysis of the data.

     If, indeed, such shifts in blood pressure of the whole community
can be achieved, hypertension community programs acquire a different
meaning and become much more important than if the treatment of great

numbers of hypertensive subjects were their only result. In fact, although the achievement of high treatment rates is the aim of present hypertension community control programs, the attainment of this aim should be considered only as an intermediate step. Life-long drug treatment of some 15% of the population should not be the definitive goal. High drug usage in the community is close to abusage. Eventually, the whole community as a socio-biological entity should shift towards the lower end of the blood pressure distribution. This goal is hopefully achievable without the administration of potent chemicals.

REFERENCES

1. M. I. Roemer, A world perspective on health care in the twentieth century, Journal of Public Health Policy, 1: 370-378 (1980).
2. A. Doyle, Australian National Blood Pressure Study, Scientific Meeting of the International Society of Hypertension, Mexico City (Feb. 21-24, 1982).

COMPREHENSIVE CARDIOVASCULAR COMMUNITY CONTROL

PROGRAM IN THE PHILIPPINES

Santiago V. Guzman*, Jose V. Yason, Jr.*,
Jaime S. Vizcayno*, Esperanza I. Cabral*
and Juan P. Estrada**

*Research Division, Philippine Heart Center for Asia
**Ministry of Health

In collaboration with the Ministry of Health (MOH), the Philippine Heart Center for Asia (PHCA) initiated in 1977 feasibility studies on community control of rheumatic fever-rheumatic heart disease[1] and, a year later, on hypertension and stroke[2], utilizing primary health personnel of MOH. The encouraging results obtained and the experiences gained from these studies logically lead us to embark on feasibility studies in comprehensive cardiovascular community control program (CCCCP).

THE RHEUMATIC FEVER - RHEUMATIC HEART DISEASE (RF-RHD)
COMMUNITY CONTROL PROGRAM IN A RURAL AREA (PANGASINAN)

The general objectives of the control program are:

a) to promote early diagnosis and treatment of rheumatic fever and rheumatic heart disease occurring in a defined area of the province of Pangasinan, utilizing the primary health care personnel of the Ministry;
b) to establish an RF-RHD registry in the area; and
c) to promote secondary prevention of rheumatic fever.

The primary health workers including nurses and physicians were initially given training on the epidemiology, etiopathogenesis, clinical manifestations and on prophylaxis of RF-RHD before the program started. Posters, strategically placed in health centers, churches and market places were used for the education of the public.

607

After two years of operation, we demonstrated that the utilization of the primary health care personnel in the early recognition of rheumatic fever-rheumatic heart disease was very gratifying as judged by the number of referrals made by them and their ability to detect murmurs. Midwives alone referred nearly half of 472 referrals made during the period, and their specificity in the recognition of murmurs was 100%, although they missed the presence of a murmur in 8% of cases.

In addition, these midwives carried out the administration of the prophylaxis in 70.8% of the cases. The adherence of patients to a long-term program of subsidized chemoprophylaxis in a non-subsidized program.

HYPERTENSION AND STROKE COMMUNITY CONTROL PROGRAM

The pilot project has the following objectives:

a)   to find an applicable way of control of hypertension and stroke within the existing delivery system of medical care;
b)   to determine the feasibility of community-based hypertension and stroke control in rural areas of the Philippines; and
c)   to evaluate the effect of long-term intervention of the knowledge, attitude and behavior on the cardiovascular health of the population.

The communities involved are part of the area covered in the RF-RHD community control program already described, involving 25,000 individuals in each of the study areas and a reference community.

As in the RF-RHD program, the existing primary health care personnel is being utilized. Baseline screening gave a prevalence rate for hypertension (i.e. 160/95 mm Hg or above) of 7% in both communities. Patients identified to be hypertensive in the study area were given antihypertensive therapy through their service of choice (i.e. through the hypertension clinic established by the program, or through their own physicians). Intensive public education, as well as education of practitioners in the area is being done. A stroke surveillance and registry is also being initiated. The control area will participate in all evaluative activities but will not have an active intervention program.

Evaluation of the project will be based on mortality and morbidity statistics, and for this purpose, periodic screening of the target populations will be carried out after three, five, and ten years.

COMPREHENSIVE CARDIOVASCULAR COMMUNITY CONTROL PROGRAM

The results in the community control program of RF-RHD and hypertension and stroke utilizing the existing primary health workers is very encouraging. The logical step is to unify these single disease projects into a comprehensive cardiovascular community control program. Such a program is now being conducted jointly by the PHCA and MOH in two rural areas north of Manila. Basically, it entails the study of two sets of communities;.one representing the intervention area and the other as the reference. Baseline epidemiological survey as well as survey on the knowledge, attitude and practices (KAP) of the people are being done in both sets of communities.

Active community intervention will be carried out mainly through an educational approach. Hypertension being the most prevalent, will be the main target in the prevention and control program although the other CVD will be taken up also. The major risk factors to be controlled are cigarette smoking and salt intake. Morbidity and mortality registers will be set up in both communities.

After a period of five years, KAP, prevalence and risk factors surveys will be done for comparison with the results of the baseline survey.

The Ministry of Health is now developing pilot studies to make primary health care as the foundation of the national health service system. It is envisioned that CCCCP will be integrated into PHC.

REFERENCES

1. J. S. Vizcayno, MD, J. P. Estrada, MD, C. K. Galsim, MD, J. V. Yason, Jr. MD, I. C. de Guzman, MD, M. Marmot, PhD, S. V. Guzman, MD, The RF-RHD Control Program in Pangasinan: a Preliminary Report, Phil. J. of Cardiol. 6: 77 (1978).
2. E. A. Icasas-Cabral, MD, D. M. Castro, MD, J. Estrada, MD, A. Casipit, MD, G. Padilla, MD, S. V. Guzman, MD, A Hypertension and Stroke Control Program in Rural Philippine Community, Phil. J. of Cardiol. 10: 75 (1980).

PREVENTION OF CARDIOVASCULAR DISEASES

WHO PROGRAMME

Z. Pisa* and K. Günther**

* WHO, Geneva
**GDR

The World Health Organization has concentrated in its cardiovascular disease activities specifically on those areas where international collaboration and coordination was essential. For that
reason the area of epidemiology and prevention and control of different cardiovascular diseases became very soon much preferred field
in all WHO activities. Starting with prevalence and incidence population surveys, preparation of teaching materials (among which "Cardiovascular Survey Methods: Methodology" by G. Rose and H. Blackburn
(1968) was the most important publication) and intensive training
program in epidemiology and prevention of cardiovascular diseases
were essential. Later, WHO has initiated in collaboration with many
centers, aided by its trainees, more systematic epidemiological research to assess the extent of the program of cardiovascular diseases
in different countries, both industrial and developing, as well as
entered the field of intervention trials. The project on myocardial
infarction as well as stroke community registers carried out in the
early 70's became the basis of presently formulated project on "The
monitoring of the incidence and determinants of cardiovascular diseases in populations". It will help to provide the reasons for the
different trends in the incidence of cardiovascular diseases and
specifically coronary heart disease and cerebrovascular stroke in
different populations. The clofibrate trial has provided beside its
scientific results, new stimulants for and considerations about the
ethical aspects connected with the application of long term drug
therapies.

The wide network of collaborating institutions with epidemiological skills in the field of cardiovascular diseases provided the
possibility of developing and initiating community control programs
of different cardiovascular diseases.

From this background the symposium aimed at highlighting the
successes as well as the mistakes and problems encountered while
carrying different projects.

Professor G. Rose, London, the chief coordinator of the "WHO
European trial in the multi-factorial prevention of coronary heart
disease" discussed general problems of international trials and their
possibility to give the answer to the major question "does prevention
really work?". He stressed that the controlled intervention trial
provides more scientifically important evidence because of its unbiased quantitative and experimental set-up. However, it still does
not provide unambiguous nor universal conclusions. Different trials
produced often different answers and results can depend on local
circumstances. The advantage of international collaboration is the
increase in trials size and its statistical power. The important
lesson was that beside adhering to the standardized protocol to
achieve the comparability of the results and standardization of the
methods of data acquisition, provision for external quality control
of data has to be made. The successful collaboration however, also
depends on an accumulated mutual understanding between investigators
who know each other and who are used to working together. The role
of WHO set a scientific and ethical standard which influenced the
investigators, the subjects and the sponsors.

The hypertension control in populations was discussed by Dr T.
Strasser, WHO, Geneva. The concept of community control of disease
rests on a defined community as a social, biological entity. The
modern community disease control programs require full participation
of the individuals, family, different sections of community including
health services. The WHO hypertension control program initiated by
the Organization in 1972 aimed at assessing whether community control
of hypertension is feasible and effective in various circumstances,
such as socialized or private medical care and in individual and developing countries. The control of hypertension in the population
is feasible and effective. It leads to diminution of non-treated
hypertensive subjects. The major changes in the percentage of treated
population were registered specifically in the very beginning of the
project. The proportion of hypertensive subjects whose blood pressure
has been brought under control - had been normalized - increased
considerably during the project accompanied by the decrease in the
group of severe blood pressure elevations. The proportion of mild
hypertension within the cohort increased due to the fact that the
number of subjects with higher elevations of blood pressure moved
down due to treatment.

The systematic hypertension control program effects the blood
pressure of the whole community. That means that the mean blood
pressure of the population studied is shifted to the biological normality. In such a way hypertension community control programs acquire
a different meaning and become much more important from public health

point of view and health of the community as such. However, the study
has also shown that life-long drug treatment of some 15% of the population should not be the definitive goal. Questions have been raised
if high drug usage in the community is not an abuse.

Collaboration between the town of Kaunas, USSR, and WHO is of
long-lasting tradition. Originally, a Kaunas-Rotterdam multi-factor
preventive trial has been initiated coordinated by Dr I. Glasunov
(WHO, Geneva), who was the speaker in the symposium. The population
of Kaunas participated in other WHO activities such as myocardial
infarction and the stroke registers, rehabilitation and secondary
prevention of myocardial infarction patients, and recently in the
project on comprehensive control of non-communicable diseases as well
as in the project on the monitoring of the incidence and determinants
of cardiovascular diseases (MONICA Project). This collaboration provided great experience for the Kaunas medical community as well as
for WHO. Kaunas is one of the population areas where, for example,
the myocardial infarction community register is being continued since
1971 until now. Therefore, its experience is of great value for the
planning of the MONICA Project. Kaunas on the other hand serves to
the public health service in the USSR as a public health laboratory
specifically in studies in prevention of cardiovascular diseases and
other non-communicable diseases.

Dr S. Guzman and his collaborators, Manila, Philippines, have
discussed the problems of the establishment of comprehensive cardiovascular control program in a developing country. Feasibility studies
on community control of rheumatic fever and rheumatic heart disease
demonstrated that existing primary health care workers were able to
recognise the disease with reasonable accuracy and were able to institute secondary prophylaxis in rheumatic heart disease programs on the
level of peripheral health units. Later, encouraged by these results
the community study was extended to control of hypertension and stroke.
Screening for elevated blood pressure was done by primary health care
workers and hypertensives discovered were registered. Medications
were given under physicians' supervision and regular follow up and
surveys were done again by primary health care workers. This project
showed the feasibility of the community control programs to be carried
out in developing countries when the role of the health personnel at
different levels is appropriately identified and proper training is
introduced. These programs increase the health education of the
public and improve the surveillance in the community for cardiovascular diseases. The community control programs in cardiovascular
diseases are now being integrated into the primary health care programs
of the Ministry of Health. In such a way it is expected that the
prevention and control of cardiovascular diseases will become an integral part of the health care programs of the public health service.

A new concept of primary prevention of cardiovascular disease in
developing countries was presented by Dr S. Dodu, WHO, Geneva. "Primordial prevention" expressed the need to take appropriate action at
an early stage aiming to prevent the emergence or entrenchment of

those social, economic and cultural backgrounds that have been shown
to contribute to the high incidence of certain diseases in industrial
populations. Some preliminary approaches have already been done and
analysis of the country's situation have shown that in many developing
countries realistic priorities for the primordial prevention of cardiovascular diseases will at best be restricted at the present time to
smoking and hypertension control. The challenge of a broader based
approach to primordial prevention is more likely to be accepted in
the middle income developing countries where the cardiovascular and
other diseases of "affluence" are emerging as a public health problem
and where major risk factors are beginning to be established in the
community at large and not merrily in the urban elite. Definite plans
have been drafted by the World Health Organization to promote this
approach and show by example of a few countries that it is feasible.

In its concluding remarks, the co-chairman, Dr Z. Pisa, WHO,
Geneva, has stressed the importance of the work done by WHO and by
other investigators in promoting and testing different methods to
make the prevention and control of cardiovascular diseases a part of
daily medical practice in countries with different social and economic
structures. The problem of cardiovascular diseases is too extensive
and emerging quite strongly now in developing countries that without
prevention the problem cannot be tackled and controlled effectively.
The lack of present acceptance of preventive programs is very often
more in the resistance and traditions of the medical profession and
its identification of prevention in populations with control of infectious diseases. Prevention of cardiovascular diseases is nevertheless
more than medicine requiring the collaboration of different sections
in the community involving also nutrition, city planning, agriculture,
finances and others.

The present WHO strategy to prevention of cardiovascular diseases
is based on three approaches: the first one and most important is the
"population approach". It aims at altering the mass characteristics
of life-style and environment which are underlying causes of cardiovascular diseases (for example coronary heart disease), or in low incidence populations preventing the developing of such precuros (primary
prevention). The second approach is the identification of individuals
with elevated risk factor levels and helping to modify these risk factors. This is a traditional approach in preventive efforts in the
field of cardiovascular diseases as is the third approach, namely
preventing the recurrence and progression of the disease - secondary
prevention.

In the "population approach" the attempt is to shift the distribution curves of precursors and determinants of cardiovascular diseases in the whole population to the biological normality. Its importance is specifically stressed by the fact that the highest number of
cases for instance of myocardial infarction is around the mean values
of the population's risk factor levels, in spite of the fact that the
risk of an individual itself increases with the increase in the level

of these factors. Further consideration for population strategy is based on the fact that artherosclerotic changes in the vessels start early in life. The population approach is specifically important in smoking control as well as in the approach to nutrition.

This strategy and its implementation through community control programs is of great significance and exceeds the importance and implications of cardiovascular diseases only. Examples of the cardiovascular control programs and preventive strategies are being now considered and adapted to the programs of other non-communicable diseases as well.

The work WHO could not be done without the enthusiasm and support of individual investigators, centers and Governments. WHO is most thankful to all those who are collaborating with it in their support.

INTEGRATED PREVENTION WITHIN PRIMARY HEALTH CARE

K. H. Gunther, P. Piorkowski, Renate Bohm, W. Handreg
and H. Braun

Cardiology Section, Medical Department
Hospital Charite, DDR-1040 Berlin
Schumannstrasse 20/21, GDR

After the "World Health Day 1972" with the slogan "Your Heart is Your Health", announced by WHO and ISC, considerable effort has been undertaken world-wide to control the major cardiovascular diseases, especially by preventive measures. Taking increasingly into consideration that cardiovascular disease is a social epidemic spreading from man to man and to women, from parent to child, and from culture to culture it became obvious: there are life habits that have to be changed. On this way, it might be possible to keep those diseases from appearing, stopping them when already going on, and even reversing their progression. But this is not a simple vaccination like in some communicable diseases!

Health starts in families. Home doctors, therefore, play a very important role joined by their nurses. They are able to detect easily people with elevated risk, provide them with the necessary preventive information, and make regular check-ups of what is going on, individually and on a community level. Being aware of that and of the fact that cardiovascular disease is a general public health problem in the German Democratic Republic as well as in other highly industrialized countries a model of prevention[1,2] has been tested integratable into the primary health care system of the country.

MATERIAL AND METHODS

The study was performed in the County of Cottbus, an energy production area based on brown coal mines. The study population incidentally screened within the daily practice of 24 General Practitioners comprised 6465 subjects, 2930 men and 3535 women, within the age limits of 30 and 50 years, i.e. working people. They came to their doctors for different reasons and were checked for the main risk factors of coronary heart disease, additionally.

Before starting the study, doctors and nurses were trained in measuring blood pressure. Cholesterol determination has also been standardized from taking the blood samples until the laboratory which is working in coordination with the WHO Reference Lab. in Prague. The number of cigarettes per day has been registered by a short question- naire for self-administration in which the Rose Questionnaire was partly included. In addition, some social factors were obtained on the basis of a national standard; some of those results have been re- ported already elsewhere[3].

Screening and prevention procedures were connected closely to get a high patients' compliance. The first step of treatment was without any (additional) drug, only giving information and advice to each individual, using printed material on smoking, hypertension, hypercholesterolemia, (physical inactivity and overweight). Inter- vention was started from 1 cigarette/day, blood pressure 140/90 mm Hg or 220 mg% cholesterol, i.e. borderline-ranges included. The patients were asked for a second visit to tell him/her the results at least. If there was a smoker consultation has been provided during the first visit. People with elevation of cholesterol or blood pressure, being classified during the second visit, then got preven- tive advice. (People with overweight or physical inactivity were only advised if one of the main risk factors was found, supporting non- medical treatment.)

RESULTS

Within the first, "hygienic" period a considerable shift took place in hypertensives. Three months after screening the prevalences had been diminished roughly by one third in both age and sex groups (Table 1). Simultaneously, a similar reduction could be seen with the prevalences of hypercholesterolemia, more pronounced in the age group 40-49 years concerning both sexes. In contrast, borderline hypertension prevalences did not change very much obviously due to the fact that a lot of hypertensives entered this group and only few (borderline) hypertensives reached the normal range of blood pressure. If looking at overweight nearly nothing changed, thus, indicating that losing weight cannot be a main reason for diminution of hyper- tension and hypercholesterolemia in the first period of intervention.

A second check-up, after 18 months, unfortunately showed that the gain was mostly lost with the exception of the severest hyper- tensive (Table 2 a/b) who got profit from the additional therapy provided during the second period by drugs. Their prevalence dimin- ished already during the "hygienic period" and further decreased

Table 1. Prevalence reduction by hygienic approach only within
          3 months.

Age groups	30 – 39		40 – 49		
Sex	males	females	males	females	
Hypertension[1]	21.9	18.9	31.3	32.7	
	14.8	11.6	23.4	23.0	per cent
Hypercholesterol[2]	21.1	12.8	27.2	20.8	
	17.4	9.2	21.5	14.0	

1) Definition acc. to WHO: 160/95 mm Hg or more
2) Serum cholesterol: 260 mg per cent or more

Table 2 a/b. Two step hypertension control within primary health care.

Prevalence changes:	Normotension	Borderline-H	Hypertension[1]
Males (n = 2340)[2]			per cent
Incidental screening	40.7	32.3	12.3 + 14.7
After hygienic approach	49.9	30.8	9.2 + 10.1
After drugs additionally	41.1	33.4	21.2 + 4.3
Females (n = 3037)[3]			
Incidental screening	43.1	30.5	10.3 + 16.1
After hygienic approach	54.6	27.7	7.2 + 10.5
After drugs additionally	46.8	32.5	17.8 + 2.9

1) Definitions acc. to WHO, but the hypertension group has been
    divided into those with blood pressures of 160/95-199/109 and
    those with 200/110 mm Hg or more.
2) Dropout 590 cases (20 per cent) after 18 ms.
3) Dropout 498 cases (14 per cent) after 18 ms.

considerably during the "medical period". They again shifted, however, only to blood pressures being still hypertensive since borderline hypertension increased not very much at long-term.

DISCUSSION AND SUMMARY

     Prevention doesn't need special diagnostics. Home doctors,
therefore, can perform the necessary basic examinations standardized
within the daily practice. This allows a definition of individual

risk and provides the basis for interventional measures which should
be first non-medical.

It is of strategical interest from the primary care point of
view to know that prevalence of hypertension and hypercholesterolemia
may remarkably be reducing within a few weeks, not being decidable
whether this is due to a large regression to the mean or, at least
partly, induced by the preventive information and check-up. That
leads the GP to a much lesser number of risk people to be treated at
length and serves to avoid a misuse of drugs which is, on the other
hand, an essential condition for a good patients' compliance.

The study shows, however, that doctor's compliance is not a
constant. GPs being primarily prone to use non-medical treatment
may lose their interest with the guidance by the District Cardiologist
is getting weaker. Then they return to their traditional, i.e. therapeutical way of practice, and the same may occur with the population.

In future it will be of high interest to get a) in general reliable basic prevalence data being comparable on a national and even
international level, b) more implementable hygienic approaches, at
least as first step of control of the main risk factors, c) systemic
medical and public education in prevention and, last but not least,
d) improved doctors' and patients' compliance.

REFERENCES

1. A. C. Arntzenius, F. H. Epstein, K. H. Gunther, M. Kornitzer,
   J. Menard and I. Strasser, Preventing coronary heart disease,
   A guide for the practising physician, European Society of
   Cardiology, Van Gorcum, Assen, The Netherlands (1978).
2. K. H. Gunther, P. Piorkowski, R. Bohm, H. Braun and W. Handreg,
   Integrierte Pravention der Herz-Kreislauf-Krankheiten, Ein
   Modell fur die allgemeine medizinische Grundbetreuung, Dt.
   Gesundh. -Wesen 35: 1893 (1980).
3. P. Piorkowski, K. H. Gunther, H. Harig, W. Handreg and H. Braun,
   Social factors' correlation with coronary heart disease risk
   in a rural community of the GDR, Activitas Nervosa Superior,
   Prague (1983), in press.
4. Z. Fejfar and J. N. Morris, How to prevent heart disease, World
   Health, 4 (1972).

MULTIPLE RISK FACTOR INTERVENTION TRIAL:

6 YEAR RISK FACTOR CHANGES

Lewis H. Kuller

Department of Epidemiology, Graduate School of Public
University of Pittsburgh
Pittsburgh PA 15261

The Multiple Risk Factor Intervention Trial completed the follow
up of the participants on February 28, 1982. This report describes
the results of the changes in risk factors. Some of the data to be
presented is still preliminary as final tabulations of the risk factor
changes are being completed.

The design of the Multiple Risk Factor Intervention Trial has
been published. A monograph describing basic intervention methods and
preliminary risk factor changes has also recently been published.
The methods will be briefly reviewed. The basic goal was to determine
whether death rates for coronary heart disease could be reduced by
a special intervention program aimed at reducing the serum cholesterol,
blood pressure and cigarette smoking. Men were selected on the basis
of a risk score distribution determined from the Framingham study.
The risk score included the men's serum cholesterol, blood pressure
and cigarette smoking. Initially men in the upper 15% of risk were
eligible. After about one third of the screening had been completed,
this was changed to the upper 10% of risk. The men were between the
ages of 30 to 57 at entry to the trial and were free of clinical heart
disease based on a history of myocardial infarction, positive Rose
questionnaire or EKG evidence of myocardial infarction. The men were
also to be free of other life threatening disorders. They had to be
willing to participate in a six year intervention trial and at least
attempt to make the risk factor changes which were proposed for the
special intervention group.

The men were recruited in the community from available resources.
No attempt was made to select a random sample of any defined population. Twenty-two clinical centers in the United States participated
in the trial.

Table 1. Risk Factor Levels at each Screening Visit for Men Random-
          ized to the Trial and Compared with All Men at First Screen.

Eligible Randomized	DBP	Cholesterol[a]	Percent Smokers
Screen 1	99.9	253.7	63.7
Screen 2	91.2	240.3	61.7
Screen 3	90.7	N.A.	59.2
All Screenees	84.0	214.6	36.8

[a]Screen 1 is serum and Screen 2 is plasma

    The men had three preliminary examinations prior to randomization.
The first screening examination included the measurement of blood
pressure, serum cholesterol, and cigarette smoking behavior. These
measurements were used to determine a risk score for eligibility for
a second screen which included a physical examination and further evaluation of the individuals' health status. Finally, a third screening
examination was done for those men still eligible which included a
Bruce type submaximal exercise test as well as a behavioral evaluation
prior to randomization. At the initial screen, 361,662 were seen.
From the initial screenees, 7.1% were eligible for second screen and
3.6% or 12,866 men were ultimately randomized into special intervention
(6,428) and usual care (6,438). The risk factor levels of the men
randomized to the trial as compared to all men screened is shown in
Table 1.

    By the time the men were randomized to the trial at third screen,
there had already been a substantial change in the risk factor levels
especially for blood pressure and cholesterol. The primary reason
for this decrease was probably regression to the mean. Other factors
included changes made by the men prior to randomization and differences
between plasma about 4 mg lower than serum cholesterol levels. At the
time of randomization, the special intervention and usual care men
were very similar for nearly all risk factors.

    The development of the intervention process has been published.
Men randomized to usual care were referred back to their physicians,
contacted every 4 months to determine their vital status, and evaluated annually including a physical examination and measurement of risk
factors.

    The initial plan of intervention for those men randomized to
special intervention was an intensive group intervention program which
usually lasted about 10 sessions. During these 10 sessions, there
was a structured program aimed at smoking cessation, changes in dietary

intake of cholesterol and saturated fat, and various aspects of the diagnosis and management of hypertension. Following the initial 10 week sessions, the men were placed in a follow up program based on their initial risk factor levels and changes during the intensive intervention. All special intervention men were seen at least every 4 months for evaluation of their risk factor levels and continued counseling. Many were seen more often. The special intervention participants also had an annual examination identical to that of the usual care men.

The specific goals of the intervention program were established prior to the trial and have been previously published. An important point to note is that little change in risk factors was expected among the usual care men.

The study has been very successful in maintaining the participation of the men. Only 7.2% of the special intervention and 9.1% of the usual care participants were not seen for their sixth annual exam. The result of the risk factor changes and morbidity to be published subsequently are, therefore, based on a very high level of ascertainment unusual for trials of this length and complexity. Very few participants were lost to follow up.

The Hypertension Treatment Protocol for special intervention participants was based on the Stepped Care model used in the Hypertension Detection and Follow up Program. Men were classified as having hypertension at baseline if the average of their second and third screen blood pressure was equal to or greater than 90 or if they were being treated for hypertension at the time of randomization.

Based on these criteria, 2,757 (42.8%) of the special intervention participants had a diastolic blood pressure greater than 90 at baseline and 1,261 (19.6%) were on drug treatment for hypertension, a total of 4,018 (62.4%) hypertensives. A participant normotensive at baseline could later be defined as hypertensive if at one of the four month visits, he had a blood pressure level greater than 89 and at a repeat confirmation visit usually one to four weeks later, it was still above 89.

Every special intervention participant defined by the criteria above was eligible to be given a goal blood pressure for the trial. The goal was based on the blood pressure level at the time of a confirmation visit. It was a diastolic blood pressure of 89 mm Hg or 10 mm Hg less than the average diastolic blood pressure at that visit. Men who had been previously on drug treatment prior to randomization and had a diastolic blood pressure less than 90 were given a goal of 80 mm Hg.

At 72 months, approximately two thirds of the special intervention participants had a goal blood pressure established. Their

mean blood pressure at baseline was 94.2 mm and at 72 months, 81.2 mm.
Approximately two thirds had a blood pressure less than goal and 88%
had a diastolic blood pressure less than 90 mm.

The mean blood pressure for all of the special intervention participants at year 6 was 80.5 compared to 83.6 for usual care men, a
difference of 3.1 mm. This difference includes both the normotensive
(Table 2) and hypertensive participants. The differences between
special intervention and usual care participants were directly related
to the level of the baseline blood pressure, about 1 mm for those
with screen 1 levels less than 95 mm Hg and 4.9 mm for those with
a screen 1 diastolic greater than 105. The number of special intervention participants prescribed drug therapy rose from 44.5% at 12
months to 58.2% at year 6. For usual care men the percentage rose
from 30.3% at 12 months to 47.0% at year 6. The use of drug therapy
for hypertension was directly related to the baseline blood pressure
level. However, even among those with a baseline diastolic blood
pressure less than 90 mm, 26% of special intervention and 18% of usual
care men were on drug therapy for hypertension by year 6.

The mean serum cholesterol level at first screen was 253 mg%,
and the mean plasma cholesterol level at second screen was 240 mg%
At entry the men repeated an average about 2,500 kilocalories, 14.0
from saturated fat and 450 mg of cholesterol in their diet. Approximately 7.4% of the calories were derived from alcoholic beverages.

Table 2.   Risk Factor Changes Between Baseline and Year 6
           Special Intervention and Usual Care

	SI Baseline	Year 6	UC Baseline	Year 6	SI-UC Diff.
Serum cholesterol	254	236	254	240	−4 mg
LDL cholesterol	160	149	162	153	−4 mg
HDL cholesterol	42	42	42	42	0 mg
Triglycerides	192	198	192	199	−1 mg
Diastolic blood pressure	91	81	91	84	−3 mm
Reported cigarette smokers (per cent)	64	32	64	45	−13

The Nutrition Program was aimed at a reduction of saturated fat and cholesterol and total calories for weight reduction for those men whose weight was greater than 1.15 above their ideal weight. The initial dietary plan included reduction of saturated fat to less than 10% of calories, dietary cholesterol to less than 300 mg, and an increase in polyunsaturated fats to 10% of calories. In 1976, the amount of saturated fat was further reduced to 8% and dietary cholesterol to 250 mg per day.

At the end of 6 years, the serum cholesterol had decreased to 235.5 mg/dl for the special intervention and 240.3 for the usual care, a 4.8 mg/dl difference (Table 2). This difference in cholesterol was greatest for men with high initial levels of serum cholesterol, 2.7 mg/dl for those with screen 1 cholesterol 220-239 mg/dl and a 10.6 mg/dl difference between special intervention and usual care for those with cholesterol greater than 300 mg%.

Lipoproteins were measured at second screen and every two years following randomization. The mean baseline LDL cholesterol was 160 mg%. It had dropped to 148.7 mg/dl for special intervention and 152.9 for usual care by year 6 (a 4.2 mg/dl difference). The HDL cholesterol averaged 42 mg% at second screen and was approximately the same at year 6. Preliminary analysis has determined that a decrease in saturated fat and weight loss contributed to the decline of LDL cholesterol while alcohol intake, weight change and cigarette smoking were primary determinants of the HDL cholesterol levels (Table 2).

The smoking cessation program urged all special intervention participants to quit smoking. Initially no effort was made to change the smoking habits of men who smoked only pipes and cigars. As noted, about 60% of the participants smoked cigarettes at baseline (Table A). The dose and change of cigarettes smoking was monitored by questionnaire including information about number of cigarettes, brand and inhalation characteristics and objective changes in serum thiocyanate levels and expired air carbon monoxide levels (Table 2).

At the end of 6 years, 49.6% of the special intervention and 29.1% of the usual care reported that they had quit smoking cigarettes. The thiocyanate adjusted quit percentage was 46.1% for special intervention and 28.5% for usual care. The quit for special intervention men was greatest within the first 4 months following randomization but was maintained throughout the trial. There was a substantial increase in the usual care quit percentage as the trial progressed from only 11% at year one to close to 30% at year six.

The quit percentage was inversely related to the number of cigarettes smoked at first screen, ranging for special intervention men from 68.6% for those smoking 1-19 cigarettes to 40% for those smoking 2 or more packs per day. The differences between special intervention and usual care were also inversely related to the number of cigarettes at first screen.

Many men quit smoking for a period of time and then started again.
Of the 1,399 special intervention men who quit smoking between randomization and the four month visit in year one, 36.5% were smoking at
the time of their sixth annual examination. Therefore, the reported
quit percentage represents a balance between current quitters and men
who started to smoke again. Interestingly, it appeared that men who
quit smoking later in the trial were more likely to start smoking
again.

Not all of the men in the trial had the same distribution of risk
factors. Most had at least 2 of the 3 major risk factors present.
The simultaneous intervention on different risk factors had important
effects on risk factor changes especially the use of drug therapy
for the treatment of hypertension. For special intervention men,
hypertension drug treatment tended to blunt the cholesterol lowering
effects of the qualitative dietary and weight changes. A combination
of diuretic therapy with weight gain or even weight stability was associated with substantial increase in plasma triglyceride levels.
Hypertensive cigarette smokers had the least favorable change in their
serum cholesterol levels. Reduction of alcohol intake was urged in
order to reduce both calories and blood pressure levels but this may
also have resulted in lowering of the HDL cholesterol levels for some
men. Weight loss enhanced the qualitative dietary changes for cholesterol lowering effect but some cigarette smokers who quit gained weight.

Overall, the special intervention men did reasonably well in
terms of their risk factor modification. Practically all normalized
their blood pressure using pharmacological therapy. Over 40% had quit
smoking by year 6. The cholesterol reduction was not as large as
expected but for the hypercholesterolemic group was similar to that
noted in other studies. The changes in usual care participants, however, were far greater than expected. This was especially true for
the treatment for hypertension, for the reduction of serum cholesterol
and somewhat for the changes in cigarette smoking. The overall difference between special intervention and usual care especially early
in the trial were, therefore, less than planned. However, the maintenance of the changes in risk factors among the special intervention
participants and their continued participation in the trial was unex-
pectedly strong and so by the end of the trial, the observed differences in risk factor changes although notachieving the goals approached
those initially expected.

MULTIFACTOR PREVENTION OF ISCHEMIC HEART DISEASE

(A COOPERATIVE SURVEY)

L. V. Chazova, I. S. Glazunov, Z. I. Yanushkevicius,
S. B. Domarkene, E. I. Zborovsky, R. A. Katzenovich,
K. Kh. Makjmudov, T. S. Meymanaliev, O. V. Lakutin,
V. V. Naumova and R. F. Fomina

Cardiology Research Centre, Academy of Medical Sciences
Moscow, USSR

Prevention of ischemic heart disease and control of arterial hypertension is a most important task of health care in the USSR, since the implementation of this task is sure to result in decreasing morbidity and mortality. A lot has been done to the effect for the past years in this country, but there still exists a number of theoretical and practical problems, which are presently being worked at.

Since 1977 the USSR Cardiology Research Center has been guiding a cooperative survey of multifactorial prevention of ischemic heart disease (IHD). It is aimed at: 1) elucidating a possibility of reducing IHD morbidity and mortality by primary prevention - affecting such risk factors as arterial hypertension (AH), hypercholesterolemia (HC), smoking (S), excess body weight (EBW), low physical activity (LPA), and by secondary prevention; 2) working out a schedule of primary and secondary IHD prevention measures which can be put into practice within the framework of the existing health service.

The survey is being carried out among 40-59 year old randomized male population. According to the schedule (Figure. I) it involves three groups of population: an active intervention group and two control ones. The first group was subjected to examination, which includes the use of questionnaires to reveal angina of effort, possible myocardial infarction, intermittent claudication, chronic pulmonary diseases as well as smoking habits and physical activity level; registration of a 12-lead ECG with subsequent evaluation according to Minnesota code; measurement of AP (twice); biochemical determination of blood cholesterol content; anthropometry (height, weight, skinfold thickness).

627

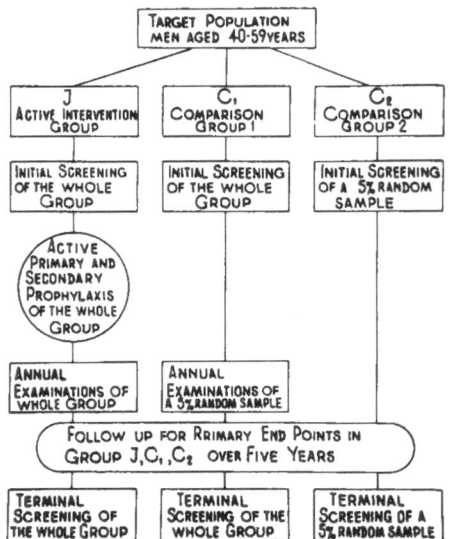

Fig. 1.   General study design.

IHD and risk factors were established on the basis of the following criteria;

1) IHD — myocardial infarction (MI) in the anamnesis, I-I, I-2
category alterations in ECG and (or) documented MI. (The diagnosis
in each case is decided upon by the consultative committee on the
basis of criteria used in WHO "Myocardial Infarction Register");
angina of effort — the corresponding WHO questionnaire; painless form
(in the absence of MI and angina of effort — ECG alterations (type
1-3; 4-1,2,3; 5-1,2,3; 6-1,2; 7-1; 8-3 of Minnesota code).

2) AH — diastolic arterial pressure (DP) of 95 mm Hg or higher;
any DP on the background of hypotensive drug therapy for the last 2
weeks.

3) Smoking — regular smoking of at least one cigarette a day.

4) Hypercholesterolemia — blood cholesterol of 260 mg% or more.

5) EBW — $\dfrac{\text{weight (kg)}}{\text{height}^2\text{(m)}}$ index equal to or exceeding 30.

6) LPA — sedentary work for 5 and more hours a day and active
leisure of less than 10 h a week.

After a screening and a classification of patients the first group (active intervention) is subjected to active primary and secondary IHD prevention measures. The latter are being carried out on the basis of maximal involvement of the existing health service personnel. The second group (I control) undergoes the same examination as the first one; the obtained data are handed over to practising physicians; preventive measures are taken according to the usual procedure. In the third group (II control) a list of the population is made and only a 5% random selection is examined and subsequently subjected to routine preventive measures. The whole of the first group and a 5 or 10% random selection from the second are seen annually while the third group is not examined at all.

The minimal follow-up period is 5 years. During the whole period we register mortality and new cases of MI and brain stroke in all three groups.

Besides, dynamics of risk factor levels, new cases of angina of effort, ischemic ECG alterations, temporary and permanent disability, and some other health indices are analyzed in the I and II group at annual examinations.

When the follow-up period is over the whole of the first two groups and a 5-10% random selection from the third are examined.

The results of the survey will be evaluated by comparing the number of the following dead points in three groups:

```
major points     - new cases of MI
                 - brain stroke
                 - IHD mortality
                 - total mortality;
secondary points - risk factor levels
                 - new cases of stable disablement due to IHD
                   and brain stroke
                 - new cases of angina of effort and ischemic
                   ECG alterations.
```

The following centers collaborate in the survey: USSR Cardiology Research Center and Kaunas Medical Institute (since 1977), Belorussian Scientific Research Institute (SRI) of Cardiology in Minsk (since 1979), Kirgizian SRI of Cardiology in Frunze and Uzbek SRI of Cardiology in Tashkent (since 1981), Kharkov branch of Ukrainian Strashesko SRI of Cardiology (since 1982).

The population observed in each center in all three groups ranges from 9,000 to 16,000. In Frunze, Tashkent and Kharkov primary examination of the selected groups is not over yet: the total number of people observed is 71,000: 23,000 have been examined by now in all centers; 12,000 have been assigned to a program of special intervention.

The survey is conducted according to a common plan and protocol using unified examination techniques. For a better coordination of efforts a special committee incorporating the representatives of all centers was set up. All cases involving major final points of the survey are considered by an intercenter consultative body which makes it easier to unify the evaluation of results.

Before starting the program the members of the teams from all the centers had a special training course and all the examination techniques were standardized (questionnaires, AP measurement, ECG coding). In the course of the survey training and control standardization is annually repeated which makes it possible to compare the data obtained by various centers.

This report analyzes and compares the tentative data of male population screening in 5 cities (Moscow, Kaunas, Minsk, Tashkent and Frunze) and the tentative results of special intervention toward altering the risk factors in Moscow, Kaunas and Minsk.

The analysis and comparison of IHD and risk factors spread were made on the basis of random selections with a 65-69% response (Moscow - 6737, Kaunas - 5929, Minsk - 1806, Tashkent - 1284, Frunze - 4719).

According to the primary examination data (Figure. 2) only 17-25.3% of the subjects observed had neither IHD nor the risk factors. The lowest number was in Moscow (17%) and the highest - in Tashkent (25.3%) (Kaunas - 21.5%, Minsk - 22.5%, Frunze - 20.5%). From 64 to 68% of the subjects observed had one or more risk factors, and half of them had two or more. At the time of the examination from 8.6-15% had IHD and brain stroke record in the anamnesis. Moscow accounted for the largest number of such cases (15%), Tashkent - for the fewest (8.6%) (Kaunas - 11.5%, Minsk - 13.2%, Frunze - 11.5%).

Thus, in the 5 cities of the Soviet Union from 75% to 83% of 40-59 year old men observed needed primary and secondary preventive measures.

The distribution of IHD incidence was as follows: Moscow (14.5%) Minsk (12.6%), Kaunas (10.9%), Frunze (10.3%), Tashkent (8.4%). It is of interest that major differences are registered in the incidence of such forms of IHD as myocardial infarction (from 1.1% in Tashkent to 3.7% in Moscow: Kaunas - 2.7%, Minsk - 2.5%, Frunze - 1.5% and angina of effort (from 2.8% in Tashkent to 6.5% in Moscow; Kaunas - 2.5%; Minsk - 4%; Frunze - 3.4%). At the same time there is a lesser variety in the incidence of painless IHD form (from 4.4% in Moscow to 6.1% in Minsk). Moscow is distinguished both by a considerable spread of IHD and the domination of its painful forms (10.1% of MI and angina pectoris of 14.5%). In Kaunas, Tashkent, Frunze and Minsk painless IHD either prevails or insignificantly

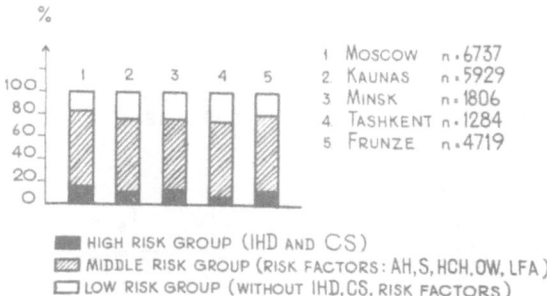

Fig. 2. Prevalence of the three risk groups.

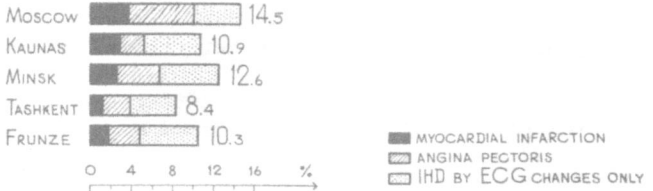

Fig. 3. IHD prevalence in examined populations.

differs from the incidence of painful forms. There are subjects in
MI group who have only ECG signs (1-1, 1-2 according to Minnesota
code) without MI in the anamnesis.

The distribution of the risk factors (Figure. 4) was as follows:
the incidence of AH varied from 22.5% (Minsk) to 27.9% (Moscow)
(Kaunas - 23.9%, Tashkent - 25.0%, Frunze - 25.2%); smoking - from
42.9% (Kaunas) to 52.3% (Tashkent) (Moscow - 46.2%, Minsk - 51.8%,
Frunze - 48.0%); HH - from 20.0% (Frunze) to 26.8% (Tashkent) (Moscow
- 21.1%, Kaunas - 24.2%, Minsk - 23.6%); EBW - from 8.4% (Frunze) to
21.2% (Kaunas), (Moscow - 9.8%, Minsk - 13.7%, Tashkent - 19.9%); LPA
- from 11.5% (Kaunas) to 22% (Frunze) (Moscow - 21.0%, Minsk - 11.9%,
Tashkent - 13.7%).

The above mentioned variety in the incidence of IHD and risk
factors is quite natural since the people assigned to the program
live in different geographical and climatic conditions, and have
their own national peculiarities and traditions, eating habits, etc.

The incidence of IHD and risk factors turned out to be rather
high in all the cities which proves the necessity of the most active
primary and secondary preventive measures. For example, in Tashkent
IHD incidence is the lowest, while the spread of risk factors is
practically the same or even higher than in other cities. That

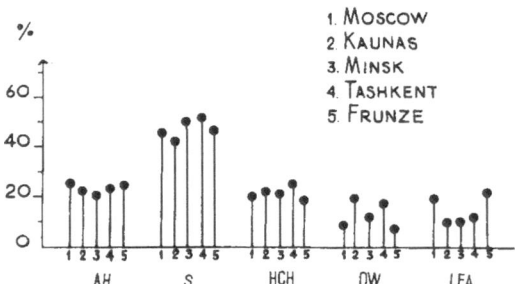

Fig. 4.   Prevalence of risk factors in examined populations.

indicates a possibility of the rise in the incidence of IHD in Tashkent if timely intervention does not alter the risk factors.

Preventive measures in the active intervention group are carried out by specially trained health service personnel and scientific research centers.

The intervention program in each center may have its local characteristic features if it keeps to basic common principles. These are as follows: 1) maximally differentiated approach to all patients; 2) mostly non-medicamental preventive measures against smoking, hypercholesterolemia, excess body weight and low physical activity; 3) medicamental therapy conditioned by the state of each patient in the group of subjects with AH and IHD.

In Moscow, Kaunas and Minsk the annual examinations of random samples selected from the same group of people who passed 3 examinations (primary, after 1 and 2 years of follow-up) elucidated the dynamics of risk factor levels on the background of intervention.

During the first two years AH, smoking and hypercholesterolemia dropped in all three centers. AH decreased by 7.8% in Moscow, by 6.1% in Kaunas and by 9.8% in Minsk (Figure. 5). The decrease in the spread of AH is accompanied by significant lowering of mean levels of systolic and diastolic AP in populational groups. Even in the first year the number of people subjected to effective treatment considerably increased: Moscow (to 48%); Kaunas (to 51%); Minsk (to 37.7%).

Smoking (Figure. 6) in Moscow, Kaunas and Minsk dropped by 7.9%, 8.1%, 14.8%, respectively. In subjects who gave up smoking external breathing indices (spirometry data) and tolerance to physical load (cycloergometry data) significantly improved even during the first year.

In Moscow, Kaunas and Minsk hypercholesterolemia (Figure. 6) decreased by 4%, 4.9% and 8.4% respectively.

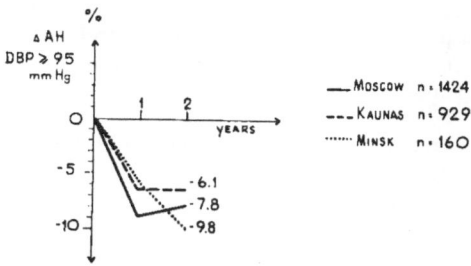

Fig. 5. Dynamics of the prevalence of risk factors in the active
         prophylaxis group (Figure 5,6,7).

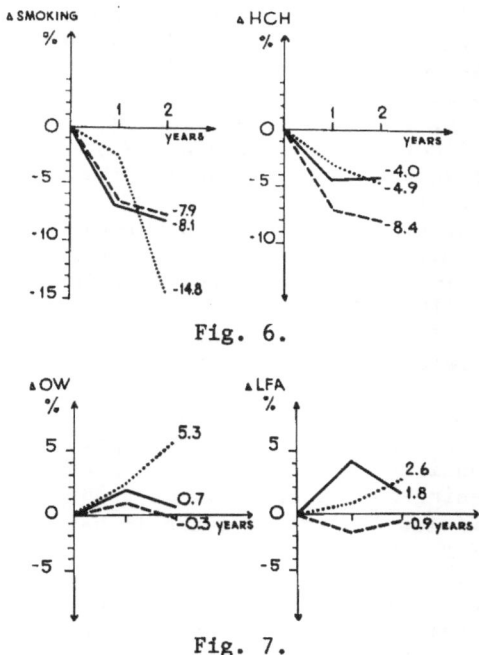

Fig. 6.

Fig. 7.

    As far as excess body weight and low physical activity are
concerned, different trends were observed in 3 centers. The first
year in all three centers saw an increase in the number of people
with EBW: in Moscow and Minsk - by 2.8%, in Kaunas - by 0.7%. During
the second year in Moscow and Kaunas the trend to weight reduction
appeared: in Kaunas EBW dropped below the baseline and in Moscow
returned to it. At the same time EBW increased in Minsk.

    No doubt, it is still too early to estimate the efficacy of
preventive measures. It needs a longer observation of a larger

population and a thorough comparison with the control. This report
constitutes an attempt to demonstrate the trends in the dynamics of
major risk factors that were found in the first years of multifactor
program inplementation.

The survey continues and its results will be evaluated and
summed up in the future.

REFERENCES

1. L. V. Chazova, I. S. Glazunov, A. M. Shishova, S. P. Oleinikov,
   M. B. Balavadze et al. The results of the cardiological
   survey of men in one of the precincts of a district out-
   patient clinic in Moscow. Ther. Arc., N 9, p.31-33. (1977)
2. S. P. Oleinikov, E. S. Glazunov, L. V. Chazova, V. J. Lisitsyn,
   A. M. Shishova et al. Smoking and IHD prevention. Cor. et
   vasa, N 2, p.81-88. (1979)
3. I. S. Glazunov, L. V. Chazova, A. V. Baubinene, R. Prokhorskas,
   et al. Multifactorial IHD prevention program (the data of
   the cooperative survey in Moscow and Kaunas). Kardiologija,
   N 7, p.31-34. (1980)
4. L. V. Chazova, M. B. Balavadze, I. S. Glazunov, S. P. Oleinikov,
   A. M. Shishova, A. D. Deev. Preventive examination of 40-59
   year old men in one of the Moscow districts. Kardiologija, N
   2, p.79-83. (1981)
5. S. P. Oleinikov, I. S. Glazunov, L. V. Chazova Smoking habits in
   different male and female age groups. Ther.Acc., N 2, P.111-
   115. (1981)
6. L. V. Chazova, M. B. Balavadze, I. S. Glazunov, N. J. Mordashova,
   I. M. Trincher, Zh.P. Pryakhina The application of standard
   WHO questionnaire to detect angina pectoris at mass population screening Ther.Acc., N 5, p.33-38 (1981).
7. Z. I. Yanushkevicius Control of ischemic heart disease in
   Lithuanian SSR. Kardiologija, N 9, p.5-9. (1981)
8. A. V. Baubinene, S. B. Domarkene, J. Klumbene, Ja. Kuprenite, I.
   Misyavichene et al. Experimental preventive and prospective
   epidemiological studies of ischemic heart disease in Kaunas.
   Kardiologija, N 9, p.75-80. (1981)
9. A. M. Shishova, L. V. Chazova, I. S. Glazunov The results of a
   2-year treatment of AH patients under conditions of an out-
   patient clinic. USSR Cardiology Research Center Bul., N 1,
   p.79-83. (1982)
10. V. L. Gromov, S. S. Dobo, L. V. Chazova The proportion of major
    risk factors and physical load tolerance in healthy subjects
    and IHD patients. Ther.Acc., N 5, p.32-36. (1982)
11. WHO. Myocardial Infarction Community Registers, Copenhagen,
    p.157-160. (1976)
12. G. A. Rose, H. Blackburn Cardiovascular Survey Methods. Geneva,
    (1968)

EFFECT OF DIET AND SMOKING INTERVENTION

ON THE INCIDENCE OF CORONARY HEART DISEASE

I. Hjermann

Oslo Study. Medical Outpatient Clinic
Ullevaal Hospital
Oslo 1, Norway

Improved hospital care has lowered hospital mortality from acute coronary heart disease (CHD). However, the goal of a sizeable reduction in the prevalence of CHD in young and middle age can only be achieved by postponing or preventing the disease. Intervention trials have been carried out in order to be able to demonstrate that such prevention is possible. These trials have not shown unequivocal results, except for the beneficial effect of antihypertensive treatment on prevention of stroke.

No intervention trials on healthy middle aged subjects at high risk of CHD have earlier been carried out. The purpose of our trial was to find out whether the lowering of high levels of blood lipids by dietary changes and the cessation of smoking, if maintained for many years, would reduce the incidence of first attacks of CHD in men aged 40-50 years.

All Oslo men aged 40-50 years were invited to a screening for coronary risk factors.[1] 65% (16202 men) attended the screening and from this cohort men with high risk were selected for a controlled trial[2] if they had serum cholesterol levels (mean of two measurements) of 7.5 - 9.8 mmol/1, coronary risk score (based on cholesterol levels, smoking habits and blood pressure) in the upper quartile of the distribution, and systolic blood pressure (mean of two measurements) below 150 mm Hg. A full clinical examination and exercise ECG was performed. Those with cardiovascular disease, diabetes, cancer, disabling disease, psychopathological disease and those already on lipidlowering diet were all excluded before randomization.

1232 men satisfied the inclusion criteria and were randomized to the intervention (n=604) and control group (n=628).

Table 1 shows that the groups were well comparable before start.
The men in the intervention group were all subjected to dietary advice in order to lower their elevated blood lipids. Antismoking advice was given to all smokers. Dietary advice was given individually
and based on each man's diet record, on body weight, serum cholesterol
and triglyceride levels and his general background. For those with
high serum cholesterol, without elevated triglyceride levels, the
diet change mainly consisted of a reduction in saturated fat. In
addition total energy intake was reduced in those who also had elevated triglycerides. The wives of the subjects in the intervention
group were invited in groups of 30-40 together with their husbands .
for diet and smoking information. Other risk factors were not subjected to intervention.

Follow-up examinations were made every 6 months in the intervention group and every 12 months in the controls. A short clinical
examination was made, 12 had ECG recorded, and at each follow-up the
men in the intervention group were asked about their eating and
smoking habits. A cholesterol curve was made for each man and shown
to him.

Follow-up compliance was good. Only 1 control subject and 9
subjects from the intervention group refused to attend at the final
exercise - ECG examination. For only 5 subjects of those still alive
at the end of the observation period, information was lacking.

An attempt was made to separate the effects on CHD incidence of
reducing cigarette consumption and of reducing serum cholesterol.
The analysis included a Cox proportional hazard model with the following explanatory variables: change in serum cholesterol, change
in cigarette consumption, initial serum cholesterol, initial cigarette
consumption and initial age. An extensive statistical analysis has
been made elsewhere.[3]

The cardiovascular events counted were fatal and non-fatal myocardial infarction, sudden death and stroke. All events were diagnosed by a diagnostic board not involved in the study and ignorant
of the group to which the men belonged. Detailed diagnostic criteria
had been listed before the start of the trial.

Results. The effects on serum cholesterol and smoking are shown
in Figures 1 and 2. Before randomization, 3 determinations of serum
cholesterol were made. As can be seen from the figures, the pre-
randomization level of these two risk factors were similar. Immediately after randomization, the efforts started to lower serum
cholesterol and cigarette consumption in the intervention group.

In the intervention group there was a reduction of 17% of mean
serum cholesterol from screening to first follow-up. The mean difference in serum cholesterol between the groups during the study was

Table 1. Comparability of Study Groups before Trial

	Intervention group (n=604)	Control group (n=628)
Sex	Male	Male
Age (mean and range;yr)	45.2(40-49)	45.2(40-49)
History/symptoms of CHD	None	None
Mean daily cigarette consumption	13.0	12.5
Smokers (%)	79.1	79.6
Body weight*(kg)	77.3±10.3	78.2±9.8
Height (cm)	177.4±6.0	176.9±6.3
Serum cholesterol*(mg/dl)		
Screening examination	328.2±26.9	329.2±27.5
1st re-examination	322.7±27.6	322.5±28.9
Range (mean of these 2 examinations)	290-379	290-379
Serum triglycerides*(mmol/1)		
Screening examination	2.80±1.5	2.84±1.5
1st re-examination	2.21±0.9	2.25±1.1
SBP (mm Hg)	<150	<150
% with SBP≥150 mm Hg and/or DBP≥98 mm Hg at screening	23	20
Sedentary workers (%)	50	48
Diet score*	14.8±6.1	14.1±6.1

*Value±1 SD. Subjects were non-fasting at the screening
examination and fasting at the 1st re-examination.
SBP=systolic blood pressure; DBP=diastolic blood pressure.

13%. Tobacco consumption (expressed as number of cigarettes per man
per day) fell about 45% more in the intervention group than in the
controls. However, only 25% of the smokers in the intervention
group completely stopped smoking as compared with 17% in the control
group.

Mean of fasting and non-fasting serum triglycerides levels was
20% and 25% lower in the intervention group than in the controls
during the trial. In a subgroup of good diet responders it was
shown[4] that the ratio of high density lipoprotein (HDL) cholesterol
to the other serum cholesterol fractions after 4 years of intervention
was 66% higher than in controls matched with respect to initial HDL
cholesterol, triglycerides, cholesterol, body weight, cigarette
smoking, level of physical activity and diet score, all recorded before randomization.

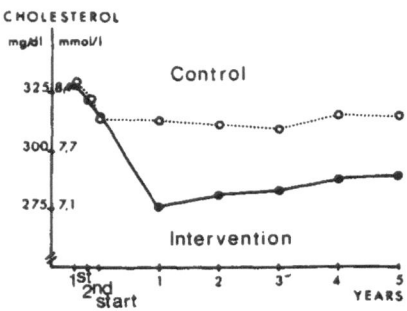

Fig. 1.   Intervention effect on serum cholesterol.   Oslo Study.

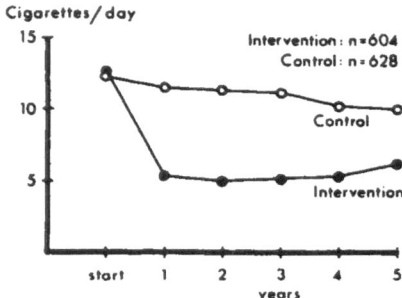

Fig. 2.   Intervention effect on cigarette smoking. Pipe smoking
         is included: 50g pipe tobacco/week equals 7 cigarettes/
         day. Oslo Study.

    The incidence of fatal and non-fatal MI and sudden death is
shown in Figure 3 as a life table. The difference between the intervention and control group is significant, p = 0.03, two-tailed test,
(one-tailed test should also be accepted). In Table 2 the different
cardiovascular events in the two groups are listed. The endpoints
sudden death, sudden coronary death, major CHD (sudden coronary
death + MI) and total cardiovascular events show significant differences between the two groups. Table 3 shows no significant difference for total mortality but a trend is present in the same
direction as for the cardiovascular events. It should be emphasized
that the trial was not dimensioned for showing differences in mortality. When evaluating the trial, it is important to note that
the trend for mortality is in the same direction as the difference
in CHD-incidence. And if a one-tailed test is used (which should be
acceptable for this trial), the difference between the groups for
total coronary death is also significant.

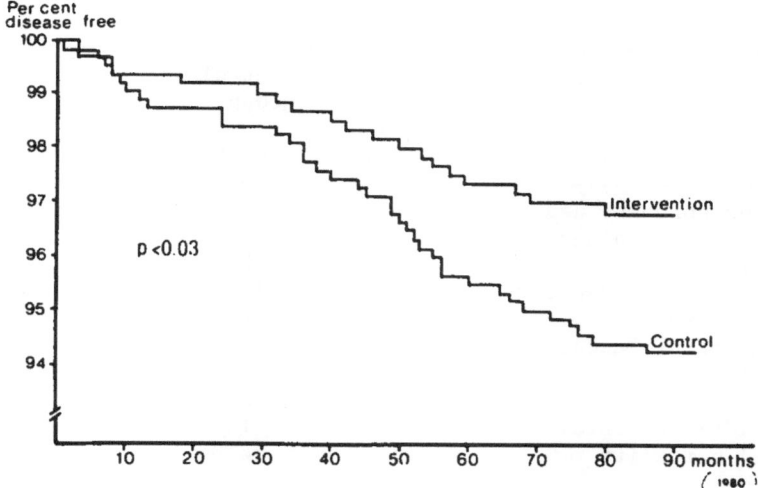

Fig. 3. Life table analysis of CHD (fatal and non-fatal myocardial infarction and sudden death) in intervention and control groups. Oslo Study.

Table 2. Cardiovascular Events

	Intervention group (n=604)		Control group (n=628)		
	No events	Rate (per thousand)	No events	Rate (per thousand)	p*
Sudden coronary death	3	5	11	18	..
Sudden unexplained death	0	..	1	2	..
Sudden coronary + unexplained death	3	5	12	19	0.024
Fatal MI	3	5	2	3	..
Fatal MI + sudden death	6	10	14	22	0.086
Non-fatal MI	13	22	22	35	0.153
Total coronary events	19	31	36	57	0.028
Fatal stroke	2	3	1	2	..
Non-fatal stroke	1	2	2	3	..
Total cardiovascular events	22	36	39	62	0.038
Bypass surgery	1	2	3	5	..

*By two-tailed test.

Table 3.   Mortal Events

	Inter-vention group (n=604)	Control group (n=628)	p
Sudden coronary death	3	11	0.024
Sudden unexplained death	0	1	..
Fatal MI	3	2	..
Fatal MI + sudden death	6	14	0.086
Fatal stroke	2	1	..
Total cardiovascular events	8	15	0.168
Cancer deaths	5	8	..
Suicide/accidental death	3	1	
Total mortality	16	24	0.246

The two risk factors influenced in this study was smoking and eating habits. Physical activity not influenced, as assessed by a questionnaire.

The men in the intervention group were examined and subjected to intervention every 6 months, but because of capacity problems the controls were examined only every 12 months. This difference between the groups in frequency of medical contact might have favored the intervention group, if a feeling general attention had a reassuring effect. On the other hand, the more frequent medical contact in the intervention group might have led to increased reporting of symptoms and more events may have been diagnosed.

It is important to find out to what extent each of the two factors influenced in this trial was responsible for the observed difference in incidence. As mentioned, a multivariate statistical model was used in an attempt to separate the two factors. Changes in serum cholesterol appeared to correlate more closely with CHD incidence than did the change in cigarette consumption. The statistical model predicted that the changes in serum cholesterol accounted for about 60% of the reduction in CHD incidence, whereas, most optimistically, the cigarette factor accounted for 25%.

Thus, although a substantial reduction in cigarette consumption was achieved during the trial, it was not large enough to create a significant reduction in risk. The statistical power of the trial was, in this respect, too low. The effect of change in smoking was also less than predicted from earlier observational studies in Oslo. It is possible that observational studies have over-estimated the decline in risk of CHD brought about by reducing (not quitting)

cigarette smoking. This is in accordance with an earlier monofac-
torial, controlled trial on smoking reduction.[5]

It is concluded that in healthy men aged 40-49, at high risk of
CHD advice to change eating habits and to stop smoking significantly
reduced the incidence of first event of major CHD. Statistical
multivariate analysis indicate that the reduction in incidence in
the intervention group is correlated with the reduction in serum
cholesterol and to a lesser extent with smoking reduction.

REFERENCES

1. P. Leren, E. M. Askevold, O. P. Foss, A. Frøili, D. Grymyr,
    A. Helgeland, I. Hjermann, I. Holme, P. G. Lund-Larsen,
    and K. R. Norum, Cardiovascular disease in middle-aged and
    young Oslo men. The Oslo Study. Monograph, Acta.Med.Scand.,
    suppl.588 (1975).
2. I. Hjermann, K. Velve Byre, I. Holme, and P. Leren, Effect of
    diet and smoking intervention on the incidence of coronary
    heart disease. Report from the Oslo Study Group of a ran-
    domized trial in healthy men, Lancet, II:1303 (1981).
3. I. Holme, On the separation of the effect of antismoking and
    lipidlowering diet on incidence of acute myocardial in-
    farction in high risk men. The Oslo Study. J.Oslo City Hosp.
    32:31 (1982).
4. I. Hjermann, S. C. Enger, A. Helgeland, I. Holme, P. Leren, and
    K. Trygg, The effect of dietary changes on high density
    lipoprotein cholesterol. The Oslo Study, Am.J.Med., 66:105
    (1979).
5. G. Rose and P. J. S. Hamilton, A randomized controlled trial of
    the effect on middle aged men of advice to stop smoking,
    J.Epidemiol.Commun.Hlth., 32:275 (1978).

THE PRESENT STATUS OF CARDIOVASCULAR MEDICINE IN AFRICA

Oladipo O. Akinkugbe

Department of Medicine
University of Ibadan
Ibadan, Nigeria

The three dominant groups of cardiovascular conditions in Africa today are: Hypertension, Rheumatic Heart Disease and the Cardiomyopathies (including Endomyocardial Fibrosis). Less common are congenital heart disease, cor pulmonale, pericarditis, the arrhythmias, anaemia or beriberi heart disease, ventricular aneurysms and idiopathic aortitis. It is worthy of note that Ischaemic Heart Disease remains distinctly uncommon among indigenous African communities, although sporadic cases are now beginning to emerge in the higher socio-economic strata of certain urban populations[1-3].

Hypertension in Africa forms part of a world-wide aetiopathogenic problem. In the majority of African populations (rural and urban) mean blood pressure rises with age and the prevalence rate of arterial pressure differs little from that in black and white communities in other parts of the world[4-10]. However, pockets of population exist in Africa and elsewhere, notably in the rural setting, in whom the blood pressure does not appear to rise with age[11-14]. Most reported studies relate this phenomenon to diet, life-style and the environment. Much has been made of the preliminary observations that when Masai tribesmen in the rural north of Kenya were recruited into the army and migrated to urban Nairobi, their gain in weight was followed some months later by a gradual rise in mean arterial pressures, and that these pressures fell in those who subsequently returned to their former habitat on demobilization[15].

The lifestyle in most African cities is undergoing remarkable transformation. Although the role of such acknowledged risk factors as atherosclerosis, tobacco, alcohol, lack of exercise, diet and salt in the genesis of hypertension is still to be critically assessed in the context of Africa, there is little doubt that the natural history

of hypertension continues to be affected by the changing socio-economic circumstances of those communities.

Cardiac ischaemic complications are as rare as cerebrovascular
are common[16],[17]. The low incidence of certain atherosclerotic risk
factors may be partly responsible for this apparent immunity of black
communities to heart attacks - relatively low levels of plasma triglycerides, cholesterol and high-density-lipoprotein cholesterol as
compared with whites[18],[19]. Haemorrhagic cerebrovascular complications
occur more frequently in blacks than in whites; this is probably attributable to the height of the blood pressure itself[20]. The apparent
rarity of severe retinopathy in the hypertensive African constitutes
yet another conundrum[21].

Hormonal studies have been undertaken in several biracial population groups but the results are often difficult to interpret[22],[23].
Renin suppression is a common finding in black hypertensive populations
but sympathetic activity as determined by plasma levels of noradrenaline is inconsistent. Studies in blacks outside Africa have confirmed
lower levels of dopamine β-hydroxylase than in whites, but its significance remains doubtful[24].

Another area worthy of more attention is the role of sodium and
potassium[25-27]. It is clear that dietary salt excess alone cannot be
held as a major contributory factor to hypertension in black Africa,
nor can its lack be directly related to the low prevalence of hypertension in certain defined tribal societies on the continent[22]. Of
more interest in recent times are observations on the cellular transport of sodium and potassium in normotensive and hypertensive black
communities[28]. These communities have a significantly reduced ouabain-
insensitive sodium/potassium pump activity compared to white normotensives, implying a diminished cellular capacity to eliminate sodium.
Differences have also been observed in urinary sodium/potassium ratios
as between blacks and whites[29]. All these suggest a genetic basis
and much further work needs to be done to unravel any cause-effect
relationships.

Rheumatic Heart Disease (RHD), an eminently preventable condition
constitutes a major cause of cardiovascular morbidity and mortality
in developing countries[30]. It occurs in a significantly higher proportion of children and adolescents in Africa than in industrialized
societies. Refinements in the clinical diagnosis of complicating
arrhythmias or established valvular disease (phonocardiography,
echocardiography, catheterisation, coronary arteriography etc.) are
still confined to very few cardiological centers in Africa - within
or attached to Teaching Hospitals. So also are such specialized procedures as cardiac pacing, valve replacement, coronary bypass and open
heart surgery. The major thrust in the control of RHD is obviously
the integration, however modest, of preventive measures with national
and primary health care programs[31]. Infective endocarditis complicating known RHD needs to be distinguished from the persistent fever

in RHD itself, coexistence of RHD with haemoglobinopathy, or fever
following urological instrumentation. Staph. aureus is more commonly
encountered than Strept. viridans, or there may be such unusual
organisms as Strept. faecalis, Haemophilus parainfluenza, Pseudomonas,
Klebsiella and Escherichia coli[32]. Primary sites of infection include
skin and scalp sepsis, osteomyelitis or pyomyositis.

Classification of the Cardiomyopathies has only recently been
tidied up, and the conflict of terminology that has always bedevilled
the subject is now hopefully resolved[33]. Congestive (dilated) cardiomyopathy is easily the dominant type of myocardial disease of unknown
cause on the African continent. Alcohol, malnutrition and hypokalaemia have been variously blamed as aetiological factors but evidence
remains unconvincing[34-36]. Peripartal cardiomyopathy[37] is but a facet
of this "congestive" variety, and its descriptive appellation merely
signifies its occurrence in or around pregnancy, often in situations
associated with volume overload or vitamin deficiency. Toxoplasma[38]
or Coxsackie B viruses[39] are infections often associated with the
presence of congestive cardiomyopathy, but the new classification
rightly places these infections in the category of "Specific heart
muscle disease of known cause". The relationship between cardiomyopathy and hypertension has often led some investigators to regard
congestive cardiomyopathy as synonymous with hypertensive heart failure[40], but haemodynamic studies would seem to refute such hypothesis.

Restricted cardiomyopathy manifests in the tropical milieu essentially as Endomyocardial Fibrosis (EMF)[41]. Some would regard
Loeffler's cardiomyopathy as an early phase of EMF, and have even
attempted to rename EMF "Eosinophilic endomyocardial disease"[42].

Health care systems in Africa, beset as they are by the burden
of infectious disease, are yet to be fully alive to the problems that
cardiovascular diseases are destined to pose in the coming decades.
The answers to many of the intricate problems in the aetiology and
pathogenesis of hypertension, ischaemic heart disease and cardiomyopathy in Africa will come, not through superficial surveys of populations or half-hearted and poorly supported haemodynamic studies,
but through well-ordered, in-depth clinical experimental and epidemiological application. Inter-regional scientific collaboration is thus
vital as the ultimate realization of these goals.

REFERENCES

1. H. C. Seftel. The rarity of coronary heart disease in South
      African blacks. S. Afr. Med. J., 54:99, 1978.
2. A. O. Falase, T. O. Cole and B. O. Osuntokun. Myocardial infarc-
      tion in Nigerians. Trop. Geogr. Med., 25:147, 1973.
3. G. V. Mann, A. Spoerry, M. Gray and D. Jarashow. Atherosclerosis
      in the Masai. Amer. J. Epidemiol., 95:26, 1972.

4. O. O. Akinkugbe and O. A. Ojo. Arterial pressures in rural and
    urban populations in Nigeria. Brit. Med. J., 2:222, 1969.
5. G. W. Comstock. An epidemiologic study of blood pressure levels
    in a biracial community in the Southern United States. Amer.
    J. Hygiene, 65:271, 1957.
6. W. E. Miall, E. H. Kass, J. Ling and K. L. Stuart. Factors influ-
    encing arterial pressure in the general population in Jamaica.
    Brit. Med. J., ii:497, 1962.
7. A. C. Ikeme, F. J. Bennett and K. Somers. The cardiovascular
    status of middle-aged and elderly Ugandan Africans. E. Afr.
    Med. J., 51:409, 1974.
8. S. Hatano, Hypertension in Japan: in:"Epidemiology of Hypertension"
    ed. O. Paul, Florida Symposium Specialists, 1975.
9. I. Prior. Cardiovascular epidemiology in New Zealand and the
    Pacific. New Zealand Med. J., 80:245, 1974.
10. F. H. Epstein and R. D. Eckhoff. The epidemiology of high blood
    pressure - geographic distributions and etiological factors.
    In: Epidemiology of Hypertension: Proceedings of an Inter-
    national Symposium eds. J. Stamler, R. Stamler and T. N. Pul-
    lman. New York: Grune and Stratton, 1967.
11. A. S. Truswell, B. M. Kennelly, J. D. L. Hansen and R. B. Lee.
    Blood pressures of Kung bushmen in Northern Botswana. Amer.
    Heart J., 84:5, 1972.
12. I. Maddocks. Blood pressure in Melanesians. Med. J. Australia,
    1:1123, 1967.
13. S. Padmavati and S. Gupta. Blood pressure studies in rural and
    urban groups in Delhi. Circulation 19:395, 1959.
14. A. G. Shaper, D. H. Wright and J. Kyobe. Blood pressure and body
    build in three nomadic tribes of Northern Kenya. E. Afr. Med.
    J., 46:273, 1969.
15. A. G. Shaper. Cardiovascular disease in the tropics III. Brit.
    Med. J., iii:805, 1972.
16. J. R. Billinghurst. Analysis of neurological admissions to Mulago
    Hospital, Kampala 1965-66. E. Afr. Med. J., 43:566, 1966.
17. B. O. Osuntokun, E. L. Odeku and A. Adeloye. Cerebrovascular
    accidents in Nigerians: A study of 348 patients. W. Afr.
    Med. J., 18:160, 1969.
18. R. R. Frerichs, S. R. Srinivasan, L. S. Webber and G. S. Berenson.
    Serum cholesterol and triglyceride levels in 3446 children
    from a biracial community. The Bogalusa Heart Study. Circulation
    54:302, 1976.
19. S. R. Srinivasan, R. R. Frerichs, L.S. Webber and G. S. Berenson.
    Serum lipoprotein profile in children from a biracial community.
    The Bogalusa Heart Study. Circulation 54:309, 1976.
20. Y. K. Seedat and J. Reddy. The clinical pattern of hypertension
    in the South African black population: a study of 1000 patients
    Afr. J. Ed. Sci., 5:1, 1976.
21. O. O. Akinkugbe. The rarity of severe hypertensive retinopathy
    in the African. Amer. J. Med., 45:401, 1968.

22. P. S. Sever, D. Gordon, W. S. Peart and P. Beighton. Blood
    pressure and its correlates in urban and tribal Africa.
    Lancet, ii:60, 1980.
23. W. S. Peart. Concepts in Hypertension: The Croonian Lecture.
    J. Royal Coll. Phys. London. 14:141, 1979.
24. A. W. Voors, G. S. Berenson, E. R. Datferes, L. S. Webber and
    W. E. Shuler. Racial differences in blood pressure control.
    Science, 204:1091, 1979.
25. L. K. Dahl. Possible role of chronic excess salt consumption in
    the pathogenesis of essential hypertension. Amer. J. Cardiol.
    8:571, 1961.
26. L. B. Page. Epidemiologic evidence on the aetiology of human
    hypertension and its possible prevention. Amer. Heart J.
    91:527, 1976.
27. F. C. Luft, C. E. Grim, J. T. Higgins Jr. and M. H. Weinberger.
    Differences in response to sodium administration in normoten-
    sive white and black subjects. J. Lab. Clin. Med. 90:555,
    1977.
28. A. F. Aderounmu and L. A. Salako. Abnormal cation composition
    and transport in erythrocytes from hypertensive patients.
    Eur. J. Clin. Invest., 9:369, 1979.
29. G. R. Meenly and H. D. Battarbee. High sodium, low potassium
    environment and hypertension. Amer. J. Cardiol., 28:768,
    1979.
30. P. G. D'Arbela. Rheumatic heart disease and infective endocar-
    ditis: the problem in cardiological practice in Africa in:
    Cardiovascular Disease in Africa, O. O. Akinkugbe ed. Ciba-
    Geigy, Basle, 1976.
31. B. L. Agrawal. Rheumatic heart disease unabated in developing
    countries. Lancet, 2:910, 1981.
32. O. Ogunbi, H. O. Fadahunsi, I. Ahmed, A. Animasahun, S. O. Daniel,
    D. U. Onuoha and L. Q. O. Ogunbi. An epidemiological study
    of rheumatic fever and rheumatic heart disease in Lagos,
    Nigeria. In: Cardiovascular Disease in Africa, O. O. Akink-
    ugbe ed. Ciba-Geigy, Basle, 1976.
33. Brit. Heart Journal. Report of the WHO/ISFC task force on the
    definition and classification of cardiomyopathies. 44:672,
    1980.
34. H. C. Seftel. Cardiomyopathies in the Johannesburg Bantu: Part
    II Aetiology of idiopathic cardiomegaly. S. Afr. Med. J.,
    46:1823, 1972.
35. U. Basile, B. O. Osuntokun, A. O. Falase and M. A. Aladetoyinbo.
    Thiamine deficiency and idiopathic cardiomegaly in Nigerian
    adults. Afr. J. Med. Sci., 4:465, 1973.
36. Z. Fejfar. Cardiomyopathies: An international problem.
    Cardiologia, 52:9, 1968.
37. N. McD. Davidson and E. H. O. Parry. Peripartum cardiac failure
    p.199. In: Cardiovascular disease in the Tropics eds. A. G.
    Shaper, M. S. R. Hutt and Z. Fejfar. Levenham Press, Suffolk.

38. A. O. Falase, A. Fabiyi and E. O. Ogunba. Idiopathic cardiomeg-
    aly in Ibadan revisited. In: Cardiovascular Disease in
    Africa ed. O. O. Akinkugbe. Ciba-Geigy, Basle. p.37, 1976.

39. G. Cambridge, C. G. C. MacArthur, A. P. Waterson, J. R. Goodwin
    and C. M. Oakley. Antibodies to Coxsackie B viruses in con-
    gestive cardiomyopathy. Brit. Heart J., 41:692, 1979.

40. I. F. Brockington. Debate: That congestive cardiomyopathy is
    really hypertensive heart disease in disguise. Postgrad.
    Med. J., 48:778, 1972.

41. E. H. O. Parry and D. G. Abrahams. The natural history of endo-
    myocardial fibrosis. Quart. J. Med., (NS) 34:383, 1965.

42. I. F. Brockington and E. G. J. Olsen. Loeffler's endocarditis
    and Davies' endomyocarditis. Amer. Heart J., 85:308, 1973.

CHAGAS' CARDIOMYOPATHY

Armenio Costa Guimaraes

Professor of Cardiology
Faculty of Medicine
Federal University of Bahia, Brazil

Chagas' disease is restricted to the American continent and has been identified from the southern United States to Argentina[1]. Its epidemiology is related to poor housing in the rural communities and to trypanosoma cruzi infected triatominae. Less frequently the disease may be transmitted through blood transfusion, congenitally or by accident in the laboratory[2]. It is estimated that a total of 7 million people are infected[3].

Chagas' cardiomyopathy, however, is highly prevalent only in Argentina, Brazil and Venezuela. In Bahia, Brazil, at the University Hospital, it is responsible for 42.4% of all cardiac deaths. In a few cases, it may be preceded, 10 to 30 years ago, by an acute myocarditis with complete recovery in 90.0% of the cases and death in 10.0%. Forty six percent of such cases occur in the first decade of life[4].

Basic pathologic changes are related to a diffuse chronic myocarditis. The degree of involvement of the ventricular myocardium and/or the excitation-conduction system of the heart is a major determinant of the type of clinical presentation. Extensive myocardial damage leads to progressive dilatation of the heart with congestive heart failure (CHF). Lesions of the excitation-conduction system are common and give rise to the rhythm and conduction disturbances frequently seen in this condition[5].

The clinical presentation of chronic Chagas' cardiomyopathy comprehends asymptomatic patients with electrocardiographic changes and no cardiomegaly to patients with symptomatic cardiac arrhythmias and/or CHF[6]. These latter patients are more common (71.1%) between the 3rd and the 5th decades of life, with a 2.7 male to female ratio (Table 1). Complete right bundle branch block (CRBBB), isolated or

649

Table 1. Sex and age distribution in Chagas' cardiomyopathy[a]

Age yrs.	11-20	21-30	31-40	41-50	51-60	>60	Total
Male	13	16	12	20	9	3	73
Female	1	8	8	7	2	1	27
Total	14	24	20	27	11	4	100

[a]Data of 100 patients who died with advanced Chagas' cardiomyopathy at the University Hospital, Bahia, Brazil.

associated with left anterior hemiblock (LAHB), is the most frequent and characteristic ECG abnormality, occurring in 30 to 60% of the cases[7].

Ten percent or less of patients with Chagas' cardiomyopathy may present with total A-V block, requiring pacemaker implantation[8]. In those with a normal or mildly enlarged heart this procedure seems to improve survival in addition to symptomatic control. Improvement of survival, however, doesn't occur in some patients with a moderately to severely enlarged heart, whose CHF shows a progressive downhill course immediately after pacemaker implantation. In order to understand how the heart of these patients responds to ventricular pacing, 9 of them were studied in our laboratory. They were divided in 2 groups according to their left ventricular end-diastolic pressure (LVED): Group I - 5 patients, LVED from 10.5 to 14.9 mm Hg, mean 12.7 mm Hg; Group II - 4 patients, LVED from 20.8 to 26.6 mm Hg, mean 23.5 mm Hg (Table 2). During pacing, G.I. patients showed a uniform LVED decrease between idioventricular rate and 100 b/min pacing rate, ranging from 3.7 to 11.8 mm Hg, mean 9.0 mm Hg. In G.II, LVED decreased in 3 patients, reaching normal values in nos. 1 and 3 (10.5 and 13.2 mm Hg) and remaining elevated in no. 2 (22.3 mm Hg); in patient no. 4 it rose from 25.8 to 32.5 mm Hg. The lowest LVED was reached at pacing rates equal or above 80 b/min in all but patient no. 5 (G.I.), in whom it happens at 70 b/min. Although the still limited number of patients studied, this data suggests the following: 1) artificial pacing seems to improve left ventricular function of total A-V block chagasic patients with a normal, mildly or moderately elevated LVED; 2) this improvement seems to be maximal at pacing rates equal or above 70 b/min; 3) in patients with severely elevated LVED, left ventricular function doesn't improve or may even become worse. Based on still very limited data, it has been claimed that 50 b/min is the best pacing rate for these latter patients[9]. Our data doesn't confirm this assertion, but further studies using larger series of patients are necessary to clarify this important point.

Table 2. Hemodynamic data in chagasic total A-V block[a]

Groups	Patient No.	Basal HR (b/min)	Basal LVED (mmHg)	Pacing (b/min) LVED (mmHg) 60	70	80	90	100	LVED Gradient Basal-100 (b/min)
I	1	33	13.4	4.4	4.0	4.3	2.1	1.6	11.8
	2	20	11.2	7.2	7.2	6.2	5.2	3.3	7.9
	3	30	10.5	6.8	6.6	6.3	6.1	6.8	3.7
	4	32	13.5	9.8	5.1	6.2	3.3	1.8	11.7
	5	35	14.9	4.6	2.1	3.6	3.8	4.8	10.1
II	1	27	20.8	13.4	10.5	9.5	9.5	10.5	10.3
	2	25	26.6	20.7	20.7	19.2	19.2	22.3	4.3
	3	20	20.8	16.3	14.9	12.4	11.3	13.2	7.6
	4	32	25.8	22.5	23.2	21.7	24.1	32.5	-6.7

[a]Left ventricular end-diastolic pressure (LVED) response to pacing rates 60 to 100b/min of 9 patients divided in Groups I and II according LVED basal level

Ventricular arrhythmias are one of the major problems to deal with in patients with Chagas' cardiomyopathy. In endemic areas sudden death is a common cause of death among young and middle aged adults. The presence of these arrhythmias doesn't keep any relationship with heart size; patients with normal heart size may present with life threatening ventricular arrhythmias.

Although there are no definitive data for identification of high risk sudden death patients with this condition, the presence of couplets or salvos in the standard ECG has been considered as an indication for permanent antiarrhythmic treatment. In this regard the sensitivity of the 12 leads ECG with a 30" V_1 rhythm strip was compared with that of the 24:00 hs Holter monitoring[10], a high sensitive technique but too much expensive and time consuming to be used on a large scale basis, especially in rural communities. Three groups of chagasic patients were studied: Group I - normal ECG (N = 43); Group II - conduction defects but no ventricular premature beats (VPB's) (N = 29); Group III - one or more VPB's (N = 16). Age ranged from 18 to 55 years, mean 38.4 years; there were 27 females and 12 males. The number of couplets and salvos in the 24:00 hs. Holter increases sharply from Groups I and II to G.III (Table 3). In G.I., the number of couplets ranged from 1 to 7, mean 1.7, in G.II from 1 to 38; mean 9.4, and in G.III from 2 to 5.749, mean 563.1. Salvos occurred only once in G.I. and G.II patients, but in G.III ranged from 1 to 855, mean 76.1. Based in these findings, it was possible to evaluate the predictive value of the 12 leads ECG in relation to the 24:00 hs Holter (Table 4). So, in G.I. patients 11.6% will have chance to present with couplets or salvos in the 24:00 hs Holter, in G.II 24.1%, and in G.III 92.0%. Then, the existence of couplets and/or salvos should be strongly suspected in chagasic patients with one or more VPB's in the standard ECG.

Low adherence to treatment secondary to poor socio-economic conditions, and drug selection make antiarrhythmic treatment a difficult task. Any drug that decreases contractility or conduction should be avoided or used with utmost precaution in this condition, especially in patients with a dilated heart.

At the present moment, amiodarone is the most useful drug for the treatment of VPB's in Chagas' cardiomyopathy. Its efficiency and safety has been documented elsewhere[11] and in our laboratory in 25 patients[12], divided in Group I, 19 patients with at least couplets in the one hour sedentary ECG, and Group II, 6 patients with the same arrhythmia only on exercise. In G.I., after 10 days of 600mg daily of oral amiodarone, the mean total number of VPB's decreased from 393.4 to 52.5 (p<0.01), and remained stable until the end of the study, on the 22nd day. In G.II, this number decreased from 65.2 to 2.2 (p<0.05) during this latter period of time (Table 5). From the qualitative stand-point, amiodarone was able to suppress the more

Table 3. Ventricular premature beats (VPB's) in Chagas' cardiomyopathy

	GROUP[b]					
	I(N=43)		II(N=29)		III(N=25)	
	C	S	C	S	C	S
Range	1-3	1	1-38	1	2-5,740	1-855
Mean	1.7	1	9.4	1	563.1	76.1

[a]Frequency of couplets (C) and salvos (S) of VPB's in the 24:00 hs Holter monitoring of 97 patients.

[b]Groups selected according the 12 leads ECG with a 30 seconds V_1 rhythm strip: G.1 = normal ECG; G.II = conduction disturbance, no VPB's; G.III = VPB's

Table 4. Predictive value of the standard ECG in Chagas' cardiomyopathy[a]

VPB's[b]	VPB's in the 24:00 hs Holter		
	G.I.(%)	G.II.(%)	G.III(%)
At least 1	36(83.7)	26(90.0)	25(100.0)
Couplets (C)	3(7.0)	7(24.1)	23(92.0)
Salvos (S)	2(4.7)	1(3.4)	16(64.0)
C + S	5(11.6)	7(21.4)	23(92.0)

[a]Same groups as in Table 3.

[b]Number and type of VPB's in the 12 leads ECG with a 30 seconds V_1 rhythm strip.

Table 5. Antiarrhythmic action of oral amiodarone (600 mg daily) in Chagas' cardiomyopathy

Treatment Day	Mean total of VPB's[a]			Extrassystolic Index	$\left(\%\dfrac{\text{mean total VPB's}}{\text{mean total QRS}}\right)$	
	Range	Mean	SD	Range	Mean	SD
GROUP I (N $\doteq$ 19)						
Before	90–1,044	393.4	249.8	2.0–23.0	10.1	6.8
10th	0–278	52.5[b]	97.3	0–10.6	1.8[b]	3.6
22nd	0–603	69.9	160.3	0–21.6⁻	2.5	0.7
GROUP II (N = 6)						
Before	35–177	65.3	55.3	2.7–19.2	9.7	6.0
22nd	0–8	2.2[c]	3.5	0–1.2	0.3[c]	0.5

[a]VPB's were counted in one hour of sedentary ECG monitoring (paper speed of 10min/sec) in Group I and during bicyclergometer exercise test in G.II.

[b]$p < 0.01$
[c]$p < 0.05$

complex forms of VPB's (R/T, couplets and salvos), both at rest and on exercise, in all but one G.I. patient, who still showed couplets on exercise even after further 10 days of 800 mg of amiodarone per day.

Amiodarone also decreased significantly the heart rate (p<0.01) and increased significantly the QT interval (p<0.05), but didn't cause any change in the PR interval whatsoever. In one patient with recurrent ventricular tachycardia this amiodarone induced sinus bradycardia was so marked that required pacemaker implantation in order to continue drug administration. In general, drug tolerance has been good, except for a patient with severe partial loss of vision after 3 months on a 600 mg daily dosage, but who recovered completely after withdrawal of the drug.

The treatment of advanced CHF in Chagas' cardiomyopathy is another challenge for the clinician. These patients are very sensitive to digitalis, so, usually, only half to one third of the regular dosage can be employed. The use of vasodilators, specially prazosin, has been of great help in management of such patients. Nevertheless, diuretics continue to be the basis of anti-congestive treatment, with refractory patients showing a very good response to the association of furosemide, hydrochlorothiazide and spirolactone.

Another great problem concerns the natural history of seropositive individuals without or with ECG changes like bundle branch block or primary ST-T wave changes and a good functional heart. The potential risk of severe heart disease in these individuals has created serious problems regarding employment opportunities.

Finally, the greatest challenge will be the eradication of the disease through better socio-economic conditions for the rural inhabitants and through a triatominae extermination program in order to keep the houses free of the vectors of the diseases.

REFERENCES

1. M. P. Barreto. Epidemiologia, in: Typranosoma cruzi e Doenca de Chagas, Z. Brener and Z. Andrade, eds. Guanabara Koogan, Rio de Janeiro (1979).
2. J. C. P. Dias. Mecanismos de Transmissao, in: Trypanosoma Cruzi e Doenca de Chagas, Z. Brener and Z. Andrade, eds., Gunabara Koogan, Rio de Janeiro (1979).
3. World Health Organization Technical Report Series no. 202. Chagas' Disease: report of a study group. World Health Organization, Geneve (1960).
4. A. Rassi, C. Borges, J. M. Rezende, O. Carneiro, J. Salum,I.B. Ribeiro and O. H. Paula, Fase aguda da doenca de Chagas: aspectos clínicos observados em 19 casos. Rev. Goiana Med. 4: 161 (1958).

5. Z. A. Andrade, S. G. Andrade, G. B. Oliveira and D. R. Alonso,
    Histopathology of the conducting tissue of the heart in Chagas'
    myocarditis, Am. Heart. J., 93: 316 (1978).
6. A. Prata, Z. Andrade and A. Guimaraes. Chagas' Heart Disease,
    in: Cardiovascular Disease in the Tropics, A. G. Shaper, M. S.
    D. Hutt and Z. Fejfar, eds., British Medical Association,
    London (1974).
7. M. B. Rosembaum and A. J. Alvarez. The electrocardiogram in
    chronic chagastic myocarditis, Am. Heart J., 50:492 (1955).
8. F. S. Laraja, E. Dias, G. Nobrega and S. Miranda. Chagas'
    disease. A clinical epidemiologic and pathology study.
    Circulation, 14: 1035 (1956).
9. D. S. Kormann, H. C. Araujo, J. C. Bembom, V. F. Fontes, H. M.
    Magalhaes and A. D. Jatene. Marca-passo cardiaco de frequencia
    baixa em chagasicos com grande cardiomegalia, Arq. Bras. Cardiol
    28 (Supl. II): 302 (1975).
10. J. H. Maguire, N. B. Ramos, O. O. Santana, E. C. Almeida and A.
    C. Guimaraes, Comparacao do eletrocardiograma convencional com
    o eletrocardiograma dinamico na avaliacao das arritmias na
    doenca de Chagas, Arq. Bras. Cardiol., 37 (Supl. I): 82 (1981).
11. M. B. Rosembaum, P. A. Chiale, M. S. Halpern, G. J. Nau, A. Tam-
    bussi, J. Przybylski, J. O. Lazari and M. V. Elizari. Clinical
    efficacy of amiodarone as an antiarrhythmic agent, Amer. J.
    Cardiol., 38: 934 (1976).
12. E. C. Almeida, A. C. Guimaraes and J. Maguire; Uso do cloridrato
    de amiodarona na forma arritmica da miocardite cronica chag-
    asica, Arq. Bras. Cardiol., 37: 10 (1981).

CARDIOVASCULAR DISEASE IN DEVELOPING COUNTRIES

RHEUMATIC HEART DISEASE

S. Padmavati*, Vineeta Vishvbandhu**,
Vijay Gupta** and K. Prakash***

*Director, National Heart Institute, New Delhi
**Research Officer, All India Heart Foundation, New Delhi
***Associate Professor and Head of Dept. of Microbiology
Lady Hardinge Medical College, New Delhi

PREVALENCE

Since World War II, published literature points to a high prevalence of RHD in developing countries, which contribute to two thirds of the world population. Rheumatic heart disease is the commonest type in children and adolescents and one of the most frequent in adults. For many parts of Latin America (Brazil, Chile, Columbia, Guatemala, Mexico, Panama, Peru), the West Indies, in the Middle East (Algeria, Cyprus, Egypt, Morocco, Sudan), in Ethiopia, Nigeria, Senegal, Iran, Pakistan, India, Burma, Hongkong, Indonesia, Thailand, Sri Lanka and Mongolia this holds true[1].

The sources of data unfortunately for RHD are mostly from surveys in vulnerable groups such as school children and not from autopsy or death statistics, as the latter are unreliable or unobtainable in these countries. Hospital statistics point to RHD accounting for 22 to 50 percent of all cardiac cases. In school children the prevalence ranges from 6 to 22 per 1000. The position is similar to what is obtained in Western countries e.g. the UK and USA at the turn of the century[1].

The incidence of acute rheumatic fever declined in the West long before the antibiotic era. The incidence of acute RF in developing countries is not clearly known because such patients do not reach hospital except in the cities. The symptoms of acute RF are no different from that described in Western literature, in those that reach hospital[2].

657

It has been pointed out that RHD in the developing countries shows special clinical features, viz. accelerated course, multi-valvular lesions, congestive heart failure, severe tricuspid insufficiency and "juvenile mitral stenosis". The Jones' criteria appears to be as applicable in developing countries as in the West[2].

NATIONAL AND INTERNATIONAL PROGRAMS FOR RHEUMATIC FEVER CONTROL

In recent years developing countries, with and without the aid of WHO have made co-ordinated or individual efforts for the study and control of the problem of RF and RHD.

A collaborative study involving seven centres was conducted between 1972 and 1979 with WHO collaboration[3,4,5]. A similar program was followed in Latin-American countries during the years 1975-1976. A WHO meeting on the "Community control of RF and RHD" was held in New Delhi in 1979. An Indo-US Conference-Workshop on "Rheumatic Fever in the 1980's" was held in 1981 in New Delhi, India under the auspices of the Indian Council of Medical Research, All India Heart Foundation and the National Heart Lung and Blood Institute (USA)[6].

A national program for control of RF and RHD was started in Japan in 1969. A South-East Asia RF and RHD Prevention Conference was held in Japan in 1973. At the present time three countries - Japan, Indonesia and the Philippines are carrying out a cooperative study for isolation of streptococci, their grouping and typing, from the throats of school children during various seasons and for determination of prevalence of RF and RHD[7].

India has its own programs for RF control, some of the results of which will be discussed later in this paper. These programs started in 1966 are:

- A collaborative study on prevalence of RHD in school children.
- A secondary prophylaxis pilot program for RF and RHD.
- A RF criteria study.
- A longitudinal study on 2000 children at 6 monthly intervals for evidence of streptococcal infection, RF and RHD: factor analysis of prevalence, evaluation of current methods of surveillance and research into alternative approaches for control.

STUDIES IN INDIA

Prevalence

It is believed that there are some 6 to 8 million children in India with RF and RHD today. The prevalence from school surveys is 6 to 11 per 1000 with a national average of 6 per 1000. Delhi has

the highest figure of 11 per 1000 school children between 5 and 15
years. Hospital admissions account for 33 to 50 percent of all heart
cases. Surveys in adult populations point to a figure of 123 to 200
per 1,000,000. The differences in clinical and epidemiological features between developed and developing countries has been brought out
in recent publications[1,4].

Table 1. RHD in India , Age and Sex distribution of 885 cases.

Age Group	Male	Female	Total
Up to 5 yrs.	–	–	–
5-9 yrs.	97	47	144 (16.3%)
10-14 yrs.	323	215	538 (60.8%)
15-19 yrs.	86	84	170 (19.2%)
20 yrs. and above	19	14	33 (3.7%)
Total	525 (59.37%)	360 (40.7%)	885

Table 2. RHD in India, Socio-economic Status of 885 cases.

Income group	No. of Patients	% age
100 or less	6 ⎤	
101 - 300	293 ⎟	81.1
301 - 500	358 ⎟	
501 - 700	61 ⎦	
701 - 1000	112	12.7
1001 - 1500	38	4.3
1501 - 2000	15	1.7
2000 and above	2	.2
Total	885	100.0

Table 3. RHD in India, Rheumatic Manifestations and Rheumatic
          Recurrences.

Total No. of Cases	885	
	First Attacks	Recurrence
Arthritis	323 (36.5%)	169 (19.1%)
Acute Carditis	247 (27.9%)	131 (14.8%)
Chorea	40 (4.5%)	17 (1.9%)
Subcutaneous nodules	14 (1.6%)	9 (1.0%)
Polyarthralgia	406 (45.9%)	352 (39.8%)
Erythema marginatum	Nil	Nil

Table 4. RHD in India, Applicability of Jones' Criteria.

	No. of cases	% age
Total No. of cases	885	
I. Patients satisfying Jones' criteria.	514	58.1%
a. Two or more major criteria	96	10.9%
b. One major with two minor criteria.	418	47.2%
II. Patients not satisfying Jones' criteria.	371	41.9%

Epidemiological and Clinical Features

The facts given in the following paragraphs are from a group
of 885 children being followed up at the present time in Delhi. These
children were referrals from School Health Services, general practitioners or hospital discharges. The age distribution was highest
in the 10 to 14 year group. The sexes showed a slight male prepon-
derance. The socio-economic status was the lowest income group in
80 percent of patients. Rheumatic manifestation in first attacks and
recurrences followed the same pattern with polyarthralgia in the majority followed by arthritis and acute carditis. Nodules and Chorea
were infrequent and no case of erythema marginatum was seen.

Table 5. RHD in India, Break-down of 885 Cases by Severity of Disease*

	No. of cases	% age
Group I		
Arthritis & Chorea	121	13.7%
Group II		
Carditis alone or associated with arthritis, Chorea.	396	44.7%
Group III		
With no CHF or carditis	321	
With CHF alone	41	
With CHF & carditis	2	
With carditis alone	4	
Total	368	41.6%
Total	885	

*Ref. Circulation 32,457. 1965.

Table 6. RHD in India, Valvular Lesions in 885 Cases.

Valvular Lesion	Male	Female	Total
MS	79	50	129 (14.6%)
MR	211	120	331 (37.4%)
MS + MR	88	74	162 (18.3%)
AR	9	8	17 (1.9%)
Combined aortic & mitral valve lesion	75	50	125 (14.1%)
No valvular lesion	63	58	121 (13.7%)
Total	525	360	885 (100.0%)

The Jones' criteria were applicable in 58 percent of patients
with 11 percent showing two major criteria and 47 one major and two
minor criteria. Nearly 42 percent of patients did not satisfy the
Jones' criteria on admission to the study but in view of the low
economic status of most of these patients it is possible that minor
illness was not taken note of.

The severity of disease on entrance into the study was Group III
in 42·percent, Group II in 45 percent and Group I (with no carditis)
in 13 percent according to the criteria used in the UK-USA combined
trial[8].

Of the valvular lesions, the order of frequency was mitral insufficiency followed by MS and MI, pure MS and combined mitral and
aortic valvular lesions. Lone A I was present only in a small number.
2 percent of patients had a familial pattern with two or more members
of a family being affected.

LABORATORY DATA

Throat Cultures

Beta haemolytic streptococci was isolated in 211 out of 885 cases
on entry into the study (23.9 percent). The largest number of cases
were of Group A, 91 (43.13 percent), followed by Group G, 83 (39.34
percent).

Table 7.   RHD in India, Beta Haemolytic Streptococci Isolations in
           885 Cases.

Group	No. of Cases	Total isolations	Serological Groups			
			A	B	C	G
Regular	703	133 (18.92%)	57 (42.86%)	2	20	54 (40.60%)
Irregular	182	78 (42.89%)	34 (43.59%)	3	12	29 (37.19%)
Total	885	211 (23.89%)	91 (43.13%)	5	32	83 (39.34%)

The dominant T types were 3/13/B-3264 followed by 5/11/12/27/44 and 8/25/Imp.19.

M typing could only be done in 20 percent of Group A strains, most of whom were positive for serum opacity reaction. This last is believed to be an epidemiological marker. M-types isolated were 1, 3,11,12,22,31,60,52,56,63 and 28. No prevalent M types were found.

Table 8. RHD in India, ASO Titre/Beta Haemolytic Streptococci in 885 Cases

Clinical Groups	No. of Cases	ASO Levels			
		200	200–400	400–596	596 & above
I. RHD cases without isolations of Beta-haemolytic streptococci	674	409	179	66	20
II. RHD cases with isolations of Beta haemolytic streptococci.	211	133	56	15	7
Isolations:					
A	91	91	25	9	5
B	5	4	1	–	–
C	32	24	7	1	–
G	83	53	23	5	2

Serology

High ASO titres were obtained in 343 cases (38.8 percent). In 265 cases (29.9 percent) there was no positive throat culture. With the use of both ASO and ADnase-B estimations it was possible to detect 578 (65.3 percent) cases of streptococcal infection whereas by the use of ASO alone this was possible only in 38.8 percent and by the use of ADnase-B alone only in 235 (26.5 percent) cases. Antipolysaccharide antibodies showed high values in 60 percent of cases with valvular involvement.

IMMUNOLOGIC STUDIES

T & B Lymphocytes

Peripheral blood T & B lymphocytes were studied in cases of acute
RF (36), chronic RHD (25), acute streptococcal pharyngitis (37) and
in 24 normal controls. A distinct depression of T cells was observed
in cases of acute RF and acute streptococcal pharyngitis (P<.05).
Statistically significant elevation of B cells was noted in acute RF
RHD and acute streptococcal pharyngitis cases.

A positive humoral response was seen in cases who had elevation
of B cells in acute RF and RHD cases. No such correlation could be
made out in cases of acute streptococcal pharyngitis[9].

HLA Mapping

HLA mapping was done in 22 cases of acute RF and RHD and 18 normal controls. DR typing showed 55 percent cases of RHD, RF to be
positive for 885 sera-DR specificity undefined. In the normal population of the same age group this type of genetic marker was seen in
16.6 percent. The HLA types reported from other centers in India for
cases of acute RF showed HLA-A 28 in 48.2 percent (14.4 percent in
controls), HLA B 5 in 48.2 percent (28.8 percent in controls), HLA-B
18 in 14.8 percent (4.4 percent in controls). This work is being
continued in a larger number of cases.

VALIDATION OF JONES' CRITERIA

In 162 cases with acute major manifestations (carditis, polyarthritis, nodules, chorea and arthralgia) studied at Delhi, ESR and
ASO elevation were present in 98.6 percent to 92.6 percent of patients
with carditis, polyarthritis and chorea and in 100 percent of patients
with subcutaneous nodules. In the case of arthralgia, when accompanied by a rise of ASO and ESR in patients with previous RHD, it was
considered a significant symptom of RF. Immunologic studies in these
patients have not yielded any new facts.

Seasonal Throat Culture

In a study of 2000 children being carried out now, throat swabs
in summer and winter months showed a significant difference in five
consecutive surveys, being nearly double in winter months. (P =
<0.01). This is an important pointer to control measures which may
have to be taken for primary prophylaxis.

Table 9.   RHD in India, Seasonal Incidence of B-Haemolytic Streptococci   along with Group-wise Break-up.

Season	No. of Specimens	Isolation	Serological Groups				
			A	B	C	G	
Winter'79	2034	357* (17.6%)	207 (10.2%)	8 (0.4%)	52 (2.6%)	90* (4.4%)	
Summer'80	2034	217* (10.5%)	94 (4.6%)	9 (0.4%)	54 (2.7%)	60* (2.9%)	
Winter'80	2034	369* (18.2%)	192 (9.4%)	10 (0.5%)	63 (3.1%)	104* (5.2%)	
Summer'81	2034	224* (11.1%)	104 (5.1%)	1 (0.05%)	55 (2.7%)	64* (3.1%)	
Winter'81	2034	338* (16.6%)	165 (8.1%)	– –	55 (2.7%)	118* (5.8%)	

*p = 0.01

COLLABORATIVE STUDY IN ASIA

A similar study has been carried out in 3 countries of South-East Asia (Japan, Indonesia and the Philippines) under a cooperative study in school children between 6 and 8 years of age from 1977. The prevalence of Group A streptococci using identical methods was 10 to 40 percent and was similar among the participating countries. It was significantly higher during the rainy months in Indonesia and the Philippines and high in winter in Japan. A higher prevalence was observed also in the lower income groups in Indonesia and the Philippines during the rainy season. Group A accounted for the largest number of streptococci isolated. There was a variation in predominant T types in the three countries and during the different seasons.

The prevalence of RF was 0.8 to 1 per 1000 in Indonesia and the Philippines and well below 0.1 per 1000 in Japan.

The low prevalence of RF and RHD in Japan compared with the higher rates in Indonesia and the Philippines in spite of the same isolation rates of streptococci in the throat raised questions regarding host response and virulence of bacteria.

CONTROL OF RHEUMATIC FEVER AND RHEUMATIC HEART DISEASE

Primary Prevention

In the Indian experience primary prevention still remains the ideal goal but is hard of achievement, because of the large population involved and the lack of medical facilities over the greater part of the country, in rural and semi-rural areas.

One method of primary prophylaxis to be attempted in India is seasonal prophylaxis of all school children during the months of peak streptococcal infection which may vary in different parts of the country.

The difficulty of recognising streptococcal infection except by culture stresses the need for a quick method of recognising such infection.

SECONDARY PREVENTION

Pilot studies at Delhi and at Hyderabad have conclusively shown the feasibility of secondary prevention even in a developing country.

Prophylaxis has been given in the Delhi clinic regularly from 1966 onwards. In 1975 a change was made from 4-weekly to 3-weekly injections. The differences in the number of positive throat cultures

Table 10. RHD in India, Streptococcal Infection and
           Rheumatic Recurrence.

	1966-75		1976-81	
	No.	Rate/pt.year	No.	Rate/pt.year
No. of patient years	1656.16	-	3062.5*	-
Positive throat culture	263	0.15	133	0.04
Raised ASO	257	0.155	206	0.06
No. of cases with raised ASO & positive Group A throat culture	118	0.07	22	0.007
Rheumatic recurrences	21	0.012	3	0.0009

*No. of patient years with 3 weekly Penicillin injections.

Table 11. RHD in India, Cost of Chemoprophylaxis

Drug	Cost per child per year	
	US $	Rupees
1. Penicillin Benzathine (injection 3 weekly)	5	42.00
2. Penicillin G oral	18	142.00
3. Penicillin V oral	15	102.00
4. Sulpha oral	2.4	15.30
5. Erythromycin	65	520.00

raised ASO and of rheumatic recurrences showed very significant differences suggesting the efficacy of 3-weekly as opposed to 4-weekly injections even in children[5].

Lessons that have been learnt from our own experience have been:

a) the need for early start between 5 and 9 years, when the disease is relatively mild and which makes allowances for a longer follow up as many children drop out of school between 12 and 15 years of age.
b) 3-weekly instead of 4-weekly injections in children.
c) assiduous follow up with the help of social workers of all patients who do not come to clinic regularly.

The minimum staff needed for such a clinic and the cost involved of Penicillin injections and other chemoprophylactic agents have been worked out and do not appear formidable.

Injections are preferable to oral tablets because of poor adherence to the regimen in children of the poor social classes due to overcrowded living conditions.

Another encouraging factor has been the results of a collaborative study carried out under WHO auspices in seven centers. This showed that control projects as outlined in the WHO protocol are feasible in developing countries and that even with the follow up rate of around 50 percent and only half of these receiving regular prophylaxis the gains achieved are considerable.

"These benefits are related to the level of prophylaxis, so that while full prophylaxis is obviously desirable, imperfect prophylaxis is better than none at all. Thus, the difficulties associated with establishing a full rheumatic fever control program should not deter authorities from building up similar programs with lower co-efficients of efficiency, since they will also yield considerable benefits[5]."

The most important problem is the extension of the rheumatic fever prophylaxis program to cover the entire population. In India two methods are being tried, one through the school health services and the other through the Primary Health Care centers. The first method has also been tried in the Philippines and the second in Cyprus[6].

DISCUSSION

Considering the urgency and magnitude of the problem there is need for research in the following areas:

1. A quick method for identifying streptococcal infection without throat culture using perhaps monoclonal fluorescent antibodies.

2. A fool proof method for clinical diagnosis of acute RF.
3. Biologic markers indicating rheumatogenic potential or lack thereof, other than serotypes as in M 5 and M 4 strains.
4. The comparative efficiency of Penicillin injections given through school health services and primary health centers.
5. Efficacy in raising serum Penicillin levels of brands of benzathine Penicillin currently in use.
6. A cooperative study to document the incidence and nature of reactions to Penicillin in children.
7. Trial of seasonal primary prophylaxis.

There is need for education among all sections of the population including doctors and parents on the relationship between sore throat and heart disease.

There is also need for improvement in surgical facilities for RHD especially mitral stenosis by open and closed technics, for causes of restenosis and thrombogenicity of prosthetic valves. Better tissue or biological valves which do not need anticoagulation and suitable for children should be sought.

SUMMARY

1. There is a high prevalence of RF and RHD in children and young adults in the developing countries.
2. The special features in developing countries are severe disease, multi-valvular lesions, TR, CHF, juvenile MS, frequent hospital admissions and high morbidity and mortality.
3. Primary prevention is ideal but difficult of achievement. Seasonal primary prophylaxis may be feasible.
4. Secondary chemoprophylaxis remains the best weapon at the present time. Recent collaborative studies have shown encouraging results, and even submaximal prophylaxis is worthwile.
   Early start between 5 and 9 years of age, 3-weekly injections and close follow up yields excellent results. The cost of staff and drugs are not exorbitant. The scheme is eminently feasible in developing countries. Its incorporation into the health care delivery system either through primary health care centers or school health services, would ensure universal coverage.
5. Suggestions for future research include identification of biologic markers for rheumatogenic potential, diagnosis of streptococcal infection without culture and a test for definite clinical diagnosis of acute RF. The relative merits of the school health or primary health care systems for secondary and primary prophylaxis and improvement of surgical facilities and methods are other areas for research.

REFERENCES

1. S. Padmavati. Rheumatic fever and rheumatic heart disease in
   developing countries, Bulletin of WHO 56(4), 543-550 (1978).
2. S. K. Sanyal, M. K. Thapar, S. H. Ahmed, V. Hooja, P. Tawari.
   The initial attack of RF during childhood in North-India -
   A prospective study of the clinical profile. Circulation
   32:664 (1974).
3. Community Control of rheumatic heart disease in developing countries. 1, WHO chronicle, 34:336-345 (1980).
4. Community Control of rheumatic heart disease in developing countries. 2, WHO chronicle, 34:389-395 (1980).
5. T. Strasser, N. Dondog, A. El Kholy, R. Gharagozloo, V. V. Kalbian,
   O. Ogunbi, S. Padmavati, K. Stuart, E. Dowd and A. Bekessy.
   Community control of rheumatic fever and rheumatic heart
   disease: report of a WHO International Cooperative Project.
   Bulletin of WHO, 59(2):285-294 (1981).
6. Proceedings of Indo-US Conference Workshop "Rheumatic Fever in
   the 1980's" March, 1981, New Delhi (under publication).
7. International cooperative study on Streptococcal infection
   Rheumatic fever and rheumatic heart disease in Asia - Results
   of 4 yrs. Cooperative study (1977-81).
8. The Natural History of Rheumatic Fever and Rheumatic Heart Disease: Circulation 32:457 (1965).
9. K. Prakash, P. K. Bhatnagar, K. B. Sharma. Peripheral blood T
   and B Lymphocytes during Acute Rheumatic Fever, rheumatic heart
   disease and streptococcal pharyngitis (in press).

LONG-TERM RESULTS OF CORONARY REHABILITATION:

RATIONALE, IMPLEMENTATION AND SIGNIFICANCE OF PROGRAMS

Nanette K. Wenger

Professor of Medicine (Cardiology)
Emory University School of Medicine
Director - Cardiac Clinics
Grady Memorial Hospital
Atlanta, Georgia

INTRODUCTION

Rehabilitative programs are based on the concept that many patients with symptomatic coronary disease can and should return to a productive and active life. In the United States, particularly during the past decade, this rehabilitative approach has been progressively incorporated into traditional medical care. Because rehabilitation should begin at the onset of the acute illness and continue during the long-term care of the patient, the primary physician has a pivotal role in initiating and coordinating rehabilitative efforts.

A major component of rehabilitation involves activity: early ambulation during the hospitalization and subsequent prescriptive exercise training after discharge from the hospital. The second component is education of the patient and family, including the provision of a variety of counseling services as warranted.

EARLY AMBULATION

In recent years there has been unequivocal documentation of the safety of early ambulation for appropriately selected and supervised patients with acute myocardial infarction. There has been no increase in the complications of infarction; indeed, some studies suggest a more favorable outcome with this approach.

The major benefits of early ambulation are evident in the short-term. These include prevention of the deconditioning effects of protracted immobilization at bed rest, decrease in pulmonary atelectasis

and thromboembolic complications, and lessening of the anxiety and
depression commonly associated with myocardial infarction; the reassurance offered by the performance of progressive physical activity
improves the patient's self-confidence and self-image.

Early ambulation permits the patient's functional capacity to
be reliably ascertained at pre-discharge exercise testing; it enables
the current shorter hospital stay with its saving in medical care
costs. Because physiologic and emotional deconditioning has been
limited the functional status of the patient is improved at the time
of discharge from the hospital; this is reported to facilitate an
earlier and more complete return to work.

EXERCISE TRAINING AFTER MYOCARDIAL INFARCTION

Convalescent Physical Activity

Physical activity during convalescence is designed to increase
endurance to a level which will enable a prompt return to work and/or
to usual preinfarction activities. In the United States, over 85%
of patients with an uncomplicated infarction, employed at the onset
of illness, currently return to work within 2 to 3 months, typically
resuming their former job. Walking is the major activity during convalescence, with patients monitoring their pulse rate response to exercise. Ideally, patients should enter a supervised (and often a
hospital-based) progressive activity program within the first month
after infarction. The pre-discharge exercise test is often used for
the initial exercise prescription. When this is not available, the
symptomatic, heart rate, and electrocardiographic response to an
exercise regimen can guide the level of recommended activity. In
addition to the safety features of a supervised and intermittently
monitored exercise regimen, the group setting provides emotional support and facilitates educational efforts and counseling.

Individualized Prescriptive Exercise Training

After convalescence, individualized prescriptive physical activity
is designed to enhance cardiovascular function. When the patient has
recovered and typically has attained sufficient endurance to return
to work (commonly within 4 to 8 weeks after infarction), more intensive
exercise training can be undertaken; the exercise prescription is based
on results of a sign-symptom limited exercise test. Patients typically
exercise at least 2 or 3 times weekly, preferably on nonsuccessive
days; exercise sessions are 30-45 minutes in duration, including warm-
up and cool-down periods. The target heart rate intensity of 70-85%
of the highest level safely achieved at exercise testing corresponds
to 60-78% of the peak oxygen uptake, an effective yet safe range
within which to stimulate aerobic metabolism.

An ideal regimen initially involves medically-supervised exercise
to enable exercise guidance, increase motivation and reassurance, and
insure care for cardiovascular emergencies; as exercise performance
and fitness improve, medical supervision can be decreased. The ultimate goal is reasonable independence in exercising; this mandates a
weaning, initially from the monitored setting and subsequently from
the ritualization of formal exercise training, with progressive involvement in an exercise setting that is social, pleasurable, convenient, and appropriate.

The characteristic design of supervised exercise regimens entails
a 5- to 10-minute warm-up period of stretching and a range of motion
exercises, a 15- to 20-minute aerobic or endurance component which
may consist of walk-run sequences, stationary bicycle exercise, arm
exercises and calisthenics, and aerobic games. The final 5- to 10
minute cool-down segment involves a gradual decrease in exercise intensity. Exercise recommendations for unsupervised home exercise
vary considerably, but in the United States are the pattern of care
for about half of patients for whom an exercise regimen is recommended.
Some initial home exercise instructions involve progressive walking
and walk-jog sequences, others use a stationary bicycle and/or a
variety of community-based aerobic activities and sports.

Serial assessment of exercise capacity is recommended at 3- to
6-month intervals to document performance changes, permit revision
of the exercise prescription, and/or define the need for changes in
the medical regimen. Patients who attain a 7- to 8-met level of performance are often progressed to an unsupervised or minimally supervised exercise setting; this typically occurs within 3 to 6 months
after infarction.

An important benefit of exercise training is a decrease in myocardial oxygen requirement for any submaximal task, allowing the
patient to function farther from the ischemic threshold in usual daily
activities; this enables an increased intensity and duration of work
and a reduction in chest pain symptoms by increasing the exercise
threshold for angina. Because the energy requirement for any task
is a lesser percent of this increased physical work capacity, patients
perceive less exertion as they work, which they describe as improved
"endurance". The hemodynamic determinants of this increase in functional capacity include an increase in maximal cardiac output and
oxygen consumption, a decrease in resting heart rate, a lesser increase
in heart rate and systolic blood pressure for any level of submaximal
work, and more rapid return to normal of the exercise heart rate.
Peripheral oxygen extraction by working muscle improves, as does the
redistribution of cardiac output; both further decrease the demand
for oxygen transport. There is currently little or no evidence that
short-term, modest-intensity exercise improves intrinsic myocardial
performance, especially in older individuals with significant coronary
disease.

Neither is there evidence that exercise training alters the
coronary collateral circulation in man, either as detected angiographically or by myocardial perfusion studies. It remains controversial whether exercise training affects the incidence or severity
of cardiac arrhythmias. Exercise training has not been shown to alter
the natural history of coronary atherosclerotic heart disease – the
recurrence of myocardial infarction or the incidence of coronary death.
However, recent studies suggest that fatal reinfarction is decreased.

Serum triglyceride levels decrease with exercise training, but
the effect on total serum cholesterol is not predictable; high-density
lipoprotein cholesterol increases. Long-term effects on fibrinolysis
and platelet function are inconclusive. Exercise may exert a beneficial effect on coronary disease by modifying other more powerful
coronary risk factors: discontinuation of cigarette smoking, weight
reduction, favorable dietary alterations, blood pressure control etc.
Psychosocial benefits are that patients who exercise often feel better,
have improvement in self-confidence and self-esteem, show less depression and dependency on standard psychometric tests, and appear better
able to tolerate life crises.

PATIENT AND FAMILY EDUCATION

Education of the patient and family is designed to provide the
information about coronary disease and its management that enables
patients to assume some responsibility for continuing health care.
During the hospitalization, a variety of health professionals can
readily institute an educational program. However, if the benefits
are to be maintained, the recommendations for care and their implementation must be reinforced after return home.

The patient education curriculum should include a brief review
of normal cardiac structure and function and of the atherosclerotic
process causing coronary obstruction; this forms the basis for subsequent recommendations for care. Prevalent myths regarding the precipitation of myocardial infarction must be dispelled. Prescriptive
components – dietary changes, cigarette smoking cessation, physical
activity, etc. – are explained,defining the rationale for each and
offering suggestions for effecting the changes; community resources
that may be helpful should be identified. Discussions should include
advice about resumption of sexual activity, response to new or recurrent symptoms, control of associated diseases, and return to work.
All medications should be reviewed in detail. Additionally, in many
hospitals cardiopulmonary resuscitation is taught to families of
myocardial infarction survivors; family counseling addresses lifestyle
adjustments necessary during convalescence, focusing on averting unnecessary invaliding of the patient.

Patients who understand their disease and the rationale for
management have improved ability and motivation to cooperate in re-

ommendations for care; since many components of the care of coronary patients involve a lifetime change in habits, intensive education appears appropriate.

SUMMARY

Effective rehabilitation can enable survivors of myocardial infarction or patients after coronary bypass surgery to return rapidly to a relatively normal lifestyle; patients with angina pectoris may be kept at work or at desired leisure activities. A plan of care must be designed to help the patient achieve realistically optimal physiologic improvement, attain an acceptable level of self-care, and to resume a useful activity level in the home and/or work environment. The majority of patients who recover from myocardial infarction can achieve a functional capacity adequate to perform most moderate personal, occupational, and recreational activities. The rehabilitative approach should limit the economic impact of the illness on the patient, family, and community through a shortened hospital stay, deemphasis of invalidism, a decreased need for convalescent care, and an earlier and more complete return to work. The risk of recurrent coronary events and the incidence of late complications of myocardial infarction may be lessened by a secondary prevention program. Ideally, rehabilitation is incorporated into the traditional care during the hospitalization for myocardial infarction or coronary bypass surgery, involves the patient's family and social environment as a support system, and continues in the office of the patient's physician and/or in a variety of community facilities.

REFERENCES

1. N. K. Wenger, H. K. Hellerstein, H. W. Blackburn and S. J. Castranova. Physician practice in the management of patients with uncomplicated myocardial infarction - changes in the past decade. Circulation 65:421 (1982).
2. Report of the Task Force on Cardiovascular Rehabilitation, National Heart and Lung Institute: Needs and opportunities for rehabilitating the coronary heart disease patient, December 15, 1974, Washington DC, Department of Health, Education and Welfare Publication (NIH) 75-750.
3. N. K. Wenger and H. K. Hellerstein (eds). "Rehabilitation of the Coronary Patient", John Wiley & Sons, Inc., New York (1978).
4. B. Saltin, G. Blomqvist, J. H. Mitchell, R. L. Johnson, K. Wildenthal and C. B. Chapman. Response to exercise after bed rest and after training. Circulation 37-38 (Suppl. 7):1 (1968).
5. "The Exercise Standards Book", American Heart Association, 70-041-A, Dallas, Texas (1979).
6. L. W. Shaw. Effects of a prescribed supervised exercise program on mortality and cardiovascular morbidity in patients after a

myocardial infarction. The National Exercise and Heart Disease Project. Am. J. Cardiol. 48:39 (1981).

7. Subcommittee on Exercise/Rehabilitation: Standards for supervised cardiovascular exercise maintenace programs. Circulation 62: 669A (1980).

8. J. M. R. Detry, M. Rousseau and L. A. Brasseur. Early Hemodynamic adaptations to physical training in patients with healed myo- cardial infarction. Eur. J. Cardiol. 2/3:307 (1975).

9. L. Wilhelmsen, H. Sanne, D. Elmfeldt, G. Grimby, G. Tibbins and H. Wedel. A controlled trial of physical training after myo- cardial infarction: Effects on risk factors, nonfatal rein- farction, and death. Prev. Med. 4:491 (1975).

10. V. Kallio, H. Hamalainen, J. Hakkila and O. Luurila. Reduction in sudden deaths by a multifactoral intervention program after acute myocardial infarction. Lancet 2:1091 (1979).

11. B. A. Kushnir, K. M. Fox, I. W. Tomlinson and C. P. Aber. The effect of a pre-discharge consultation on the resumption of work, sexual activity, and driving following acute myocardial infarction. Scand. J. Rehab. Med. 8:155 (1976).

12. N. K. Wenger: Rehabilitation of the patient with symptomatic coronary disease, in: "The Heart", J. W. Hurst, ed., 5th ed, McGraw-Hill, New York, p. 1149 (1982).

LONG-TERM RESULTS OF CORONARY REHABILITATION:

FACTORS AND REASONS FOR SUCCESS AND FAILURE

H. Denolin

Laboratoire de Recherches Cardiologiques
Centre de Cardiologie du Travail
Hopital Universitaire St Pierre.
Bruxelles (Belgium)

The short term benefits of rehabilitation after myocardial infarction are now well documented, such as shorter hospitalization, improvement of physical capacity by training, psychological effects and earlier return to work.

Unfortunately, the long term studies failed to demonstrate a significant benefit of a comprehensive rehabilitation program or of a supervised physical training, on morbidity and mortality in randomized studies.

A few studies reported in the past encouraging results in cases of exercise rehabilitation after myocardial infarction, but these studies were not randomized and the exercise protocol as well as the duration of follow up were generally not specified.

If we consider the effects of physical exercise training as a secondary prevention measure in patients who have survived a myocardial infarction, we find several prospective randomized trials, in the United States, in Canada and in Europe.

In the US the National Heart Disease Project was proceeded to evaluate the effects of regularly performed medically prescribed exercise in male survivors of MI, who were assigned by randomization to either an exercise group or a non treated group[1]. This trial was effective in inducing a physiological training effect, at least for a short time. A reduction in mortality of 37% was observed in the exercise group; there is no suggestion of a benefit in cardiovascular morbidity. The number of patients is low (651) and some of them enter the program 36 months after MI; the observed reduction in mortality was not significantly different.

In Canada, in the Ontario Exercise-Heart Collaborative study[2], a total number of 751 patients was divided in 2 groups submitted to high intensity exercise or to low intensity exercise; the drop out was very high in the 2 groups and the rate of recurrence was not significantly different between the groups.

In Europe, the studies of SANNE, KENTALA, PALATSI and KALLIO, with a number of patients around 300 to 400, demonstrate some benefit in the trained group but again the difference with the control group were not significant[3].

In Europe also, as a result of several years preparatory work, WHO coordinated study or exercise training and comprehensive secondary prevention was designed: this study was aimed at assessing the effectiveness of comprehensive rehabilitation in reducing recurrent MI and cardiovascular mortality[4,5]. Patients under the age of 65 with definite MI, treated in hospital, were admitted to the study. The intervention measures were to be applied according to the best knowledge in each individual center; the follow up period was 3 years; the main end points were death and morbidity, but physical working capacity, changes in the quality of life and reduction in risk factors were used as additional criteria. The total number of patients (3,118) coming from 19 centers were divided into two groups by randomization.

Considering the end points, the pooling of all data is quite impossible, related to local attitudes or other reasons. If we consider the 17 centers with a sufficient number of patients in the treated and control group: 13 have a mortality experience which favors the rehabilitation group, but the difference in reinfarction is not significant. There were big intercenter differences in return to work. In most of the centers the physical capacity is improved.

Finally, from all these studies it appears that none of the trials showed a statistically significant difference in total mortality between the exercise and control groups; some showed a trend in favor of the exercise group. There was also only a little effect on the incidence of reinfarction[2,3].

The same type of doubtful answer is observed when other secondary prevention methods are used, such as long term prescription of anti-arrhythmias drugs, lipid lowering drugs and diet, anticoagulant drugs, platelet active drugs, beta-blocking drugs, and others. The only attitude for which a strongly positive result is observed is the suppression of smoking habits[3-7].

In conclusion, all these studies failed, till now, to provide a clear answer to the question whether a comprehensive program could reduce mortality or morbidity after MI in the long run.

Should such a conclusion appear as a condemnation of our rehabilitation programs: of course not, it is probably only a demonstration that our trials are not well conducted.

The reasons for this are numerous: low number of patients in most of the studies; insufficient definition of the patients, from the physiological and psycho-social point of view; compliance of the patients to the program; drop out; drop in related to a scattering of the knowledge; unadapted level of training; therapeutic local traditions and use of different drugs for secondary prevention; local organization; technical resources, cost of programs, economical resources, role of surgery etc.

A good conclusion is presented by R. Shepard: "Pessimists may conclude that a control study to determine the influence of exercise upon the rate of reinfarction is logistically impossible ... optimists might attempt to meet the requirement of long numbers by pooling data from various current controlled studies, ignoring obvious differences of philosophy and protocol".

But from a scientific point of view, the only satisfactory course is to regard existing experients as pilot trials[6]...

I could not conclude on the success or the failure of cardiac rehabilitation in the long run, but only stress the difficulties in an evaluation of the comprehensive post coronary care programs generally adapted.

Important changes in the therapeutic approach to MI have appeared during the last 2 decades. The current attitudes have modified the way of life and the perspectives of our patients: most of those with a good clinical condition reintegrate easily the family and the professional life and even if it is not ascertained that their life expectation is improved, the quality of their life is. But we have to accept that, in spite of excellent results at short time, the progressive changes in our attitude are based on empiricism and that most of the hypotheses on which our actual programs are based, are neither proved or disproved.

More research is needed, especially for what concern the implementation of an optimal comprehensive program. Such programs should include exercise, for the reason that, at least, it brings up a positive psychological and physiological improvement.

REFERENCES

1. L. W. Shaw. Effects of a prescribed supervised Exercise program on mortality and cardiovascular morbidity in patients after a myocardial infarction. Am. J. Cardiol. 48,39 (1981).
2. T. Kavanagh. Evidence to date for the beneficial effect of exercise following myocardial infarction. in: Controversies in Cardiac Rehabilitation, Mathes and Halhuber eds. Springer Verlag, Berlin (1982).

3. S. G. May, K. A. Eberlein, C. D. Furberg, E. R. Passamani and
    D. L. Demets. Secondary prevention after myocardial infarc-
    tion: a review of long-term trials. Progress in C. V. Dis.
    24,331 (1982).
4. WHO, European Office. Study on the effects of rehabilitation and
    comprehensive secondary prevention in patients after acute
    myocardial infarction. To be published.
5. V. Kallio. Evaluation of earlier study: Europe in:Physical Con-
    ditioning and Cardiovascular rehabilitation. L. S. Cohen,
    M. B. Mock and I. Ringquist, eds. John Wiley and Sons. New York
    (1981).
6. R. J. Shepard. Evaluation of earlier studies: Canada in: Physical
    Conditioning and Cardiovascular rehabilitation. L. S. Cohen
    M. B. Mock and I. Ringquist, eds. John Wiley and Sons. New
    York (1981).
7. Secondary prevention in myocardial infarction survivors. Joint
    Recommendations. Circulation, 65,216 A (1982).

THE ECONOMIC EFFECTS OF CARDIAC REHABILITATION:

PRINCIPLES, METHODS AND PROBLEMS OF EVALUATION

Veikko Kallio

The Rehabilitation Research Center of the
Social Insurance Institution
Peltolantie 3, SF-20720 Turku 72, Finland

Two major indicators of successful rehabilitation are social integration of the patient and return to meaningful and productive activities. The economic effects of rehabilitation - both costs and benefits - may often be difficult and even impossible to calculate with any precision. Improvement of quality of life, such an important goal for rehabilitation, is not easily transferable to monetary units. Nevertheless, attempts have and should be made to evaluate rehabilitation activities even from economical points of view. It will help to direct investments of limited resources available for development of rehabilitation services[1].

In order to give a general overview of changes in the cost of burden of both health and sickness attributable to various diseases, some data from the USA are presented in Table 1. It shows the percent distribution of costs attributable to the three leading diagnostic categories in 1930 and 1975[2]. It can be seen that the cost of sickness, in particular, has increased remarkably as regards cardiovascular diseases, while the cost of premature deaths has increased less in this diagnostic group compared to accidents, poisoning and violence, and neoplasms. It remains to be seen how the downward trend in cardiovascular mortality will affect these figures.

As regards the overall economic burden of diseases of the circulatory system an estimation has been presented indicating that 1.7% of the adjusted Gross National Product was claimed by these diseases in the USA in 1975.[2] There is good reason to believe that the situation is similar in many industrialized countries in Europe.

Together with the development of public health policy and measures to combat cardiovascular diseases the importance of rehabilitation has increased rapidly. This may be due to several factors,

Table 1. Cost burden of death and sickness by disease in 1930 and
          1975 in the USA[2].
          (Percent distribution)

	Cost of premature deaths		Cost of sickness	
	1930	1975	1930	1975
Diseases of the circulatory system	12.9	22.4	8.3	15.1
Accidents, poisoning and violence	14.6	30.2	14.2	9.8
Neoplasms	4.9	14.8	1.2	1.9

such as increased demand for these services and emphasis on high-
quality after-care. Measures should be resorted to in order to
develop rehabilitation services in the most cost-effective manner.

Evaluation of the effects of rehabilitation depends on whether
the impact is analyzed from the point of view of an individual or of
society. These two different view points, subjective and objective
need, must be taken into account when evaluating the overall economic
effect of rehabilitation.

As rehabilitation represents an important field of social policy,
methods used in social policy research can be applied in the evaluation
of the economic effects of rehabilitation measures. Cost-benefit
analysis and cost effectiveness analysis have both been used for evaluation. Cost-benefit analysis was originally developed for evaluation
of physical investments in order to provide information required for
economically efficient decision making[1]. In the 1960s it was recognized that many social expenditures could reasonably be considered
investments and along with this development cost-benefit analysis
was being increasingly applied to social programs. Since its sole
concern is economic efficiency, cost-benefit analysis cannot be used
alone in decision making concerning complex programs such as rehabilitation. It is thus merely a method to provide information about the
problems and not the method to solve them.

Cost-effectiveness analysis on the other hand can be applied
when the economic effects cannot be easily measured or they cannot
be made commensurable. Cost-effectiveness analysis is particularly
useful in problem areas such as public health when the output cannot
be measured in terms of market price. The effectiveness can be evaluated for instance by increase in years of life or decrease in days
due to inability to work. A typical example of this type of approach

is as follows: it has been calculated that the average expected
duration of life of a new-born boy in Finland would increase by 6.8
years if all cardiovascular diseases could be abolished[3].

Typical problems in cost-benefit analysis of rehabilitation are
presented in the following:

- calculation of direct costs to persons and families such as loss
  in earnings, loss in production efficiency, added costs etc.
- calculation of costs to industry such as loss in product and work
  time
- calculation of secondary or indirect costs such as loss in taxable
  revenue, loss in productivity, continuing costs of medical and
  other services etc.
- calculation of the capital cost
- calculation in monetary value of the increase in social welfare and
  quality of life resulting from rehabilitation
- differences in patient groups with regard to life expectancy

In spite of apparent problems of evaluation cost-benefit analysis
has been applied in some studies on cardiac patients published
recently. The economic impact of coronary by-pass surgery and subsequent rehabilitation was analyzed by Liddle[4]. The patients provided
information by completing a questionnaire concerning pre- and post-
operative salaries, disability payments, costs of medical care, and
return to work. Of 607 questionnaires submitted to patients 90% were
returned. Among all reporting patients 75% returned to employment
within the first 6 postoperative months. Cost-benefit analysis of
the 153 patients not working before the operation but who returned
to work after the operation is shown in Table 2. The patients are
divided into 5 groups according to years worked after the operation
by the time of follow up study. The average 1-year salary was in all
groups at least somewhat higher than total cost of care. If these
disabled patients had not undergone operation and had been rehabili-
tated and returned to work, the indirect costs caused by lost working
years, disability payments etc. would have exceeded the costs of
operation and rehabilitation by many times.

Table 3 shows the cost-production relationship of the 152 men
who were working preoperatively and returned to work. In all subgroups formed according to years worked after operation, total cost
of care was substantially less than their reported annual salary.
The annual salary after operation compares well with that before the
surgery.

Crosby et al.[5] have presented their series of 66 patients who
underwent aneurysmectomy and revasularization and were encouraged to
participate in individual physical rehabilitation postoperatively.
The average follow-up was 20 months. Full employment increased from
33% preoperatively to 63% postoperatively, and total disability rate

Table 2. Cost-production relationship in 153 patients incapacitated for work before coronary by-pass operation but working after operation[4].

Number of patients	Years worked	Average income per year and cost in US dollars		
		Disability payment before operation	Salary after operation	Total cost of care
30	< 1	1492	16467	15436
70	1 – 5	830	16257	14256
39	5 – 8	790	16705	13076
13	8 – 10	783	19461	12443
1	> 10	0	25000	10000

Table 3. Cost-production relationship in 152 patients working both before and after coronary by-pass operation[4].

Average income per year and cost in US dollars.

N	Year worked after operation	Salary before operation	Salary after operation	Total cost of care
20	< 1	19400	19550	12785
67	1 - 5	18708	20410	13166
51	5 - 8	15892	19421	11785
14	8 - 10	17857	22500	11959

decreased from 60% preoperatively to 29% postoperatively. When the
employment capability was used as an indication of improvement after
surgery, the results were even more favorable.

When the economic impact of the procedure in the community in
terms of improvement in income, decrease in disability payments and
reduction in tax revenues was calculated, the positive balance was
such as to allow the cost of the procedure to be paid back over 1.68
years.

The authors emphasize the need of aggressive physical and vocational rehabilitation programs for patients undergoing expensive
cardiac operations in order to make them cost effective.

In some studies[6,7] the return to work after myocardial infarction
has been reported to be relatively low or 42 or 44%, respectively.
There is evidence from literature indicating that return to work can
be improved by active rehabilitation programs[7,8] although essential
differences between countries exist even in this respect.

We have analyzed the individual economic impact of return to work
in a material of men under 65 years who were treated in hospital because of acute myocardial infarction. The patients were randomly allocated in two groups: one with a comprehensive rehabilitation program
and the other with ordinary services. All patients provided information by filling in a questionnaire concerning return to work and
the salary or disability payment before and one year after the myocardial infarction. Return to work was almost similar in both groups
of 58 and 55% respectively. There were, however, other positive effects which we consider worthy of investment required for the rehabilitation program[9,10,11,12]. Furthermore, the patients of the rehabilitation group who returned to work paid back in taxes the costs of
the comprehensive rehabilitation program for all patients in about
1 year.

The effect on income of return to work is presented in Table 4.
The results refer to patients who were working before the myocardial
infarction. The pre-infarct salary was given an index value of 100
and the subsequent salries and disability payments were calculated
as percentages of the pre-infarct salary. The average salary one
year after the myocardial infarction was almost on the pre-infarct
level, while the patients who were not working experienced a considerable economic loss which was bigger than expected. From the
community point of view, the economic impact of not working after the
myocardial infarction is substantial due to disability payments, lost
taxes, inability to pay for medical treatments etc.

In our experience about 20% of men with acute myocardial infarction below the age of 65 receive disability payments at the time of
the acute event. It is extremely rare for these patients to return

Table 4. Effect of return to work, disability or old age pension on income 1 year after myocardial infarction. (Kallio et al., unpublished data)*.

	Number	Mean age	Income index
Patients employed before the acute myocardial infarction	226	51.9	100
Work status one year after infarction			
– Patients returned to work	108	49.0	97
– Patients on disability pension	83	53.7	35
– Patients on old age pension	8	63.7	52
– Deaths or no income data	27	–	–

*Index figures refer to salary before the new infarction

to work in spite of an active rehabilitation program. Vocational rehabilitation seems, therefore, best indicated in patients who are employed when they get their myocardial infarction.

It can be concluded that rehabilitation measures which improve the working capacity and especially return to work are cost-effective particularly if all costs incurred by permanent disability are taken into account. New studies are, however, needed especially on patients with coronary heart disease in order to develop the most cost-effective organization and program of rehabilitation. Finally, many effects provided by cardiac rehabilitation cannot be measured in terms of economic benefit. These effects are at least as important and worth striving for as the economic gain.

REFERENCES

1. M. Berkowitz, V. Englander, J. Rubin and J. D. Worral,"An Evaluation of Policy-Related Rehabilitation Research", Praeger Publishers Inc., New York (1975).
2. S. J. Mushkin, "Biomedical Research: Costs and Benefits", Ballinger Publishing Company, Cambridge, Massachesetts (1979).
3. A. Mattila and K. Rosendahl. Factors affecting life expectancy, Acta Soc. Med. Scand., Suppl. 1 (1969).
4. H. V. Liddle, Perspectives in coronary artery surgery, J. Thorac. Cardiovasc. Surg. 81:1-10 (1981).
5. I. K. Crosby, H. A. Wellons, R. P. Martin, D. Schuch and W. H. Muller. Employability - a new indication for aneurysmectomy and coronary revascularization, Circulation 62:Suppl.1:79-83 (1980).

6. U. Vuopala. Resumption of work after myocardial infarction in northern Finland, Acta Med. Scand., Suppl. 530 (1972).

7. H. J. Stijns, A. Corniere, L. De Backer and H. De Geest. Physical rehabilitation in hospital and at home for patients after an acute myocardial infarction, Rehabilitation 94:31 (1975).

8. K. Scaller, A. Gutschker and W. G. Geissler. Ergebnisse und Probleme bei der beruflichen Rehabilitation Herzinfarktkranker, Z. Gesamte Hyg. 23:599 (1977).

9. V. Kallio, H. Hämäläinen, J. Hakkila and O. J. Luurila. Reduction in sudden deaths by a multifactorial intervention program after acute myocardial infarction, Lancet 2:1091-1094 (1979).

10. H. Hämäläinen, "Kammioperäisten rytmihäiriöiden esiintyminen ja ennusteellinen merkitys sydäninfarktin jälkeen," (English Summary: Occurrence and Prognostic Significance of Ventricular Arrhythmias. A Follow-up Study after Acute Myocardial Infarction and Rehabilitation.), Publications of the Social Insurance Institution AL:18. Turku (1982).

11. R-L. Karvetti, "Ravitsemusneuvonnan vaikutus sydäninfarktipotilaiden ruoankäyttöön ja ravinnonsaantiin", (English Summary: The Effect of Nutrition Education on the Diet and Nutrient Intake of Myocardial Infarction Patients.), Publications of the Social Insurance Institution AL:10, Turku (1979).

12. S. Laaksovirta, "Sydäninfarktipotilaan kuntoutusura", (English Summary: The Rehabilitation Career of the Myocardial Infarction Patient.), Publications of the Social Insurance Institution AL:20, Turku (1982) (in print).